Malignant Mesothelioma

Malignant Mesothelioma

Editors

Joanna Kopecka
Daniel L. Pouliquen

MDPI • Basel • Beijing • Wuhan • Barcelona • Belgrade • Manchester • Tokyo • Cluj • Tianjin

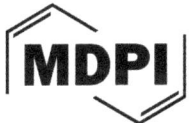

Editors
Joanna Kopecka
Department of Oncology
University of Torino
Torino
Italy

Daniel L. Pouliquen
ICO Cancer Center, Inserm UMR 1232 (CRCINA)
University of Angers
Angers
France

Editorial Office
MDPI
St. Alban-Anlage 66
4052 Basel, Switzerland

This is a reprint of articles from the Special Issue published online in the open access journal *Cancers* (ISSN 2072-6694) (available at: www.mdpi.com/journal/cancers/special_issues/Ma-Me).

For citation purposes, cite each article independently as indicated on the article page online and as indicated below:

LastName, A.A.; LastName, B.B.; LastName, C.C. Article Title. *Journal Name* **Year**, *Volume Number*, Page Range.

ISBN 978-3-0365-2368-2 (Hbk)
ISBN 978-3-0365-2367-5 (PDF)

© 2021 by the authors. Articles in this book are Open Access and distributed under the Creative Commons Attribution (CC BY) license, which allows users to download, copy and build upon published articles, as long as the author and publisher are properly credited, which ensures maximum dissemination and a wider impact of our publications.

The book as a whole is distributed by MDPI under the terms and conditions of the Creative Commons license CC BY-NC-ND.

Contents

About the Editors vii

Daniel L. Pouliquen and Joanna Kopecka
Malignant Mesothelioma
Reprinted from: *Cancers* 2021, 13, 3447, doi:10.3390/cancers13143447 1

Giovanni Cugliari, Chiara Catalano, Simonetta Guarrera, Alessandra Allione, Elisabetta Casalone, Alessia Russo, Federica Grosso, Daniela Ferrante, Clara Viberti, Anna Aspesi, Marika Sculco, Chiara Pirazzini, Roberta Libener, Dario Mirabelli, Corrado Magnani, Irma Dianzani and Giuseppe Matullo
DNA Methylation of *FKBP5* as Predictor of Overall Survival in Malignant Pleural Mesothelioma
Reprinted from: *Cancers* 2020, 12, 3470, doi:10.3390/cancers12113470 5

Giovanni Cugliari, Alessandra Allione, Alessia Russo, Chiara Catalano, Elisabetta Casalone, Simonetta Guarrera, Federica Grosso, Daniela Ferrante, Marika Sculco, Marta La Vecchia, Chiara Pirazzini, Roberta Libener, Dario Mirabelli, Corrado Magnani, Irma Dianzani and Giuseppe Matullo
New DNA Methylation Signals for Malignant Pleural Mesothelioma Risk Assessment
Reprinted from: *Cancers* 2021, 13, 2636, doi:10.3390/cancers13112636 19

Raunak Shrestha, Noushin Nabavi, Stanislav Volik, Shawn Anderson, Anne Haegert, Brian McConeghy, Funda Sar, Sonal Brahmbhatt, Robert Bell, Stephane Le Bihan, Yuzhuo Wang, Colin Collins and Andrew Churg
Well-Differentiated Papillary Mesothelioma of the Peritoneum Is Genetically Distinct from Malignant Mesothelioma
Reprinted from: *Cancers* 2020, 12, 1568, doi:10.3390/cancers12061568 33

Marcella Barbarino and Antonio Giordano
Assessment of the Carcinogenicity of Carbon Nanotubes in the Respiratory System
Reprinted from: *Cancers* 2021, 13, 1318, doi:10.3390/cancers13061318 45

Alex Dipper, Nick Maskell and Anna Bibby
Ancillary Diagnostic Investigations in Malignant Pleural Mesothelioma
Reprinted from: *Cancers* 2021, 13, 3291, doi:10.3390/cancers13133291 63

Gabriele Moretti, Paolo Aretini, Francesca Lessi, Chiara Maria Mazzanti, Guntulu Ak, Muzaffer Metintaş, Cecilia Lando, Rosa Angela Filiberti, Marco Lucchi, Alessandra Bonotti, Rudy Foddis, Alfonso Cristaudo, Andrea Bottari, Alessandro Apollo, Marzia Del Re, Romano Danesi, Luciano Mutti, Federica Gemignani and Stefano Landi
Liquid Biopsies from Pleural Effusions and Plasma from Patients with Malignant Pleural Mesothelioma: A Feasibility Study
Reprinted from: *Cancers* 2021, 13, 2445, doi:10.3390/cancers13102445 77

Joëlle S. Nader, Alice Boissard, Cécile Henry, Isabelle Valo, Véronique Verrièle, Marc Grégoire, Olivier Coqueret, Catherine Guette and Daniel L. Pouliquen
Cross-Species Proteomics Identifies CAPG and SBP1 as Crucial Invasiveness Biomarkers in Rat and Human Malignant Mesothelioma
Reprinted from: *Cancers* 2020, 12, 2430, doi:10.3390/cancers12092430 91

Kalyani B. Karunakaran, Naveena Yanamala, Gregory Boyce, Michael J. Becich and Madhavi K. Ganapathiraju
Malignant Pleural Mesothelioma Interactome with 364 Novel Protein-Protein Interactions
Reprinted from: *Cancers* **2021**, *13*, 1660, doi:10.3390/cancers13071660 111

Melanie Vogl, Anna Rosenmayr, Tomas Bohanes, Axel Scheed, Milos Brndiar, Elisabeth Stubenberger and Bahil Ghanim
Biomarkers for Malignant Pleural Mesothelioma—A Novel View on Inflammation
Reprinted from: *Cancers* **2021**, *13*, 658, doi:10.3390/cancers13040658 141

Francesca Napoli, Angela Listì, Vanessa Zambelli, Gianluca Witel, Paolo Bironzo, Mauro Papotti, Marco Volante, Giorgio Scagliotti and Luisella Righi
Pathological Characterization of Tumor Immune Microenvironment (TIME) in Malignant Pleural Mesothelioma
Reprinted from: *Cancers* **2021**, *13*, 2564, doi:10.3390/cancers13112564 165

Martina Schiavello, Elena Gazzano, Loredana Bergandi, Francesca Silvagno, Roberta Libener, Chiara Riganti and Elisabetta Aldieri
Identification of Redox-Sensitive Transcription Factors as Markers of Malignant Pleural Mesothelioma
Reprinted from: *Cancers* **2021**, *13*, 1138, doi:10.3390/cancers13051138 183

Luka Brcic, Alexander Mathilakathu, Robert F. H. Walter, Michael Wessolly, Elena Mairinger, Hendrik Beckert, Daniel Kreidt, Julia Steinborn, Thomas Hager, Daniel C. Christoph, Jens Kollmeier, Thomas Mairinger, Jeremias Wohlschlaeger, Kurt Werner Schmid, Sabrina Borchert and Fabian D. Mairinger
Digital Gene Expression Analysis of Epithelioid and Sarcomatoid Mesothelioma Reveals Differences in Immunogenicity
Reprinted from: *Cancers* **2021**, *13*, 1761, doi:10.3390/cancers13081761 199

Kazuhiro Kitajima, Mitsunari Maruyama, Hiroyuki Yokoyama, Toshiyuki Minami, Takashi Yokoi, Akifumi Nakamura, Masaki Hashimoto, Nobuyuki Kondo, Kozo Kuribayashi, Takashi Kijima, Seiki Hasegawa and Koichiro Yamakado
Response to Immune Checkpoint Inhibitor Therapy in Patients with Unresectable Recurrent Malignant Pleural Mesothelioma Shown by FDG-PET and CT
Reprinted from: *Cancers* **2021**, *13*, 1098, doi:10.3390/cancers13051098 215

Dong-Seok Lee, Andrea Carollo, Naomi Alpert, Emanuela Taioli and Raja Flores
VATS Pleurectomy Decortication Is a Reasonable Alternative for Higher Risk Patients in the Management of Malignant Pleural Mesothelioma: An Analysis of Short-Term Outcomes
Reprinted from: *Cancers* **2021**, *13*, 1068, doi:10.3390/cancers13051068 231

Emanuela Di Gregorio, Gianmaria Miolo, Asia Saorin, Elena Muraro, Michela Cangemi, Alberto Revelant, Emilio Minatel, Marco Trovò, Agostino Steffan and Giuseppe Corona
Radical Hemithoracic Radiotherapy Induces Systemic Metabolomics Changes That Are Associated with the Clinical Outcome of Malignant Pleural Mesothelioma Patients
Reprinted from: *Cancers* **2021**, *13*, 508, doi:10.3390/cancers13030508 241

Haitang Yang, Duo Xu, Zhang Yang, Feng Yao, Heng Zhao, Ralph A. Schmid and Ren-Wang Peng
Systematic Analysis of Aberrant Biochemical Networks and Potential Drug Vulnerabilities Induced by Tumor Suppressor Loss in Malignant Pleural Mesothelioma
Reprinted from: *Cancers* **2020**, *12*, 2310, doi:10.3390/cancers12082310 257

Dario P. Anobile, Paolo Bironzo, Francesca Picca, Marcello F. Lingua, Deborah Morena, Luisella Righi, Francesca Napoli, Mauro G. Papotti, Alessandra Pittaro, Federica Di Nicolantonio, Chiara Gigliotti, Federico Bussolino, Valentina Comunanza, Francesco Guerrera, Alberto Sandri, Francesco Leo, Roberta Libener, Pablo Aviles, Silvia Novello, Riccardo Taulli, Giorgio V. Scagliotti and Chiara Riganti
Evaluation of the Preclinical Efficacy of Lurbinectedin in Malignant Pleural Mesothelioma
Reprinted from: *Cancers* **2021**, *13*, 2332, doi:10.3390/cancers13102332 277

Rupesh Kotecha, Raees Tonse, Muni Rubens, Haley Appel, Federico Albrecht, Paul Kaywin, Evan W. Alley, Martin C. Tom and Minesh P. Mehta
Meta-Analysis of Survival and Development of a Prognostic Nomogram for Malignant Pleural Mesothelioma Treated with Systemic Chemotherapy
Reprinted from: *Cancers* **2021**, *13*, 2186, doi:10.3390/cancers13092186 291

Sean Dulloo, Aleksandra Bzura and Dean Anthony Fennell
Precision Therapy for Mesothelioma: Feasibility and New Opportunities
Reprinted from: *Cancers* **2021**, *13*, 2347, doi:10.3390/cancers13102347 307

About the Editors

Joanna Kopecka

I received my PhD degree from the University of Turin, Italy, in 2013. My research focuses on the basis of chemoresistance and immunoresistance of cancer cells. In particular, I am interested in finding new therapeutic approaches to target resistant cancer cells, using both pharmacological and molecular biology tools. I have co-authored more than 50 scientific papers, abstracts and reviews.

Daniel L. Pouliquen

Following a Pharm.D and a specialized degree in clinical biochemistry (1984, Rennes, France), I worked on the characterization and applications of new NMR contrast agents for proton MRI, and then extended NMR relaxometry to the study of water states and dynamic properties in protein solutions, biofluids, normal preneoplastic and neoplastic tissues and organisms under development (seeds, fish eggs, embryos). This led to investigations on quantitative and qualitative changes in the different water phases in mitochondria and implications of diet in the biophysics of water in tissues during carcinogenesis. The beneficial effects of combinations of phytochemicals were observed for the prevention of some experimental models of cancers in laboratory rodents. I also established a biocollection of cell lines and experimental models of malignant mesothelioma in immunocompetent rats. With this background, I presently work on biomarkers of cancer invasiveness by quantitative proteomics.

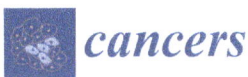

Editorial

Malignant Mesothelioma

Daniel L. Pouliquen [1,*] and Joanna Kopecka [2,*]

1. Université d'Angers, Inserm, CRCINA, F-44000 Nantes, France
2. Department of Oncology, University of Turin, 10126 Turin, Italy
* Correspondence: daniel.pouliquen@inserm.fr (D.L.P.); joanna.kopecka@unito.it (J.K.)

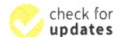

Citation: Pouliquen, D.L.; Kopecka, J. Malignant Mesothelioma. *Cancers* 2021, 13, 3447. https://doi.org/10.3390/cancers13143447

Received: 1 July 2021
Accepted: 6 July 2021
Published: 9 July 2021

Publisher's Note: MDPI stays neutral with regard to jurisdictional claims in published maps and institutional affiliations.

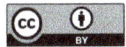

Copyright: © 2021 by the authors. Licensee MDPI, Basel, Switzerland. This article is an open access article distributed under the terms and conditions of the Creative Commons Attribution (CC BY) license (https://creativecommons.org/licenses/by/4.0/).

Malignant mesothelioma (MM) is a rare and aggressive cancer, related to chronic inflammation and oxidative stress caused mainly by exposure to asbestos. Although this mineral has been banned for decades in many countries, epidemiologists predict the MM epidemic will last past 2040, raising many concerns in public health given its late diagnosis, dismal prognosis, and lack of current efficient therapies. To deal with this situation, important breakthroughs have recently been made in the understanding of MM's complex biology and the carcinogenic process of the different patterns of the disease. Examples of these include the development of new biomarkers and the deciphering of gene-environment interactions, molecular mechanisms of invasiveness, deregulated pathways, altered expression of miRNAs, DNA damage repair or metabolic profiles. From this recent research, MM's aggressive and chemoresistant character appears linked to a polyclonal malignancy, and heterogeneity in molecular alterations. Given these improvements, new therapeutic strategies are being explored to solve the double challenge faced by clinicians. The first is to reduce tumor development and its wasting consequences as soon as possible, without resistance and with limited toxicity. The second is to stimulate recognition of tumor cells by induction of a specific immune response.

In this Special Issue, 168 authors representing 71 affiliations from 13 countries over three continents have made 19 contributions, and it is a great privilege and pleasure for the editors to introduce this collective work which summarizes important insights in this field of research. As MM is mostly related to genetic and epigenetic alterations caused by prolonged exposure to asbestos fibers, in the search for a noninvasive prognosis test, Cugliari et al. showed the potential predictive value of DNA methylation changes in white blood cells as a MM survival biomarker [1], and investigated differences between MM cases and asbestos-exposed cancer-free controls [2]. Another important question concerns the discrimination between MM and benign proliferation of mesothelial cells (also frequently treated by surgery), for which Shresta et al. propose a genomic differential characterization [3]. Although asbestos has been banned in many countries, epidemiologists predict the MM epidemic will probably last over 2040 as new environmental risks, such as carbon nanotubes, are emerging, as reviewed by Barbarino et al. [4]. The diagnosis of MM could now benefit from the developments of ancillary tests, as reviewed by Dipper et al. [5]. Moretti et al. also analyzed tumor biopsy and liquid biopsies from a set of patients and demonstrated that most mutated DNA can be detected into pleural fluids [6].

Fortunately, the last few years have also been characterized by important breakthroughs in improving our understanding of MM's complex biology and in identifying biomarkers which could help early diagnosis and prognosis of this cancer. To limit potential sources of bias in the identification of such biomarkers, Nader et al. conducted cross-species proteomic analyses on three different MM sources [7]. To understand the role of the genes that relate to this disease, Karunakaran et al. constructed a MM interactome and identified five repurposable drugs targeting the interactome proteins [8]. Since immune therapy emerged as a promising treatment alternative, Vogl et al. reviewed the role of inflammatory parameters [9], and Napoli et al. examined the contribution of the tumor immune microenvironment [10]. As redox-sensitive transcription factors regulate cellular antioxidant defense, Schiavello et al. presented their potential as predictive biomarkers [11].

The involvement of the immune system is crucial in MM development and progression, however, as MM consists of different histological subtypes varying in aggressiveness, an important understanding of the biological background of its escape mechanisms was provided by Brcic, Mathilakathu et al. [12]. With the development of immune checkpoint therapy, Kitajima et al. also demonstrated how hybrid imaging modalities could contribute to therapy response assessment and predict prognosis [13]. Among other treatment strategies, Lee et al. showed how minimally invasive surgery may help manage short-term outcomes of patients with MM [14], while Di Gregorio et al. revealed how metabolomic changes are associated with clinical outcomes following radical hemithoracic radiotherapy [15]. In the search for new targets, Yang et al. demonstrated that the exploration of aberrant biochemical networks and potential drug vulnerabilities induced by tumor suppressor loss provide interesting prospects for the treatment of MM [16]. Moreover, Anobile, Bironzo et al. evaluated the preclinical efficacy of a new marine-derived anticancer drug in patient-derived samples of MM [17]. Finally, Kotecha, Tonse et al. provided baseline comparative values in their review of survival of MM patients treated with systemic therapy combinations for locally, advanced, or metastatic disease [18], and Dulloo et al. reviewed new opportunities in molecular strategy therapy for this cancer [19].

Malignant mesothelioma still represents a devastating disease, and the final goal of all our research efforts is to provide prolonged survival with maintained quality of life to patients. The 19 articles contained in this Special Issue, which cover multiple and complementary aspects of this research, might contribute to reach this goal in the future, while opening interesting prospects for improving both the early diagnosis and treatment of this cancer. This collective work is also a good illustration of continued collaboration between disciplines and research teams all over the world, which could provide a basis for the emergence of new ideas and concepts in this field.

Funding: This research received no external funding.

Conflicts of Interest: The authors declare no conflict of interest.

References

1. Cugliari, G.; Catalano, C.; Guarrera, S.; Allione, A.; Casalone, E.; Russo, A.; Grosso, F.; Ferrante, D.; Viberti, C.; Aspesi, A.; et al. DNA methylation of *FKBP5* as predictor of overall survival in malignant pleural mesothelioma. *Cancers* **2020**, *12*, 3470. [CrossRef] [PubMed]
2. Cugliari, G.; Allione, A.; Russo, A.; Catalano, C.; Casalone, E.; Guarrera, S.; Grosso, F.; Ferrante, D.; Sculco, M.; La Vecchia, M.; et al. New DNA methylation signals for malignant pleural mesothelioma risk assessment. *Cancers* **2021**, *13*, 2636. [CrossRef] [PubMed]
3. Shrestha, R.; Nabavi, N.; Volik, S.; Anderson, S.; Haegert, A.; McConeghy, B.; Sar, F.; Brahmbhatt, S.; Bell, R.; Le Bihan, S.; et al. Well-differentiated papillary mesothelioma of the peritoneum is genetically distinct from malignant mesothelioma. *Cancers* **2020**, *12*, 1568. [CrossRef] [PubMed]
4. Barbarino, M.; Giordano, A. Assessment of the carcinogenicity of carbon nanotubes in the respiratory system. *Cancers* **2021**, *13*, 1318. [CrossRef] [PubMed]
5. Dipper, A.; Maskell, N.; Bibby, A. Ancillary diagnostic investigations in malignant pleural mesothelioma. *Cancers* **2021**, *13*, 3291. [CrossRef] [PubMed]
6. Moretti, G.; Aretini, P.; Lessi, F.; Mazzanti, C.M.; Ak, G.; Metintas, M.; Lando, C.; Filiberti, R.A.; Lucchi, M.; Bonotti, A.; et al. Liquid biopsies from pleural effusions and plasma from patients with malignant pleural mesothelioma: A feasibility study. *Cancers* **2021**, *13*, 2445. [CrossRef] [PubMed]
7. Nader, J.S.; Boissard, A.; Henry, C.; Valo, I.; Verrièle, V.; Grégoire, M.; Coqueret, O.; Guette, C.; Pouliquen, D.L. Cross-species proteomics identifies CAPG and SBP1 as crucial invasiveness biomarkers in rat and human malignant mesothelioma. *Cancers* **2020**, *12*, 2430. [CrossRef] [PubMed]
8. Karunakaran, K.B.; Yanamala, N.; Boyce, G.; Becich, M.J.; Ganapathiraju, M.K. Malignant pleural mesothelioma interactome with 364 novel protein-protein interactions. *Cancers* **2021**, *13*, 1660. [CrossRef] [PubMed]
9. Vogl, M.; Rosenmayr, A.; Bohanes, T.; Scheed, A.; Brndiar, M.; Stubenberger, E.; Ghanim, B. Biomarkers for malignant pleural mesothelioma—A novel view on inflammation. *Cancers* **2021**, *13*, 658. [CrossRef] [PubMed]

10. Napoli, F.; Listi, A.; Zambelli, V.; Witel, G.; Bironzo, P.; Papotti, M.; Volante, M.; Scagliotti, G.; Righi, L. Pathological characterization of tumor immune microenvironment (TIME) in malignant pleural mesothelioma. *Cancers* **2021**, *13*, 2564. [CrossRef] [PubMed]
11. Schiavello, M.; Gazzano, E.; Bergandi, L.; Silvagno, F.; Libener, R.; Riganti, C.; Aldieri, E. Identification of redox-sensitive transcription factors as markers of malignant pleural mesothelioma. *Cancers* **2021**, *13*, 1138. [CrossRef] [PubMed]
12. Brcic, L.; Mathilakathu, A.; Walter, R.F.H.; Wessolly, M.; Mairinger, E.; Beckert, H.; Kreidt, D.; Steinborn, J.; Hager, T.; Christoph, D.C.; et al. Digital gene expression analysis of epithelioid and sarcomatoid mesothelioma reveals differences in immunogenicity. *Cancers* **2021**, *13*, 1761. [CrossRef] [PubMed]
13. Kitajima, K.; Maruyama, M.; Yokoyama, H.; Minami, T.; Yokoi, T.; Nakamura, A.; Hashimoto, M.; Kondo, N.; Kuribayashi, K.; Kijima, T.; et al. Response to immune checkpoint inhibitor therapy in patients with unresectable recurrent malignant pleural mesothelioma shown by FDG-PET and CT. *Cancers* **2021**, *13*, 1098. [CrossRef] [PubMed]
14. Lee, D.-S.; Carollo, A.; Alpert, N.; Taioli, E.; Flores, R. VATS pleurectomy decortication is a reasonable alternative for higher risk patients in the management of malignant pleural mesothelioma: An analysis of short-term outcomes. *Cancers* **2021**, *13*, 1068. [CrossRef] [PubMed]
15. Di Gregorio, E.; Miolo, G.; Saorin, A.; Muraro, E.; Cangemi, M.; Relevant, A.; Minatel, E.; Trovo, M.; Steffan, A.; Corona, G. Radical hemithoracic radiotherapy induces systemic metabolomics changes that are associated with the clinical outcome of malignant pleural mesothelioma patients. *Cancers* **2021**, *13*, 508. [CrossRef]
16. Yang, H.; Xu, D.; Yang, Z.; Yao, F.; Zhao, H.; Schmid, R.A.; Peng, R.-W. Systematic analysis of aberrant biochemical networks and potential drug vulnerabilities induced by tumor suppressor loss in malignant pleural mesothelioma. *Cancers* **2020**, *12*, 2310. [CrossRef]
17. Anobile, D.P.; Bironzo, P.; Picca, F.; Lingua, M.F.; Morena, D.; Righi, L.; Napoli, F.; Papotti, M.G.; Pittaro, A.; Di Nicolantonio, F.; et al. Evaluation of the preclinical efficacy of Lurbinectedin in malignant pleural mesothelioma. *Cancers* **2021**, *13*, 2332. [CrossRef]
18. Kotesha, R.; Tonse, R.; Rubens, M.; Appel, H.; Albrecht, F.; Kaymin, P.; Alley, E.W.; Tom, M.C.; Mehta, M.P. Meta-analysis of survival and development of a prognostic nomogram for malignant pleural mesothelioma treated with systemic chemotherapy. *Cancers* **2021**, *13*, 2186. [CrossRef] [PubMed]
19. Dulloo, S.; Bzura, A.; Fennell, D.A. Precision therapy for mesothelioma: Feasibility and new opportunities. *Cancers* **2021**, *13*, 2347. [CrossRef] [PubMed]

Article

DNA Methylation of *FKBP5* as Predictor of Overall Survival in Malignant Pleural Mesothelioma

Giovanni Cugliari [1,*], Chiara Catalano [1], Simonetta Guarrera [2,3], Alessandra Allione [1], Elisabetta Casalone [1], Alessia Russo [1], Federica Grosso [4], Daniela Ferrante [5,6], Clara Viberti [1], Anna Aspesi [7], Marika Sculco [7], Chiara Pirazzini [8], Roberta Libener [9], Dario Mirabelli [10,11,†], Corrado Magnani [5,6,11,†], Irma Dianzani [7,11] and Giuseppe Matullo [1,11,12,*]

1. Department of Medical Sciences, University of Turin, 10126 Turin, Italy; chiara.catalano@unito.it (C.C.); alessandra.allione@unito.it (A.A.); elisabetta.casalone@unito.it (E.C.); alessia.russo@unito.it (A.R.); clara.viberti@unito.it (C.V.)
2. Italian Institute for Genomic Medicine, IIGM, 10060 Candiolo, Italy; simonetta.guarrera@iigm.it
3. Candiolo Cancer Institute, FPO-IRCCS, 10060 Candiolo, Italy
4. Division of Medical Oncology, SS. Antonio e Biagio General Hospital, 15121 Alessandria, Italy; federica.grosso@unipo.it
5. Unit of Medical Statistics, Department of Translational Medicine, University of Piemonte Orientale, 28100 Novara, Italy; daniela.ferrante@med.uniupo.it (D.F.); corrado.magnani@med.uniupo.it (C.M.)
6. Cancer Epidemiology Unit, CPO-Piemonte, 28100 Novara, Italy
7. Department of Health Sciences, University of Piemonte Orientale, 28100 Novara, Italy; anna.aspesi@med.uniupo.it (A.A.); marika.sculco@med.uniupo.it (M.S.); irma.dianzani@med.unipmn.it (I.D.)
8. Department of Experimental, Diagnostic and Specialty Medicine (DIMES), University of Bologna, 40126 Bologna, Italy; chiara.pirazzini5@unibo.it
9. Pathology Unit, SS. Antonio e Biagio General Hospital, 15122 Alessandria, Italy; rlibener@ospedale.al.it
10. Cancer Epidemiology Unit, Department of Medical Sciences, University of Turin, 10126 Turin, Italy; dario.mirabelli@gmail.com
11. Interdepartmental Center for Studies on Asbestos and Other Toxic Particulates "G. Scansetti", University of Turin, 10126 Turin, Italy
12. Medical Genetics Unit, AOU Città della Salute e della Scienza, 10126 Turin, Italy
* Correspondence: giovanni.cugliari@unito.it (G.C.); giuseppe.matullo@unito.it (G.M.)
† Disclosure: C.M.: D.M.: expert witness in court trials for asbestos related diseases.

Received: 9 October 2020; Accepted: 18 November 2020; Published: 21 November 2020

Simple Summary: Our study is the first one to investigate DNA methylation changes in white blood cells (WBCs) from easily accessible peripheral blood as malignant pleural mesothelioma (MPM) survival biomarker. The Cox proportional hazards regression model highlighted that the methylation status of the CpG dinucleotide cg03546163 is an independent marker of prognosis in MPM patients with a better performance than traditional inflammation-based scores such as lymphocyte-to-monocyte ratio (LMR). Biological validation and replication showed that epigenetic changes at the *FKBP5* gene were robustly associated with overall survival (OS) in MPM cases. The identification of simple and valuable prognostic markers for MPM will enable clinicians to select patients who are most likely to benefit from aggressive therapies and avoid subjecting non-responder patients to ineffective treatment.

Abstract: Malignant pleural mesothelioma (MPM) is an aggressive tumor with median survival of 12 months and limited effective treatments. The scope of this study was to study the relationship between blood DNA methylation (DNAm) and overall survival (OS) aiming at a noninvasive prognostic test. We investigated a cohort of 159 incident asbestos exposed MPM cases enrolled in an Italian area with high incidence of mesothelioma. Considering 12 months as a cut-off for OS, epigenome-wide association study (EWAS) revealed statistically significant (p value = 7.7×10^{-9}) OS-related differential methylation of a single-CpG (cg03546163), located in the 5′UTR region of the *FKBP5* gene. This is an independent marker of prognosis in MPM patients with a better performance than traditional inflammation-based scores such as lymphocyte-to-monocyte ratio (LMR). Cases with DNAm < 0.45 at the cg03546163 had significantly poor survival compared with those showing DNAm ≥ 0.45 (mean: 243 versus 534 days; p value< 0.001). Epigenetic changes at the *FKBP5* gene were robustly associated with OS in MPM cases. Our results showed that blood DNA methylation levels could be promising and dynamic prognostic biomarkers in MPM.

Keywords: malignant pleural mesothelioma; asbestos exposure; DNA methylation; lymphocyte-to-monocyte ratio; epigenome-wide analysis; survival analysis

1. Introduction

Malignant pleural mesothelioma (MPM) is an aggressive tumor. The disease usually develops after a long latency (20–40 years) following asbestos exposure [1]. Although MPM is considered a rare malignancy (prevalence 1–9/100,000), about 40,000 deaths have been estimated to occur each year globally [2,3]. The World Health Organization estimates that 125 million people annually around the world are exposed to asbestos. The International Agency for Research on Cancer confirmed that all fibrous forms of asbestos are carcinogenic to humans, causing mainly mesothelioma, respiratory-tract tumors, mesothelioma, and cancer at other tissue sites [4].

The prognosis of MPM is poor with a median survival of about 12 months from the diagnosis [5].

Generally, the first-line treatment is a combination of a multitargeted anti folate (pemetrexed or raltitrexed) drug and a platinum compound (cisplatin or carboplatin) [6] Currently, only a single randomized trial demonstrated an increase in survival time when comparing cisplatin and pemetrexed versus cisplatin alone [7]; unfortunately, most patients became resistant to this treatment and relapsed rapidly. No oncogenic driver has been identified and molecular pathways leading to MPM have not yet been clearly determined. Other therapeutic strategies such as immunotherapy are promising but require further investigation and improvement [8].

Recent research on the pathogenesis of MPM indicated that (i) both genetic and epigenetic alterations contribute to asbestos-induced tumorigenesis [9,10], (ii) inflammation-based prognostic scores that include lymphocyte counts are associated with survival [11].

MPM has a low frequency of protein-altering mutations (~25 mutations per tumor), compared to many other tumors [12]. Moreover, germline mutations in different genes mainly involved in DNA damage repair confer moderate-to-high genetic risk of MPM development [13]. The BAP1-tumor predisposition syndrome is the most studied genetic condition associated with MPM development and is caused by mutations in the BRCA1-associated protein 1 (*BAP1*) gene [13].

In the last 10 years, epigenetic markers, such as DNA methylation (DNAm) and microRNAs (miRNAs), have gained popularity as possible early diagnostic and prognostic biomarkers in cancer research, including MPM. While genetic markers may differ from case to case in most cancer patients (i.e., each patient may carry a different mutation within the same gene), different subjects show variable levels of epigenetic biomarkers in specific target regions and different tissues depending on disease status [14].

DNA methylation is one of the epigenetic factors [15] that can be altered in cancer tissues. However, regarding mechanisms and clinical outcome of epigenetic derangements in MPM, less information is available [16,17] Although DNAm is stable, it can be modified throughout life by several factors such as ageing, lifestyle, environmental exposures, and diseases. It thus represents an adaptive phenomenon linking environmental factors and the development of pathologic phenotypes such as cancers. DNAm changes are considered to possibly play a role in MPM progression, and have therefore been suggested as a potential tool for prognosis [18].

The fact that epigenetic modifications, unlike genetic changes, are potentially reversible, may open new perspectives for patient clustering and novel therapeutic options. A reliable prognostic biomarker that offers high sensitivity and specificity would be a major advancement for MPM. Blood-based biomarkers that have been explored in MPM include megakaryocyte potentiating factor (an alternative cleavage product of the mesothelin precursor protein) [19], and Fibulin 3 which is also found in pleural fluid, and whose high levels appear to correlate with advanced disease [20].

Considering clinical end-point, low pleural fluid glucose and high C-reactive protein and pleural thickening represent the main prognosis factors [21]. Recent studies confirm that using also a combination of epigenetic alterations as biomarkers is more informative with respect to an only genetic approach on overall survival (OS) [17].

This study was undertaken with the goal of better characterizing the MPM OS evaluating the potential predictive value of peripheral blood DNAm profiles. The second goal was the comparison of the DNAm prognostic performance with the broadly used lymphocyte-to-monocyte ratio (LMR) method.

2. Results

2.1. Epigenome-Wide Association Study (EWAS)

EWAS revealed a statistically significant hypo-methylated single-CpG (cg03546163) in the *FKBP5* gene in the low survival group after Bonferroni post-hoc correction (Figure 1).

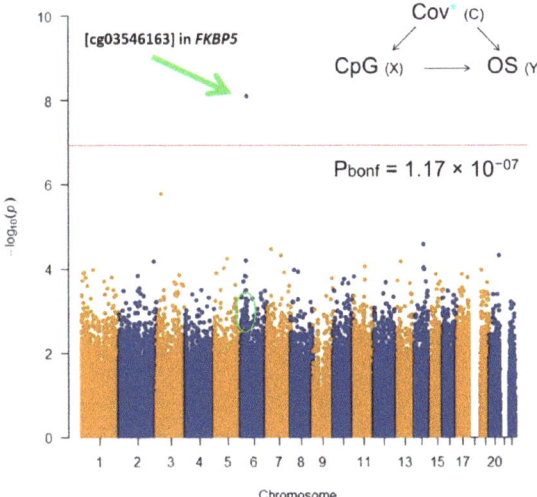

Figure 1. Manhattan plot for epigenome-wide association study (EWAS) test on 450k single CpGs. Overall survival was used as dependent variable considering 12 months as cut-off adjusting for age, gender, histological subtype, asbestos exposure, WBCs estimation, population stratification, and technical variability. Bonferroni post hoc line highlights statistically significant differences on OS at single CpG level.

Bootstrap was computed to estimate the measures of accuracy, using random sampling methods.

The other five CpGs in the *FKBP5* gene showed hypomethylation in poor MPM survivors, with unadjusted p value < 0.05 (Table 1); instead, no CpGs in the *FKBP5* gene showed statistically significant hypermethylation in poor MPM survivors.

Table 1. Differential DNAm analyses of the *FKBP5* gene ordered by effect size (low survival group was used as reference). Information about single CpGs including location-related values and model outputs (effect size, standard error, *p* values).

TargetID	CHR	UCSC RefGene Group	Enhancer	Probe Start	Probe End	Closest TSS	Distance Closest TSS	Closest TSS Gene Name	Effect Size	SE	*p* value	Bonferroni	Significance
cg03546163	6	5'UTR;5'UTR;5'UTR;5'UTR	NA	35654313	35654363	35656691	2329	FKBP5	0.12	0.02	7.71E-09	0.003280418	*§
cg00052684	6	5'UTR	TRUE	35694195	35694245	35696396	2152	FKBP5	0.04	0.02	0.014589031	1	*
cg00130530	6	5'UTR;TSS1500;TSS1500;TSS1500	NA	35657152	35657202	35656718	-483	FKBP5	0.03	0.01	0.001490825	1	*
cg19226017	6	TSS1500;Body	NA	35697185	35697235	35696396	-788	FKBP5	0.03	0.01	0.021639194	1	*
cg08915438	6	TSS1500;Body	NA	35697709	35697759	35696396	-1362	FKBP5	0.02	0.01	0.050779639	1	
cg14642437	6	5'UTR;5'UTR;5'UTR;5'UTR	NA	35652471	35652521	35656691	4171	FKBP5	0.02	0.01	0.030718193	1	*
cg25114611	6	TSS1500;Body	NA	35696820	35696870	35696396	-473	FKBP5	0.02	0.01	0.080435168	1	
cg16052510	6	Body;Body;Body;Body	TRUE	35603093	35603143	35656691	53549	FKBP5	0.01	0.01	0.201783727	1	
cg03591753	6	5'UTR	NA	35659141	35659191	35656718	-2422	FKBP5	0.01	0.01	0.071287867	1	
cg23416081	6	5'UTR	TRUE	35693573	35693623	35696396	2824	FKBP5	0.01	0.01	0.300181524	1	
cg19014730	6	5'UTR;5'UTR;5'UTR;5'UTR	TRUE	35635985	35636035	35656691	20707	FKBP5	0.01	0.01	0.510924063	1	
cg20813374	6	5'UTR;TSS1500;TSS1500;TSS1500	NA	35657130	35657180	35656718	-461	FKBP5	0.01	0.01	0.538622493	1	
cg07061368	6	5'UTR;5'UTR;5'UTR;5'UTR	TRUE	35631736	35631786	35656691	24956	FKBP5	0.01	0.01	0.440719926	1	
cg08636224	6	5'UTR;TSS1500;TSS1500;TSS1500	NA	35657871	35657921	35656718	-1202	FKBP5	0.00	0.00	0.18248273	1	
cg01294490	6	TSS200;TSS200;5'UTR;TSS1500	NA	35656906	35656956	35656718	-187	FKBP5	0.00	0.01	0.421300242	1	
cg07485685	6	5'UTR;Body	NA	35696060	35696110	35696396	336	FKBP5	0.00	0.00	0.847941933	1	
cg14284211	6	Body;Body;Body;Body	TRUE	35570224	35570274	35656691	86468	FKBP5	0.00	0.01	0.974334781	1	
cg17030679	6	5'UTR;Body;1stExon	NA	35696300	35696350	35696396	97	FKBP5	0.00	0.00	0.955719442	1	
cg08622770	6	5'UTR;5'UTR;5'UTR;5'UTR	NA	35655764	35655814	35656691	928	FKBP5	0.00	0.00	0.939904147	1	
cg00140191	6	5'UTR;5'UTR;5'UTR;5'UTR	NA	35656193	35656243	35656691	450	FKBP5	0.00	0.00	0.882388191	1	
cg00610228	6	5'UTR;Body	NA	35695934	35695984	35696396	463	FKBP5	0.00	0.00	0.87376216	1	
cg07633853	6	Body;Body;Body;Body	TRUE	35569421	35569471	35656691	87221	FKBP5	0.00	0.01	0.965427693	1	
cg10300814	6	Body;Body;Body;Body	TRUE	35565066	35565116	35480646	-84469	TULP1	0.00	0.00	0.620677997	1	
cg16012111	6	TSS200;TSS200;TSS200;5'UTR	NA	35656758	35656808	35656718	-39	FKBP5	0.00	0.00	0.519047184	1	
cg06937024	6	5'UTR;Body	NA	35695440	35695490	35696396	908	FKBP5	0.00	0.00	0.135004544	1	
cg08586216	6	5'UTR;5'UTR;5'UTR;5'UTR	TRUE	35612301	35612351	35656691	44341	FKBP5	0.00	0.00	0.105631333	1	
cg17085721	6	5'UTR;5'UTR;5'UTR;5'UTR	TRUE	35645291	35645341	35656691	11351	FKBP5	0.00	0.00	0.211582562	1	
cg02665568	6	Body;Body;Body	NA	35544468	35544518	35480646	-63821	TULP1	-0.01	0.01	0.294757699	1	
cg15929276	6	5'UTR	TRUE	35687456	35687506	35696396	8940	FKBP5	-0.01	0.01	0.455969031	1	
cg06087101	6	Body;3'UTR;Body;Body	NA	35551882	35551932	35480646	-71285	TULP1	-0.02	0.02	0.203783874	1	

Low survival group was set as reference. Adjustment covariates: age, gender, asbestos exposure, histological subtype, smoke, population stratification, WBCs estimation, and technical variability. *: statistically significant at *p* value< 0.05; §: statistically significant at Bonferroni and FDR post hoc adjustments.

2.2. Survival Analysis

CpG sites and LMR were considered as predictors in the regression model. Categorical variables (quantile information) were used.

Cox model was computed considering the same list of covariates included in the EWAS. Patients with DNAm < 0.45 at the cg03546163 had significantly poorer survival compared with subjects with DNAm ≥ 0.45 (mean, 243 versus 534 days; p value < 0.001). Survival at the 1st and the 3rd Quartiles was 135 versus 209 days and 401 versus 842 days, respectively, comparing patients with single CpG DNAm < 0.45 with those with single CpG DNAm ≥ 0.45. The multivariate analysis showed that cg03546163 DNAm at *FKBP5* was independently associated with OS. Kaplan–Meier curves revealed that a decrease of methylation at cg03546163 (<0.45) was significantly associated with worse OS (HR = 2.14 p value < 0.0001) (Figure 2a).

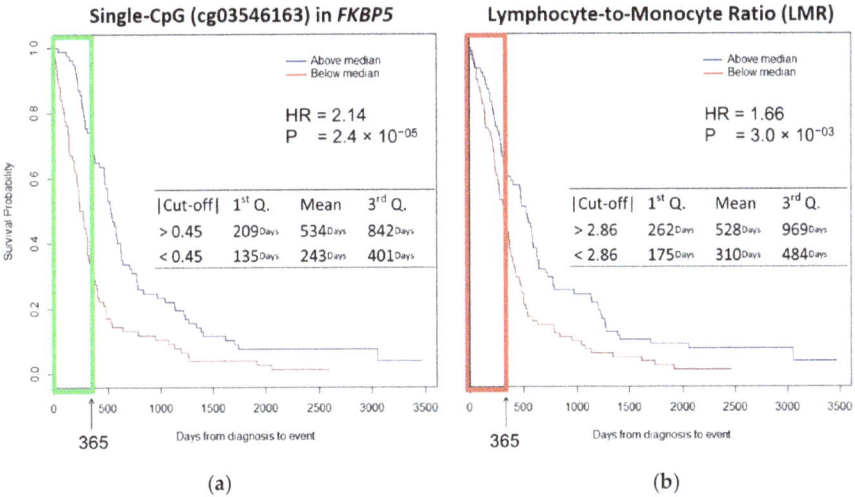

Figure 2. K-M survival curves show (**a**) cg03546163: patients with a DNAm < 0.45 had significantly poor survival compared with a DNAm ≥ 0.45 (mean, 243 versus 534 days; p value < 0.001); (**b**) LMR: patients with values < 2.86 had significantly poor survival compared with patients with values ≥ 2.86 (mean, 310 versus 528 days; p value < 0.001). cg03546163 is an independent marker of prognosis in patients with MPM and performs better than LMR ($HR_{cg03546163}$ = 2.14 vs HR_{LMR} = 1.66).

Patients with LMR < 2.86 had significantly poorer survival compared with patients with LMR ≥ 2.86 (mean, 310 versus 528 days; p value < 0.001). Survival at 1st Quartile was 175 versus 262 days whereas at 3rd Quartile was 484 versus 969 days comparing patients with LMR < 2.86 with those with LMR > 2.86. LMR was independently associated with OS: Kaplan–Meier curves showed that decreased LMR (<2.86) was significantly associated with decreased OS (HR = 1.66; p value < 0.01) (Figure 2b).

Histological subtype (epithelioid versus non-epithelioid), smoking status (current, never, and former), and asbestos exposure showed no statistically significant results on survival.

2.3. Validation and Replication

The statistically significant association between cg03546163 DNAm and OS was confirmed in an independent sample of patients (replication) and using a different targeted DNAm analysis technique (validation). A sample of 133 MPM cases (58 low survivors and 75 high survivors) was recruited and stratified in low and high OS considering the same cut-off (365 days).

The same model used for the discovery phase was performed. Patients with below median OS had significantly lower DNAm at the cg03546163 compared with those with above median OS (mean, 188 versus 786 days; p value < 0.001). The 1st Quartile was 113 versus 482 days and the 3rd Quartile was 262 versus 862 days comparing patients with DNAm difference (reference above median OS, MD: −0.04, 95%CI: −0.07|−0.01, p value: 0.04) at the cg03546163. The multivariate analysis confirmed that cg03546163 DNAm at *FKBP5* was independently associated with OS.

3. Discussion

A growing number of studies reported on the identification of epigenetic prognostic biomarkers in several cancers [17,22].

This study focused on the exploration of epigenetic factors related to MPM survival in MPM incident cases from Piedmont (Italy), a region with a well-documented history of asbestos exposure [23].

More than 450k methylation sites were evaluated in DNA from whole blood looking for new insights related to overall survival in MPM. The main result was the hypomethylation of a single CpG (cg03546163) in the 5′ UTR region of the FKBP5 gene in patients with poorer survival compared to patients with longer survival; it also showed to be an independent marker of prognosis in MPM patients. This result was replicated in a different series of patients belonging to the same cohort using the Sequenom Quantitative DNAm analysis.

In general, a combination of epigenetic and clinical factors is under investigation in clinical prognosis and survival, including tumor histology, gender, hemoglobin level, platelet and white blood cell count, and lactate dehydrogenase level [24].

Recently, due to the important role of inflammation in the development of MPM, several studies investigated the effect of inflammation-based biomarkers on the prognosis [11,22]. We selected the LMR for the comparison because its performance was previously reported to be higher than other inflammation-based markers in MPM [25].

To validate the prognostic value of the observed CpG methylation site, we compared our result with the LMR score.

Kaplan–Meier survival curves for MPM patients highlighted cg03546163 methylation at FKBP5 gene as a prognostic factor superior to the LMR score.

The FKBP Prolyl Isomerase 5 (FKBP5), also known as FK506 binding protein 51 (FKBP51), is a member of the immunophilin protein family, which contributes to the immunoregulation and to the basic cellular processes involving protein folding and trafficking. Together with other members of the FKBPs family, this protein participates in transcriptional complexes and acts as a co-transcription factor.

Although no studies have investigated the methylation of *FKBP5* as prognostic factor in MPM, a growing number of whole-blood studies investigated its DNA methylation levels in order to explain the impact of environmental stress in the etiology and treatment of several diseases [26]. Interestingly, in a recent study on the Behcet's disease (BD) hypomethylation in the 5′UTR region (including cg03546163) of FKBP5 characterized cases was demonstrated and it was strongly associated with high gene expression, suggesting a possible role of DNA methylation in the pathogenesis [27].

Other five single CpGs at FKBP5 showed hypomethylation in poor survivors: this evidence supports the potential overall contribution of *FKBP5* methylation on the patient classification by OS.

In several human cancer tissues, a relevant role for FKBP5 in sustaining cancer cell growth and aggressiveness has been documented. In particular, for glioma [28], prostate cancer and melanoma [29] a strict correlation between protein abundance and aggressiveness has been demonstrated.

Probably, the relationship between FKBP5 and tumor progression and aggressiveness, is represented by its implication in NF-kB and AKT signaling pathways, with key roles in tumorigenesis and response to antineoplastic chemotherapy [30].

Moreover, a well characterized antiapoptotic effect is mediated by NF-κB transcription factors and FKBP5 has documented antiapoptotic effects: recent studies hypothesized that FKBP5 could promote inflammation, by activating the master immune regulator NF-kB, after an epigenetic upregulation due to aging and stress [31,32].

Previous studies conducted on various cancer types, showed that upregulation of FKBP5 gene expression is associated with drug resistance [33]. In a study on an ovarian cancer cell line, the upregulation of FKBP5 increased the resistance to chemotherapeutic agents, whereas the gene silencing sensitized ovarian cancer cells to taxol [34]. In the present study we could not evaluate FKBP5 gene expression due to the lack of available RNA, which was not collected in the study. However, this should be further addressed and verified in future studies.

One study demonstrated that overexpression of FKBP5 increased the chemosensitivity through the AKT pathway [31]. A similar study supported this observation making FKBP5 an effective biomarker for sensitivity to chemotherapy; patient responses to chemotherapy may be determined by the variation in FKBP5 levels [35].

Limitation of the Study

Being able to identify the direction of causality will greatly aid in determining the usefulness of epigenetic variation.

Leukocyte DNA methylation could mainly represent a nonspecific marker related to a general inflammatory status due to the presence of a tumor rather than a specific MPM biomarker and further studies should be carried out to support our findings.

As additional limitation, we had therapy information only for a small subset of patients and we could not test treatment-specific OS differences in relation to FKBP5 methylation levels.

4. Material and Methods

4.1. Study Population

Study subjects belong to a wider ongoing collaborative study on MPM, which is actively enrolling MPM cases in the municipalities of Casale Monferrato (Piedmont region, Italy), an area with an exceptionally high incidence of mesothelioma caused by widespread asbestos exposure for locals, both occupational and environmental, due to the asbestos-cement Eternit plant that was operational until 1986 [36]. Additional MPM cases were recruited in the main hospitals of the municipalities of Turin, Novara, and Alessandria (Piedmont region, Italy). The study included incident MPM cases diagnosed between 2000 and 2010 after histological and/or cytological confirmation of MPM diagnosis [37,38].

No peritoneal cases were considered with the aim to better identify epigenetics characteristics of MPM.

In the present study, 159 MPM cases belonging to a larger case–control study with genetic [10,39] and blood DNAm data [9] were selected according to the following criteria: (i) availability of good quality DNA at the time of the analyses and (ii) asbestos exposure above the background level, as defined in [40]. An additional 133 independent samples from the same cohort were included for the validation/replication analyses.

Descriptive information of MPM patients are shown in Table 2. Median survival (365 days) was used as cut-off value to stratify patients in high and low survivors.

No differences in categorical (center, gender, smoke, histotype) and continuous (asbestos exposure, WBCs composition) variables among low and high survivors were found.

Our study complies with the Declaration of Helsinki principles and conforms to ethical requirements. All volunteers signed an informed consent form at enrollment. The study protocol was approved by the Ethics Committee of the Italian Institute for Genomic Medicine (prot.n.CE-2015-GM-2, 30/10/2015, HUGEF, Turin, Italy).

4.2. Exposure Assessment

For all subjects, occupational history and lifestyle habits information were collected through interviewer-administered questionnaires filled out at enrollment during a face-to-face interview.

Job titles were coded according to the International Standard Classification of Occupations [40] and according to the Statistical Classification of Economic Activities in the European Community.

Frequency, duration, and intensity of exposure were estimated, then a cumulative exposure index was computed. The evaluation of asbestos exposure (occupational, environmental, and domestic) was conducted by an experienced occupational epidemiologist. For the selection criteria and descriptive evaluation, asbestos exposure doses (fibers/mL years) were rank transformed to remove skewness.

Table 2. Descriptive information of MPM patients. Median survival (365 days) was used as cut-off value to stratify patients in high and low survivors.

Categorical Variable	Level	Low OS ($n = 79$)		High OS ($n = 80$)	
		N	%	N	%
Centre	Casale	50	63.3	46	57.5
	Torino	29	36.7	34	42.5
Gender	Males	59	74.7	50	62.5
	Females	20	25.3	30	37.5
Smoke	Current	20	26.3	8	10.3
	Former	24	31.6	29	37.2
	Never	32	42.1	41	52.6
Histotype	Epithelioid	44	55.7	61	76.3
	Sarcomatoid	14	17.7	2	2.5
	Biphasic	17	21.5	11	13.8
	Undefined	2	2.5	1	1.3
	Not known	2	2.5	5	6.3
Continuous Variable	**Level**	**Low OS**		**High OS**	
		Mean	SD	Mean	SD
Overall Survival (days)		198.7	101.6	957.8	698.7
Age (years)		67.7	12.4	67.5	9.6
Asbestos Exp. (norm)		1.4	1.5	1.5	1.9
CD8T (%)		2.9	4.5	3	3.4
CD4T (%)		6.8	5.3	8.8	5.4
Natural Killer (%)		4.9	4.9	6.3	4.1
B cell (%)		6.1	2.8	6.4	2.7
Monocytes (%)		8.1	4.1	7.6	4.4
Granulocytes (%)		75	13	72	10

Asbestos exposure (occupational, environmental, and domestic) was normalized considering frequency, duration, and intensity.

4.3. Blood DNAm Analysis

Genomic DNA was extracted from whole blood collected in EDTA by an on-column DNA purification method (QIAamp DNA Blood Mini Kit, QIAGEN GmbH, Germany), according to manufacturer's instructions. DNA integrity was checked by an electrophoretic run in standard TBE 0.5× buffer on a 1% low melting agarose gel (Sigma-Aldrich GmbH, Schnelldorf, Germany); DNA purity and concentration were assessed by a NanoDrop 8000 Spectrophotometer (Thermo Fisher Scientific Inc., Waltham, MA, USA). Five hundred nanograms of genomic DNA for each sample were bisulfite treated (EZ-96 DNA Methylation-Gold Kit, Zymo Research Corporation, Irvine, CA, USA) to convert un-methylated cytosine to uracil. Cases were randomly and blindly distributed across conversion plates.

The Infinium HumanMethylation450 BeadChip (Illumina Inc., San Diego, CA, USA) was used to measure the methylation level of more than 485,000 individual CpG loci at a genome-wide resolution [41].

Twelve samples were analyzed on each BeadChip. As a "position effect" was reported for Illumina Methylation BeadChips, each sample position on the BeadChip was completely random as well. We further verified the randomization of the position on each BeadChip was effective by checking for a position effect, and we found no occurrence of it. BeadChips were processed according to manufacturer protocols. Data were inspected with the dedicated GenomeStudio software v2011.1 with Methylation module 1.9.0 (Illumina Inc., San Diego, CA), and quality checked as previously described [42].

4.4. Beta-Value Extraction

Raw DNAm data were analyzed with the R package (methylumi'). The average methylation value at each locus was computed as the ratio of the intensity of the methylated signal over the total signal (un-methylated + methylated) [43]. Beta-values represent the percentage of methylation at each individual CpG locus, ranging from 0 (no methylation) to 1 (full methylation).

We excluded from the analyses (i) single Beta-values with detection p value ≥ 0.01; (ii) CpG loci with missing Beta-values in more than 20% of the assayed samples; (iii) CpG loci detected by probes containing SNPs with MAF ≥ 0.05 in the CEPH (Utah residents with ancestry from northern and western Europe, CEU) population; (iv) samples with a global call rate $\leq 95\%$. Lastly, CpGs on chromosomes X and Y were excluded from the analysis.

4.5. Batch Effect, Population Stratification, and White Blood Cell Estimations

To account for methylation assay variability and batch effects, we corrected all differential methylation analyses for "control probes" principal components (PCs). Using PCs assessed by principal component analysis of the BeadChip's built-in control probes as a correction factor for statistical analyses of microarray data is a method that allows to account for the technical variability of several steps in the DNAm analysis, from the bisulfite conversion to BeadChip processing [44].

Geographic origins of subjects may influence DNAm profiles. To consider this source of potential bias, we took advantage of the whole genome genotyping dataset from the same subjects from our previous study [10]. The first PCs calculated based on genome-wide genotyping were shown to correlate with different geographic origins of people [45,46].

WBC subtype percentages calculated based on genome-wide methylation data [47] for each subject were extracted. This method quantifies the normally mixed composition of leukocytes beyond what is possible by simple histological or flow cytometric assessments. In a diverse array of diseases and following numerous immune-toxic exposures, leukocyte composition will critically inform the underlying immune-biology to most chronic medical conditions. Then, it is necessary to extract and control for the percentage of involved WBCs with the aim to infer about a functional biological pathway.

LMR score was calculated from the DNAm-estimated WBCs by dividing the total lymphocyte count by the monocyte count.

4.6. Statistical Analyses

Epigenome-Wide Association Study

Association test was used to analyze the mean differences (MD) at single-CpG methylation between low and high survival. Multiple regression analysis adjusted for age, gender, histological subtype, asbestos exposure, smoke, estimated WBCs, population stratification (first 2 PCs) and technical variability (first 10 PCs) was implemented. For multiple comparisons tests, Bonferroni p value ≤ 0.05 was considered statistically significant.

Using random sampling methods, bootstrap was implemented to estimate the measures of accuracy defined in terms of bias, variance, confidence intervals, and prediction error. Bootstrap is also an appropriate way to control and check the stability of the results. The bias-corrected and accelerated (BCa) bootstrap interval was calculated with regard to single CpGs.

4.7. Survival Analysis

The survival time was determined as the time between the date of diagnosis and the date of death. If patients were still alive at the last follow-up (2016), survival was defined as the time from the date of diagnosis until June 2016. The time and the median event times with 95% confidence intervals were estimated according to the Kaplan–Meier method. The proportional hazards regression model was used for both the univariate and multivariate analyses (Cox model).

Comparison of OS curves was performed using two-tailed log-rank tests with a 0.05 level of significance. Only variables with p value < 0.1 in the univariate analysis were included in the final model for the multivariate analysis. In the Cox regression analysis, the backward conditional method (stepwise-AIC) was used. LMR and CpG sites were considered as predictors in regression model.

4.8. Statistical Power

To ensure a power of the study greater than 80% (two-tailed test at 0.05 alpha error), only CpGs with mean difference (MD) of Beta-value between low and high survival of ≥ |0.035| were selected. Covariates were included step-by-step in sensitivity analysis to validate the association output considering effect size, standard error, 95% confidence interval and p value variations.

CpGs with Bonferroni p value ≤ 0.05 underwent gene set enrichment analysis to identify pathways potentially affected by MPM related methylation changes.

All statistical analyses were conducted using the open source software R (4.0.2).

4.9. Validation and Replication

Sequenom MassARRAY for the DNAm signal validation and replication was used. In detail, the EpiTYPER assay (Sequenom) uses a MALDI-TOF mass spectrometry-based method to quantitatively assess the DNA methylation state of CpG sites of interest [48]. DNA (500 ng) was bisulfite-converted using the EZ-96 DNA Methylation Kit (Zymo Research) with the following modifications: incubation in CT buffer for 21 cycles of 15 min at 55 °C and 30 s at 95 °C, elution of bisulfite-treated DNA in 100 µL of water. The treatment converts unmethylated Cytosine into Uracil, leaving methylated Cytosine unchanged. In this way, variations in the sequence are produced depending on DNA methylation status of the original DNA molecule.

PCR amplification, treatment with SAP solution, and Transcription/RNase A cocktails were performed according to the protocol provided by Sequenom and the mass spectra were analyzed by EpiTYPER analyzer (Sequenom, San Diego, CA, USA). As the MassARRAY assay is unable to discriminate between CpGs located at close vicinity to each other in the sequence, the close neighboring CpGs were analyzed as "Units", i.e., the measured methylation level is the average of the methylation levels of the CpGs cumulatively analyzed within the Unit. In the case of cg03546163 the measured methylation level is the average between two CpG sites located very close (Figure S1).

The amplicon for cg03546163 (chr6:35,654,364) encompasses 196bp (chr6:35,654,222-chr6:35,654,418 (GRCh37/hg19)) and PCR was performed on 10 ng of converted DNA using the following primers:

- cg03546163_10FW: aggaagagagTTTTTGTTTAGGATGAATTAGTTTGG;
- cg03546163_T7RV: cagtaatacgactcactatagggagaaggctAAAAACTACAATCTTATCCAATTCCTTT.

5. Conclusions

Our results suggest the potential use of DNAm analysis in blood to develop noninvasive tests for prognostic evaluation in MPM; our study is the first to demonstrate that a single CpG in *FKBP5* gene is an independent marker of prognosis in patients with MPM and is superior to the LMR inflammation-based prognostic score. The identification of simple and valuable prognostic markers for MPM will enable clinicians to select patients who are most likely to benefit from aggressive therapies and avoid subjecting nonresponder patients to ineffective treatment. Moreover, epigenetic modifications such as DNAm are potentially reversible and can open new perspectives for epigenetic therapies in MPM. Knowledge of epigenetic changes has provided new therapeutic opportunities against cancer. To allow better approach of cancer cell inhibitory strategies, the understanding of molecular mechanisms that underlie cellular DNA epigenetic alterations may be useful. In this context, we reported epigenetic deregulations in blood samples from MPM patients in relation to OS, paving the road to both patients' stratification and the possible discovery of new combined therapeutic options in MPM. Studies of a large population are needed to investigate the relationship between prognostic markers and treatment regimens. The usage of methylation alterations in clinical specimens as biomarkers could be recognized. Noninvasively obtained, methylation-based biomarkers detected in blood cells from cancer patients offer significant practical advantages, being promising and dynamic prognostic markers.

Supplementary Materials: The following are available online at http://www.mdpi.com/2072-6694/12/11/3470/s1, Figure S1. Locations of cg03546163 (CpG2, in bold) and a second CpG site very close (CpG1, in red), investigated by Sequenom MassARRAY.

Author Contributions: Conceptualization, G.C., G.M., C.M., D.M., I.D. and F.G.; methodology, G.C., G.M. and S.G.; software, G.C.; validation, G.C., G.M., A.A. (Alessandra Allione), A.R., E.C. and C.P.; formal analysis, G.C.; investigation, G.C., G.M., S.G., A.A. (Alessandra Allione), A.R., E.C. and C.C.; resources, G.C., G.M., C.M., D.M., I.D., F.G., C.V., D.F., A.A. (Anna Aspesi), M.S. and R.L.; data curation, G.C., C.M., D.M., I.D., F.G., C.P., C.V., D.F., A.A. (Anna Aspesi), M.S. and R.L.; writing—original draft preparation, G.C.; writing—review and editing, G.C., G.M., C.M., D.M., I.D., F.G., S.G., A.A. (Alessandra Allione), A.R., E.C., C.C., C.P., C.V., D.F., A.A. (Anna Aspesi), M.S. and R.L.; visualization, G.C., G.M., S.G., A.A. (Alessandra Allione), A.R., E.C., C.C., C.P., C.V., D.F., A.A. (Anna Aspesi), M.S. and R.L.; supervision, G.C. and G.M.; project administration, G.C. and G.M.; funding acquisition, G.M., C.M., D.M., I.D. and F.G. All authors have read and agreed to the published version of the manuscript.

Funding: The research leading to these results has received funding from AIRC under IG 2018—[ID. 21390 project—P.I. GM] and partly by the HERMES (Hereditary Risk in MESothelioma) Project, funded by the offer of compensation to the inhabitants of Casale Monferrato deceased or affected by mesothelioma (to I.D. and C.M.). and the Ministero dell'Istruzione, dell'Università e della Ricerca—MIUR project "Dipartimenti di Eccellenza 2018–2022" (n° D15D18000410001, to GM) to the Department of Medical Sciences, University of Turin.

Acknowledgments: The authors wish to thank all the patients contributing to this research, Caterina Casadio and Ezio Piccolini for their past clinical contribution and Paolo Garagnani for the Sequenom analysis supervision.

Conflicts of Interest: The authors declare that they have no competing interest.

References

1. Sekido, Y. Molecular pathogenesis of malignant mesothelioma. *Carcinogenesis* **2013**, *34*, 1413–1419. [CrossRef]
2. Rossini, M.; Rizzo, P.; Bononi, I.; Clementz, A.; Ferrari, R.; Martini, F.; Tognon, M.G. New Perspectives on Diagnosis and Therapy of Malignant Pleural Mesothelioma. *Front. Oncol.* **2018**, *8*, 91. [CrossRef]
3. Furuya, S.; Chimed-Ochir, O.; Takahashi, K.; David, A.; Takala, J. Global Asbestos Disaster. *Int. J. Environ. Res. Public Health* **2018**, *15*, 1000. [CrossRef]
4. Straif, K.; Benbrahim-Tallaa, L.; Baan, R.; Grosse, Y.; Secretan, B.; El Ghissassi, F.; Bouvard, V.; Guha, N.; Freeman, C.; Galichet, L.; et al. A review of human carcinogens—Part C: Metals, arsenic, dusts, and fibres. *Lancet Oncol.* **2009**, *10*, 453–454. [CrossRef]
5. Curran, D.; Sahmoud, T.; Therasse, P.; Van Meerbeeck, J.; Postmus, P.E.; Giaccone, G. Prognostic factors in patients with pleural mesothelioma: The European Organization for Research and Treatment of Cancer experience. *J. Clin. Oncol.* **1998**, *16*, 145–152. [CrossRef] [PubMed]
6. Jassem, J.; Ramlau, R.; Santoro, A.; Schuette, W.; Chemaissani, A.; Hong, S.; Blatter, J.; Adachi, S.; Hanauske, A.; Manegold, C. Phase III Trial of Pemetrexed Plus Best Supportive Care Compared with Best Supportive Care in Previously Treated Patients with Advanced Malignant Pleural Mesothelioma. *J. Clin. Oncol.* **2008**, *26*, 1698–1704. [CrossRef] [PubMed]
7. Vogelzang, N.J.; Rusthoven, J.J.; Symanowski, J.; Denham, C.; Kaukel, E.; Ruffie, P.; Gatzemeier, U.; Boyer, M.; Emri, S.; Manegold, C.; et al. Phase III Study of Pemetrexed in Combination with Cisplatin Versus Cisplatin Alone in Patients with Malignant Pleural Mesothelioma. *J. Clin. Oncol.* **2003**, *21*, 2636–2644. [CrossRef] [PubMed]
8. Yap, T.A.; Aerts, J.G.; Popat, S.; Fennell, D.A. Novel insights into mesothelioma biology and implications for therapy. *Nat. Rev. Cancer* **2017**, *17*, 475–488. [CrossRef] [PubMed]

9. Guarrera, S.; Viberti, C.; Cugliari, G.; Allione, A.; Casalone, E.; Betti, M.; Ferrante, D.; Aspesi, A.; Casadio, C.; Grosso, F.; et al. Peripheral Blood DNA Methylation as Potential Biomarker of Malignant Pleural Mesothelioma in Asbestos-Exposed Subjects. *J. Thorac. Oncol.* **2019**, *14*, 527–539. [CrossRef]
10. Matullo, G.; Guarrera, S.; Betti, M.; Fiorito, G.; Ferrante, D.; Voglino, F.; Cadby, G.; Di Gaetano, C.; Rosa, F.; Russo, A.; et al. Genetic Variants Associated with Increased Risk of Malignant Pleural Mesothelioma: A Genome-Wide Association Study. *PLoS ONE* **2013**, *8*, e61253. [CrossRef] [PubMed]
11. Tanrikulu, A.C.; Abakay, A.; Komek, H.; Abakay, O. Prognostic value of the lymphocyte-to-monocyte ratio and other inflammatory markers in malignant pleural mesothelioma. *Environ. Health Prev. Med.* **2016**, *21*, 304–311. [CrossRef] [PubMed]
12. Guo, G.; Chmielecki, J.; Goparaju, C.; Heguy, A.; Dolgalev, I.; Carbone, M.; Seepo, S.; Meyerson, M.; Pass, H.I. Whole-Exome Sequencing Reveals Frequent Genetic Alterations in BAP1, NF2, CDKN2A, and CUL1 in Malignant Pleural Mesothelioma. *Cancer Res.* **2014**, *75*, 264–269. [CrossRef] [PubMed]
13. Betti, M.; Aspesi, A.; Sculco, M.; Matullo, G.; Magnani, C.; Dianzani, I. Genetic predisposition for malignant mesothelioma: A concise review. *Mutat. Res.* **2019**, *781*, 1–10. [CrossRef] [PubMed]
14. Gai, W.; Sun, K. Epigenetic Biomarkers in Cell-Free DNA and Applications in Liquid Biopsy. *Genes* **2019**, *10*, 32. [CrossRef]
15. Moore, L.D.; Le, T.; Fan, G. DNA Methylation and Its Basic Function. *Neuropsychopharmacology* **2013**, *38*, 23–38. [CrossRef]
16. Bononi, A.; Napolitano, A.; Pass, H.I.; Yang, H.; Carbone, M. Latest developments in our understanding of the pathogenesis of mesothelioma and the design of targeted therapies. *Expert Rev. Respir. Med.* **2015**, *9*, 633–654. [CrossRef]
17. Vandermeers, F.; Sriramareddy, S.N.; Costa, C.; Hubaux, R.; Cosse, J.-P.; Willems, L. The role of epigenetics in malignant pleural mesothelioma. *Lung Cancer* **2013**, *81*, 311–318. [CrossRef]
18. Ferrari, L.; Carugno, M.; Mensi, C.; Pesatori, A.C. Circulating Epigenetic Biomarkers in Malignant Pleural Mesothelioma: State of the Art and critical Evaluation. *Front. Oncol.* **2020**, *10*, 445. [CrossRef]
19. Creaney, J.; Yeoman, D.; Demelker, Y.; Segal, A.; Musk, A.; Skates, S.J.; Robinson, B.W. Comparison of Osteopontin, Megakaryocyte Potentiating Factor, and Mesothelin Proteins as Markers in the Serum of Patients with Malignant Mesothelioma. *J. Thorac. Oncol.* **2008**, *3*, 851–857. [CrossRef]
20. Creaney, J.; Dick, I.M.; Meniawy, T.M.; Leong, S.L.; Leon, J.S.; Demelker, Y.; Segal, A.; Musk, A.W. (Bill); Lee, Y.C.G.; Skates, S.J.; et al. Comparison of fibulin-3 and mesothelin as markers in malignant mesothelioma. *Thorax* **2014**, *69*, 895–902. [CrossRef]
21. Tanrikulu, A.C.; Abakay, A.; Kaplan, M.A.; Küçüköner, M.; Palanci, Y.; Evliyaoglu, O.; Sezgi, C.; Sen, H.; Carkanat, A.I.; Kirbas, G. A Clinical, Radiographic and Laboratory Evaluation of Prognostic Factors in 363 Patients with Malignant Pleural Mesothelioma. *Respiration* **2010**, *80*, 480–487. [CrossRef] [PubMed]
22. Costa-Pinheiro, P.; Montezuma, D.; Henrique, R.; Jerónimo, C. Diagnostic and prognostic epigenetic biomarkers in cancer. *Epigenomics* **2015**, *7*, 1003–1015. [CrossRef] [PubMed]
23. Comba, P.; D'Angelo, M.; Fazzo, L.; Magnani, C.; Marinaccio, A.; Mirabelli, D.; Terracini, B. Mesothelioma in Italy: The Casale Monferrato model to a national epidemiological surveillance system. *Annali Istituto Superiore Sanità* **2018**, *54*, 139–148.
24. Pass, H.I.; Giroux, D.; Kennedy, C.; Ruffini, E.; Cangir, A.K.; Rice, D.; Asamura, H.; Waller, D.; Edwards, J.; Weder, W.; et al. The IASLC Mesothelioma Staging Project: Improving Staging of a Rare Disease Through International Participation. *J. Thorac. Oncol.* **2016**, *11*, 2082–2088. [CrossRef]
25. Yamagishi, T.; Fujimoto, N.; Nishi, H.; Miyamoto, Y.; Hara, N.; Asano, M.; Fuchimoto, Y.; Wada, S.; Kitamura, K.; Ozaki, S.; et al. Prognostic significance of the lymphocyte-to-monocyte ratio in patients with malignant pleural mesothelioma. *Lung Cancer* **2015**, *90*, 111–117. [CrossRef]
26. Argentieri, M.A.; Nagarajan, S.; Seddighzadeh, B.; Baccarelli, A.A.; Shields, A.E. Epigenetic Pathways in Human Disease: The Impact of DNA Methylation on Stress-Related Pathogenesis and Current Challenges in Biomarker Development. *EBioMedicine* **2017**, *18*, 327–350. [CrossRef]
27. Yu, H.; Du, L.; Yi, S.; Wang, Q.; Zhu, Y.; Qiu, Y.; Jiang, Y.; Li, M.; Wang, D.; Wang, Q.; et al. Epigenome-wide association study identifies Behçet's disease-associated methylation loci in Han Chinese. *Rheumatology* **2019**, *58*, 1574–1584. [CrossRef]

28. Yamaguchi, I.; Nakajima, K.; Shono, K.; Mizobuchi, Y.; Fujihara, T.; Shikata, E.; Yamaguchi, T.; Kitazato, K.; Sampetrean, O.; Saya, H.; et al. Downregulation of PD-L1 via FKBP5 by celecoxib augments antitumor effects of PD-1 blockade in a malignant glioma model. *Neuro-Oncology Adv.* **2020**, *2*, vdz058. [CrossRef]
29. Romano, S.; Simeone, E.; D'Angelillo, A.; D'Arrigo, P.; Russo, M.; Capasso, M.; Lasorsa, V.A.; Zambrano, N.; Ascierto, P.A.; Romano, M.F. FKBP51s signature in peripheral blood mononuclear cells of melanoma patients as a possible predictive factor for immunotherapy. *Cancer Immunol. Immunother.* **2017**, *66*, 1143–1151. [CrossRef]
30. Li, L.; Lou, Z.; Wang, L. The role of FKBP5 in cancer aetiology and chemoresistance. *Br. J. Cancer* **2010**, *104*, 19–23. [CrossRef]
31. Staibano, S.; Mascolo, M.; Ilardi, G.; Siano, M.; De Rosa, G. Immunohistochemical analysis of FKBP51 in human cancers. *Curr. Opin. Pharmacol.* **2011**, *11*, 338–347. [CrossRef] [PubMed]
32. Zannas, A.S.; Jia, M.; Hafner, K.; Baumert, J.; Wiechmann, T.; Pape, J.C.; Arloth, J.; Ködel, M.; Martinelli, S.; Roitman, M.; et al. Epigenetic upregulation of FKBP5 by aging and stress contributes to NF-kappaB-driven inflammation and cardiovascular risk. *Proc. Natl. Acad. Sci. USA* **2019**, *116*, 11370–11379. [CrossRef] [PubMed]
33. Romano, M.F.; Avellino, R.; Petrella, A.; Bisogni, R.; Romano, S.; Venuta, S. Rapamycin inhibits doxorubicin-induced NF-kappaB/Rel nuclear activity and enhances the apoptosis of melanoma cells. *Eur. J. Cancer* **2004**, *40*, 2829–2836. [CrossRef] [PubMed]
34. Sun, N.-K.; Huang, S.-L.; Chang, P.-Y.; Lu, H.-P.; Chao, C.C.-K. Transcriptomic profiling of taxol-resistant ovarian cancer cells identifies FKBP5 and the androgen receptor as critical markers of chemotherapeutic response. *Oncotarget* **2014**, *5*, 11939–11956. [CrossRef] [PubMed]
35. Romano, S.; D'Angelillo, A.; Romano, M.F. Pleiotropic roles in cancer biology for multifaceted proteins FKBPs. *Biochim. Biophys. Acta* **2015**, *1850*, 2061–2068. [CrossRef] [PubMed]
36. Ferrante, D.; Bertolotti, M.; Todesco, A.; Mirabelli, D.; Terracini, B.; Magnani, C. Cancer Mortality and Incidence of Mesothelioma in a Cohort of Wives of Asbestos Workers in Casale Monferrato, Italy. *Environ. Health Perspect.* **2007**, *115*, 1401–1405. [CrossRef]
37. Dianzani, I.; Gibello, L.; Biava, A.; Mirabelli, D.; Terracini, B.; Magnani, C. Polymorphisms in DNA repair genes as risk factors for asbestos-related malignant mesothelioma in a general population study. *Mutat. Res.* **2006**, *599*, 124–134. [CrossRef]
38. Betti, M.; Ferrante, D.; Padoan, M.; Guarrera, S.; Giordano, M.; Aspesi, A.; Mirabelli, D.; Casadio, C.; Ardissone, F.; Ruffini, E.; et al. XRCC1 and ERCC1 variants modify malignant mesothelioma risk: A case—Control study. *Mutat. Res. Mol. Mech. Mutagen.* **2011**, *708*, 11–20. [CrossRef]
39. Betti, M.; Casalone, E.; Ferrante, D.; Aspesi, A.; Morleo, G.; Biasi, A.; Sculco, M.; Mancuso, G.; Guarrera, S.; Righi, L.; et al. Germline mutations in DNA repair genes predispose asbestos-exposed patients to malignant pleural mesothelioma. *Cancer Lett.* **2017**, *405*, 38–45. [CrossRef]
40. Ferrante, D.; Mirabelli, D.; Tunesi, S.; Terracini, B.; Magnani, C. Pleural mesothelioma and occupational and non-occupational asbestos exposure: A case—control study with quantitative risk assessment. *Occup. Environ. Med.* **2016**, *73*, 147–153. [CrossRef]
41. Bibikova, M.; Barnes, B.; Tsan, C.; Ho, V.; Klotzle, B.; Le, J.M.; Delano, D.; Zhang, L.; Schroth, G.P.; Gunderson, K.L.; et al. High density DNA methylation array with single CpG site resolution. *Genomics* **2011**, *98*, 288–295. [CrossRef] [PubMed]
42. Bibikova, M.; Lin, Z.; Zhou, L.; Chudin, E.; Garcia, E.W.; Wu, B.; Doucet, D.; Thomas, N.J.; Wang, Y.; Vollmer, E.; et al. High-throughput DNA methylation profiling using universal bead arrays. *Genome Res.* **2006**, *16*, 383–393. [CrossRef] [PubMed]
43. Du, P.; Zhang, X.; Huang, C.-C.; Jafari, N.; Kibbe, W.A.; Hou, L.; Lin, S.M. Comparison of Beta-value and M-value methods for quantifying methylation levels by microarray analysis. *BMC Bioinform.* **2010**, *11*, 587.
44. Lehne, B.; Drong, A.W.; Loh, M.; Zhang, W.; Scott, W.R.; Tan, S.-T.; Afzal, U.; Scott, J.; Jarvelin, M.-R.; Elliott, P.; et al. A coherent approach for analysis of the Illumina HumanMethylation450 BeadChip improves data quality and performance in epigenome-wide association studies. *Genome Biol.* **2015**, *16*, 37. [CrossRef] [PubMed]
45. Campanella, G.; Polidoro, S.; Di Gaetano, C.; Fiorito, G.; Guarrera, S.; Krogh, V.; Palli, D.; Panico, S.; Sacerdote, C.; Tumino, R.; et al. Epigenetic signatures of internal migration in Italy. *Int. J. Epidemiol.* **2014**, *44*, 1442–1449. [CrossRef]

46. Di Gaetano, C.; Voglino, F.; Guarrera, S.; Fiorito, G.; Rosa, F.; Di Blasio, A.M.; Manzini, P.; Dianzani, I.; Betti, M.; Cusi, D.; et al. An Overview of the Genetic Structure within the Italian Population from Genome-Wide Data. *PLoS ONE* **2012**, *7*, e43759. [CrossRef]
47. Houseman, E.A.; Accomando, W.P.; Koestler, D.C.; Christensen, B.C.; Marsit, C.J.; Nelson, H.H.; Wiencke, J.K.; Kelsey, K.T. DNA methylation arrays as surrogate measures of cell mixture distribution. *BMC Bioinform.* **2012**, *13*, 86. [CrossRef]
48. Ehrich, M.; Nelson, M.R.; Stanssens, P.; Zabeau, M.; Liloglou, T.; Xinarianos, G.; Cantor, C.R.; Field, J.K.; Boom, D.V.D. Quantitative high-throughput analysis of DNA methylation patterns by base-specific cleavage and mass spectrometry. *Proc. Natl. Acad. Sci. USA* **2005**, *102*, 15785–15790. [CrossRef]

Publisher's Note: MDPI stays neutral with regard to jurisdictional claims in published maps and institutional affiliations.

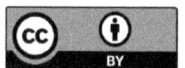

© 2020 by the authors. Licensee MDPI, Basel, Switzerland. This article is an open access article distributed under the terms and conditions of the Creative Commons Attribution (CC BY) license (http://creativecommons.org/licenses/by/4.0/).

Article

New DNA Methylation Signals for Malignant Pleural Mesothelioma Risk Assessment

Giovanni Cugliari [1,*], Alessandra Allione [1], Alessia Russo [1], Chiara Catalano [1], Elisabetta Casalone [1], Simonetta Guarrera [2,3], Federica Grosso [4], Daniela Ferrante [5,6], Marika Sculco [7], Marta La Vecchia [7], Chiara Pirazzini [8], Roberta Libener [9], Dario Mirabelli [10,11], Corrado Magnani [5,6,11], Irma Dianzani [7,11] and Giuseppe Matullo [1,11,12,*]

1. Department of Medical Sciences, University of Turin, 10126 Turin, Italy; alessandra.allione@unito.it (A.A.); alessia.russo@unito.it (A.R.); chiara.catalano@unito.it (C.C.); elisabetta.casalone@unito.it (E.C.)
2. Italian Institute for Genomic Medicine, IIGM, 10060 Candiolo, Italy; simonetta.guarrera@iigm.it
3. Candiolo Cancer Institute, FPO-IRCCS, 10060 Candiolo, Italy
4. Mesothelioma Unit, Azienda Ospedaliera SS. Antonio e Biagio e Cesare Arrigo, 15121 Alessandria, Italy; federica.grosso@uniupo.it
5. Medical Statistics, Department of Translational Medicine, University of Eastern Piedmont, 28100 Novara, Italy; daniela.ferrante@med.uniupo.it (D.F.); corrado.magnani@med.uniupo.it (C.M.)
6. Cancer Epidemiology Unit, CPO-Piemonte, 28100 Novara, Italy
7. Department of Health Sciences, University of Eastern Piedmont, 28100 Novara, Italy; marika.sculco@uniupo.it (M.S.); marta.lavecchia@uniupo.it (M.L.V.); irma.dianzani@med.uniupo.it (I.D.)
8. IRCCS Istituto delle Scienze Neurologiche di Bologna, 40126 Bologna, Italy; chiara.pirazzini5@unibo.it
9. Department of Integrated Activities Research and Innovation–Azienda Ospedaliera SS. Antonio e Biagio e Cesare Arrigo, 15122 Alessandria, Italy; rlibener@ospedale.al.it
10. Cancer Epidemiology Unit, Department of Medical Sciences, University of Turin, 10126 Turin, Italy; dario.mirabelli@cpo.it
11. Interdepartmental Center for Studies on Asbestos and Other Toxic Particulates "G. Scansetti", University of Turin, 10126 Turin, Italy
12. Medical Genetics Unit, AOU Città della Salute e della Scienza, 10126 Turin, Italy
* Correspondence: giovanni.cugliari@unito.it (G.C.); giuseppe.matullo@unito.it (G.M.)

Simple Summary: Our study investigated DNA methylation differences in easily accessible white blood cells (WBCs) between malignant pleural mesothelioma (MPM) cases and asbestos-exposed cancer-free controls. A multiple regression model highlighted that the methylation level of two single CpGs (cg03546163 in *FKBP5* and cg06633438 in *MLLT1*) are independent MPM markers. The epigenetic changes at the *FKBP5* and *MLLT1* genes were robustly associated with MPM in asbestos-exposed subjects. Interaction analyses showed that MPM cases and cancer-free controls showed DNAm differences which may be linked to asbestos exposure.

Abstract: Malignant pleural mesothelioma (MPM) is a rare and aggressive neoplasm. Patients are usually diagnosed when current treatments have limited benefits, highlighting the need for noninvasive tests aimed at an MPM risk assessment tool that might improve life expectancy. Three hundred asbestos-exposed subjects (163 MPM cases and 137 cancer-free controls), from the same geographical region in Italy, were recruited. The evaluation of asbestos exposure was conducted considering the frequency, the duration and the intensity of occupational, environmental and domestic exposure. A genome-wide methylation array was performed to identify novel blood DNA methylation (DNAm) markers of MPM. Multiple regression analyses adjusting for potential confounding factors and interaction between asbestos exposure and DNAm on the MPM odds ratio were applied. Epigenome-wide analysis (EWAS) revealed 12 single-CpGs associated with the disease. Two of these showed high statistical power (99%) and effect size (>0.05) after false discovery rate (FDR) multiple comparison corrections: (i) cg03546163 in *FKBP5*, significantly hypomethylated in cases (Mean Difference in beta values (MD) = −0.09, 95% CI = −0.12 | −0.06, $p = 1.2 \times 10^{-7}$), and (ii) cg06633438 in *MLLT1*, statistically hypermethylated in cases (MD = 0.07, 95% CI = 0.04 | 0.10, $p = 1.0 \times 10^{-6}$). Based on the interaction analysis, asbestos exposure and epigenetic profile together may improve MPM risk assessment. Above-median asbestos exposure and hypomethylation of cg03546163 in *FKBP5*

(OR = 20.84, 95% CI = 8.71 | 53.96, $p = 5.5 \times 10^{-11}$) and hypermethylation of cg06633438 in *MLLT1* (OR = 11.71, 95% CI = 4.97 | 29.64, $p = 5.9 \times 10^{-8}$) genes compared to below-median asbestos exposure and hyper/hypomethylation of single-CpG DNAm, respectively. Receiver Operation Characteristics (ROC) for Case-Control Discrimination showed a significant increase in MPM discrimination when DNAm information was added in the model (baseline model, BM: asbestos exposure, age, gender and white blood cells); area under the curve, AUC = 0.75; BM + cg03546163 at *FKBP5*. AUC = 0.89, 2.1×10^{-7}; BM + cg06633438 at *MLLT1*. AUC = 0.89, 6.3×10^{-8}. Validation and replication procedures, considering independent sample size and a different DNAm analysis technique, confirmed the observed associations. Our results suggest the potential application of DNAm profiles in blood to develop noninvasive tests for MPM risk assessment in asbestos-exposed subjects.

Keywords: malignant pleural mesothelioma; asbestos exposure; DNA methylation; epigenome-wide analysis; interaction analysis

1. Introduction

Mesothelioma has a long latency period, usually emerging 20–40 years after asbestos exposure [1]. Malignant pleural mesothelioma (MPM) is rare (prevalence 1–9/100,000), but the corresponding annual death toll worldwide is still estimated at about 40,000 [2,3]. Each year, 125 million people are exposed to asbestos, according to a World Health Organization report [4]. The International Agency for Research on Cancer confirmed that all fibrous forms of asbestos are carcinogenic to humans. The main outcome of exposure is mesothelioma, but cancer at other sites, such as respiratory-tract tumors, are moderately frequent [4]. Previous in vitro studies have demonstrated the cytotoxic effects of asbestos fibers [5,6].

A significant association between MPM and asbestos exposure has been reported, showing a clear, increasing trend in the odds ratio (OR) with increasing cumulative exposure among subjects exposed to over 10 fiber/mL-years [7]. Another study reported that the incidence of malignant mesothelioma (MM) was strongly associated with the proximity of one's residence to an asbestos exposure source [8].

DNA methylation (DNAm) is an epigenetic mechanism involved in gene expression regulation. In particular, dysregulation of promoter DNAm and histone modification are epigenetic mechanisms involved in human malignancies [9].

According to recent papers, both DNAm and genetic alterations may contribute to MPM tumorigenesis [10–15]. Whereas the genome remains consistent throughout one's lifetime, factors like ageing, lifestyle, environmental exposures and diseases can modify DNAm. The adaptive nature of DNAm means that it can be used to link environmental factors to the development of pathologic phenotypes such as cancers. Fasanelli et al. observed an association between exposure to tobacco and site-specific CpG methylation. They also used peripheral blood DNA to evaluate the importance of these epigenetic alterations in the aetiology of lung cancer [16].

There is less information on the mechanisms and clinical outcomes of epigenetic derangements in MPM [17–19]. Several studies have evaluated DNAm alterations in MM samples [20–22], but few of them focused on DNAm alteration in blood as a circulating marker. Fischer et al. examined serum DNAm of nine gene-specific promoters from MM cases [23]. A more recent paper identified hypomethylation of a single CpG in *FKBP5* in whole blood cells as a predictor of overall survival in MPM cases [13]. Guarrera et al. evaluated methylation levels in DNA from whole blood leukocytes as potential diagnostic markers for MPM and found a differential methylation between asbestos-exposed MPM cases and controls, mainly in genes related to the immune system [11]. The identification of reliable DNAm biomarkers with high sensitivity and specificity for MPM risk assessment would be a major advancement.

This study was undertaken with the goal to identify new biomarkers for MPM risk assessment and to determine if peripheral blood DNAm profiles have any predictive value. The second goal was to evaluate the interaction effect of asbestos exposure with DNAm on MPM risk. Currently, there are no sensitive testing methods available for the screening of asbestos-exposed individuals who are at high risk of developing MPM. Thus, the identification of reliable MPM diagnostic biomarkers in peripheral blood might provide a tool for detecting the disease at an early stage.

2. Results

2.1. Epigenome-Wide Association Study (EWAS)

CpGs (445,254) passed quality control procedures and were considered for statistical analyses. EWAS revealed two statistically significant differentially methylated single-CpGs between case and control groups: cg03546163 in the *FKBP5* gene (Mean Difference in beta values (MD) = 0.09, 95% CI = $-0.12 | -0.06$, $p = 1.2 \times 10^{-7}$, $p = 0.028$) and cg06633438 in the *MLLT1* gene (MD = 0.07, 95% CI = $0.04 | 0.10$, $p = 1.0 \times 10^{-6}$, $p = 0.049$) after False Discovery Rate (FDR) post hoc correction (Figure 1; Table 1).

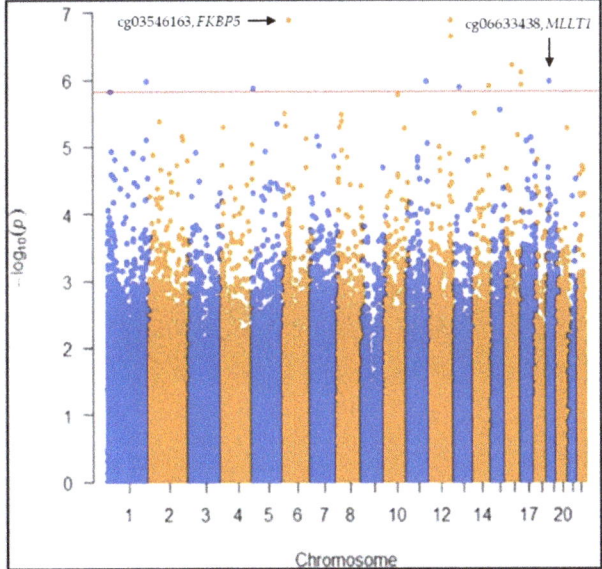

Figure 1. Manhattan plot for EWAS test on 450 k single CpGs. Single-CpG DNAm was used as dependent variable adjusting for age, gender, White blood cells (WBCs: monocytes, granulocytes, natural killer, B cells, CD4+ T and CD8+ T) estimation, population stratification and technical variability. FDR post hoc line highlights statistically significant differences between cases and controls at single CpG level.

Another 10 CpGs showed hypo/hypermethylation in MPM considering FDR < 0.05 but not effect size (MD) cut off $\geq |0.05|$ (Table 1).

Bootstrap was computed to estimate measures of accuracy using random sampling methods. The bias-corrected and accelerated (BCa) bootstrap interval was calculated for cg03546163 in *FKBP5* (95% CIBCa = $-0.16 | -0.10$, z0 = -0.008, a = 0.002) and cg06633438 in *MLLT1* (95% CIBCa = $-0.06 | -0.1$, z0 = -0.011, a = 0.0004) genes, confirming the robustness of the results considering the sample under study.

Table 1. Differential DNAm analyses ordered by effect size. Information about single-CpGs, including location-related values and model outputs (effect size, standard error, p values).

Probe ID	Chr	Map Position	Gene Symbol	Ucsc Refgene Group	Snp Probe	Effect Size	Standard Error	p Value	Fdr	Significance
cg02869235	12	124726864			rs73223527	0.058	0.011	1.3×10^{-7}	0.028	*§
cg03546163	6	35654363	FKBP5	5'UTR		−0.089	0.016	1.3×10^{-7}	0.028	*§⋔
cg02353048	12	124718401				0.033	0.006	2.2×10^{-7}	0.032	*§
cg06633438	19	6272158	MLLT1	Body		0.069	0.014	1.0×10^{-6}	0.049	*§⋔
cg18860329	13	43354421	C13orf30	TSS1500		0.050	0.010	1.3×10^{-6}	0.049	*§
cg19782190	14	103487004	CDC42BPB	Body		0.043	0.009	1.2×10^{-6}	0.049	*§
cg06834916	5	95610				0.037	0.008	1.4×10^{-6}	0.049	*§
cg09479650	16	85578516			rs4843449	0.037	0.007	1.2×10^{-6}	0.049	*§
cg26680989	16	85560739			rs80332660	0.036	0.007	7.6×10^{-7}	0.049	*§
cg25409554	1	234871422				0.034	0.007	1.1×10^{-6}	0.049	*§
cg01201399	16	30793389	ZNF629	Body		0.030	0.006	6.1×10^{-7}	0.049	*§
cg17283266	11	111717611	ALG9	Body		−0.030	0.006	1.1×10^{-6}	0.049	*§

Control group was set as reference. Adjustment covariates: age, gender, population stratification, WBCs (monocytes, granulocytes, natural killer, B cells, CD4+ T and CD8+ T) estimation and technical variability. *: statistically significant at p value < 0.05; §: statistically significant at FDR post hoc adjustments. ⋔: statistically significant at beta = 0.01.

Statistically significant differences in MD between cases and controls were found in the WBCs estimated (monocytes, $p = 6.0 \times 10^{-3}$; granulocytes, $p = 2.2 \times 10^{-16}$; B cells, $p = 1.1 \times 10^{-12}$; NK cells, $p = 3.6 \times 10^{-4}$; CD4+ T, $p = 2.2 \times 10^{-16}$; CD8+ T, $p = 6.8 \times 10^{-11}$; Naïve CD4T, $p = 0.012$; Naïve CD8T, $p = 7.0 \times 10^{-3}$).

In order to assess if smoking status, classified as current, former and never-smokers, could modify DNAm profiles, we performed a multivariate regression analysis with the same model used for the discovery phase. No evidence of methylation differences linked to different smoking levels was found for any of the twelve statistically significant CpGs.

2.2. Receiver Operation Characteristics (ROC) for Case-Control Discrimination

The baseline model (BM) including age, gender, asbestos exposure and WBCs was compared with BM adding the DNAm levels of cg03546163 or cg06633438. Receiver Operation Characteristics 8ROC9 curves showed a significant increase in MPM discrimination when DNAm information was added in the model (Table 2).

Table 2. Disease discrimination test considering (AUC) comparison between baseline model and models additionally including single-CpG.

Model	AUC	DeLong's Test
BM (asbestos exposure, age, gender and WBCs)	0.75	Reference
BM + cg03546163 (FKBP5)	0.89	2.1×10^{-7}
BM + cg06633438 (MLLT1)	0.89	6.3×10^{-8}

Models are shown as baseline model (BM) or BM + Single CpG DNAm. AUC Differences between considered model and BM were estimated with the DeLong's test.

2.3. Interaction Analysis

CpG sites and asbestos exposure were considered as predictors of MPM risk in the interaction model. Categorical variables (quantile information) were used considering median values.

We tested the interaction between asbestos exposure and DNAm levels at cg03546163 in *FKBP5* and cg06633438 in *MLLT1*.

Considering cg03546163 in *FKBP5*, DNA hypermethylation and low asbestos exposure levels were used as references, while for cg06633438 in *MLLT1*, DNA hypomethylation and low asbestos exposure levels were set as references (Table 3).

The OR was estimated as the relationship between the combination of single-CpGs DNAm levels and asbestos exposure quantile, and the reference (low median asbestos exposure and hypermethylation status for cg03546163, or hypomethylation status for cg06633438). Age, gender, population stratification, and WBCs were included in the GLM (family = binomial) to adjust the interaction effect.

Table 3. Interaction between asbestos exposure and single CpG DNAm on the MPM Odds ratios.

DNAm	Asbestos Exposure	OR	Std. Error	95% CI	p Value
cg03546163 (FKBP5)					
Hypo	Low	2.79	1.51	1.26 | 6.33	0.013
Hyper	High	7.21	1.54	3.17 | 17.27	4.6×10^{-6}
Hypo	High	20.84	1.59	8.71 | 53.96	5.5×10^{-11}
cg06633438 (MLLT1)					
Hyper	Low	1.29	1.63	0.70 | 3.81	0.258
Hypo	High	7.27	1.55	3.17 | 17.65	5.3×10^{-6}
Hyper	High	11.71	1.57	4.97 | 29.64	5.9×10^{-8}

Reference for cg03546163 in *FKBP5*: hypermethylation and low asbestos exposure levels; Reference for cg06633438 in *MLLT1*: hypomethylation and low asbestos exposure levels.

The relationship between asbestos exposures and single-CpG DNAm levels was evaluated. An increase of one unit of asbestos exposure (rank transformed fibers/mL years) was related to the *FKBP5* gene ($\beta = -0.016$, 95% CI = $-0.031 \mid -0.001$, $p = 0.044$) and *MLLT1* gene ($\beta = -0.014$, 95% CI = $0.001 \mid 0.026$, $p = 0.035$) methylation level variations.

Strong association between asbestos exposure and MPM risk, considering dichotomous distribution of asbestos exposure, was found (OR = 6.11, 95% CI = 3.73 \| 10.20, $p = 1.8 \times 10^{-12}$). Quartile distribution of asbestos exposure was evaluated to estimate the potential incremental association with MPM risk (1st quartile: used as reference; 2nd quartile: OR = 1.83, 95% CI = 0.93 \| 3.69, $p = 0.09$; 3rd quartile: OR = 6.63, 95% CI = 3.30 \| 13.81, $p = 2.1 \times 10^{-7}$; 4th quartile: OR = 11.00, 95% CI = 5.26 \| 24.30, $p = 7.3 \times 10^{-10}$).

2.4. Validation and Replication

For the replication and validation approaches, an independent sample of 140 MPM cases and 104 cancer-free asbestos-exposed controls from the same areas were considered, using a targeted DNAm analysis technique.

The direction and magnitude of the association was consistent for cg03546163 and cg06633438 DNAm. Patients showed significantly lower DNAm at cg03546163 (MD = -0.061, 95% CI = $-0.087 \mid -0.036$, $p = 4.5 \times 10^{-6}$) and higher DNAm at cg06633438 (MD = 0.024, 95% CI = 0.061 \| 0.013, $p = 4.0 \times 10^{-2}$) compared with controls. A multivariate analysis confirmed that DNAm at cg03546163 in *FKBP5* and cg06633438 in *MLLT1* were independently associated with MPM detection.

3. Discussion

In the present study, we used a whole genome microarray approach to investigate DNAm in WBCs from MPM cases and asbestos-exposed cancer-free controls from a region with a history of asbestos exposure (Piedmont, Italy) [10] in order to identify new noninvasive epigenetic markers related to MPM. The identification of reliable MPM diagnostic biomarkers in peripheral blood might improve risk assessment.

We observed hypomethylation of CpG cg03546163, located in the 5' UTR region of *FKBP5* gene, in MPM cases compared to controls.

Epigenetic activation of the FKBP Prolyl Isomerase 5 (*FKBP5*) gene has been shown to be associated with increased stress sensitivity and the risk of psychiatric disorders [24]. *FKBP5* is an immunophilin and has an important role in immunoregulation and in protein folding and trafficking. It plays a role in transcriptional complexes and acts as a cotranscription factor, along with other proteins in the *FKBP* family [25]. The suggestion of a possible role of *FKBP5* in the development and progression of different types of cancer has stemmed from several studies. In particular, high protein expression has been linked to either suppression or promotion of tumour growth, depending on tumour type and microenvironment [26,27].

FKBP5 is involved in the NF-kB and AKT signaling pathways, both of which are implicated in tumorigenesis [28]. Notably, NF-kB appears to be frequently constitutively activated in malignant tumours and involved in the modulation of genes linked to cell motility, neoangiogenesis, proliferation and programmed cell death [29]. An epigenetic upregulation of *FKBP5* could promote NF-kB activation [30]. STAT3-NFkB activity is involved in chemoresistance in MM cells [31], and NFkB was shown to be constitutively active as a result of asbestos-induced chronic inflammation [32].

CpG cg06633438 located in the body region of the *MLLT1* gene was hypermethylated in cases compared to controls.

The *MLLT1* gene encodes the ENL protein, a histone acetylation reader component of the super elongation complex (SEC), which promotes transcription at the elongation stage by suppressing transient pausing by the polymerase at multiple sites along the DNA. In acute myeloid leukemia, *MLLT1* regulates chromatin remodeling and gene expression of many important proto-oncogenes [31]. Yoshikawa and colleagues suggested that mesothelioma may be the consequence of the somatic inactivation of chromatin-remodeling complexes and/or histone modifiers, including *MLLT1* [30].

In mesothelioma patients with short-term recurrence after surgery, frequent 19p13.2 loss was reported. This region encompasses several putative tumor suppressors or oncogenes, including *MLLT1* [32].

Interestingly, *MLLT1* and *FKBP5* showed opposite behavior, increasing and decreasing DNAm levels, respectively, in relation to MPM. This finding could reflect the opposite expression profiles of the two genes among all the different subtypes of white blood cells in normal human hematopoiesis, as reported in the Blood Spot database (http://servers.binf.ku.dk/bloodspot/, accessed on 26 May 2021) (Figure 2) [33].

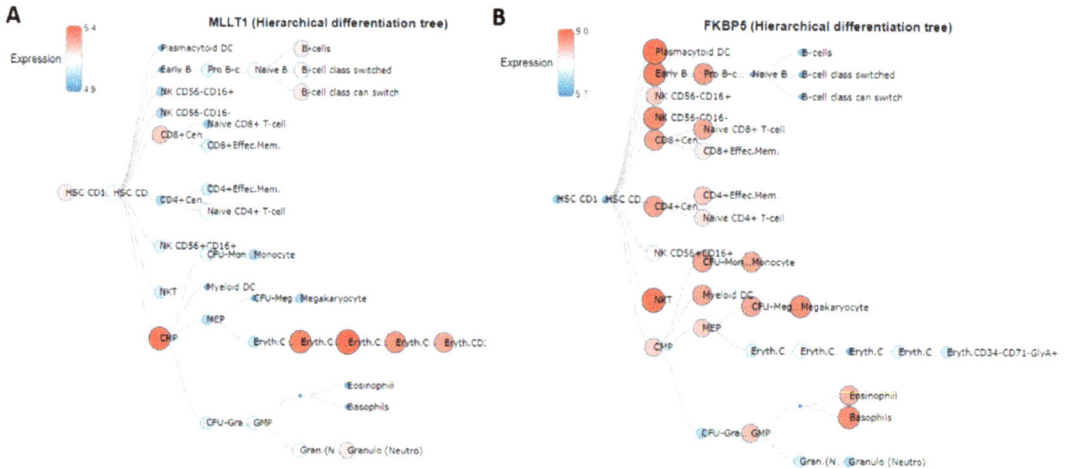

Figure 2. Expression profiles in normal human haematopoiesis. *MLLT1* (**A**) and *FKBP5* (**B**) expression profiles in normal human haematopoiesis as reported in the Blood Spot database (http://servers.binf.ku.dk/bloodspot/, accessed on 26 May 2021).

Our interaction analysis showed that considering DNAm levels at *FKBP5* and *MLLT1* genes together with asbestos exposure levels may help to better define MPM risk for asbestos-exposed subjects.

Six single-CpGs showed differential methylation in patients, including those located in *C13orf30, CDC42BPB, ZNF629* and *ALG9* genes; the other six were not annotated to named genes. *ALG9* is a glycogene whose reduced expression has been described during the epithelial-to-mesenchymal transition, an essential process also involved in cancer progression [34]. The *CDC42BPB* gene is ubiquitously expressed in mammals and encodes a serine/threonine protein kinase, a member of the MRCK family [35]. The role of MRCKs in cytoskeletal reorganization during cell migration and invasion has been characterized [36]. The biological function of *C13orf30* and *ZNF629*, a DNA-binding transcription factor, is still to be established.

MPM cases and asbestos-exposed controls showed different proportions of estimated WBCs, which may denote the crucial implication of the immune system. It is known that in cancer, including mesothelioma, the immune system is affected [37], and there is evidence that asbestos directs antigen overstimulation, and that reactive oxygen species production induces functional changes in WBCs [38]. Indeed, in MPM cases, we showed a reduction of estimated CD4+ and CD8+ T lymphocytes, suggesting a weaker adaptive immune system [39]. This may reflect the possible occurrence of functional changes in WBC subtypes in MPM [40,41].

The need for reliable biomarkers is of extreme relevance for a disease such as MPM, which is characterized by the accumulation and persistence of asbestos fibers in the lungs, leading to a long latency period before clear clinical signs of the tumor are detectable. Several biomarkers for early MPM detection (e.g., mesothelin, osteopontin and fibulin-3) have been proposed so far; however, some of them are still under investigation [42]. In this context, DNAm changes in easily-accessible WBCs may provide a useful tool to better assess MPM risk in asbestos-exposed subjects.

Our findings that DNAm levels in single-CpGs in *FKBP5* and *MLLT1* genes are independent markers of MPM in asbestos-exposed subjects suggest the potential use of blood DNAm analysis as a noninvasive test for MPM detection.

Some somatic gene alterations in lung cancer have been linked to tobacco smoke, but few data are available on the role of asbestos fibers: Andujar and colleagues investigate the mechanism of P16/CDKN2A alterations in lung cancer including asbestos-exposed patients. P16/CDKN2A gene inactivation in asbestos-exposed non-small-cell lung carcinoma (NSCLC) cases, a tumor independent of tobacco smoking but associated with asbestos exposure, mainly occurs via promoter hypermethylation, loss of heterozygosity and homozygous deletion, suggesting a possible relationship with an effect of asbestos fibers [43].We observed epigenetic deregulations in the blood of MPM patients compared to that of cancer-free controls, suggesting the potential use of DNAm for risk stratification among asbestos-exposed individuals.

If this observation can be verified in prospectively collected samples, it may be possible to use CpGs methylation to further improve MPM risk estimation for subjects with occupational and/or environmental asbestos exposure.

Limitation of the Study

Leukocyte DNAm may be a nonspecific marker related to a general, tumour-induced inflammatory status rather than a specific MPM biomarker. Further studies are therefore needed to support our findings.

One main limitation of the functional interpretation of our results is that all our cases had already developed MPM at recruitment: thus, our findings likely reflect disease status rather than being markers of the dynamic processes leading to MPM onset. The lack of MPM tissue from the same subjects also poses major constraints to the functional interpretation of our findings.

Notwithstanding the above limitations, the discrimination between MPM cases and asbestos-exposed cancer-free controls improved when DNAm levels were considered together with asbestos exposure levels.

4. Material and Methods

4.1. Study Population

Study subjects were part of a wider, ongoing collaborative study, which is actively enrolling MPM cases and cancer-free controls in the municipality of Casale Monferrato (Piedmont Region, Italy). This area was chosen due to its exceptionally high incidence of mesothelioma, caused by widespread occupational and environmental asbestos exposure originating from the Eternit asbestos-cement plant, which was operational until 1986 [44]. Additional MPM cases and cancer-free controls were recruited from other main hospitals of the Piedmont Region (in the municipalities of Turin, Novara and Alessandria). The ongoing collaborative study includes MPM cases diagnosed between incident MPM cases diagnosed between 2000 and 2010 after histological and/or cytological confirmation, and matched controls [45].

The present study included 159 MPM cases and 137 cancer-free controls from a larger case-control study, all of whom had genetic and blood DNAm data [46], good quality DNA at the time of the analyses, and information on asbestos exposure above the background level, as defined in Ferrante et al. [47]. MPM cases and asbestos-exposed cancer-free controls were matched by date of birth (±18 months) and gender. An additional 244 (140 MPM cases and 104 cancer-free controls) independent samples from the same case-control study were included for validation/replication analyses.

Tables 4 and 5 shows the descriptive characteristics of controls and cases (Min, 1st Q, Median, Mean, 3rd Q and Max) that were considered in the statistical analysis (gender, age, asbestos exposure and WBC estimates: monocytes, granulocytes, natural killer, B cells, CD4+ T and CD8+ T). Asbestos exposure (occupational, environmental and domestic) was normalized considering frequency, duration and intensity. Smoking status (current, former and never smokers) is also explained in Table 6.

Table 4. Descriptive characteristics of cancer-free control group.

Variable	Controls (Male 100, Female 37)					
	Min	1st Q	Median	Mean	3rd Q	Max
Age	41.60	57.41	65.65	64.59	72.63	90.94
Asbestos exposure	−2.71	−0.97	−0.48	−0.44	0.09	1.73
Monocytes	0.00	0.05	0.06	0.07	0.08	0.26
Granulocytes	0.36	0.54	0.60	0.62	0.68	0.99
Natural Killer	0.00	0.04	0.07	0.08	0.11	0.29
B cells	0.00	0.07	0.09	0.09	0.11	0.19
CD4+ T	0.00	0.10	0.14	0.14	0.19	0.35
CD8+ T	0.00	0.03	0.06	0.07	0.10	0.23

Minimum (Min), First Quartile (1st Q), Median, Mean, Third Quartile (3rt Q) and Maximum (Max) of variables related to cancer-free controls.

Table 5. Descriptive characteristics of MPM group.

Variable	Cases (Male 113, Female 50)					
	Min	1st Q	Median	Mean	3rd Q	Max
Age	33.90	61.19	68.68	67.59	75.17	90.80
Asbestos exposure	−2.71	−0.21	0.39	0.37	0.98	2.94
Monocytes	0.00	0.05	0.07	0.08	0.10	0.20
Granulocytes	0.37	0.67	0.74	0.74	0.81	1.03
Natural Killer	0.00	0.02	0.05	0.06	0.08	0.23
B cells	0.00	0.05	0.06	0.06	0.08	0.16
CD4+ T	0.00	0.03	0.07	0.08	0.11	0.22
CD8+ T	0.00	0.00	0.02	0.03	0.04	0.22

Minimum (Min), First Quartile (1st Q), Median, Mean, Third Quartile (3rt Q) and Maximum (Max) of variables related to MPM cases.

Table 6. Descriptive characteristics of smoking status stratified by disease.

Smoking Habits	Cases (163)		Controls (137)	
	n	%	n	%
Current smokers	29	17.79	30	21.90
Former smokers	54	33.13	60	43.80
Never smokers	75	46.01	47	34.31

n and % of the three levels of smoking status stratified by disease.

Our study complied with the Declaration of Helsinki principles and conformed to ethical requirements. All volunteers signed an informed consent form at enrollment. The study protocol was approved by the Ethics Committee of the Italian Institute for Genomic Medicine (IIGM, Candiolo, Italy).

4.2. Exposure Assessment

Information on occupational history and lifestyle habits were collected from all subjects through interviewer-administered questionnaires, which were completed during face-to-face interviews at enrollment. Job titles were coded in two ways according to the International Standard Classification of Occupations [47] and the Statistical Classification of Economic Activities in the European Community.

A cumulative exposure index was computed considering frequency, duration and intensity of asbestos exposure. Occupational, environmental and domestic asbestos exposure were evaluated by an experienced occupational epidemiologist [47], and exposure doses (fibers/mL years) were rank-transformed to remove skewness.

4.3. Blood DNAm Analysis and Beta-Value Extraction

DNAm levels were measured in DNA from whole blood collected at enrollment using the Infinium HumanMethylation450 BeadChip (Illumina, San Diego, CA, USA). For blood DNAm analysis (including quality control) please refer to the previous work of the same group [11].

We used the R package 'methylumi' to analyze DNAm data. The average methylation value at each locus was computed as the ratio of the intensity of the methylated signal over the total signal (unmethylated + methylated) [48]. Beta-values ranging from 0 (no methylation) to 1 (full methylation) represent the percentage of methylation at each individual CpG locus.

We excluded the following from the analyses: (i) single beta-values with a p-value for detection ≥ 0.01; (ii) CpG loci that had missing beta-values in more than 20% of the assayed samples; (iii) CpG loci detected by probes containing single nucleotide polymorphisms (SNPs) with MAF ≥ 0.05 in the CEPH (Utah residents with ancestry from northern and western Europe, CEU) population; and iv) samples with a global call rate $\leq 95\%$. We also excluded CpGs on chromosomes X and Y.

4.4. Batch Effect, Population Stratification and White Blood Cells Estimations

All differential methylation analyses were corrected for "control probes" Principal Components (PCs) to account for variability and batch effects in methylation assays. We used PCs assessed by principal component analysis of the BeadChip's built-in control probes as a correction factor for statistical analyses of microarray data. This method allows researchers to account for the technical variability in the different steps in DNAm analysis, from bisulfite conversion to BeadChip processing [49].

An individual's geographic origins may influence DNAm profiles, which could potentially introduce bias. To take this into consideration, we took advantage of the available data from our previous study, which includes a genome-wide genotyping dataset from the same study subjects [50]. When genome-wide genotyping was used to calculate the first PCs, they were shown to correlate with different geographic origins [51].

For each subject, we extracted WBC subtype percentages, estimated based on genome-wide methylation data. This method provides quantification of the composition of leukocytes than can be achieved by simple histological or flow cytometric assessments, with an admissible range of variability [52].

4.5. Statistical Analyses

4.5.1. Epigenome-Wide Association Study

An association test was used to analyze the mean differences (MD) in single-CpG methylation between MPM cases and asbestos-exposed cancer-free controls. We performed multiple regression analysis adjusted for age, gender, estimated WBCs (monocytes, granulocytes, natural killer, B cells, CD4+ T and CD8+ T), population stratification (first 2 PCs) and technical variability (first 10 PCs). For multiple comparison tests, a FDR p value ≤ 0.05 was considered statistically significant.

Bootstrapping was performed using random sampling methods to estimate the measures of accuracy defined in terms of bias, variance, confidence intervals and prediction error. Bootstrapping can also be applied to control and check the results for stability. The bias-corrected and accelerated (BCa) bootstrap interval was calculated with regard to single CpGs.

ROC for Case-Control Discrimination was implemented, and the AUC metric was applied to estimate the predictive performance of a binary classification (cases/controls). The baseline model (BM) included age, gender, asbestos exposure and WBCs, and was compared with the BM after adding the DNAm levels of statistically significant, single-CpGs at EWAS. AUC differences between BMs before and after the addition of DNAm levels were estimated with DeLong's test.

4.5.2. Statistical Power

To ensure a study power greater than 99% (two-tailed test at $\alpha = 0.05$ and $\beta = 0.01$), only CpGs with a MD between cases and controls $\geq |0.05|$ were selected.

Covariates were included step-by-step in a sensitivity analysis to validate the association output considering effect size, standard error, 95% confidence interval and p value variations.

Gene set enrichment analyses were carried out on CpGs with a False Discovery Rate p value (P_{FDR}) ≤ 0.05 to identify pathways that may be affected by MPM-related changes in methylation.

All statistical analyses were conducted using the open source software R (4.0.2).

4.5.3. Interaction Analysis

Logistic regression was used to analyze the relationship between CpGs and asbestos exposure in MPM risk (odds ratio), adjusting for age, gender, SNP PCs and WBCs estimates. Asbestos exposure was classified as above-median or below-median, and CpG methylation was categorized as above-median or below-median.

MPM risk for a given CpG level and asbestos exposure was expressed by OR_{ij}, where i indicates the asbestos exposure (below-median or above-median) and j indicates the CpG (above-median or below-median). Considering the direction of the effect, the same approach was used: for hypomethylated CpGs, above-median was used as the reference level, whereas below-median was used for hypermethylated CpGs.

Subjects with below-median asbestos exposure and reference-level CpG DNAm were considered the baseline group, and their MPM risk was coded as $OR_{00} = 1$. Interaction was analyzed with respect to both additive and multiplicative models based on the ORs obtained by logistic regression.

Synergistic interaction (positive interaction) implies that the combined action of two factors in an additive model is greater than the sum of their individual effects. Antagonistic interaction, on the other hand, means that when two factors are present in an additive model, the action of one reduces the effect of the other.

Multivariable logistic regression models were used to explore any deviations from a multiplicative model, including asbestos exposure, CpG and the corresponding interaction term (CpG × exposure). All models were adjusted for age, gender, SNP PCs, technical covariates and WBCs estimates. p-values < 0.05 were considered statistically significant.

4.6. Validation and Replication

DNAm signal validation and replication was done by the EpiTYPER MassARRAY assay (Agena Bioscience). This assay uses a MALDI-TOF mass spectrometry-based method to quantitatively assess the DNA methylation state of the CpG sites of interest [53]. DNA (500 ng) was bisulfite-converted as indicated in Section 4.3.

PCR amplification, treatment with SAP solution and Transcription/RNase A cocktails were performed according to the manufacturer's instructions, and the mass spectra were analyzed by an EpiTYPER analyzer. The MassARRAY assay cannot discriminate between CpGs located in close proximity in the sequence, so instead, the close neighboring CpGs are analyzed as "Units", i.e., the measured methylation level is the average of the methylation levels of the CpGs cumulatively analyzed within the Unit. In the case of cg03546163, the measured methylation level is the average between two CpG sites located in very close proximity (Figure S1). For cg06633438, the two adjacent signals were considered, since the results for the model did not differ for effect size, standard error, 95% CI or p value (Figure S2).

Supplementary Materials: The following are available online at https://www.mdpi.com/article/10.3390/cancers13112636/s1, Figure S1: Location of cg03546163 investigated by EpiTYPER MassARRAY, Figure S2: Location of cg06633438 investigated by EpiTYPER MassARRAY.

Author Contributions: Conceptualization, G.C., G.M., C.M., D.M., I.D. and F.G.; methodology, G.C.; software, G.C.; validation, G.C., A.A. and C.P.; formal analysis, G.C.; investigation, G.C., G.M., S.G., A.A., A.R., E.C. and C.C.; resources, G.C., G.M., C.M., D.M., I.D., F.G., D.F., M.S., M.L.V. and R.L.; data curation, G.C., C.M., D.M., I.D., F.G., C.P., D.F., M.S., M.L.V. and R.L.; writing—original draft preparation, G.C., S.G., A.A., A.R., E.C. and C.C.; writing—review and editing, G.C., G.M., C.M., D.M., I.D., F.G., S.G., A.A., A.R., E.C., C.C., C.P., D.F., M.S., M.L.V. and R.L.; visualization, G.C., G.M., S.G., A.A., A.R., E.C., C.C., C.P., D.F., M.S., M.L.V. and R.L.; supervision, G.C. and G.M.; project administration, G.C. and G.M.; funding acquisition, G.M., C.M., D.M., I.D. and F.G. All authors have read and agreed to the published version of the manuscript.

Funding: The research leading to these results received funding from AIRC under IG 2018-ID. 21390 project (to G.M.), from the HERMES (Hereditary Risk in MESothelioma) Project funded by the offer of compensation to the inhabitants of Casale Monferrato deceased or affected by mesothelioma (to I.D. and C.M.), and from the Ministero dell'Istruzione, dell'Università e della Ricerca–MIUR project "Dipartimenti di Eccellenza 2018–2022" (n° D15D18000410001, to G.M.) to the Department of Medical Sciences, University of Torino.

Institutional Review Board Statement: Ethics approval and consent to participate: The study protocol was approved by the Ethics Committee of the Italian Institute for Genomic Medicine (IIGM, Candiolo, Italy).

Informed Consent Statement: Informed consent was obtained from all subjects involved in the study.

Data Availability Statement: The methylation of single individuals cannot be published due to informed consent limitations.

Acknowledgments: The authors wish to thank all the patients contributing to this research, Caterina Casadio and Ezio Piccolini for their past clinical contribution and Paolo Garagnani for the Sequenom analysis supervision.

Conflicts of Interest: The authors declare that they have no competing interest.

References

1. Sekido, Y. Molecular pathogenesis of malignant mesothelioma. *Carcinogenesis* **2013**, *34*, 1413–1419. [CrossRef]
2. Rossini, M.; Rizzo, P.; Bononi, I.; Clementz, A.; Ferrari, R.; Martini, F.; Tognon, M.G. New Perspectives on Diagnosis and Therapy of Malignant Pleural Mesothelioma. *Front. Oncol.* **2018**, *8*, 91. [CrossRef] [PubMed]
3. Furuya, S.; Chimed-Ochir, O.; Takahashi, K.; David, A.; Takala, J. Global Asbestos Disaster. *Int. J. Environ. Res. Public Health* **2018**, *15*, 1000. [CrossRef] [PubMed]
4. Straif, K.; Benbrahim-Tallaa, L.; Baan, R.; Grosse, Y.; Secretan, B.; El Ghissassi, F.; Bouvard, V.; Guha, N.; Freeman, C.; Galichet, L.; et al. A review of human carcinogens—Part C: Metals, arsenic, dusts, and fibres. *Lancet Oncol.* **2009**, *10*, 453–454. [CrossRef]
5. Jaurand, M.C. Mechanisms of fiber-induced genotoxicity. *Environ. Health Perspect.* **1997**, *105*, 1073–1084.
6. Kelsey, K.T.; Yano, E.; Liber, H.L.; Little, J.B. The in vitro genetic effects of fibrous erionite and crocidolite asbestos. *Br. J. Cancer* **1986**, *54*, 107–114. [CrossRef]
7. Iwatsubo, Y.; Pairon, J.C.; Boutin, C.; Ménard, O.; Massin, N.; Caillaud, D.; Orlowski, E.; Galateau-Salle, F.; Bignon, J.; Brochard, P. Pleural mesothelioma: Dose-response relation at low levels of asbestos exposure in a French population-based case-control study. *Am. J. Epidemiol.* **1998**, *148*, 133–142. [CrossRef] [PubMed]
8. Howel, D.; Arblaster, L.; Swinburne, L.; Schweiger, M.; Renvoize, E.; Hatton, P. Routes of asbestos exposure and the development of mesothelioma in an English region. *Occup. Environ. Med.* **1997**, *54*, 403–409. [CrossRef] [PubMed]
9. Kanherkar, R.R.; Bhatia-Dey, N.; Csoka, A.B. Epigenetics across the human lifespan. *Front. Cell Dev. Biol.* **2014**, *2*, 49. [CrossRef] [PubMed]
10. Ferrante, D.; Bertolotti, M.; Todesco, A.; Mirabelli, D.; Terracini, B.; Magnani, C. Cancer mortality and incidence of mesothelioma in a cohort of wives of asbestos workers in Casale Monferrato, Italy. *Environ. Health Perspect.* **2007**, *115*, 1401–1405. [CrossRef]
11. Guarrera, S.; Viberti, C.; Cugliari, G.; Allione, A.; Casalone, E.; Betti, M.; Ferrante, D.; Aspesi, A.; Casadio, C.; Grosso, F.; et al. Peripheral Blood DNA Methylation as Potential Biomarker of Malignant Pleural Mesothelioma in Asbestos-Exposed Subjects. *J. Thorac. Oncol.* **2019**, *14*, 527–539. [CrossRef]
12. Matullo, G.; Guarrera, S.; Betti, M.; Fiorito, G.; Ferrante, D.; Voglino, F.; Cadby, G.; Di Gaetano, C.; Rosa, F.; Russo, A.; et al. Genetic variants associated with increased risk of malignant pleural mesothelioma: A genome-wide association study. *PLoS ONE* **2013**, *8*, e61253. [CrossRef]
13. Cugliari, G.; Catalano, C.; Guarrera, S.; Allione, A.; Casalone, E.; Russo, A.; Grosso, F.; Ferrante, D.; Viberti, C.; Aspesi, A.; et al. DNA Methylation of FKBP5 as Predictor of Overall Survival in Malignant Pleural Mesothelioma. *Cancers* **2020**, *12*, 3470. [CrossRef]
14. Betti, M.; Aspesi, A.; Sculco, M.; Matullo, G.; Magnani, C.; Dianzani, I. Genetic predisposition for malignant mesothelioma: A concise review. *Mutat. Res.* **2019**, *781*, 1–10. [CrossRef]
15. Guo, G.; Chmielecki, J.; Goparaju, C.; Heguy, A.; Dolgalev, I.; Carbone, M.; Seepo, S.; Meyerson, M.; Pass, H.I. Whole-exome sequencing reveals frequent genetic alterations in BAP1, NF2, CDKN2A, and CUL1 in malignant pleural mesothelioma. *Cancer Res.* **2015**, *75*, 264–269. [CrossRef]
16. Fasanelli, F.; Baglietto, L.; Ponzi, E.; Guida, F.; Campanella, G.; Johansson, M.; Grankvist, K.; Johansson, M.; Assumma, M.B.; Naccarati, A.; et al. Hypomethylation of smoking-related genes is associated with future lung cancer in four prospective cohorts. *Nat. Commun.* **2015**, *15*, 10192. [CrossRef] [PubMed]
17. Moore, L.D.; Le, T.; Fan, G. DNA methylation and its basic function. *Neuropsychopharmacology* **2013**, *38*, 23–38.
18. Bononi, A.; Napolitano, A.; Pass, H.I.; Yang, H.; Carbone, M. Latest developments in our understanding of the pathogenesis of mesothelioma and the design of targeted therapies. *Expert. Rev. Respir. Med.* **2015**, *9*, 633–654. [CrossRef] [PubMed]
19. Vandermeers, F.; Neelature, S.; Costa, C.; Hubaux, R.; Cosse, J.P.; Willems, L. The role of epigenetics in malignant pleural mesothelioma. *Lung Cancer* **2013**, *81*, 311–318. [CrossRef] [PubMed]
20. Zhang, X.; Tang, N.; Rishi, A.K.; Pass, H.I.; Wali, A. Methylation profile landscape in mesothelioma: Possible implications in early detection, disease progression, and therapeutic options. *Methods Mol. Biol.* **2015**, *1238*, 235–247. [PubMed]
21. Goto, Y.; Shinjo, K.; Kondo, Y.; Shen, L.; Toyota, M.; Suzuki, H.; Gao, W.; An, N.; Fujii, M.; Murakami, H.; et al. Epigenetic profiles distinguish malignant pleural mesothelioma from lung adenocarcinoma. *Cancer Res.* **2009**, *69*, 9073–9082. [CrossRef] [PubMed]
22. Christensen, B.C.; Houseman, E.A.; Poage, G.M.; Godleski, J.J.; Bueno, R.; Sugarbaker, D.J.; Wiencke, J.K.; Nelson, H.H.; Marsit, C.J.; Kelsey, K.T. Integrated profiling reveals a global correlation between epigenetic and genetic alterations in mesothelioma. *Cancer Res.* **2010**, *70*, 5686–5694. [CrossRef]
23. Fischer, J.R.; Ohnmacht, U.; Rieger, N.; Zemaitis, M.; Stoffregen, C.; Kostrzewa, M.; Buchholz, E.; Manegold, C.; Lahm, H. Promoter methylation of RASSF1A, RARbeta and DAPK predict poor prognosis of patients with malignant mesothelioma. *Lung Cancer* **2006**, *54*, 109–116. [CrossRef]
24. Matosin, N.; Halldorsdottir, T.; Binder, E.B. Understanding the molecular mechanisms underpinning gene by environment interactions in psychiatric disorders: The FKBP5 model. *Biol. Psychiatry* **2018**, *83*, 821–830. [CrossRef] [PubMed]
25. Kang, C.B.; Hong, Y.; Dhe-Paganon, S.; Sup Yoon, H. FKBP family proteins: Immunophilins with versatile biological functions. *Neurosignals* **2008**, *16*, 318–325. [CrossRef]
26. Li, L.; Lou, Z.; Wang, L. The role of FKBP5 in cancer aetiology and chemoresistance. *Br. J. Cancer* **2011**, *104*, 19–23. [CrossRef] [PubMed]

27. Romano, S.; D'Angelillo, A.; Romano, M.F. Pleiotropic roles in cancer biology for multifaceted proteins FKBPs. *Biochim. Biophys. Acta* **2015**, *1850*, 2061–2068. [CrossRef]
28. Staibano, S.; Mascolo, M.; Ilardi, G.; Siano, M.; De Rosa, G. Immunohistochemical analysis of FKBP51 in human cancers. *Curr. Opin. Pharmacol.* **2011**, *11*, 338–347. [CrossRef] [PubMed]
29. Zannas, A.S.; Jia, M.; Hafner, K.; Baumert, J.; Wiechmann, T.; Pape, J.C.; Arloth, J.; Ködel, M.; Martinelli, S.; Roitman, M.; et al. Epigenetic upregulation of FKBP5 by aging and stress contributes to NF-kappaB-driven inflammation and cardiovascular risk. *Proc. Natl. Acad. Sci. USA* **2019**, *116*, 11370–11379. [CrossRef]
30. Yoshikawa, Y.; Sato, A. Biallelic germline and somatic mutations in malignant mesothelioma: Multiple mutations in transcription regulators including mSWI/SNF genes. *Int. J. Cancer* **2015**, *136*, 560–571. [CrossRef]
31. Zhou, J.; Ng, Y.; Chng, W.J. ENL: Structure, function, and roles in hematopoiesis and acute myeloid leukemia. *Cell Mol. Life Sci.* **2018**, *75*, 3931–3941. [CrossRef] [PubMed]
32. Canino, C.; Luo, Y.; Marcato, P.; Blandino, G.; Pass, H.I.; Cioce, M. STAT3-NFkB/DDIT3/CEBPbeta axis modulates ALDH1A3 expression in chemoresistant cell subpopulations. *Oncotarget* **2015**, *6*, 12637–12653. [CrossRef]
33. Bagger, F.O.; Kinalis, S.; Rapin, N. BloodSpot: A database of healthy and malignant haematopoiesis updated with purified and single cell mRNA sequencing profiles. *Nucleic Acids Res.* **2019**, *47*, 881–885. [CrossRef] [PubMed]
34. Schins, R.P.; Donaldson, K. Nuclear Factor Kappa-B Activation by Particles and Fibers. *Inhal. Toxicol.* **2000**, *12*, 317–326. [CrossRef]
35. Tan, Z.; Lu, W.; Li, X.; Yang, G.; Guo, J.; Yu, H.; Li, Z.; Guan, F. Altered N-Glycan expression profile in epithelial-to-mesenchymal transition of NMuMG cells revealed by an integrated strategy using mass spectrometry and glycogene and lectin microarray analysis. *J. Proteome Res.* **2014**, *13*, 2783–2795. [CrossRef] [PubMed]
36. Kale, V.P.; Hengst, J.A.; Desai, D.H.; Dick, T.E.; Choe, K.N.; Colledge, A.L.; Takahashi, Y.; Sung, S.S.; Amin, S.G.; Yun, J.K. A novel selective multikinase inhibitor of ROCK and MRCK effectively blocks cancer cell migration and invasion. *Cancer Lett.* **2014**, *354*, 299–310. [CrossRef]
37. Tanrikulu, A.C.; Abakay, A.; Komek, H.; Abakay, O. Prognostic value of the lymphocyte-to-monocyte ratio and other inflammatory markers in malignant pleural mesothelioma. *Environ. Health Prev. Med.* **2016**, *21*, 304–311. [CrossRef]
38. Zhao, Z.S.; Manser, E. PAK and other Rho-associated kinases—Effectors with surprisingly diverse mechanisms of regulation. *Biochem. J.* **2005**, *386 Pt 2*, 201–214. [CrossRef]
39. Nishimura, Y.; Kumagai-Takei, N.; Matsuzaki, H.; Lee, S.; Maeda, M.; Kishimoto, T.; Fukuoka, K.; Nakano, T.; Otsuki, T. Functional alteration of natural killer cells and cytotoxic T lymphocytes upon asbestos exposure and in malignant mesothelioma patients. *Biomed. Res. Int.* **2015**, *2015*, 238431. [CrossRef]
40. Maeda, M.; Nishimura, Y.; Kumagai, N.; Hayashi, H.; Hatayama, T.; Katoh, M.; Miyahara, N.; Yamamoto, S.; Hirastuka, J.; Otsuki, T. Dysregulation of the immune system caused by silica and asbestos. *J. Immunotoxicol.* **2010**, *7*, 268–278. [CrossRef]
41. Miura, Y.; Nishimura, Y.; Katsuyama, H.; Maeda, M.; Hayashi, H.; Dong, M.; Hyodoh, F.; Tomita, M.; Matsuo, Y.; Uesaka, A.; et al. Involvement of IL-10 and Bcl-2 in resistance against an asbestos-induced apoptosis of T cells. *Apoptosis* **2006**, *11*, 1825–1835. [CrossRef]
42. Cristaudo, A.; Bonotti, A.; Guglielmi, G.; Fallahi, P.; Foddis, R. Serum mesothelin and other biomarkers: What have we learned in the last decade? *J. Thorac. Dis.* **2018**, *10*, 353–359. [CrossRef] [PubMed]
43. Andujar, P.; Wang, J.; Descatha, A.; Galateau-Sallé, F.; Abd-Alsamad, I.; Billon-Galland, M.A.; Blons, H.; Clin, B.; Danel, C.; Housset, B.; et al. p16INK4A inactivation mechanisms in non-small-cell lung cancer patients occupationally exposed to asbestos. *Lung Cancer* **2010**, *67*, 23–30. [CrossRef] [PubMed]
44. Dianzani, I.; Gibello, L.; Biava, A.; Giordano, M.; Bertolotti, M.; Betti, M.; Ferrante, D.; Guarrera, S.; Betta, G.P.; Mirabelli, D.; et al. Polymorphisms in DNA repair genes as risk factors for asbestos-related malignant mesothelioma in a general population study. *Mutat. Res.* **2006**, *599*, 124–134. [CrossRef]
45. Betti, M.; Ferrante, D.; Padoan, M.; Guarrera, S.; Giordano, M.; Aspesi, A.; Mirabelli, D.; Casadio, C.; Ardissone, F.; Ruffini, E.; et al. XRCC1 and ERCC1 variants modify malignant mesothelioma risk: A case-control study. *Mutat. Res.* **2011**, *708*, 11–20. [CrossRef] [PubMed]
46. Betti, M.; Casalone, E.; Ferrante, D.; Aspesi, A.; Morleo, G.; Biasi, A.; Sculco, M.; Mancuso, G.; Guarrera, S.; Righi, L.; et al. Germline mutations in DNA repair genes predispose asbestos-exposed patients to malignant pleural mesothelioma. *Cancer Lett.* **2017**, *405*, 38–45. [CrossRef] [PubMed]
47. Ferrante, D.; Mirabelli, D.; Tunesi, S.; Terracini, B.; Magnani, C. Pleural mesothelioma and occupational and non-occupational asbestos exposure: A case-control study with quantitative risk assessment. *Occup. Environ. Med.* **2016**, *73*, 147–153. [CrossRef]
48. Du, P.; Zhang, X.; Huang, C.C.; Jafari, N.; Kibbe, W.A.; Hou, L.; Lin, S.M. Comparison of Beta-value and M-value methods for quantifying methylation levels by microarray analysis. *BMC Bioinform.* **2010**, *11*, 587. [CrossRef]
49. Lehne, B.; Drong, A.W.; Loh, M.; Zhang, W.; Scott, W.R.; Tan, S.T.; Afzal, U.; Scott, J.; Jarvelin, M.R.; Elliott, P.; et al. A coherent approach for analysis of the Illumina HumanMethylation450 BeadChip improves data quality and performance in epigenome-wide association studies. *Genome Biol.* **2015**, *16*, 37. [CrossRef]
50. Campanella, G.; Polidoro, S.; Di Gaetano, C.; Fiorito, F.; Guarrera, S.; Krogh, V.; Palli, D.; Panico, S.; Sacerdote, C.; Tumino, R.; et al. Epigenetic signatures of internal migration in Italy. *Int. J. Epidemiol.* **2015**, *44*, 1442–1449. [CrossRef]

51. Di Gaetano, C.; Voglino, F.; Guarrera, S.; Fiorito, G.; Rosa, F.; Di Blasio, A.M.; Manzini, P.; Dianzani, I.; Betti, M.; Cusi, D.; et al. An overview of the genetic structure within the Italian population from genome-wide data. *PLoS ONE* **2012**, *7*, e43759. [CrossRef] [PubMed]
52. Houseman, E.A.; Accomando, W.P.; Koestler, D.C.; Christensen, B.C.; Marsit, C.J.; Nelson, H.H.; Wiencke, J.K.; Kelsey, K.T. DNA methylation arrays as surrogate measures of cell mixture distribution. *BMC Bioinform.* **2012**, *13*, 86. [CrossRef] [PubMed]
53. Ehrich, M.; Nelson, M.R.; Stanssens, P.; Zabeau, M.; Liloglou, T.; Xinarianos, G.; Cantor, C.R.; Field, J.K.; van den Boom, D. Quantitative high-throughput analysis of DNA methylation patterns by base-specific cleavage and mass spectrometry. *Proc. Natl. Acad. Sci. USA* **2005**, *102*, 15785–15790. [CrossRef] [PubMed]

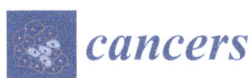

Article

Well-Differentiated Papillary Mesothelioma of the Peritoneum Is Genetically Distinct from Malignant Mesothelioma

Raunak Shrestha [1,2,3], Noushin Nabavi [1,4], Stanislav Volik [1], Shawn Anderson [1], Anne Haegert [1], Brian McConeghy [1], Funda Sar [1], Sonal Brahmbhatt [1], Robert Bell [1], Stephane Le Bihan [1], Yuzhuo Wang [1,2,4], Colin Collins [1,2,*] and Andrew Churg [5,*]

[1] Vancouver Prostate Centre, Vancouver, BC V6H 3ZH, Canada; raunakman.shrestha@ucsf.edu (R.S.); nabavinoushin@gmail.com (N.N.); svolik@prostatecentre.com (S.V.); sanderson@prostatecentre.com (S.A.); ahaegert@prostatecentre.com (A.H.); brian.mcconeghy@ubc.ca (B.M.); fsar@prostatecentre.com (F.S.); sonal.brahmbhatt2001@gmail.com (S.B.); rbell@prostatecentre.com (R.B.); slebihan@prostatecentre.com (S.L.B.); ywang@bccrc.ca (Y.W.)
[2] Department of Urologic Sciences, University of British Columbia, Vancouver, BC V5Z 1M9, Canada
[3] Department of Radiation Oncology, University of California San Francisco, San Francisco, CA94143, USA
[4] Department of Experimental Therapeutics, BC Cancer Agency, Vancouver, BC V5Z 1L3, Canada
[5] Department of Pathology, Vancouver General Hospital, Vancouver, BC V5Z 1M9, Canada
* Correspondence: ccollins@prostatecentre.com (C.C.); achurg@mail.ubc.ca (A.C.)

Received: 17 May 2020; Accepted: 11 June 2020; Published: 13 June 2020

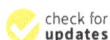

Abstract: Well-differentiated papillary mesothelioma (WDPM) is an uncommon mesothelial proliferation that is most commonly encountered as an incidental finding in the peritoneal cavity. There is controversy in the literature about whether WDPM is a neoplasm or a reactive process and, if neoplastic, whether it is a variant or precursor of epithelial malignant mesothelioma or is a different entity. Using whole exome sequencing of five WDPMs of the peritoneum, we have identified distinct mutations in *EHD1*, *ATM*, *FBXO10*, *SH2D2A*, *CDH5*, *MAGED1*, and *TP73* shared by WDPM cases but not reported in malignant mesotheliomas. Furthermore, we show that WDPM is strongly enriched with C > A transversion substitution mutations, a pattern that is also not found in malignant mesotheliomas. The WDPMs lacked the alterations involving *BAP1*, *SETD2*, *NF2*, *CDKN2A/B*, *LASTS1/2*, *PBRM1*, and *SMARCC1* that are frequently found in malignant mesotheliomas. We conclude that WDPMs are neoplasms that are genetically distinct from malignant mesotheliomas and, based on observed mutations, do not appear to be precursors of malignant mesotheliomas.

Keywords: well-differentiated papillary mesothelioma; WDPM; malignant mesothelioma; DNA sequencing; mutation

1. Introduction

Well-differentiated papillary mesothelioma (WDPM) is a morphologically distinctive papillary proliferation of mesothelial cells that is most commonly encountered as an incidental finding in the peritoneal cavity, and less often in the pleural cavity, pericardium, and tunica vaginalis. These lesions may be single or multiple but by definition do not invade the underlying stroma and usually behave in a benign or indolent fashion, sometimes persisting for many years [1]. However, the nature of WDPM is disputed, with theories ranging from a reactive non-neoplastic process to a benign tumor, to a variant and/or precursor of epithelial malignant mesotheliomas [2]. To add further confusion, unequivocal invasive malignant mesotheliomas can have areas that mimic WDPM. Since malignant mesotheliomas are aggressive tumors, the distinction from WDPM is important, but WDPMs are sometimes treated with debulking cytoreductive surgery followed by hyperthermic intraperitoneal chemotherapy (HIPEC) as if they were mesotheliomas [3].

Genome-wide sequencing analyses of malignant mesotheliomas have revealed frequently observed genomic aberrations such as loss of function mutation and/or copy number alterations/deletion of *BAP1*, *SETD2*, *CDKN2A*, and *NF2* [4–6]. Studies analyzing WDPM using DNA sequencing technology are limited. Case studies have reported WDPMs with somatic mutation of *E2F1* [7], heterozygous loss of *NF2* [8], and germline *BAP1* mutation [9], which if correct would suggest that they may be variants of malignant mesothelioma. Nevertheless, using immunohistochemistry (IHC) and fluorescence in situ hybridization (FISH), Lee et al. demonstrated that, unlike in malignant mesothelioma, both *BAP1* and *CDKN2A* are intact and respective proteins are expressed in WDPMs [10]. More recently, Stevers et al. [11] performed genomic profiling of 10 WDPMs and found that they harbored *TRAF7* or *CDC42* mutually exclusive missense mutations.

To shed further light on this question we performed an extensive genomic characterization of a cohort of five WDPMs of the peritoneum.

2. Results

2.1. Histopathological Features of WDPM

We assembled a cohort of five incidentally identified WDPM cases in the peritoneum detected during surgery for another process and all were solitary lesions. All of these five cases had the typical features described for WDPM [12], i.e., a papillary architecture with a single layer of covering bland mesothelial cells and myxoid cores in the papillae (Figure 1).

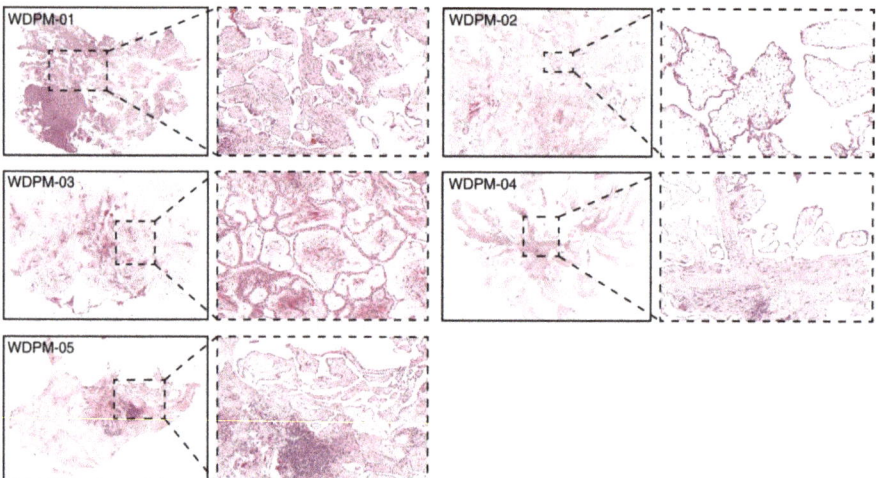

Figure 1. Histopathology of five WDPM cases used for the study. Microphotographs of histological features of WDPM stained using haematoxylin and eosin (H&E). The panel under the dotted box represents the magnified section of the photomicrographs at ×20. The lesion sites/sizes were peritoneum, site not specified, for cases WDPM-01 (3 mm), WDPM-02 (6 mm), WDPM-03 (4 mm), WDPM-04 mesentery (4 mm), and WDPM-05 omentum (4 mm).

2.2. Mutational Landscape of WDPM

We performed high-coverage whole exome sequencing of five WDPMs from formalin-fixed and paraffin embedded (FFPE) samples. We achieved a mean sequencing reads coverage of 87×–117×, with at least 20–45% of targeted bases having a coverage of 100× (Table S1). Due to papillary architecture, the tumor cellularity of the WDPM tissues was estimated to be about 50% (Table S2). Although the high coverage sequencing provides us an opportunity to detect higher proportions of mutations, the normal tissue admixture lowers the mutation detection sensitivity. To overcome this challenge, we implemented strict mutation filtering criteria as described in the Methods section and retained only high confident mutation calls for downstream analysis.

Analysis of the mutational patterns in WDPM revealed a strong enrichment of C > A transversion substitution mutation (Figure 2A). Using the software deconstructSigs [13], we evaluated the characteristic mutation patterns in WDPM against the mutational signature obtained from the COSMIC mutational signature database [14]. Intriguingly, we identified consistent patterns of nucleotide substitution mutation associated with WDPM. Notably, we found that mutational signature 24 is significantly operative in all five WDPM cases (Figure 2B). In addition to this, mutational signature 21 and 28 were also observed in the WDPM cases.

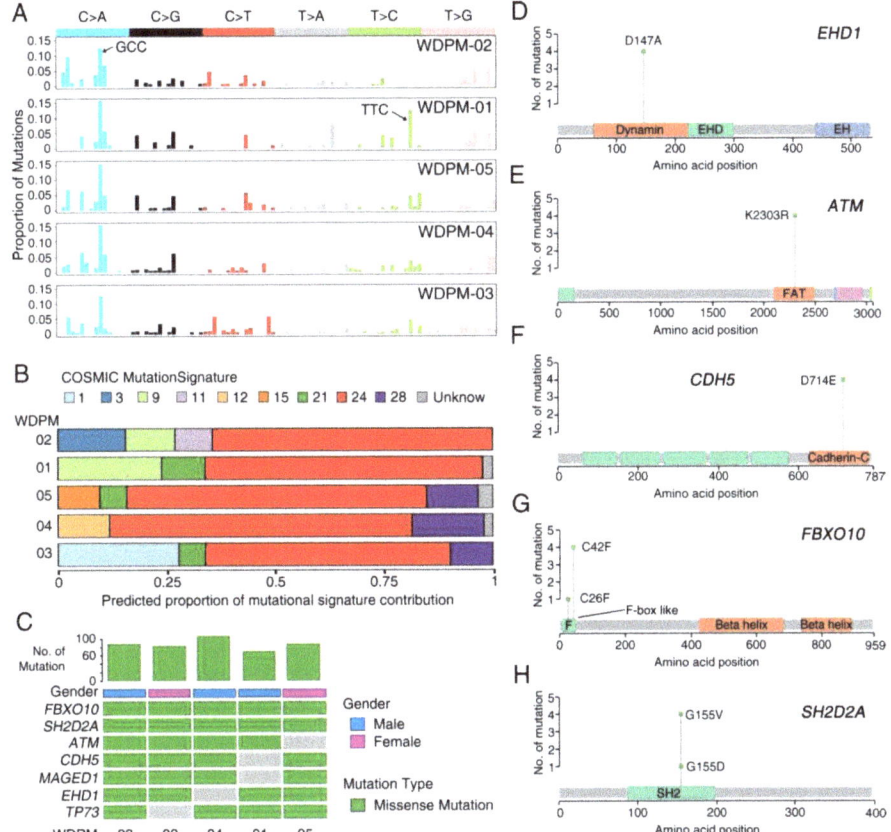

Figure 2. Landscape of mutations in WDPM. (**A**) Mutational signature present in WDPM. (**B**) Proportional contribution of different COSMIC mutational signature per sample. (**C**) Mutation status in WDPM. Top seven most recurrent mutations are represented in the figure. The bar plot on the top panel represents the total number of mutations detected in the respective WDPM. (**D–H**) Plots showing mutation distribution and the protein domains for the corresponding mutated protein.

We identified 461 unique non-silent mutations across five WDPM samples affecting 297 unique protein coding genes (Table S3). Patient WDPM-04 had the highest mutation burden and WDPM-01 had the least. Two genes—*FBXO10* and *SH2D2A*—were mutated in all five WDPM cases, again displaying consistent mutational patterns (Figure 2C). Missense mutation $EHD1^{D147A}$ in the dynamin protein domain was found in four cases (Figure 2C,D). The variant allele frequency (VAF) of $EHD1$ was in the range 29–43%, indicating its likely clonal origin (given that the tumor cellularity of the WDPM tissues were estimated to be about 50%) (Figure S1). Notably, we identified missense mutation in DNA-damage response gene ATM in four cases (Figure 2C,E). All four cases harbored ATM^{K2303R} located in the FRAP-ATM-TRRAP (FAT) domain in the ATM protein. The VAF of ATM was also in the range 25–30%, indicating its likely clonal origin (Figure S1). The gene encoding cadherin 5 ($CDH5$) harbored $CDH5^{D714E}$ mutations in its C-terminus cadherin protein domain in four cases (Figure 2C,F). The VAF of $CDH5$ was also in the range 26–38%, indicating its likely clonal origin (Figure S1). We also identified missense mutation $FBXO10^{C42F}$ in four cases and $FBXO10^{C26F}$ in one case (Figure 2C,G). Both mutation variants of $FBXO10$ were present in the F-box like protein domain. The VAF of $FBXO10$ was also in the range 24–37%, indicating its likely clonal origin (Figure S1). Similarly, we identified missense mutation $SH2D2A^{G155V}$ in four cases and $SH2D2A^{G155D}$ in one case (Figure 2C,H). These variants were located in the SH2 protein domain. The VAF of $SH2D2A$ in WDPM-04 was 69%, indicating the mutation to be clonal. The VAF of $SH2D2A$ in the rest of the four WDPMs was in the range 37–47% (Figure S1). Furthermore, we also identified mutations in $MAGED1$ and $TP73$ in each of the four WDPM cases (Figure 2C).

2.3. Copy Number Landscape of WDPM

The aggregate copy number aberration (CNA) profile of WDPM is shown in Figure S2. We observed 278 CNA events across all samples (Table S4). The CNA resulted in alterations of about 4–14% of the protein-coding genomes in the WDPM. Patient WDPM-02 had a high copy number burden and WDPM-03 had the least copy number burden (Figure S2). Overall, copy number profiles of the WDPM did not show many alterations (Figure S3). Notably, we found copy number gain of $SETDB2$ and $LAST2$ and copy number loss of $SMARCA4$ and $TRAF7$ in WDPM-02. We also found copy number loss of cancer genes such as $CCNE1$, MAF, $MAFB$, MYC, $ZNF479$, and $MGMT$ and copy number gain of $FOXA2$, $CDH10$, and $GPC5$ in at least two WDPM cases.

2.4. Signaling Pathways Dysregulated in WDPM

To identify signaling pathways dysregulated by mutated genes in WDPM, we performed pathway enrichment analysis using the KEGG [15] pathway database (see Methods section). Our analysis revealed that WDPM mutations target different signaling pathways often dysregulated in cancer (Figure 3 and Table S5) such as pathways in cancer, focal adhesion, Vascular endothelial growth factor (VEGF) signaling, Janus kinases - signal transducer and activator of transcription (JAK-STAT) signaling, Wnt signaling, P53 signaling, apoptosis, etc. We found $CDH5$ mutations target cell adhesion and the leukocyte migration pathway, $EHD1$ mutations target endocytosis, $SH2D2A$ mutations target the VEGF signaling pathway, ATM mutations target apoptosis and P53 signaling pathways, and $TP73$ targets the neurotrophin signaling and P53 signaling pathways. This indicates that the mutations identified in WDPM cases might be relevant to pathogenesis of WDPM.

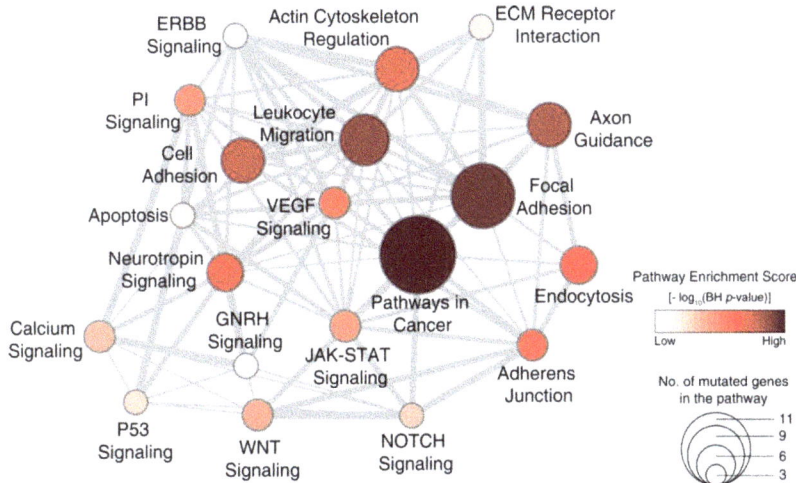

Figure 3. Signaling pathways dysregulated in WDPM. We performed pathway enrichment analysis using genes mutated in WDPM cases against the signaling pathways in the KEGG pathway database. The figure shows the top 20 pathways enriched with mutated genes in WDPM. Each circle represents a pathway, its size indicates the number of mutated genes targeting the pathway, and its color indicates the pathway enrichment score. The thickness of edges connecting two circles (pathways) is proportional to the number of mutated genes common between the two pathways. PI signaling: phosphatidylinositol signaling pathway.

2.5. WDPM is Genetically Distinct from Malignant Mesothelioma

Next, we compared the genomic profiles of WDPM with those of malignant peritoneal mesothelioma. For this, we leveraged the DNA sequencing data from two recently published peritoneal mesothelioma patient cohorts [6,16]. We first assessed the pattern of mutations in WDPM and peritoneal mesothelioma cases. Intriguingly, we observed that WDPM has a strong enrichment of C > A transversion substitution mutation (Figure 2A,B), whereas, peritoneal mesothelioma has strong enrichment of C > T transition substitution mutation (Figure S4). This mutational pattern in WDPM is different from those reported in pleural [4,5] or peritoneal [6] mesotheliomas.

Notably, we found WDPM specific mutations in *EHD1*, *FBXO10*, *CHD5*, *MAGED1*, *ATM*, and *TP73* genes that were absent in peritoneal mesothelioma (Figure 4A). Although mutations in *EHD1* and *ATM* genes were each observed in peritoneal mesothelioma, we did not find the WDPM-specific $EHD1^{D147A}$, $EHD1^{A465D}$, and ATM^{K2303R} mutations in these cases. Interestingly, in WDPM, we did not find any of the mutations in *BAP1*, *SETD2*, *TP53*, *NF2*, *CDKN2A*, and *LAST1/2* frequently observed in malignant mesotheliomas (Figure 4A). We also did not find mutations in *TRAF7* or *CDC42* in WDPM, however, *TRAF7* mutations were observed in several peritoneal mesothelioma cases. Furthermore, we evaluated the differences in the copy number status of genes between WDPM and peritoneal mesothelioma. We did not find any copy number loss in gene characteristics of malignant mesotheliomas such as *BAP1*, *SETD2*, *PBRM1*, *SMARCC1*, *CDKN2A/B*, *LATS1/2*, and *NF2* (Figure 4B). *TRAF* copy number loss was observed in one WDPM case, whereas, several peritoneal mesothelioma cases harbored *TRAF7* copy number alteration.

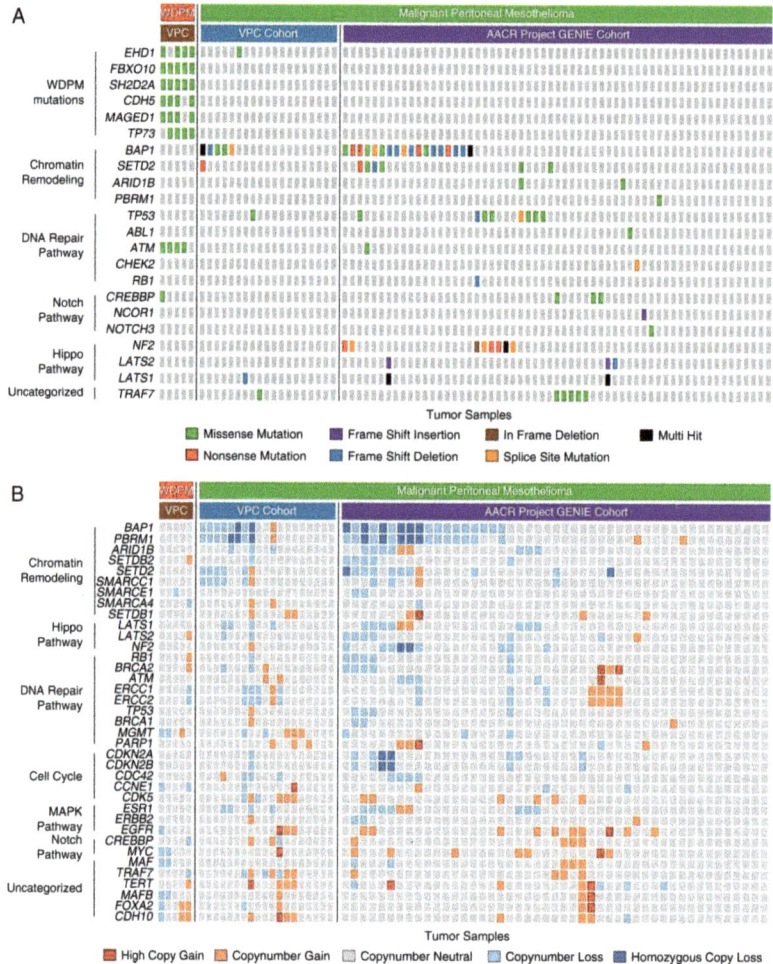

Figure 4. Genomic alterations in WDPM and peritoneal mesothelioma. We compared the genomic alteration profile of the WDPM cases to the peritoneal mesothelioma patient cohorts from two recently published studies, Vancouver Prostate Centre (VPC) cohort [6] and American Association for Cancer Research (AACR) project Genomics Evidence Neoplasia Information Exchange (GENIE) cohort [16]. (**A**) Oncoplot showing differences in mutation pattern between WDPM and peritoneal mesothelioma. Each column in the figure represents an individual cancer sample. (**B**) Oncoplot showing the copy number aberration status of WDPM and peritoneal mesothelioma. Each column in the figure represents an individual cancer sample.

3. Discussion

In this study, we investigated the genomic alterations found in a cohort of five WDPMs. The tumors analyzed here are clinically typical of the setting in which WDPM is most commonly found, i.e., as an incidental lesion discovered during surgery for another process, and all lesions were morphologically characteristic WDPM.

Overall, our results suggest that WDPM are distinctive lesions with their own set of genomic alterations. Given the number of mutations and the nature of the mutations found, including at least one tumor suppressor gene, *TP73*, and several genes that may be associated with other types of malignancy (*ATM*, *CDH5*, *MAGED1*) [17–19], WDPM clearly appears to be a functionally benign neoplasm and not a reactive process. Further, it is clear that WDPM are genetically quite different from both peritoneal and pleural mesotheliomas. Indeed, our most important finding is the lack of alterations involving *BAP1*, *SETD2*, *NF2*, *CDKN2A*, *PBRM1*, and *SMARCC1* genes consistently mutated or deleted in malignant mesotheliomas.

We found consistent mutation patterns in five WDPMs with strong enrichment of C > A transversion substitution mutation and COSMIC mutational signature 24. The WDPMs harbored distinct mutations in *EHD1*, *FBXO10*, *CHD5*, *MAGED1*, *ATM*, and *TP73* genes either in all five or at least four out of five WDPM cases. The COSMIC mutational signature 24 has been shown to be commonly found in certain liver cancers with exposure to carcinogen such as aflatoxin [20]. However, these WDPMs were incidental findings during surgery and any prior exposure to carcinogens (either aflatoxin or asbestos) is extremely unlikely. Mutations and copy number changes in *CDH5* have been previously reported in mesotheliomas [21,22] but are uncommon events and were not present in any of our reference mesothelioma datasets (Figure 3). *CHD5* is known to promote intravasation and stimulates TGF-β driven epithelial–mesenchymal transition (EMT) [23]. *EHD1* regulates the endocytic recycling process. *EHD1* is known to play a key role in transportation of receptors from endosomes into the endocytic recycling compartment (ERC) and from the ERC to the plasma membrane [24]. Moreover, *EHD1* has been associated with cell proliferation, apoptosis, metastasis, and drug resistance in breast and non-small cell lung cancer (NSCLC) [25] but has not been reported to be abnormal in malignant mesotheliomas. *FBXO10* binds to the anti-apoptotic oncoprotein BCL-2 and promotes its degradation, thereby initiating cell death in lymphomas [26]. *SH2D2A* is known to be involved in T-cell activation [27]. Mutations in *FBXO10*, *SH2D2A*, and *TP73* has not been reported in any malignant mesotheliomas.

Our study confirms a lack of copy number alterations in *BAP1*, *SETD2*, *PBRM1*, *SMARCC1*, *CDKN2A/B*, *LATS1/2*, and *NF2*. Copy number loss of *BAP1*, *SETD2*, *PBRM1*, and *SMARCC1* is often observed in peritoneal mesothelioma [6,28]. Copy number loss of *BAP1*, *CDKN2A/B*, *LAST1/2*, and *NF2* is frequently found in pleural mesothelioma [4,5].

What is surprising in our results is the absence of the TRAF7 and CDC42 alterations reported by Yu et al. [7] and Stevers et al. [11] in WDPM and by the same group in adenomatoid tumors [29]. Alterations in TRAF7 have also been reported in malignant mesotheliomas [4,16,30]. However, this does not appear to be a case of tumor misclassification, since the lesion illustrated by Stevers et al. [11] is a very typical WDPM and is identical to the tumors analyzed here. The lesions analyzed by Stevers et al. [11] were also all incidental findings and 8/10 were solitary, as were ours, and the lesions for which they had follow up did not behave in a malignant fashion.

The exact reasons for the discrepancy between our study and those of Stevers et al. [11] are unclear. It is possible that the underlying populations are genetically different, particularly given the very large and diverse immigrant population in Vancouver, Canada. The analytical approach used in these two studies was also somewhat different. Stevers et al. [11] used a targeted panel consisting of 479 cancer-related genes (UCSF500 Cancer Panel) for sequencing (Illumina HiSeq 2500), whereas we used Ion AmpliSeq™ (Thermo Fisher Scientific, Waltham, MA, USA) exome sequencing which covers 18,961 genes (Ion Proton™). The overlap in the genes examined between these two studies is given in Figure S5A. Using a targeted panel provided Stevers et al. [11] an advantage to sequence a small number of genes at a high depth (average depth = 320×, range = 33×–722×), whereas we sequenced a large number of genes at a cost of sequencing depth (average depth = 102×). Stevers et al. [11] reported 21 mutations covering 10 genes in 10 WDPM cases, whereas we identified 461 mutations covering 297 genes in 5 WDPM cases. There is no overlap of the mutated genes reported in Stevers et al. [11] and our study (Figure S5B). In fact, the UCSF500 gene panel used by Stevers et al. [11] covered only 10 mutated genes reported by our study (Figure S5C). We note that, despite high sequencing depth, no mutations in *ATM* (which was examined in the UCSF500 panel) were reported by Stevers et al. [11], whereas we identified consistent *ATM*^{K2303R} mutations in 4 out of 5 WDPM cases (Figure S5C). We did identify a few low confidence *TRAF7* mutations, but these did not pass our mutation filtering criteria (see Table S6 and Appendix A for detailed information). These differences likely indicate genomic heterogeneity in WDPM and warrants further investigation in larger patient cohort settings. Once there are sufficient cases described with consistent results, it may be possible to use a genomic approach to decide whether an equivocal case is a WDPM or a malignant mesothelioma and to base treatment on such data.

4. Materials and Methods

4.1. Patient Cohort Description and Tissue Procurement

A cohort of incidentally identified WDPM tissues (n = 5) were assembled from the surgical pathology archives at the Vancouver General Hospital. This study was approved by the Institutional Review Board of the University of British Columbia and the Vancouver Coastal Health (REB No. H15-00902 and V15-00902).

4.2. Whole Exome Sequencing

DNA from marked FFPE tissue sections (5–10 μm in thickness, ~50% WDPM cellularity) were isolated using a truXTRAC FFPE DNA Kit with Covaris Adaptive Focused Acoustics® (AFA®) technology, which enables the removal of the paraffin from the FFPE tissue in SDS buffer while simultaneously rehydrating the tissue. The samples were treated with proteinase K 0.2 mg/mL (Roche) followed by overnight incubation at 55 °C. After post-incubation in proteinase K, the samples were treated with RNAse and DNA extracted as per the truXTRAC FFPE DNA extraction protocol (cat#: 520136, Covaris, Inc., Woburn, MA, USA). The amount of DNA was quantified using Qubit® dsDNA HS Assay (Thermo Fisher Scientific).

For Ion AmpliSeq™ (Thermo Fisher Scientific) exome sequencing, 100 ng of DNA was used as input for Ion AmpliSeq™ Exome RDY library preparation, a PCR-based sequencing approach using 294,000 primer pairs (amplicon size range 225–275 bp), which covers >97% of consensus coding sequence (CCDS) (Release 12), >19,000 coding genes, and >198,000 coding exons. Libraries were prepared, quantified using qPCR, and sequenced according to the manufacturer's instructions (Thermo Fisher Scientific). Samples were sequenced on the Ion Proton System using the Ion PI™ Hi-Q™ Sequencing 200 Kit and Ion PI™ v3 chip. Two libraries were run per chip for a projected minimum coverage of 40 million reads per sample.

4.3. Single Nucleotide Variant Calling

We used Torrent Server (Thermo Fisher Scientific) for mapping aligned reads to the human reference genome hg19 (Torrent Mapping Alignment feature). Variants were identified using a Torrent Variant Caller plugin with the optimized parameters for AmpliSeq exome sequencing (Thermo Fisher Scientific). The variant call format (VCF) files from all samples were annotated using ANNOVAR [31].

To account for the low tumor cellularity in the WDPM samples and the absence of the matched control samples, we used strict mutation calls filtering criteria. Mutations were retained if (a) allele frequency (AF) < 75%, (b) read quality pass > 50%, (c) average heterozygosity < 0.1, (d) mutation calls not present in dbSNP database. We filtered out all In-Dels from our variant calls. Non-silent exonic variants including non-synonymous single nucleotide variations (SNVs), stop-codon gain SNVs, stop-codon loss SNVs, splice site SNVs, and frameshift In-Dels in coding regions were retained if they were supported by more than 50 reads. Furthermore, putative variants were manually scrutinized on the Binary Alignment Map (BAM) files through Integrative Genomics Viewer (IGV) version 2.3.25 [32]. Furthermore, due to lack of matched germline control samples from the WDPM cases, we used genomic DNA samples from blood of a cohort of peritoneal mesothelioma patients as germline control samples. We filtered out any variants that were also present in these control samples [6]. In this way, we excluded any potential germline variants as well as false positive calls and obtained highly confident variants of

WDPM. Based on the variant allele frequency (VAF), the mutations identified in WDPM were clustered into different groups using the R-package Maftools [33].

4.4. Copy Number Aberration (CNA) Calls

Copy number changes were assessed using Nexus Copy Number Discovery Edition Version 8.0 (BioDiscovery, Inc., El Segundo, CA, USA). Nexus NGS functionality with the FASST2 Segmentation algorithm was used to make copy number calls (a circular binary segmentation/hidden Markov model approach). The significance threshold for segmentation was 5×10^{-6} with a minimum of 3 probes per segment and a maximum probe spacing of 1000 between adjacent probes before breaking a segment. The log ratio thresholds for single copy gain and single copy loss were set at +0.2 and −0.2, respectively. The log ratio thresholds for homozygous gain/loss were set at +0.6 and −1.0, respectively. The tumor BAM files were processed and compared with BAM files from a normal tissue pool as reference control. Reference reads per CN point (window size) was set to 8000. We used the Genomic Identification of Significant Targets in Cancer (GISTIC) [34] algorithm in Nexus to identify significantly amplified or deleted regions across the genome. The amplitude of each aberration is assigned a G-score as well as a frequency of occurrence for multiple samples. The false discovery rate (FDR) q-value for the aberrant regions was set to a threshold of 0.15.

4.5. Mutational Signature Analysis

We used deconstructSigs [13] software, a multiple regression approach to statistically quantify the contribution of mutational signatures for each tumor. The 30 mutational signatures were obtained from the COSMIC mutational signature database [14]. Only non-silent mutations were used to obtain the mutational signatures. In brief, deconstructSigs attempts to recreate the mutational pattern using the trinucleotide mutation context from the input sample that closely resembles each of the 30 mutational signatures from the COSMIC mutational signature database. In this process, each mutational signature is assigned a weight normalized between 0 to 1 indicating its contribution. Only those mutational signatures with a weight more than 0.06 were considered for analysis.

4.6. Pathway Enrichment Analysis

The mutated genes were tested for enrichment against signaling pathways present in the KEGG [15] pathway database obtained from the Molecular Signature Database (MSigDB) v6.0 [35]. A hypergeometric test-based gene set enrichment analysis was used for this purpose (https://github.com/raunakms/GSEAFisher). A cut-off threshold of Benjamini–Hochberg (BH) corrected *p*-value < 0.01 was used to obtain the significantly enriched pathways. Only pathways that are enriched with at least three mutated genes were considered for further analysis.

4.7. Peritoneal Mesothelioma Datasets

We utilized DNA sequencing datasets of two publicly available patient cohorts of peritoneal mesothelioma—VPC cohort [6] and AACR Project GENIE Cohort [16]. We used mutation and copy number profiles from both datasets for comparison with the genomic profiles of WDPM cases. AACR GENIE project data, Version 5.0, were downloaded from https://www.synapse.org/#!Synapse:syn7222066.

5. Conclusions

We have shown that WDPM are genetically distinct from malignant mesotheliomas and in our hands have a characteristic pattern of C > A transversion substitution mutations; *EHD1*, *FBXO10*, *CHD5*, *MAGED1*, *ATM*, and *TP73* missense mutations; as well as enrichment of COSMIC mutation signature 24. Taken in conjunction with the data from Stevers et al., these findings further reinforce the idea that WDPM should not be treated in the same fashion as malignant mesotheliomas.

Supplementary Materials: The following are available online at http://www.mdpi.com/2072-6694/12/6/1568/s1, Figure S1. Distribution of variant allele frequency (VAF) in WDPM, Figure S2. Landscape of copy number alterations in WDPM, Figure S3. Copy number segments (log ratio) of WDPM samples, Figure S4. Mutational signature present in malignant peritoneal mesothelioma obtained from Shrestha et al., Genome Medicine 2019 [6], Figure S5. Comparison of Stevers et al. 2018 [11] with present study, Table S1. QC metric of whole exome sequencing, Table S2. Quality control statistics of WDPM samples, Table S3. Mutation profile of WDPM, Table S4. Copy number profile of WDPM, Table S5. Signaling Pathways dysregulated in WDPM, Table S6. Mutations in gene CDC42 and TRAF7 reported Stevers et al. 2018 [11] and the corresponding sequencing reads detected in WDPM cases in the present study.

Author Contributions: Conceptualization, R.S., N.N., C.C., and A.C.; methodology, R.S., N.N., and S.L.B.; software, R.S., S.V., S.A., and R.B.; validation, N.N., A.H., B.M., F.S., and S.B.; formal analysis, R.S. and N.N.; investigation, R.S., N.N., and A.C.; writing—original draft preparation, R.S., N.N., and A.C.; writing—review and editing, R.S., N.N., C.C., and A.C.; visualization, R.S.; supervision, S.L.B., Y.W., C.C., and A.C.; project administration, N.N., and S.L.B; funding acquisition, Y.W., C.C., and A.C. All authors have read and agreed to the published version of the manuscript.

Funding: This research was funded by BC Cancer Foundation, Mitacs, WorkSafe BC, Canadian Institutes of Health Research (CIHR), and Terry Fox Research Institute, and R.S. and N.N. were funded by Mitacs Accelerate Awards.

Conflicts of Interest: The authors declare no conflicts of interest. The funders had no role in the design of the study; in the collection, analyses, or interpretation of data; in the writing of the manuscript, or in the decision to publish the results.

Appendix A

Here we provide a detailed comparison between Stevers et al. [11] and the present study, which we label WDPM-VPC for convenience.

Stevers et al. [11] used a targeted panel of 479 cancer-related genes (UCSF500 Cancer Panel) for sequencing (Illumina HiSeq 2500 machine), whereas we used Ion AmpliSeq™ (Thermo Fisher Scientific, Waltham, MA, USA) exome sequencing, which covers 18,961 genes (Ion Proton™). The overlap in the genes examined between these two studies is given in Supplementary Figure S5A.

Using a targeted panel provided Stevers et al. [11] an advantage to sequence a small number of genes at a high depth (average depth = 320×, range = 33×–722×), whereas we sequenced a large number of genes at a cost of sequencing depth (average depth = 102×).

Stevers et al. [11] reported 21 mutations covering 10 genes in 10 WDPM cases, whereas we identified 461 mutations covering 297 genes in 5 WDPM cases. There is no overlap of the mutated genes reported in Stevers et al. [11] and our study (Supplementary Figure S5B). In fact, the UCSF500 gene panel used by Stevers et al. [11] covered only 10 mutated genes reported by our study (Supplementary Figure S5C).

Next, we analyzed the sequencing reads covering *CDC42* and *TRAF7* genes in the 5 WDPM cases in this study. Stevers et al. [11] reported two unique mutations in *CDC42* and six unique mutations in *TRAF7*. We focused on the corresponding gene regions in the WDPM cases in our study, as summarized in Supplementary Table S6.

We identified three unique very low confidence mutations in the *TRAF7* gene, one in WDPM-03 and two in WDPM-01 (Supplementary Table S6). In WDPM-03, only 16 reads (out of 111 reads) supported the $TRAF7^{Y621D}$ mutant allele. In WDPM-01, $TRAF7^{N520SD}$ was supported by 1 read (out of 102 reads), and $TRAF7^{G536S}$ was supported by 5 reads (out of 109 reads). Given that the tumor cellularity of the WDPM tissues was estimated to be about 50%, the *TRAF* mutations mentioned above were deemed very low confidence and hence did not pass our mutation filtering criteria. The rest of the *CDC42* and *TRAF7* mutated regions reported by Stevers et al. [11] were identified as wild type in the WDPM cases in this study.

Thus, within the experimental settings of our study, we do not find any high confidence mutations in *TRAF7* or *CDC42*.

References

1. Daya, D.; McCaughey, W.T. Well-differentiated papillary mesothelioma of the peritoneum. A clinicopathologic study of 22 cases. *Cancer* **1990**, *65*, 292–296. [CrossRef]
2. Butnor, K.J.; Sporn, T.A.; Hammar, S.P.; Roggli, V.L. Well-differentiated papillary mesothelioma. *Am. J. Surg. Pathol.* **2001**, *25*, 1304–1309. [CrossRef] [PubMed]
3. Deraco, M.; Nizri, E.; Glehen, O.; Baratti, D.; Tuech, J.-J.; Bereder, J.-M.; Kepenekian, V.; Kusamura, S.; Goere, D. Well differentiated papillary peritoneal mesothelioma treated by cytoreduction and hyperthermic intraperitoneal chemotherapy-the experience of the PSOGI registry. *Eur. J. Surg. Oncol.* **2019**, *45*, 371–375. [CrossRef] [PubMed]
4. Bueno, R.; Stawiski, E.W.; Goldstein, L.D.; Durinck, S.; De Rienzo, A.; Modrusan, Z.; Gnad, F.; Nguyen, T.T.; Jaiswal, B.S.; Chirieac, L.R.; et al. Comprehensive genomic analysis of malignant pleural mesothelioma identifies recurrent mutations, gene fusions and splicing alterations. *Nat. Genet.* **2016**, *48*, 407–416. [CrossRef] [PubMed]
5. Hmeljak, J.; Sanchez-Vega, F.; Hoadley, K.A.; Shih, J.; Stewart, C.; Heiman, D.; Tarpey, P.; Danilova, L.; Drill, E.; Gibb, E.A.; et al. Integrative Molecular Characterization of Malignant Pleural Mesothelioma. *Cancer Discov.* **2018**, *8*, 1548–1565. [CrossRef] [PubMed]
6. Shrestha, R.; Nabavi, N.; Lin, Y.-Y.; Mo, F.; Anderson, S.; Volik, S.; Adomat, H.H.; Lin, D.; Xue, H.; Dong, X.; et al. BAP1 haploinsufficiency predicts a distinct immunogenic class of malignant peritoneal mesothelioma. *Genome Med.* **2019**, *11*, 8. [CrossRef]
7. Yu, W.; Chan-On, W.; Teo, M.; Ong, C.K.; Cutcutache, I.; Allen, G.E.; Wong, B.; Myint, S.S.; Lim, K.H.; Voorhoeve, P.M.; et al. First somatic mutation of E2F1 in a critical DNA binding residue discovered in well-differentiated papillary mesothelioma of the peritoneum. *Genome Biol.* **2011**, *12*, R96. [CrossRef]
8. Nemoto, H.; Tate, G.; Kishimoto, K.; Saito, M.; Shirahata, A.; Umemoto, T.; Matsubara, T.; Goto, T.; Mizukami, H.; Kigawa, G.; et al. Heterozygous loss of NF2 is an early molecular alteration in well-differentiated papillary mesothelioma of the peritoneum. *Cancer Genet.* **2012**, *205*, 594–598. [CrossRef]
9. Ribeiro, C.; Campelos, S.; Moura, C.S.; Machado, J.C.; Justino, A.; Parente, B. Well-differentiated papillary mesothelioma: Clustering in a Portuguese family with a germline BAP1 mutation. *Ann. Oncol.* **2013**, *24*, 2147–2150. [CrossRef]
10. Lee, H.E.; Molina, J.R.; Sukov, W.R.; Roden, A.C.; Yi, E.S. BAP1 loss is unusual in well-differentiated papillary mesothelioma and may predict development of malignant mesothelioma. *Hum. Pathol.* **2018**, *79*, 168–176. [CrossRef]
11. Stevers, M.; Rabban, J.T.; Garg, K.; Van Ziffle, J.; Onodera, C.; Grenert, J.P.; Yeh, I.; Bastian, B.C.; Zaloudek, C.; Solomon, D.A. Well-differentiated papillary mesothelioma of the peritoneum is genetically defined by mutually exclusive mutations in TRAF7 and CDC42. *Mod. Pathol.* **2019**, *32*, 88–99. [CrossRef] [PubMed]
12. Travis, W.D.; Brambilla, E.; Müller-Hermelink, H.K.; Harris, C.C. *Pathology and Genetics of Tumours of the Lung, Pleura, Thymus and Heart*; Travis, W.D., Brambilla, E., Müller-Hermelink, H.K., Harris, C.C., Eds.; WHO Press: Lyon, France, 2004; ISBN 92 832 2418 3.
13. Rosenthal, R.; McGranahan, N.; Herrero, J.; Taylor, B.S.; Swanton, C. DeconstructSigs: Delineating mutational processes in single tumors distinguishes DNA repair deficiencies and patterns of carcinoma evolution. *Genome Biol.* **2016**, *17*, 31. [CrossRef] [PubMed]
14. Alexandrov, L.B.; Jones, P.H.; Wedge, D.C.; Sale, J.E.; Campbell, P.J.; Nik-Zainal, S.; Stratton, M.R. Clock-like mutational processes in human somatic cells. *Nat. Genet.* **2015**, *47*, 1402–1407. [CrossRef] [PubMed]
15. Kanehisa, M.; Sato, Y.; Furumichi, M.; Morishima, K.; Tanabe, M. New approach for understanding genome variations in KEGG. *Nucleic Acids Res.* **2019**, *47*, D590–D595. [CrossRef]
16. AACR Project GENIE Consortium AACR Project GENIE: Powering Precision Medicine through an International Consortium. *Cancer Discov.* **2017**, *7*, 818–831. [CrossRef]
17. Rufini, A.; Agostini, M.; Grespi, F.; Tomasini, R.; Sayan, B.S.; Niklison-Chirou, M.V.; Conforti, F.; Velletri, T.; Mastino, A.; Mak, T.W.; et al. p73 in Cancer. *Genes Cancer* **2011**, *2*, 491–502. [CrossRef]
18. Wang, X.; Gao, X.; Xu, Y. MAGED1: Molecular insights and clinical implications. *Ann. Med.* **2011**, *43*, 347–355. [CrossRef]

19. Laitman, Y.; Boker-Keinan, L.; Berkenstadt, M.; Liphsitz, I.; Weissglas-Volkov, D.; Ries-Levavi, L.; Sarouk, I.; Pras, E.; Friedman, E. The risk for developing cancer in Israeli ATM, BLM, and FANCC heterozygous mutation carriers. *Cancer Genet.* **2016**, *209*, 70–74. [CrossRef]
20. Huang, M.N.; Yu, W.; Teoh, W.W.; Ardin, M.; Jusakul, A.; Ng, A.W.T.; Boot, A.; Abedi-Ardekani, B.; Villar, S.; Myint, S.S.; et al. Genome-scale mutational signatures of aflatoxin in cells, mice, and human tumors. *Genome Res.* **2017**, *27*, 1475–1486. [CrossRef]
21. Bott, M.; Brevet, M.; Taylor, B.S.; Shimizu, S.; Ito, T.; Wang, L.; Creaney, J.; Lake, R.A.; Zakowski, M.F.; Reva, B.; et al. The nuclear deubiquitinase BAP1 is commonly inactivated by somatic mutations and 3p21.1 losses in malignant pleural mesothelioma. *Nat. Genet.* **2011**, *43*, 668–672. [CrossRef]
22. Chirac, P.; Maillet, D.; Leprêtre, F.; Isaac, S.; Glehen, O.; Figeac, M.; Villeneuve, L.; Péron, J.; Gibson, F.; Galateau-Sallé, F.; et al. Genomic copy number alterations in 33 malignant peritoneal mesothelioma analyzed by comparative genomic hybridization array. *Hum. Pathol.* **2016**, *55*, 72–82. [CrossRef] [PubMed]
23. Van Roy, F. Beyond E-cadherin: Roles of other cadherin superfamily members in cancer. *Nat. Rev. Cancer* **2014**, *14*, 121–134. [CrossRef] [PubMed]
24. Grant, B.D.; Donaldson, J.G. Pathways and mechanisms of endocytic recycling. *Nat. Rev. Mol. Cell Biol.* **2009**, *10*, 597–608. [CrossRef] [PubMed]
25. Wang, X.; Yin, H.; Zhang, H.; Hu, J.; Lu, H.; Li, C.; Cao, M.; Yan, S.; Cai, L. NF-κB-driven improvement of EHD1 contributes to erlotinib resistance in EGFR-mutant lung cancers. *Cell Death Dis.* **2018**, *9*, 418. [CrossRef] [PubMed]
26. Chiorazzi, M.; Rui, L.; Yang, Y.; Ceribelli, M.; Tishbi, N.; Maurer, C.W.; Ranuncolo, S.M.; Zhao, H.; Xu, W.; Chan, W.-C.C.; et al. Related F-box proteins control cell death in Caenorhabditis elegans and human lymphoma. *Proc. Natl. Acad. Sci. USA* **2013**, *110*, 3943–3948. [CrossRef]
27. Acuto, O.; Bartolo, V.D.; Michel, F. Tailoring T-cell receptor signals by proximal negative feedback mechanisms. *Nat. Rev. Immunol.* **2008**, *8*, 699–712. [CrossRef]
28. Yoshikawa, Y.; Emi, M.; Hashimoto-Tamaoki, T.; Ohmuraya, M.; Sato, A.; Tsujimura, T.; Hasegawa, S.; Nakano, T.; Nasu, M.; Pastorino, S.; et al. High-density array-CGH with targeted NGS unmask multiple noncontiguous minute deletions on chromosome 3p21 in mesothelioma. *Proc. Natl. Acad. Sci. USA* **2016**, *113*, 13432–13437. [CrossRef]
29. Goode, B.; Joseph, N.M.; Stevers, M.; Van Ziffle, J.; Onodera, C.; Talevich, E.; Grenert, J.P.; Yeh, I.; Bastian, B.C.; Phillips, J.J.; et al. Adenomatoid tumors of the male and female genital tract are defined by TRAF7 mutations that drive aberrant NF-kB pathway activation. *Mod. Pathol.* **2018**, *31*, 660–673. [CrossRef]
30. Sneddon, S.; Dick, I.; Lee, Y.C.G.; Musk, A.W. (Bill.; Patch, A.M.; Pearson, J.V.; Waddell, N.; Allcock, R.J.N.; Holt, R.A.; Robinson, B.W.S.; et al. Malignant cells from pleural fluids in malignant mesothelioma patients reveal novel mutations. *Lung Cancer* **2018**, *119*, 64–70. [CrossRef]
31. Wang, K.; Li, M.; Hakonarson, H. ANNOVAR: Functional annotation of genetic variants from high-throughput sequencing data. *Nucleic Acids Res.* **2010**, *38*, e164. [CrossRef]
32. Thorvaldsdóttir, H.; Robinson, J.T.; Mesirov, J.P. Integrative Genomics Viewer (IGV): High-performance genomics data visualization and exploration. *Brief. Bioinform.* **2013**, *14*, 178–192. [CrossRef] [PubMed]
33. Mayakonda, A.; Lin, D.-C.; Assenov, Y.; Plass, C.; Koeffler, H.P. Maftools: Efficient and comprehensive analysis of somatic variants in cancer. *Genome Res.* **2018**, *28*, 1747–1756. [CrossRef] [PubMed]
34. Mermel, C.H.; Schumacher, S.E.; Hill, B.; Meyerson, M.L.; Beroukhim, R.; Getz, G. GISTIC2.0 facilitates sensitive and confident localization of the targets of focal somatic copy-number alteration in human cancers. *Genome Biol.* **2011**, *12*, R41. [CrossRef] [PubMed]
35. Subramanian, A.; Tamayo, P.; Mootha, V.K.; Mukherjee, S.; Ebert, B.L.; Gillette, M.A.; Paulovich, A.; Pomeroy, S.L.; Golub, T.R.; Lander, E.S.; et al. Gene set enrichment analysis: A knowledge-based approach for interpreting genome-wide expression profiles. *Proc. Natl. Acad. Sci. USA* **2005**, *102*, 15545–15550. [CrossRef]

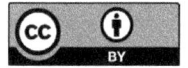

© 2020 by the authors. Licensee MDPI, Basel, Switzerland. This article is an open access article distributed under the terms and conditions of the Creative Commons Attribution (CC BY) license (http://creativecommons.org/licenses/by/4.0/).

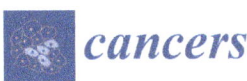

Review
Assessment of the Carcinogenicity of Carbon Nanotubes in the Respiratory System

Marcella Barbarino [1,2,*] and Antonio Giordano [1,2]

1. Department of Medical Biotechnologies, University of Siena, 53100 Siena, Italy; antonio.giordano@unisi.it
2. Sbarro Institute for Cancer Research and Molecular Medicine, Center for Biotechnology, College of Science and Technology, Temple University, Philadelphia, PA 19122, USA
* Correspondence: marcella.barbarino@unisi.it

Simple Summary: Malignant mesothelioma is an aggressive cancer of the membranes covering the lung and chest cavity (pleura) or the abdomen (peritoneum), mainly linked to asbestos exposure. Asbestos is a proven human carcinogen but its use is far from being universally banned and the forecasts on the incidence of mesothelioma over the next several years are far from optimistic. Carbon nanotubes are a promising type of nano-materials used in the field of nanotechnology for a wide range of applications. However, the similarities between asbestos and CNTs have raised many concerns about their danger and are still the subject of intense research. Keeping in mind that the asbestos tragedy could have been prevented, the aim of this study is to review the recent scientific evidence on CNTs carcinogenicity.

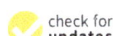

Citation: Barbarino, M.; Giordano, A. Assessment of the Carcinogenicity of Carbon Nanotubes in the Respiratory System. *Cancers* **2021**, *13*, 1318. https://doi.org/10.3390/cancers13061318

Academic Editors: Daniel L. Pouliquen and Joanna Kopecka

Received: 8 February 2021
Accepted: 11 March 2021
Published: 15 March 2021

Publisher's Note: MDPI stays neutral with regard to jurisdictional claims in published maps and institutional affiliations.

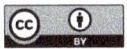

Copyright: © 2021 by the authors. Licensee MDPI, Basel, Switzerland. This article is an open access article distributed under the terms and conditions of the Creative Commons Attribution (CC BY) license (https://creativecommons.org/licenses/by/4.0/).

Abstract: In 2014, the International Agency for Research on Cancer (IARC) classified the first type of carbon nanotubes (CNTs) as possibly carcinogenic to humans, while in the case of other CNTs, it was not possible to ascertain their toxicity due to lack of evidence. Moreover, the physicochemical heterogeneity of this group of substances hamper any generalization on their toxicity. Here, we review the recent relevant toxicity studies produced after the IARC meeting in 2014 on an homogeneous group of CNTs, highlighting the molecular alterations that are relevant for the onset of mesothelioma. Methods: The literature was searched on PubMed and Web of Science for the period 2015–2020, using different combinations keywords. Only data on normal cells of the respiratory system after exposure to fully characterized CNTs for their physico-chemical characteristics were included. Recent studies indicate that CNTs induce a sustained inflammatory response, oxidative stress, fibrosis and histological alterations. The development of mesothelial hyperplasia, mesothelioma, and lungs tumors have been also described in vivo. The data support a strong inflammatory potential of CNTs, similar to that of asbestos, and provide evidence that CNTs exposure led to molecular alterations known to have a key role in mesothelioma onset. These evidences call for an urgent improvement of studies on exposed human populations and adequate systems for monitoring the health of workers exposed to this putative carcinogen.

Keywords: malignant mesothelioma; carcinogenesis; asbestos exposure; carbon nanotubes

1. Introduction

Malignant pleural mesothelioma (MPM) is an aggressive cancer of the pleural membranes covering the lungs and is strongly linked to asbestos exposure. MPM generally manifests in an advanced stage after a latency period of 30–40 years following asbestos exposure.

Asbestos is a commercial term describing a group of specific silicate minerals forming bundles of long and thin mineral fibers that, because of their intrinsic characteristic of durability and resistance to chemicals, heat and electricity, were widely used in the late 1800s with the start of the Industrial Revolution. However, as early as 1898, lung damage was described in industry workers exposed to asbestos dust [1] and in the early 1900s, the first reports documenting fibrosis [2,3] and asbestosis [4] in asbestos-exposed workers were published. Only 30 years later (1935), the first association between asbestos and lung cancer was described [5,6] and it was another 10 years passed before asbestos exposure was correlated with pleural tumors, in the work of Wedler in 1943 [7] and the doctorate thesis of Wyres in 1946 [8]. In 1977 [9] and 1987 [10], the International Agency for Research on Cancer (IARC) concluded that asbestos is a human carcinogen and that the size and shape of the fibers influence the incidence of tumors. In 2006 [11] and 2009 [12] asbestos exposure was also correlated with an increased risk of other cancers, such as laryngeal and ovarian cancer.

Currently, even though asbestos is a known carcinogen, it is not banned in about 70% of the world (Figure 1). As such, more than 100 years after the recognition of asbestos as a carcinogenic agent, the case is not yet closed (http://ibasecretariat.org/chron_ban_list.php, accessed on 2 of October 2020). Indeed, it is important to note that countries that banned asbestos a quarter of a century ago are still contributing to the worldwide toll of more than 100,000 asbestos-related deaths per year [13]. As highlighted by Terracini [13], while banning asbestos is important, that alone does not create an asbestos-free environment. It will take a very long time to ban the use of asbestos worldwide, and it will take an even longer time to end up with an environment that is completely safe from the toxic effects of asbestos. For all of these reasons, the forecasts on the incidence of mesothelioma over the next several years are far from optimistic.

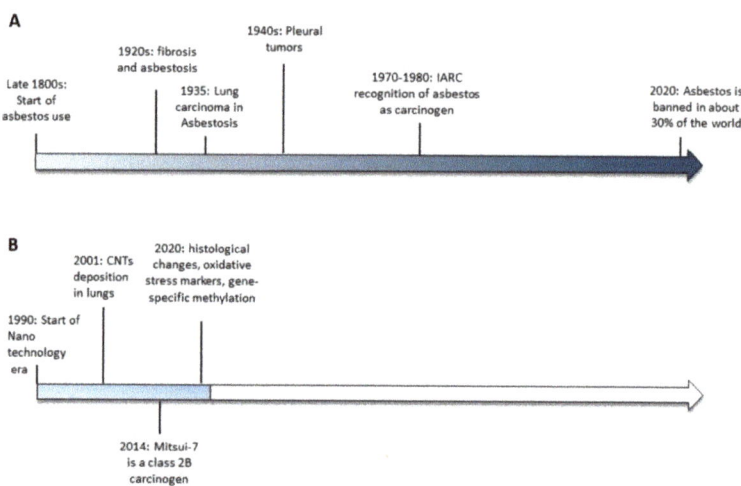

Figure 1. Timelines of the significant events leading to asbestos banning (**A**) and the available evidences of carbon nanotubes-induced toxicity (**B**).

It should also be considered that asbestos present in old constructions still represents a daily hazard to human health. There are numerous cases in which the presence of asbestos has been detected during the renovation or demolition of old buildings. The 9/11 terrorist attack in New York City to the World Trade Center, built in the 1970s, created extra exposure of asbestos, the impact of which will be known only in the coming years [14]. In the dense clouds of dust resulting from this tragic event, relevant quantities of carbon nanotubes (CNTs) produced by the high combustion temperatures were also found, along with other pollutants.

CNTs are nanomaterials composed of graphene sheets consisting of a series of carbon rings rolled into cylindrical fibers with an external measurement between 1 and 100 nm. Their fibrous particulate matter, similar to that of asbestos [15] has raised much concern about their safety for human health. In particular, growing evidence supports the idea that inhaled nanomaterials of >5 μm and with a high aspect ratio (3:1), like rod-like carbon nanotubes resembling asbestos, may cause pleural disease including mesothelioma. In 2014, the International Agency for Research on Cancer (IARC) classified the first type of CNT, the long, rigid, needle-shaped Mitsui-7, as possibly carcinogenic to humans (Group 2B) [16], while in the case of other CNTs, it was not possible to ascertain their toxicity due to lack of evidence. It is also important to consider that, together with the lack of sufficient evidence supporting CNTs' carcinogenicity, their heterogeneity in chemical and physical structures makes it difficult to generalize the available results regarding their possible hazardous effects on human health.

The present review aims to provide an overview of the recent relevant toxicity studies produced after the IARC meeting in 2014 restricting analysis on a homogeneous group of CNTs: standard materials from the Joint Repository Center (JCR) and well-characterized commercial or in-house-made CNTs produced by catalytic carbon vapor deposition (CVD). Moreover, we review the data on mesothelial and lung cells since the respiratory system is considered the main route of exposure to asbestos and CNTs due to exposure during manufacturing process or to accidental exposure. Therefore, we exclude from our analysis CNTs produced for medical purposes, which are functionalized or modified and, consequently, results obtained from cancer or other models resembling a pathological status.

This review is structured following the IARC's parameters [17] for defining an agent as a human carcinogen: induces oxidative stress; induces chronic inflammation; induces epigenetic alterations; is genotoxic; alters DNA repair or causes genomic instability; causes immortalization; alters cell proliferation, cell death, or nutrient supply; acts as an electrophile either directly or after metabolic activation; is immunosuppressive; and modulates receptor-mediated effects.

2. Methods

The literature was searched on PubMed and Web of Science for the period 2015–2020, using different combinations of the following keywords: CNT, carbon nanotubes, SWCNT, MWCNT, single-walled carbon nanotubes, multi-walled carbon nanotubes, genotoxicity, DNA damage, epigenetic, oxidative stress, inflammation, immunosuppression, immortalization, and cytotoxicity. The language was restricted to English. Only data on normal cells of the respiratory system (pleural cells, lung cells, fibroblasts, and lung macrophages) after exposure to reference material (NM-400, NM-401, NM-402, and NM-403), SWCNTs, and MWCNTs synthetized by the CVD method and fully characterized for their physicochemical characteristics (length, diameter, agglomeration, and surface area) were included in the review.

3. An Overview of Carbon Nanotubes

Thirty years ago, the IBM researcher Don Eigler moved the first individual atom using a scanning tunnelling microscope. Despite that progress, Eigler has said he is not sure about when or even if his ideas for computing will bear fruit. It was Eigler who started the era of nanotechnology, the science that is able to create and manipulate materials at the nanoscale. Nano-sized materials, defined as having at least one dimension between 1 and 100 nm, include many types of materials, different in their physicochemical properties, and used in a great variety of applications [18]. Given the immense potential of nanotechnology, the global nanotechnology market has been estimated to reach 126.8 billion U.S. dollars by 2027 [19].

The big world of nanotechnology comprises various types of nanomaterial, all differing in their chemo-physical properties. CNTs are the most promising type of nanomaterials in the industry today. They are defined as nanotubes composed of carbon, consisting of one or more cylindrical graphene layers and are classified, on the basis of the number of graphene layers, as single- or multi-walled carbon nanotubes (respectively, SWCNTs and MWCNTs). Larger MWCNTs can contain hundreds of concentric layers.

As CNTs come to be used in a wider range of products, human exposure can take place through various routes, such as local (in medical applications, such as drug delivery, cancer therapy, medical diagnostics and imaging), environmental (industrial waste or accidentally released by the final product), or pulmonary (during occupational handling or accidental exposure). The work environment is actually thought to be the principal source of human exposure to CNTs during the phases of their production, as seen for example in laboratory handling and packaging of the final product, and in this case the most plausible route of exposure to manufactured nanomaterials remains pulmonary inhalation. The inhalation of particles during their synthesis is a significant concern in the growing nanotechnology field.

Despite different governmental organizations monitoring CNT exposure in workers, there are still no standards for defining the risk levels for CNT exposure. The method of monitoring CNTs in work environments involves measurement of Elemental Carbon (EC). The National Institute for Occupational Safety and Health (NIOSH, USA), based on quantification limits and not on studies in exposed workers, recommends an exposure level of 1 $\mu g/m^3$ elemental carbon (EC) [20]. This limit, which might not be representative of a safe exposure limit, has often been found to be much lower than those measured in various industries, ranging from 2.6 $\mu g/m^3$ to 45 $\mu g/m^3$ depending on the particular workplace analyzed (handling facilities, production areas, construction sites, offices, etc.) [21,22].

The pulmonary toxicity of fibrous materials such as asbestos has been demonstrated to result from deposition (thin fibers deposit in the lungs more efficiently than thick fibers) and tissue persistence ("biopersistence" is directly related to fiber length and inversely related to dissolution and fragmentation rates). CNTs have been demonstrated to deposit in human lungs and other organs. Lung biopsies of people exposed to the dense clouds of dust during the tragic events of 9/11 in New York City have shown the presence of CNTs produced by high combustion temperatures. The first adverse health effects diagnosed were pulmonary fibrosis, and bronchiolocentric parenchymal and granulomatous diseases [14].

Carbon nanotubes, although a sub-group in the immense word of nanomaterials, comprise various substances that differ from each other in length, size, diameter, impurities, and method used for synthesis and dispersion of the final product, among other characteristics. All of these characteristics impact their biological effects, and it is now recognized that generalized conclusions about CNTs should not be drawn by extrapolating data that are available on similar, but not identical, compounds. For these reasons, we focused our analysis on the results obtained using reference CNTs (NM-400, NM-401, NM-402, and NM-403) (https://publications.jrc.ec.europa.eu/repository/bitstream/JRC91205/mwcnt-online.pdf accessed on 15 October 2020), with fully characterized commercial and in-house CNTs produced using the CVD method, which is currently one of the principal techniques used for CNT synthesis. Data regarding CNTs that had been chemically modified to alter their properties and data obtained in cancer cells were excluded from our analysis; this model is suitable for other purposes, such as drug-delivery studies, which are not the focus of this review.

We reported data relevant to assessing the potential adverse respiratory effects following the IARC's protocol for defining an agent as a human carcinogen [17]. For each group of characteristics, we analyzed data obtained from in vitro models of pleura, lung macrophages, and airway cells, from in vivo studies examining effects on the respiratory system, and from biological fluids collected from exposed workers, highlighting those results that could be relevant for mesothelioma onset.

4. Carbon Nanotubes and the Hallmarks of Cancer

4.1. Oxidative Stress, Chronic Inflammation

The oxidative potential of a particle is the intrinsic property to form reactive oxygen species (ROS). Generation of ROS and free radicals has been demonstrated to be involved in the molecular mechanisms leading to mesothelioma as well as other asbestos-related diseases. In cell-free systems, asbestos can generate free radicals and induce release of inflammatory mediators such as cytokines, growth factors, reactive oxygen and nitrogen species in neutrophils, and alveolar macrophages for incomplete/frustrated phagocytosis of fibers. At cellular level, in asbestos exposed cells, inflammation, oxidative stress, and carcinogenesis has been associated with the alteration of the iron metabolism due to iron accumulation on fibers [23]. Similarly, iron impurities in CNTs have been demonstrated to participate in increased inflammation and oxidative stress in CNTs exposed mesothelial cells, in a "dose-dependent" manner [24–26].

At the molecular level, ROS may cause different injuries, such as gene mutations and structural alterations to the DNA, leading to deregulation in cell proliferation and apoptosis. Oxidative DNA damage is often characteristic of chronic inflammation, one of the main mechanisms underlying mesothelial transformation.

During the inflammation process, the cross-talk between inflammatory cells and damaged alveolar cells has been recognized to contribute to mesothelioma pathogenesis as well as other respiratory disease like lung fibrosis and lung cancer [27,28]. Lung fibrosis manifests with excessive deposition of collagen fibers in the extracellular matrix (ECM) and remodelling of the alveolar parenchyma, leading to a progressive loss of lung function. It includes a first acute inflammation phase where inflammatory cells infiltrate the tissue, secrete proinflammatory mediators (cytokines TNFα, IL1α, IL1β, IL6, chemokine CCL2, and fibrogenic growth factors TGF-β1 and PDGF-A), and collagen is deposited in the ECM. After this early response, granulomatous fibrotic foci deposits around the lesions are detectable. Activation of fibroblasts and formation of myofibroblasts (fibroblast-to-myofibroblast transition) and epithelial-to-mesenchymal transition (EMT) of alveolar type II cells are drivers of this process [29,30]. Lung fibrosis is one of the first documented injuries to lung described in asbestos-exposed workers 2,3 and the inflammatory process leading to fibrosis has been well characterized using long, needle-like Mitsui-7 MWCNT exposure in vivo [31,32]. The role of oxidative stress in CNTs-induced lung fibrosis was demonstrated through the use of the antioxidant N-Acetyl Cysteine, which interfered with NLRP3 inflammasome activation and generation of pulmonary fibrosis in mice [33].

In both asbestos- and MWCNT-exposed workers, markers of fibrosis, profibrotic inflammatory mediators and immune markers [21,34,35], as well as dysregulation in mRNAs and target genes linked to the activation of key pathways involved in several disease outcomes (e.g., cancer, respiratory and cardiovascular disease, and fibrosis) [36] have been found. Markers of oxidative stress and mitochondrial dysfunction have also been found in exposed workers [37].

The similarity between MWCNTs and asbestos due to their inflammatory and oxidative potential has been recently demonstrated in vivo with long MWCNTs (Nanostructured & Amorphous Materials, Houston, TX, USA; University of Manchester, Manchester, UK) and long fiber amosite asbestos instilled into the pleural cavity of mice. Exposure to long fibers but not to short fibers resulted in the development and progression of inflammatory lesions along the pleura and in the increase of markers of oxidative stress and genotoxicity. All exposed animals displayed pleural lesions (mesothelial hyperplasia and fibrosis), and chronic inflammation and, in 10–25% of animals exposed to long MWCNTs, the lesions progressed to pleural mesothelioma [38]. Different results were obtained with long NM-401 and Mitsui-7 MWCNTs. In this study, toxicity and inflammation were observed only in mice exposed to short MWCNTs (NM-400, NM-402, NM-403, and MWCNTs from CheapTubes, Brattleboro, VT, USA) [39].

However, other studies in vivo have demonstrated that both long and short industrial MWCNTs induced granulomatous changes in the lungs, development of pulmonary fibrosis, and inflammation accompanied by increase in vimentin, TGF-beta, IL-1b, IL-18, and cardiac fibrotic deposition [40–44]. Commercial short MWCNTs (tangled) (Graphistrength© C100; Arkema, France) showed prolonged TNF-α release in BAL of exposed rats associated with increased collagen staining [45].

Similar results were obtained with SWCNTs (Nikkiso Co., Ltd., Tokyo, Japan), showing strong persistent pulmonary inflammation [46]. The same group also demonstrated that the shorter the length of SWCNTs is, the stronger the toxicity. Short SWCNTs (Nikkiso Co., LTD., Tokyo, Japan) with a length of 2.8 µm induced a weaker inflammatory response and pulmonary toxicity than those with a length of 0.4 µm [42].

It has also been demonstrated that chronic exposure to commercial short SWCNTs (CNI, Houston, TX, USA) induces tumor growth (subcutaneously injected) and metastasis to liver and lung through activation of EMT [47]. Cancer development (Bronchiolo-alveolar adenoma and carcinoma) was also found in 18% of mice exposed to a single intratracheal instillation of short SWCNT (Nikkiso Co., Ltd., Tokyo, Japan) [46].

For a long time, length has been considered a predictor of CNTs' adverse biological effects. However, even if this is true in some cases, many in vitro studies support the concept that the length of CNTs might not be a unique determinant of the biological response. Recently, shape and diameter have been correlated with accessibility to the macrophage interior subsequently affecting their degradation ability and, therefore, ROS production. Since alveolar clearance contributes to inhalation toxicity, the understanding of parameters predicting CNT toxicity is of crucial importance. This question has been challenged in many studies. Rigid, needle-shaped, long Mitsui-7 MWCNTs (diameter > 50 µm), which are poorly uptaken into phagosomes of alveolar macrophages, have been demonstrated to not induce ROS release. On the contrary, curved, straight, long and thin MWCNTs from different manufacturers, with diameters <20 µm which localize in vacuole-like compartments, have been demonstrated to generate intracellular ROS. For all the analyzed MWCNTs, increased levels of pro-inflammatory cytokines (IL-1α, IL-1β, MIP-1α, INF-γ, IL-18, MCP-1, and TNF-α) were found, implying that the inflammatory response might not be strictly related to the phagocytic ability of the macrophages [48]. ROS production from lung cells could be responsible for the inflammatory response of macrophages in the absence of phagocytic activity. While the rigid, straight, "needle-like" NM-401 MWCNTs, which are similar to Mitsui-7, are poorly uptaken by macrophages and do not cause an increase in NO production, lung fibroblast cells (V79) were demonstrated to be able to uptake NM-401, with 80% of fibers localized in endosomes, generating a consistent production of intracellular ROS [49]. Short NM-400 and NM-402 MWCNTs with a diameter <20 µm, are instead efficiently degraded by macrophages and induce an increase in NO accompanied by acute inflammation [50].

Markers of inflammation and oxidative stress were also studied in epithelial cells. Induction of oxidative stress have been described in lung epithelial cells exposed to NM-402 and NM-403 with values comparable to or higher than that of Mitsui-7 [51] while in BEAS-2B cells, a significant reduction in the levels of mRNA expression of pro-inflammatory cytokines IL-1β, IL-6 and IL-8 and an increase in the antioxidant HO-1 gene were found in long-term exposure (three weeks) to NM-403 [52]. However the authors associated these contradictory findings to the metal contaminants present in NM-403.

As a driver of lung fibrosis, the activation of the EMT program in lung epithelial cells by fibrous materials has been documented in four different studies in airway epithelial cells. Exposure to chrysotile asbestos, SWCNTs, Mitsui-7, and Mitsui-7-derived MWCNTs with the length reduced to 1.12 µm, at sub-toxic concentrations led to an increase in mesenchymal markers (α-smooth muscle actin, vimentin, metalloproteinases, and fibronectin), a decrease in epithelial markers (E-cadherin and β-catenin), and activation of the TGF-β–mediated signaling pathway [40,53,54].

Fibrogenic potential was also demonstrated with an in-house lung microtissue array device in airway epithelial cells exposed to non-toxic concentrations of short MWCNTs (CheapTubes.com accessed on 15th of October 2020) together with a significant increase in expression of the fibrogenic marker miR-21. These effects were not found in cells exposed to long MWCNTs [55].

All of the results reported above indicate that physico-chemical characteristics such as length and diameter could partially explain the different biological responses but, alone, might not be predictive of inflammatory response. Many variables such as the presence of CNTs of different lengths in the same preparation together with their heterogeneity in experimental settings contribute to the difficulty in predicting their inflammatory and oxidative effects. Particularly in in vivo studies (Tables 1 and 2), different route of exposure and different endpoints analyzed have been used for the evaluation of pathological parameters. Even though studies comparing the inhalation and instillation of MWCNT showed that both methods induced pulmonary inflammation [56], inhalation is more powerful in inducing inflammation [57] and should be the preferred method for studies on accidental exposure during the manufacturing process since it recreates real situations better.

Table 1. Cancer development, histological changes, and inflammatory response observed in in vivo experiments with MWCNTs.

CNTs	Length (µm); Diameter (nm)	Cancer	Histological Changes	Inflammation	Exposure Route	Ref
Mitsui-7	L: 3–5.7 D: 49–100		x	x	intratracheal instillation	[58]
Mitsui-7	L: 3–5.7 D: 49–100	bronchiolo-alveolar adenoma and adenocarcinoma	x	x	whole body inhalation	[32]
Mitsui-7	L: 5.7 ± 0.49; D: 74 (29–173)				intratracheal instillation	[39]
Short MWCNTs	L: 1.12 ± 0.05 D: 67 ± 2		x		pharyngeal aspiration	[40]
Industrial MWCNTs	L: 2–15; D: 8–15		x	x	pharyngeal aspiration	[41]
Long MWCNTs (Nikkiso similar to Mitsui-7)	L: 1–10; D: 1–20	pleural malignant mesothelioma and lung tumors			intratracheally instilled	[59]
Long MWCNTs (University of Manchester, UK)	L: 85% > 15 D: 165 + 4.7	mesothelial hyperplasia; mesothelioma	x	x	instilled into the pleural cavity	[38]
MWCNTs (Nanostructured & Amorphous Materials, USA)	L: <15; D: 125				instilled into the pleural cavity	[38]
NM-400	L: 0.85 ± 0.10; D: 11 ± 3			x	intratracheally instilled	[39]
NM-401	L: 4.0 ± 0.37; D: 67 ± 24				intratracheal instillation	[39]
NM-402	L: 1.4 ± 0.19; D: 11 ± 3		x	x	intratracheal instillation	[58]
NM-402	L: 1.4 ± 0.19; D: 11 ± 3			x	intratracheal instillation	[39]
NM-403	L: 0.4 ± 0.03; D: 12 ± 7			x	intratracheal instillation	[39]
MWCNTs Nanotechcenter Ltd.	L: 2–15; D: 8–15		x		pharyngeal aspiration	[44]
MWCNTs(Cheaptube)	L: 0.52 (±0.59); D: 20.56 (±6.94)			x	intratracheal instillation	[60]
MWCNTs(Cheaptube)	L: 0.77 (±0.35) D: 26.73 (±6.88)			x	intratracheal instillation	[60]
MWCNTs(Cheaptube)	L: 0.72 (±1.2) D: 17.22 (±5.77)			x	intratracheal instillation	[60]

Abbreviations: "x": studies that have reported a relationship between these characteristics and exposure to the material.

Table 2. Cancer development, histological changes, and inflammatory response observed in in vivo experiments with SWCNTs.

CNTs	Length (μm); Diameter (nm)	Cancer	Inflammation	Exposure Route	Ref
SWCNTs Graphistrength© C100	L: 1.06 mean; D: 11.9 mean		x	nose-only inhalation exposure	[45]
Short SWCNTs (Nikkiso & Co., LTD)	L: 0.55 ± 0.36; D: 1.4 ± 0.7	bronchiolo-alveolar adenoma and adenocarcinoma (18% of mice)		intratracheal instillation	[46]

Abbreviations: "x": studies that have reported a relationship between these characteristics and exposure to the material.

4.2. Epigenetic Alterations

It is well known that epigenetic changes in DNA and RNA play an important role in the regulation of gene expression by changing DNA accessibility to the cellular machinery, and switching on/off gene expression. As indicators of environmental insults, the study of epigenetics is a useful tool to understand disease-related mechanisms as well as serve as an indicator of disease risk. Among the epigenetic modifications affecting the genome, DNA methylation, the process by which a methyl group is added to carbon five in the cytosine pyridine ring forming 5-methylcytosine (5 mC) in DNA, is the most studied for the assessment of the potential hazard of fiber-like materials. Mesothelioma, as well other asbestos-related diseases, has been related to epigenetic changes, and the methylation changes of blood markers have been proposed as diagnostic and prognostic markers for mesothelioma [61–63]. In recent epidemiological studies in asbestos-exposed populations, a decrease in the levels of blood global 5-methylcytosine (5 mC) has been described in both healthy exposed workers and in those with benign asbestos-related disorders, confirming that global methylation could be a useful marker of asbestos exposure but, unfortunately, cannot be used as indicator of asbestos-related disease [64,65].

In MWCNT-exposed workers, changes in the methylation of specific genes mainly involved in DNA damage repair, cell cycle regulation, chromatin remodelling, and transcriptional repression (DNMT1, ATM, SKI and HDAC4 promoter) was described in a cross-sectional study [22]. Unlike with asbestos, no significant difference was found in total DNA methylation.

Hypermethylation of specific genes was also found in mice exposed to long MWCNTs (Nanostructured & Amorphous Materials, Houston, TX, USA; University of Manchester, UK) and long amosite fibers, which caused chronic inflammatory lesions or mesothelioma. Of particular importance is the epigenetic silencing of the CDKN2A locus, a well-known driver mutation in asbestos-induced mesothelioma, observed in mice exposed to both long MWCNTs and long amosite fibers [38].

Many in vitro studies have confirmed the methylation of specific genes. In 16HBE airway epithelial cells, in-house synthesized short MWCNTs and SWCNTs induced differentially methylated and expressed genes in cellular pathways related to DNA damage repair and cell cycle, with more pronounced effects in MWCNTs. No alteration of global DNA methylation was found [66]. An increased alteration on CpG sites after short -and long-term exposure has also been described for both benchmark short NM-400 MWCNTs and asbestos (CDKN1A and ATM among others) [66–70].

Together with specific gene methylation, other studies have also found a strong genome-wide DNA hypomethylation in airway epithelial cells (BEAS-2B and 16HBE) exposed to commercial short MWCNTs (CheapTubes, Brattleboro, VT, USA) and NM-400 and NM-401 [67–69,71].

It is important to note that most of the hypomethylated genes observed after two weeks of exposure to NM-401 became hypermethylated after four weeks of exposure [67], thus highlighting how time and particle type can trigger different and apparently discordant results.

In conclusion, many studies have demonstrated that change in methylation can be used as a marker of exposure to CNTs but heterogeneity of this class of nanomaterial does not allow for making generalizations. More studies are needed to expand our knowledge about epigenetic regulation of specific genes after CNT exposure. Given our current knowledge of asbestos, we know what genes are strictly linked to mesothelioma onset, and the results regarding epigenetic changes reported above suggest that CNTs could act via a similar mechanism.

4.3. Genotoxicity, Alteration in DNA Repair, and Genome Instability

Genotoxic effects can result from primary or secondary mechanisms. The first implies a direct interaction with the genetic material, the latter the oxidation of DNA by reactive oxygen/nitrogen species (ROS/RNS) generated during substance-induced inflammation. Both mechanisms could be involved in the genotoxic response elicited by MWCNTs.

Although CNTs are considered by IARC to be usually non-reactive and, for Mitsui-7 genotoxicity, have been demonstrated to act via secondary mechanisms, it cannot be excluded that defects in their structure occurring during the synthesis or functionalization could increase their reactivity [72,73]. Very recently, for long and short SWCNTs, the nucleus has been hypothesized to be the primary target site with DNA damage likely due to mechanical penetration [74].

Many studies, such as those described above, support the hypothesis that CNT genotoxicity could result from secondary mechanisms triggered by a strong inflammatory response and ROS release.

A genotoxicity study recently conducted in workers exposed to CNTs (unspecified manufacturer), revealed an 18.3% increase in telomere length and a 35.2% increase in mitochondrial DNA copy number from peripheral blood [75].

Asbestos-induced mesothelioma has been linked to polyploidization and aneuploidization, and MWCNTs seem to have similar adverse effects [76]. Chromosomal aberrations (polyploidy), and mitotic and chromosomal disruptions have been demonstrated for commercial MWCNTs (Hodogaya Chemical, Tokyo, Japan; Tokyo Chemical Industry, Tokyo, Japan; Showa Denko K.K, Tokyo, Japan), including MWCNT-7, with different length and shape (including straight fibrous, not straight fibrous (curved), and tangled MWCNTs) in Chinese hamster lung cell lines with straight fibrous being the more potent inducers of polyploidy. None of the seven MWCNTs analyzed caused structural chromosomal aberrations [76]. In the same model, NM-401 was found to be genotoxic, increasing HPRT mutant frequency [49].

In vivo experiments with long MWCNTs (Mitsui & Co. Ltd., Tokyo, Japan) showed a significant increase in DNA damage (comet assay) in the cells of lungs with straight MWCNTs but not with tangled MWCNTs. Moreover, straight MWCNTs caused an increase in DNA strand breaks in BAL cells collected after inhalation but not after pharyngeal aspiration [77]. DNA strand breaks were also observed after intratracheal instillation of straight NM-401 MWCNTs in the transgenic Muta^{TM}Mouse model. Moreover, both straight NM-401 and Mitsui-7 MWCNTs increased p53 expression predominantly in the area of fibrotic lesions (more pronounced for NM-401), and induced chronic inflammation and changes in the expression of genes linked to hallmarks of cancer. There was no evidence of a LacZ mutation [58].

Short commercial MWCNTs comprised of straight and tangled MWCNTs (Cheap-Tube, Brattleboro, VT, USA), were demonstrated to induce a dose- and time- dependent neutrophil influx in BAL and to cause DNA damage in the lungs of mice exposed by intratracheal instillation, with large MWCNTs diameter associated with increased genotoxicity (Analysis at 1, 28 and 92 days after exposure). All MWCNTs analyzed induced similar histological changes [60].

Another study using commercial short tangled MWCNTs (Graphistrength© C100; Arkema, France) did not disclose genotoxicity in lung cells or a microscopic change in the pleura. As the authors hypothesized, these effects could in part be ascribed to the formation of agglomerates that are poorly uptaken by cells [45]. However, the lack of a positive control in the experimental setting could represent a weakness in the study.

Similar results have been seen in in vitro studies. Long-term exposure of primary human airway epithelial cells (SAECs) to commercial short SWCNTs (CNI, Houston, TX, USA), long Mitsui-7 MWCNTs (Mitsui & Co., Ltd., Tokyo, Japan) and Crocidolite, and mesothelial MeT-5A cells exposed to commercial long MWCNTs (Sigma-Aldrich, St Louis, MO, USA) have demonstrated a substantial increase in DNA damage in γH2A.X foci and p53 dysregulation [54,78].

Chromosome damage and chromosome mis-segregation have also been described in airway epithelial cells chronically exposed to sub-toxic doses of short NM-400 and NM-403 MWCNTs [52], while no primary DNA damage or oxidized DNA bases have been observed in short-term experiments with NM-400, NM-401, and NM-403 [50,79,80]

Contrasting results for Micronuclei (MN) formation assay were found in NM-401-exposed cells, according to the different methods used. With the cytokinesis-blocked micronucleus assay (CBMN), authors did not observe significant increases in the frequency of micronucleated binucleated cells or induction of DNA damage by the comet assay [81]. When analyzed by flow cytometry, NM-401 at 20 and 50 µg/mL were able to increase the MN formation [79]. No genotoxic effects with the CBMN assay were detected also for NM-400, NM-402, and NM-403 [81].

Bacterial reverse mutation tests and chromosomal aberration tests, according to the Organization for Economic Co-operation and Development (OECD) Guidelines for Testing of Chemicals, were conducted on straight, long, thin MWCNTs, revealing no structural or numerical chromosomal aberrations below a concentration of 50 µg/mL following short-term exposure, both with and without metabolic activation [48]. However, this test is not suitable for studies with nanomaterials since they are not able to enter the bacterial cell wall, thus leading to the production of false-negative results.

Even though a definitive conclusion on the genotoxicity of CNTs is still impossible to draw, many results have indicated the presence of damaged DNA after exposure to CNTs. It is clear that for genotoxicity assessment, many variables, in addition to those mentioned previously, could interfere with the results. In particular, due to different responses in terms of DNA repair of different cell types, in vitro and in vivo models used represent a key factor together with the dose and time chosen for the analysis.

4.4. Immortalization, Altered Cell Proliferation, Cell Death, or Nutrient Supply

MWCNT-7 carcinogenicity has been demonstrated by different studies in mice in which the whole body has been exposed [82,83]. Nikkiso MWCNTs, which is similar to Mitsui-7, have also been demonstrated to induce pleural malignant mesothelioma and lung tumors in intratracheal instillation studies [59].

The transformation potential in vitro has been documented in different studies. After long-term exposure to commercial long MWCNTs (Sigma-Aldrich, St Louis, MO, USA), mesothelial MeT-5A cells showed features resembling a malignant transformation process and specifically an increase in cell proliferation and invasion capacity, morphology change, and DNA damage [78].

Similarly, after long-term exposure to short SWCNTs (CNI, Houston, TX, USA), Mitsui-7 (Mitsui & Co., Ltd., Tokyo, Japan) and Crocidolite asbestos, primary human small airway epithelial cells (SAECs) exhibited neoplastic and cancer stem cell-like properties, such as anchorage-independent colony formation, spheroid formation, anoikis resistance, and expression of cancer stem cell markers [54].

Altered cell proliferation was also described. Cell growth inhibition with benchmark NM-403 MWCNTs [52], and NM-400 and NM401 MWCNTs have been demonstrated in bronchial epithelial cells in long-term experiments [84] and, for NM401 and NM403, in short-term experiments without significant cytotoxicity [51].

Similar results were obtained with commercial short SWCNTs and MWCNTs (SES Research, USA; Heji, Hong Kong, China), in lung fibroblasts and in epithelial cells with short rod-like SWCNTs and straight MWCNTs showing higher toxicity [77,85,86].

Toxicity studies in macrophages mostly supported the hypothesis that rigidity and high diameters are as key factors underlying toxicity. Indeed, exposure to rigid, needle-shaped Mitsui-7 MWCNTs, and Nikkiso and NM-401 MWCNTs all induce cytotoxicity in macrophage cells while NM-400 and NM-402 did not [48,50]. However, the opposite has also been described in rat alveolar macrophages acutely exposed to highly bent, low-diameter NM-403 MWCNTs, which induced significant toxicity [87].

4.5. Immunosuppression, Modulation of Receptor-Mediated Effects, and Electrophilicity

Few data are available regarding the characteristics grouped below.

Available studies have demonstrated that CNTs can interact and activate the complement system, a key part of the immune system, and induce an early and sustained immunosuppressive response [44,88–90]. Moreover, it has been shown that SWCNT exposure in mice increases susceptibility to respiratory viral infections [91].

The ability of CNTs to act as an electrophile and then interact with cellular macromolecules, such as DNA, RNA, lipids, and proteins, has not been thoroughly investigated. It has been suggested that SWCNTs block K+ channel subunits by "plugging" the channel by virtue of the small diameter [92] and interact with TLR4 by hydrophobic interactions [93].

All of these studies suggest that the immunosuppression and modulation of the immune responses elicited by CNTs need further investigation. Indeed, an increased susceptibility to pathogens as well as immunosuppression could be a new and potentially significant mechanism of toxicity in humans.

5. Discussion

Nanotechnology is changing our world and is believed that it will improve our lives in the near future. CNTs are indeed remarkably valuable given their applications, ranging from drug delivery to electronics. Since we are at the beginning of the nanotechnology era, elucidation of the putative carcinogenicity of CNTs is also at the beginning. Intensive research is underway to understand their safety for human health and a remarkable data pool is being produced using different types of CNTs, models, methods, duration of exposure, amount of CNTs, and time points analyzed. While such heterogeneity is yielding many important results, it is, on the other hand, complicating the evaluation of the danger of CNTs. This situation well reflects the heterogeneity of this class of compounds as well as the different applications intended for their use, thereby making it particularly challenging to identify common features predicting their toxicity. It is not yet understood which aspects of carbon nanomaterials, e.g., surface areas, mass concentrations, lengths or a combination of these features or other factors, influence their toxicity. In addition, establishing criteria for preparation and dispersion, concentrations, models and methods to use, and also including reference materials, will undoubtedly play a crucial role in determining the reliability, reproducibility and comparability of data. In recent years, great improvements have been made in this direction and most non-human-based studies have reported a detailed description of the physiochemical characteristics of CNTs, the method used for their synthesis, the dispersion protocol and the percentage of the impurities present. However, despite these efforts, the lack of a complete characterization of CNT exposure in workers remains a crucial consideration. The type of CNTs varies both across companies and within them over time. Furthermore, in epidemiological studies, there is a high variability among instruments used for sampling and analysis of exposure, and there is still a low number of participants. All of these weaknesses, together with the lack of specific legislation addressing manufacturing processes for nanomaterials, make a direct comparison between studies difficult.

However, since the last IARC evaluation of CNT carcinogenicity, conducted in 2014, when enough evidence was available only for Mitsui-7, nine new studies have been performed on humans exposed to CNTs in the workplace, documenting markers of fibrosis, profibrotic inflammatory mediators, and immune markers [21,34,35,94]; epigenetic changes in genes related to DNA repair, cell cycle and repression of transcription [22]; deregulation in pathways and signaling networks linked to pulmonary and carcinogenic outcomes [36]; increase of oxidative markers in the exhaled breath condensates [37], increase in mtDNA copy number [75]; and development of respiratory allergies [95]. Recent findings in vivo have clearly indicated that CNTs induce a sustained inflammatory response and oxidative stress, and fibrosis and histological alterations have been documented in animals exposed to MWCNTs (Table 1) and SWCNTs (Table 2) by inhalation, aspiration, and tracheal instillation [32,44,58]. The development of mesothelial hyperplasia, mesothelioma, and lung tumors have been also described with SWCNTs and long fibers of both asbestos and MWCNTs [32,38,46,59] (Figure 2).

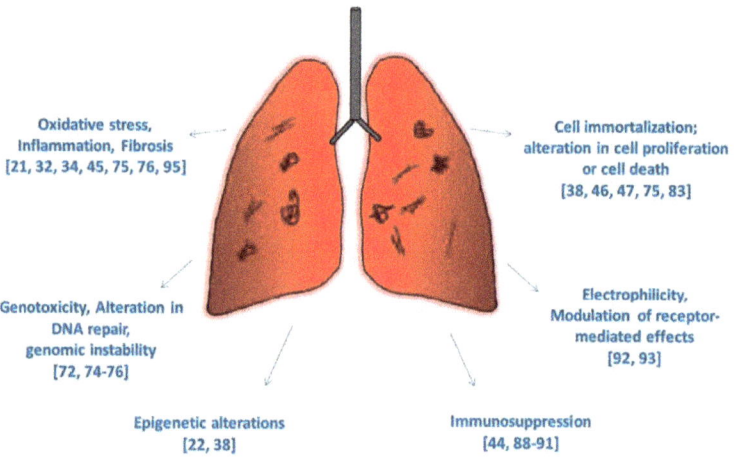

Figure 2. Hallmarks of cancer due to CNTs exposure in vivo and on human-based studies.

Less evidence is available for assessing cytotoxicity and genotoxicity and we are still far from reaching a consensus. It is nevertheless important to note that there are, however, new findings indicating DNA damage and gene-specific methylations after CNT exposure. In particular, the epigenetic silencing of the *CDKN2A* locus, a well-known driver mutation in asbestos-induced mesothelioma, has been documented in mice exposed to commercial long MWCNTs together with the loss of p16 and p19 protein expression [38].

In light of these recent studies analyzed, we agree with the need to evoke a global improvement of studies on exposed human populations as well as with the non-applicability of disproportionate precautionary measures of exposure control. However, considering the absence of any global agreement about the hazards of CNTs, we cannot take the risk creating another man-made tragedy like the case of asbestos where a century passed before its carcinogenicity was recognized, with many scientific papers defending its use to influence policy decisions on its hazards [13]. Moreover, years after its banning, we still have not achieved an asbestos-free environment and indeed the consequences thereof we still cannot predict.

Cancer is a multi-step process and, especially in the case of mesothelioma, it could takes years before it manifests itself. Fortunately, we are at the beginning of the CNT era and while we do not yet have data on the carcinogenicity of CNTs, we do have the opportunity to establish safe management of these materials. While we cannot precisely assess which modifications in the genome or in the epigenome will lead to mesothelioma onset, we do know that the long latency of malignant mesothelioma is sustained by decades of chronic inflammation in an aberrant microenvironment rich in ROS and the resulting oxidative DNA damage. We must carefully reflect on the data supporting the strong inflammatory potential of CNTs, similar to that of asbestos, as well as the data correlating CNT exposure with molecular alterations known to have a key role in mesothelioma onset

6. Conclusions

The heterogeneity of this class of substances is undoubtedly the main obstacle to reaching a consensus on their toxicity and more studies are needed to gain detailed knowledge on the effects of exposure to CNTs. We believe that future studies on CNTs toxicity must be assessed case-by-case and, on this premise, a new evaluation of the danger of CNTs for human health is urgently needed. We strongly support the need to create a repository of biological samples from CNT-exposed workers in order to monitor biologically relevant changes over time and to encourage research collaboration within different areas of expertise. In any case, an adequate system for monitoring the health of workers exposed to this putative carcinogen remains the basis on which to build future research.

Author Contributions: Conceptualization, writing—review and editing, M.B.; project administration, review, A.G. Both authors have read and agreed to the published version of the manuscript.

Funding: This work was supported by funding from the TOMA institute, Italy. The APC was funded by University of Siena, Dept. of Medical Biotechnology, Siena, Italy.

Conflicts of Interest: The authors declare no conflict of interest.

References

1. National Research Council. *Asbestiform Fibers: Nonoccupational Health Risks*; National Academies Press: Washington, DC, USA, 1984.
2. Committee on Compensation for Industrial Diseases. *Report of the Departmental Committee on Compensation for Industrial Diseases*; Wyman & Sons: London, UK, 1907.
3. Cooke, W.E. Fibrosis of the lungs due to the inhalation of asbestos dust. *BMJ* **1924**, *2*, 140–142, 147. [CrossRef]
4. Cooke, W.E. Pulmonary asbestosis. *BMJ* **1927**, *2*, 1024–1025. [CrossRef] [PubMed]
5. Gloyne, S.R. Two cases of squamous carcinoma of the lung occurring in asbestosis. *Tubercle* **1935**, *17*, 5–10. [CrossRef]
6. Lynch, K.M.; Smith, W.A. Pulmonary Asbestosis III: Carcinoma of Lung in Asbesto-Silicosis. *Am. J. Cancer* **1935**, *24*, 56–64. [CrossRef]
7. Wedler, H.-W. Asbestose und Lungenkrebs. *DMW Dtsch. Med. Wochenschr.* **1943**, *69*, 575–576. [CrossRef]
8. Wyers, H. That Legislative Measures Have Proved Generally Effective in the Control of Asbestosis. Ph.D. Thesis, University of Glasgow, Glasgow, UK, 1946.
9. International Agency Research on Cancer. *Monographs on the Evaluation of Carcinogenic Risk of Chemicals to Human*; IARC: Lyon, France, 1977.
10. Institute of Medicine (US). *Committee on Asbestos: Selected Health Effects*; National Academies Press: Washington, DC, USA, 1987.
11. Committee I of M (US). *Asbestos: Selected Cancers*; National Academies Press: Washington, DC, USA, 2006.
12. Straif, K.; Benbrahim-Tallaa, L.; Baan, R.; Grosse, Y.; Secretan, B.; El Ghissassi, F.; Bouvard, V.; Guha, N.; Freeman, C.; Galichet, L.; et al. A review of human carcinogens—Part C: Metals, arsenic, dusts, and fibres. *Lancet Oncol.* **2009**, *10*, 453–454. [CrossRef]
13. Terracini, B. Contextualising the policy decision to ban asbestos. *Lancet Planet. Health* **2019**, *3*, e331–e332. [CrossRef]
14. Wu, M.; Gordon, R.E.; Herbert, R.; Padilla, M.; Moline, J.; Mendelson, D.; Litle, V.; Travis, W.D.; Gil, J. Case Report: Lung disease in world trade center responders exposed to dust and smoke: Carbon nanotubes found in the lungs of world trade center patients and dust samples. *Environ. Health Perspect.* **2010**, *118*, 499–504. [CrossRef]
15. Donaldson, K.; Poland, C.A.; Murphy, F.A.; MacFarlane, M.; Chernova, T.; Schinwald, A. Pulmonary toxicity of carbon nanotubes and asbestos—Similarities and differences. *Adv. Drug Deliv. Rev.* **2013**, *65*, 2078–2086. [CrossRef] [PubMed]
16. Grosse, Y.; Loomis, D.; Guyton, K.Z.; Lauby-Secretan, B.; El Ghissassi, F.; Bouvard, V.; Benbrahim-Tallaa, L.; Guha, N.; Scoccianti, C.; Mattock, H.; et al. Carcinogenicity of fluoro-edenite, silicon carbide fibres and whiskers, and carbon nanotubes. *Lancet Oncol.* **2014**, *15*, 1427–1428. [CrossRef]
17. International Agency Research on Cancer. *Some Nanomaterials and Some Fibres*; IARC: Lyon, France, 2017; p. 111.
18. De Menezes, B.R.C.; Rodrigues, K.F.; Fonseca, B.C.D.S.; Ribas, R.G.; Montanheiro, T.L.D.A.; Thim, G.P. Recent advances in the use of carbon nanotubes as smart biomaterials. *J. Mater. Chem. B* **2019**, *7*, 1343–1360. [CrossRef]
19. Globe Newswire. *Global Nanotechnology Industry*; Globe Newswire: New York, NY, USA, 2020.
20. *Centre for Disease Control and Prevention: CURRENT Intelligence Bulletin 65: Occupational Exposure to Carbon Nanotubes and Nanofibers*; CDC: Atlanta, GA, USA, 2013.

21. Fatkhutdinova, L.M.; Khaliullin, T.O.; Vasil'Yeva, O.L.; Zalyalov, R.R.; Mustafin, I.G.; Kisin, E.R.; Birch, M.E.; Yanamala, N.; Shvedova, A.A. Fibrosis biomarkers in workers exposed to MWCNTs. *Toxicol. Appl. Pharmacol.* **2016**, *299*, 125–131. [CrossRef]
22. Ghosh, M.; Öner, D.; Poels, K.; Tabish, A.M.; Vlaanderen, J.; Pronk, A.; Kuijpers, E.; Lan, Q.; Vermeulen, R.; Bekaert, B.; et al. Changes in DNA methylation induced by multi-walled carbon nanotube exposure in the workplace. *Nanotoxicology* **2017**, *11*, 1195–1210. [CrossRef] [PubMed]
23. Toyokuni, S. Iron overload as a major targetable pathogenesis of asbestos-induced mesothelial carcinogenesis. *Redox Rep.* **2013**, *19*, 1–7. [CrossRef] [PubMed]
24. Cammisuli, F.; Giordani, S.; Gianoncelli, A.; Rizzardi, C.; Radillo, L.; Zweyer, M.; Da Ros, T.; Salomé, M.; Melato, M.; Pascolo, L. Iron-related toxicity of single-walled carbon nanotubes and crocidolite fibres in human mesothelial cells investigated by Synchrotron XRF microscopy. *Sci. Rep.* **2018**, *8*, 706. [CrossRef] [PubMed]
25. Muller, J.; Decordier, I.; Hoet, P.H.; Lombaert, N.; Thomassen, L.; Huaux, F.X.; Lison, D.; Kirsch-Volders, M. Clastogenic and aneugenic effects of multi-wall carbon nanotubes in epithelial cells. *Carcinogenesis* **2008**, *29*, 427–433. [CrossRef] [PubMed]
26. Kagan, V.; Tyurina, Y.; Tyurin, V.; Konduru, N.; Potapovich, A.; Osipov, A.; Kisin, E.; Schwegler-Berry, D.; Mercer, R.; Castranova, V.; et al. Direct and indirect effects of single walled carbon nanotubes on RAW 264.7 macrophages: Role of iron. *Toxicol. Lett.* **2006**, *165*, 88–100. [CrossRef]
27. Digifico, E.; Belgiovine, C.; Mantovani, A.; Allavena, P. Microenvironment and immunology of the human pleural malignant mesothelioma BT—Mesothelioma: From research to clinical practice. In *Mesothelioma*; Ceresoli, G.L., Bombardieri, E., D'Incalci, M., Eds.; Springer International Publishing: Geneva, Switzerland, 2019; pp. 69–84.
28. Mittal, V.; El Rayes, T.; Narula, N.; McGraw, T.E.; Altorki, N.K.; Barcellos-Hoff, M.H. The Microenvironment of lung cancer and therapeutic implications. *Adv. Exp. Med. Biol.* **2016**, *890*, 75–110. [CrossRef] [PubMed]
29. Dong, J.; Ma, Q. Myofibroblasts and lung fibrosis induced by carbon nanotube exposure. *Part. Fibre Toxicol.* **2016**, *13*, 1–22. [CrossRef]
30. Wang, P.; Wang, Y.; Nie, X.; Braïni, C.; Bai, R.; Chen, C. Multiwall Carbon nanotubes directly promote fibroblast-myofibroblast and epithelial-mesenchymal transitions through the activation of the TGF-β/smad signaling pathway. *Small* **2014**, *11*, 446–455. [CrossRef] [PubMed]
31. Dong, J.; Porter, D.W.; Batteli, L.A.; Wolfarth, M.G.; Richardson, D.L.; Ma, Q. Pathologic and molecular profiling of rapid-onset fibrosis and inflammation induced by multi-walled carbon nanotubes. *Arch. Toxicol.* **2014**, *89*, 621–633. [CrossRef]
32. Snyder-Talkington, B.N.; Dong, C.; Sargent, L.M.; Porter, D.W.; Staska, L.M.; Hubbs, A.F.; Raese, R.; McKinney, W.; Chen, B.T.; Battelli, L.; et al. mRNAs and miRNAs in whole blood associated with lung hyperplasia, fibrosis, and bronchiolo-alveolar adenoma and adenocarcinoma after multi-walled carbon nanotube inhalation exposure in mice. *J. Appl. Toxicol.* **2016**, *36*, 161–174. [CrossRef]
33. Sun, B.; Wang, X.; Ji, Z.; Wang, M.; Liao, Y.-P.; Chang, C.H.; Li, R.; Zhang, H.; Nel, A.E.; Xiang, W. NADPH oxidase-dependent nlrp3 inflammasome activation and its important role in lung fibrosis by multiwalled carbon nanotubes. *Small* **2015**, *11*, 2087–2097. [CrossRef]
34. Vlaanderen, J.; Pronk, A.; Rothman, N.; Hildesheim, A.; Silverman, D.; Hosgood, H.D.; Spaan, S.; Kuijpers, E.; Godderis, L.; Hoet, P.; et al. A cross-sectional study of changes in markers of immunological effects and lung health due to exposure to multi-walled carbon nanotubes. *Nanotoxicology* **2017**, *11*, 395–404. [CrossRef] [PubMed]
35. Beard, J.D.; Erdely, A.; Dahm, M.M.; de Perio, M.A.; Birch, M.E.; Evans, D.E.; Fernback, J.E.; Eye, T.; Kodali, V.; Mercer, R.R.; et al. Carbon nanotube and nanofiber exposure and sputum and blood biomarkers of early effect among U.S. workers. *Environ. Int.* **2018**, *116*, 214–228. [CrossRef]
36. Shvedova, A.A.; Yanamala, N.; Kisin, E.R.; Khailullin, T.O.; Birch, M.E.; Fatkhutdinova, L.M. Integrated Analysis of Dysregulated ncRNA and mRNA Expression Profiles in Humans Exposed to Carbon Nanotubes. *PLoS ONE* **2016**, *11*, e0150628. [CrossRef]
37. Lee, J.S.; Choi, Y.C.; Shin, J.H.; Lee, J.H.; Lee, Y.; Park, S.Y.; Baek, J.E.; Park, J.D.; Ahn, K.; Yu, I.J. Health surveillance study of workers who manufacture multi-walled carbon nanotubes. *Nanotoxicology* **2014**, *9*, 802–811. [CrossRef]
38. Chernova, T.; Murphy, F.A.; Galavotti, S.; Sun, X.-M.; Powley, I.R.; Grosso, S.; Schinwald, A.; Zacarias-Cabeza, J.; Dudek, K.M.; Dinsdale, D.; et al. Long-Fiber carbon nanotubes replicate asbestos-induced mesothelioma with disruption of the tumor suppressor gene Cdkn2a (Ink4a/Arf). *Curr. Biol.* **2017**, *27*, 3302–3314.e6. [CrossRef]
39. Knudsen, K.B.; Berthing, T.; Jackson, P.; Poulsen, S.S.; Mortensen, A.; Jacobsen, N.R.; Skaug, V.; Szarek, J.; Hougaard, K.S.; Wolff, H.; et al. Physicochemical predictors of Multi-Walled Carbon Nanotube-induced pulmonary histopathology and toxicity one year after pulmonary deposition of 11 different Multi-Walled Carbon Nanotubes in mice. *Basic Clin. Pharmacol. Toxicol.* **2018**, *124*, 211–227. [CrossRef]
40. Polimeni, M.; Gulino, G.R.; Gazzano, E.; Kopecka, J.; Marucco, A.; Fenoglio, I.; Cesano, F.; Campagnolo, L.; Magrini, A.; Pietroiusti, A.; et al. Multi-walled carbon nanotubes directly induce epithelial-mesenchymal transition in human bronchial epithelial cells via the TGF-β-mediated Akt/GSK-3β/SNAIL-1 signalling pathway. *Part. Fibre Toxicol.* **2015**, *13*, 1–19. [CrossRef]
41. Khaliullin, T.O.; Shvedova, A.A.; Kisin, E.R.; Zalyalov, R.R.; Fatkhutdinova, L.M. Evaluation of fibrogenic potential of industrial multi-walled carbon nanotubes in acute aspiration experiment. *Bull. Exp. Biol. Med.* **2015**, *158*, 684–687. [CrossRef]
42. Ema, M.; Takehara, H.; Naya, M.; Kataura, H.; Fujita, K.; Honda, K. Length effects of single-walled carbon nanotubes on pulmonary toxicity after intratracheal instillation in rats. *J. Toxicol. Sci.* **2017**, *42*, 367–378. [CrossRef]

43. Davis, G.; Lucero, J.; Fellers, C.; McDonald, J.D.; Lund, A.K. The effects of subacute inhaled multi-walled carbon nanotube exposure on signaling pathways associated with cholesterol transport and inflammatory markers in the vasculature of wild-type mice. *Toxicol. Lett.* **2018**, *296*, 48–62. [CrossRef] [PubMed]
44. Khaliullin, T.O.; Yanamala, N.; Newman, M.S.; Kisin, E.R.; Fatkhutdinova, L.M.; Shvedova, A.A. Comparative analysis of lung and blood transcriptomes in mice exposed to multi-walled carbon nanotubes. *Toxicol. Appl. Pharmacol.* **2020**, *390*, 114898. [CrossRef]
45. Pothmann, D.; Simar, S.; Schuler, D.; Dony, E.; Gaering, S.; Le Net, J.-L.; Okazaki, Y.; Chabagno, J.M.; Bessibes, C.; Beausoleil, J.; et al. Lung inflammation and lack of genotoxicity in the comet and micronucleus assays of industrial multiwalled carbon nanotubes Graphistrength© C100 after a 90-day nose-only inhalation exposure of rats. *Part. Fibre Toxicol.* **2015**, *12*, 21. [CrossRef] [PubMed]
46. Honda, K.; Naya, M.; Takehara, H.; Kataura, H.; Fujita, K.; Ema, M. A 104-week pulmonary toxicity assessment of long and short single-wall carbon nanotubes after a single intratracheal instillation in rats. *Inhal. Toxicol.* **2017**, *29*, 471–482. [CrossRef]
47. Wang, P.; Voronkova, M.; Luanpitpong, S.; He, X.; Riedel, H.; Dinu, C.Z.; Wang, L.; Rojanasakul, Y. Induction of Slug by Chronic Exposure to Single-Walled Carbon Nanotubes Promotes Tumor Formation and Metastasis. *Chem. Res. Toxicol.* **2017**, *30*, 1396–1405. [CrossRef] [PubMed]
48. Fujita, K.; Obara, S.; Maru, J.; Endoh, S. Cytotoxicity profiles of multi-walled carbon nanotubes with different physico-chemical properties. *Toxicol. Mech. Methods* **2020**, *30*, 477–489. [CrossRef]
49. Rubio, L.; El Yamani, N.; Kazimirova, A.; Dusinska, M.; Marcos, R. Multi-walled carbon nanotubes (NM401) induce ROS-mediated HPRT mutations in Chinese hamster lung fibroblasts. *Environ. Res.* **2016**, *146*, 185–190. [CrossRef] [PubMed]
50. Di Cristo, L.; Bianchi, M.G.; Chiu, M.; Taurino, G.; Donato, F.; Garzaro, G.; Bussolati, O. Chiu comparative in vitro cytotoxicity of realistic doses of benchmark multi-walled carbon nanotubes towards macrophages and airway epithelial cells. *Nanomaterials* **2019**, *9*, 982. [CrossRef] [PubMed]
51. Jackson, P.; Kling, K.; Jensen, K.A.; Clausen, P.A.; Madsen, A.M.; Wallin, H.; Vogel, U. Characterization of genotoxic response to 15 multiwalled carbon nanotubes with variable physicochemical properties including surface functionalizations in the FE1-Muta (TM) mouse lung epithelial cell line. *Environ. Mol. Mutagen.* **2014**, *56*, 183–203. [CrossRef] [PubMed]
52. Vales, G.; Rubio, L.; Marcos, R. Genotoxic and cell-transformation effects of multi-walled carbon nanotubes (MWCNT) following in vitro sub-chronic exposures. *J. Hazard. Mater.* **2016**, *306*, 193–202. [CrossRef]
53. Gulino, G.R.; Polimeni, M.; Prato, M.; Gazzano, E.; Kopecka, J.; Colombatto, S.; Ghigo, D.; Aldieri, E. Effects of chrysotile exposure in human bronchial epithelial cells: Insights into the pathogenic mechanisms of asbestos-related diseases. *Environ. Health Perspect.* **2016**, *124*, 776–784. [CrossRef] [PubMed]
54. Kiratipaiboon, C.; Stueckle, T.A.; Ghosh, R.; Rojanasakul, L.W.; Chen, Y.C.; Dinu, C.Z.; Rojanasakul, Y. Acquisition of cancer stem cell-like properties in human small airway epithelial cells after a long-term exposure to carbon nanomaterials. *Environ. Sci. Nano* **2019**, *6*, 2152–2170. [CrossRef] [PubMed]
55. Chen, Z.; Wang, Q.; Asmani, M.; Li, Y.; Liu, C.; Li, C.; Lippmann, J.M.; Wu, Y.; Zhao, R. Lung microtissue array to screen the fibrogenic potential of carbon nanotubes. *Sci. Rep.* **2016**, *6*, 31304. [CrossRef]
56. Gaté, L.; Knudsen, K.B.; Seidel, C.; Berthing, T.; Chézeau, L.; Jacobsen, N.R.; Valentino, S.; Wallin, H.; Bau, S.; Wolff, H.; et al. Pulmonary toxicity of two different multi-walled carbon nanotubes in rat: Comparison between intratracheal instillation and inhalation exposure. *Toxicol. Appl. Pharmacol.* **2019**, *375*, 17–31. [CrossRef]
57. Shvedova, A.A.; Kisin, E.; Murray, A.R.; Johnson, V.J.; Gorelik, O.; Arepalli, S.; Hubbs, A.F.; Mercer, R.R.; Keohavong, P.; Sussman, N.; et al. Inhalation vs. aspiration of single-walled carbon nanotubes in C57BL/6 mice: Inflammation, fibrosis, oxidative stress, and mutagenesis. *Am. J. Physiol. Cell. Mol. Physiol.* **2008**, *295*, L552–L565. [CrossRef]
58. Rahman, L.; Jacobsen, N.R.; Aziz, S.A.; Wu, D.; Williams, A.; Yauk, C.L.; White, P.; Wallin, H.; Vogel, U.; Halappanavar, S. Multi-walled carbon nanotube-induced genotoxic, inflammatory and pro-fibrotic responses in mice: Investigating the mechanisms of pulmonary carcinogenesis. *Mutat. Res. Toxicol. Environ. Mutagen.* **2017**, *823*, 28–44. [CrossRef]
59. Suzui, M.; Futakuchi, M.; Fukamachi, K.; Numano, T.; Abdelgied, M.; Takahashi, S.; Ohnishi, M.; Omori, T.; Tsuruoka, S.; Hirose, A.; et al. Multiwalled carbon nanotubes intratracheally instilled into the rat lung induce development of pleural malignant mesothelioma and lung tumors. *Cancer Sci.* **2016**, *107*, 924–935. [CrossRef]
60. Poulsen, S.S.; Jackson, P.; Kling, K.; Knudsen, K.B.; Skaug, V.; Kyjovska, Z.O.; Thomsen, B.L.; Clausen, P.A.; Atluri, R.; Berthing, T.; et al. Multi-walled carbon nanotube physicochemical properties predict pulmonary inflammation and genotoxicity. *Nanotoxicology* **2016**, *10*, 1263–1275. [CrossRef]
61. Sinn, K.; Mosleh, B.; Hoda, M.A. Malignant pleural mesothelioma: Recent developments. *Curr. Opin. Oncol.* **2021**, *33*, 80–86. [CrossRef]
62. Rozitis, E.; Johnson, B.; Cheng, Y.Y.; Lee, K. The Use of Immunohistochemistry, Fluorescence in situ hybridization, and emerging epigenetic markers in the diagnosis of malignant pleural mesothelioma (MPM): A review. *Front. Oncol.* **2020**, *10*, 1742. [CrossRef]
63. Ferrari, L.; Carugno, M.; Mensi, C.; Pesatori, A.C. Circulating Epigenetic biomarkers in malignant pleural mesothelioma: State of the art and critical evaluation. *Front. Oncol.* **2020**, *10*, 445. [CrossRef]
64. Yu, M.; Lou, J.; Xia, H.; Zhang, M.; Zhang, Y.; Chen, J.; Zhang, X.; Ying, S.; Zhu, L.; Liu, L.; et al. Global DNA hypomethylation has no impact on lung function or serum inflammatory and fibrosis cytokines in asbestos-exposed population. *Int. Arch. Occup. Environ. Health* **2017**, *90*, 265–274. [CrossRef]
65. Yu, M.; Zhang, Y.; Jiang, Z.; Chen, J.; Liu, L.; Lou, J.; Zhang, X. Mesothelin (MSLN) methylation and soluble mesothelin-related protein levels in a Chinese asbestos-exposed population. *Environ. Health Prev. Med.* **2015**, *20*, 369–378. [CrossRef]

66. Öner, D.; Ghosh, M.; Bové, H.; Moisse, M.; Boeckx, B.; Duca, R.C.; Poels, K.; Luyts, K.; Putzeys, E.; Van Landuydt, K.; et al. Differences in MWCNT- and SWCNT-induced DNA methylation alterations in association with the nuclear deposition. *Part. Fibre Toxicol.* **2018**, *15*, 11. [CrossRef]
67. Sierra, M.I.; Rubio, L.; Bayón, G.F.; Cobo, I.; Menendez, P.; Morales, P.; Mangas, C.; Urdinguio, R.G.; Lopez, V.; Valdes, A.; et al. DNA methylation changes in human lung epithelia cells exposed to multi-walled carbon nanotubes. *Nanotoxicology* **2017**, *11*, 857–870. [CrossRef]
68. Öner, D.; Ghosh, M.; Coorens, R.; Bové, H.; Moisse, M.; Lambrechts, D.; Ameloot, M.; Godderis, L.; Hoet, P.H. Induction and recovery of CpG site specific methylation changes in human bronchial cells after long-term exposure to carbon nanotubes and asbestos. *Environ. Int.* **2020**, *137*, 105530. [CrossRef] [PubMed]
69. Emerce, E.; Ghosh, M.; Öner, D.; Duca, R.C.; Vanoirbeek, J.; Bekaert, B.; Hoet, P.H.M.; Godderis, L. Carbon nanotube- and asbestos-induced DNA and RNA methylation changes in bronchial epithelial cells. *Chem. Res. Toxicol.* **2019**, *32*, 850–860. [CrossRef] [PubMed]
70. Ghosh, M.; Öner, D.; Duca, R.C.; Bekaert, B.; Vanoirbeek, J.A.; Godderis, L.; Hoet, P.H. Single-walled and multi-walled carbon nanotubes induce sequence-specific epigenetic alterations in 16 HBE cells. *Oncotarget* **2018**, *9*, 20351–20365. [CrossRef]
71. Chatterjee, N.; Yang, J.; Yoon, D.; Kim, S.; Joo, S.-W.; Choi, J. Differential crosstalk between global DNA methylation and metabolomics associated with cell type specific stress response by pristine and functionalized MWCNT. *Biomaterials* **2017**, *115*, 167–180. [CrossRef]
72. Bernholc, J.; Roland, C.; Yakobson, B.I. Nanotubes. *Curr. Opin. Solid State Mater. Sci.* **1997**, *2*, 706–715. [CrossRef]
73. Fukushima, S.; Kasai, T.; Umeda, Y.; Ohnishi, M.; Sasaki, T.; Matsumoto, M. Carcinogenicity of multi-walled carbon nanotubes: Challenging issue on hazard assessment. *J. Occup. Health* **2018**, *60*, 10–30. [CrossRef]
74. Jiang, T.; Amadei, C.A.; Gou, N.; Lin, Y.; Lan, J.; Vecitis, C.D.; Gu, A.Z. Toxicity of single-walled carbon nanotubes (SWCNTs): Effect of lengths, functional groups and electronic structures revealed by a quantitative toxicogenomics assay. *Environ. Sci. Nano* **2020**, *7*, 1348–1364. [CrossRef]
75. Ghosh, M.; Janssen, L.; Martens, D.S.; Öner, D.; Vlaanderen, J.; Pronk, A.; Kuijpers, E.; Vermeulen, R.; Nawrot, T.S.; Godderis, L.; et al. Increased telomere length and mt DNA copy number induced by multi-walled carbon nanotube exposure in the workplace. *J. Hazard. Mater.* **2020**, *394*, 122569. [CrossRef]
76. Sasaki, T.; Asakura, M.; Ishioka, C.; Kasai, T.; Katagiri, T.; Fukushima, S. In vitro chromosomal aberrations induced by various shapes of multi-walled carbon nanotubes (MWCNTs). *J. Occup. Health* **2016**, *58*, 622–631. [CrossRef] [PubMed]
77. Catalán, J.; Siivola, K.M.; Nymark, P.; Lindberg, H.; Suhonen, S.; Järventaus, H.; Koivisto, A.J.; Moreno, C.; Vanhala, E.; Wolff, H.; et al. In vitroandin vivogenotoxic effects of straight versus tangled multi-walled carbon nanotubes. *Nanotoxicology* **2016**, *10*, 794–806. [CrossRef] [PubMed]
78. Ju, L.; Wu, W.; Yu, M.; Lou, J.; Wu, H.; Yin, X.; Jia, Z.; Xiao, Y.; Zhu, L.; Yang, J. Different cellular response of human mesothelial cell met-5a to short-term and long-term multiwalled carbon nanotubes exposure. *BioMed Res. Int.* **2017**, *2017*, 1–10. [CrossRef] [PubMed]
79. García-Rodríguez, A.; Kazantseva, L.; Vila, L.; Rubio, L.; Velázquez, A.; Ramírez, M.J.; Marcos, R.; Hernández, A. Micronuclei detection by flow cytometry as a high-throughput approach for the genotoxicity testing of nanomaterials. *Nanomaterials* **2019**, *9*, 1677. [CrossRef] [PubMed]
80. García-Rodríguez, A.; Rubio, L.; Vila, L.; Xamena, N.; Velázquez, A.; Marcos, R.; Hernández, A. The comet assay as a tool to detect the genotoxic potential of nanomaterials. *Nanomaterials* **2019**, *9*, 1385. [CrossRef]
81. Louro, H.; Pinhão, M.; Santos, J.; Tavares, A.M.; Vital, N.; Silva, M.J. Evaluation of the cytotoxic and genotoxic effects of benchmark multi-walled carbon nanotubes in relation to their physicochemical properties. *Toxicol. Lett.* **2016**, *262*, 123–134. [CrossRef] [PubMed]
82. Dymacek, J.M.; Snyder-Talkington, B.N.; Raese, R.; Dong, C.; Singh, S.; Porter, D.W.; Ducatman, B.; Wolfarth, M.G.; Andrew, M.E.; Battelli, L.; et al. Similar and differential canonical pathways and biological processes associated with multiwalled carbon nanotube and asbestos-induced pulmonary fibrosis: A 1-year postexposure study. *Int. J. Toxicol.* **2018**, *37*, 276–284. [CrossRef]
83. Kasai, T.; Umeda, Y.; Ohnishi, M.; Mine, T.; Kondo, H.; Takeuchi, T.; Matsumoto, M.; Fukushima, S. Lung carcinogenicity of inhaled multi-walled carbon nanotube in rats. *Part. Fibre Toxicol.* **2015**, *13*, 1–19. [CrossRef]
84. Phuyal, S.; Kasem, M.; Rubio, L.; Karlsson, H.L.; Marcos, R.; Skaug, V.; Zienolddiny, S. Effects on human bronchial epithelial cells following low-dose chronic exposure to nanomaterials: A 6-month transformation study. *Toxicol. Vitr.* **2017**, *44*, 230–240. [CrossRef]
85. Ndika, J.D.T.; Sund, J.; Alenius, H.; Puustinen, A. Elucidating differential nano-bio interactions of multi-walled andsingle-walled carbon nanotubes using subcellular proteomics. *Nanotoxicology* **2018**, *12*, 554–570. [CrossRef] [PubMed]
86. Ursini, C.L.; Maiello, R.; Ciervo, A.; Fresegna, A.M.; Buresti, G.; Superti, F.; Marchetti, M.; Iavicoli, S.; Cavallo, D. Evaluation of uptake, cytotoxicity and inflammatory effects in respiratory cells exposed to pristine and -OH and -COOH functionalized multi-wall carbon nanotubes. *J. Appl. Toxicol.* **2015**, *36*, 394–403. [CrossRef]
87. Nahle, S.; Cassidy, H.; Leroux, M.; Mercier, R.; Ghanbaja, J.; Doumandji, Z.; Matallanas, D.; Rihn, B.H.; Joubert, O.; Ferrari, L. Genes expression profiling of alveolar macrophages exposed to non-functionalized, anionic and cationic multi-walled carbon nanotubes shows three different mechanisms of toxicity. *J. Nanobiotechnol.* **2020**, *18*, 1–18. [CrossRef]

88. Schubauer-Berigan, M.K.; Dahm, M.M.; Toennis, C.A.; Sammons, D.L.; Eye, T.; Kodali, V.; Zeidler-Erdely, P.C.; Erdely, A. Association of occupational exposures with ex vivo functional immune response in workers handling carbon nanotubes and nanofibers. *Nanotoxicology* **2020**, *14*, 404–419. [CrossRef]
89. Pondman, K.M.; Pednekar, L.; Paudyal, B.; Tsolaki, A.G.; Kouser, L.; Khan, H.A.; Shamji, M.H.; Haken, B.T.; Stenbeck, G.; Sim, R.B.; et al. Innate immune humoral factors, C1q and factor H, with differential pattern recognition properties, alter macrophage response to carbon nanotubes. *Nanomed. Nanotechnol. Biol. Med.* **2015**, *11*, 2109–2118. [CrossRef]
90. Huaux, F.; De Bousies, V.D.; Parent, M.-A.; Orsi, M.; Uwambayinema, F.; Devosse, R.; Ibouraadaten, S.; Yakoub, Y.; Panin, N.; Palmai-Pallag, M.; et al. Mesothelioma response to carbon nanotubes is associated with an early and selective accumulation of immunosuppressive monocytic cells. *Part. Fibre Toxicol.* **2015**, *13*, 1–10. [CrossRef]
91. Chen, H.; Zheng, X.; Nicholas, J.; Humes, S.T.; Loeb, J.C.; Robinson, S.E.; Bisesi, J.H., Jr.; Das, D.; Saleh, N.B.; Castleman, W.L.; et al. Single-walled carbon nanotubes modulate pulmonary immune responses and increase pandemic influenza a virus titers in mice. *Virol. J.* **2017**, *14*, 1–15. [CrossRef] [PubMed]
92. Park, K.H.; Chhowalla, M.; Iqbal, Z.; Sesti, F. Single-walled Carbon Nanotubes Are a New Class of Ion Channel Blockers. *J. Biol. Chem.* **2003**, *278*, 50212–50216. [CrossRef] [PubMed]
93. Mukherjee, S.P.; Bondarenko, O.; Kohonen, P.; Andón, F.T.; Brzicová, T.; Gessner, I.; Mathur, S.; Bottini, M.; Calligari, P.; Stella, L.; et al. Macrophage sensing of single-walled carbon nanotubes via Toll-like receptors. *Sci. Rep.* **2018**, *8*, 1–17. [CrossRef]
94. Kuijpers, E.; Pronk, A.; Kleemann, R.; Vlaanderen, J.; Lan, Q.; Rothman, N.; Silverman, D.; Hoet, P.; Godderis, L.; Vermeulen, R. Cardiovascular effects among workers exposed to multiwalled carbon nanotubes. *Occup. Environ. Med.* **2018**, *75*, 351–358. [CrossRef] [PubMed]
95. Schubauer-Berigan, M.K.; Dahm, M.M.; Erdely, A.; Beard, J.D.; Birch, M.E.; Evans, D.E.; Fernback, J.E.; Mercer, R.R.; Bertke, S.J.; Eye, T.; et al. Association of pulmonary, cardiovascular, and hematologic metrics with carbon nanotube and nanofiber exposure among U.S. workers: A cross-sectional study. *Part. Fibre Toxicol.* **2018**, *15*, 1–14. [CrossRef] [PubMed]

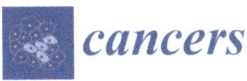

Review

Ancillary Diagnostic Investigations in Malignant Pleural Mesothelioma

Alex Dipper *, Nick Maskell and Anna Bibby

Academic Respiratory Unit, University of Bristol, Bristol BS105NB, UK; Nick.Maskell@bristol.ac.uk (N.M.); anna.bibby@bristol.ac.uk (A.B.)
* Correspondence: alex.dipper@bristol.ac.uk

Simple Summary: Malignant pleural mesothelioma (MPM) is a cancer affecting the covering of the lung (the pleura). This commonly causes a build-up of fluid around the lung, called a pleural effusion. Draining the pleural effusion can improve breathlessness and tests can be performed on the fluid. However, for most patients with MPM, a sample of tissue from the pleura, called a biopsy, is required in addition to make the diagnosis. Sometimes, due to medical conditions, frailty or personal preference, patients may not be able to have a biopsy. This review article discusses additional tests used in this situation to help doctors make a diagnosis of MPM. These techniques include tests on pleural fluid using "immunocytochemistry" methods, biomarkers and scans. Although, without a biopsy, no test in isolation can diagnose MPM, combining information from different types of tests and reviewing results among a specialist team can enable a consensus diagnosis.

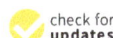

Citation: Dipper, A.; Maskell, N.; Bibby, A. Ancillary Diagnostic Investigations in Malignant Pleural Mesothelioma. *Cancers* **2021**, *13*, 3291. https://doi.org/10.3390/cancers13133291

Academic Editors: Daniel L. Pouliquen and Joanna Kopecka

Received: 10 June 2021
Accepted: 18 June 2021
Published: 30 June 2021

Publisher's Note: MDPI stays neutral with regard to jurisdictional claims in published maps and institutional affiliations.

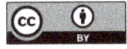

Copyright: © 2021 by the authors. Licensee MDPI, Basel, Switzerland. This article is an open access article distributed under the terms and conditions of the Creative Commons Attribution (CC BY) license (https://creativecommons.org/licenses/by/4.0/).

Abstract: For a number of patients presenting with an undiagnosed pleural effusion, frailty, medical co-morbidity or personal choice may preclude the use of pleural biopsy, the gold standard investigation for diagnosis of malignant pleural mesothelioma (MPM). In this review article, we outline the most recent evidence on ancillary diagnostic tests which may be used to support a diagnosis of MPM where histological samples cannot be obtained or where results are non-diagnostic. Immunocytochemical markers, molecular techniques, diagnostic biomarkers and imaging techniques are discussed. No adjunctive test has a sensitivity and specificity profile to support use in isolation; however, correlation of pleural fluid cytology with relevant radiology and supplementary biomarkers can enable an MDT-consensus clinico-radiological-cytological diagnosis to be made where further invasive tests are not possible or not appropriate. Diagnostic challenges surrounding non-epithelioid MPM are recognised, and there is a critical need for reliable and non-invasive investigative tools in this population.

Keywords: malignant pleural mesothelioma; pleural effusion; biomarkers

1. Introduction

Arising predominantly from the pleural or peritoneal surface (less commonly the pericardium and tunica vaginalis), mesothelioma grows insidiously, often resulting in an advanced stage at clinical presentation. Whilst research into innovative treatment options is an active area of interest and brings new hope for patients, malignant pleural mesothelioma (MPM) remains relatively refractory to conventional therapies. Consequently, prognosis is poor, with a median survival of just 9.5 months and a 3-year survival rate of 12% [1,2].

An association with asbestos was first observed in 1960 in a case series of 33 patients with pleural mesothelioma from the Asbestos Hills in the Cape Province of South Africa [3]. Today, 85% of all mesotheliomas in males are attributable to occupational asbestos exposure, with para-occupational exposure being a recognised cause in women [4]. Despite a ban on asbestos products in 52 countries by 2010 [5], the long latency period from exposure to disease (typically 30–40 years) and continued unregulated use in countries such as

India, Brazil and Russia means that MPM continues to represent a significant global health concern, with an estimated burden of 38,400 cases per year worldwide [6].

Other aetiological mechanisms include genetic predisposition, with inherited germline mutations of the BRCA 1-associated protein (BAP1) gene (a tumour suppressor gene involved in modulation of transcription and DNA repair) identified amongst families with high incidence of mesothelioma in 2011 [7]. Exposure to other elongated mineral particles (including environmental exposure to erionite and fluoro-edenite in Turkey, USA and Mexico) and ionising radiation are also implicated [8]. Pathogenic mechanisms of carcinogenesis following asbestos fibre inhalation highlight a cycle of genetic and cellular damage with chronic inflammation [2,4,9–11].

Four main histological subtypes of MPM are described; epithelioid, sarcomatoid, biphasic and desmoplastic, with epithelioid associated with the most favourable prognosis (median survival of 13 months) and sarcomatoid the least (median survival 4 months) [12]. With no established role for surgical resection outside of clinical trials [1], histological diagnosis of MPM typically relies on biopsy samples. Thoracoscopic pleural biopsy is recommended as the gold standard for investigating an undiagnosed pleural effusion where the differential includes MPM, with diagnostic yields of 95% and higher [13]. Alternatively, where contrast-enhanced thoracic computed tomography (CT) demonstrates focal areas of abnormal pleura, image-guided needle biopsy may be employed to obtain tissue [8,14,15].

There is a cohort of patients for whom frailty, medical co-morbidity or personal choice preclude the use of invasive pleural biopsy. The 2020 UK National Mesothelioma Report showed the median age of patients diagnosed with pleural mesothelioma was 76 years and that over 20% of patients had stage IV disease at diagnosis [16]. Furthermore, a multinational population-based evaluation of 9014 patients demonstrated that more than half of those diagnosed with mesothelioma were aged 70 years or older [17]. Given demographic trends, the proportion of elderly patients will continue to rise over coming decades, with increasing comorbidity further complicated by advanced stage at disease presentation. Diagnostic approaches that are tolerable to and appropriate for patients of higher age or with significant comorbidity are increasingly necessary. Additionally, a proportion of patients who are considered suitable to undergo pleural biopsy at initial assessment go on to have a protracted diagnostic pathway, with repeated procedures yielding equivocal or non-diagnostic results.

Although international guidelines do not advocate cytology-based diagnoses of MPM in patients who are fit for further diagnostic tests [1], the importance of obtaining a diagnosis for frail patients who are unable to undergo invasive procedures to obtain a biopsy is no less significant. Confirmation of a diagnosis is important for future planning and to enable patients to access financial compensation. In some regions, a multi-disciplinary team (MDT) diagnosis based on cytological, radiological and clinical information is sufficient to avoid requirements for a post-mortem examination after death [18].

In this article, we will explore and outline the most up-to-date evidence on ancillary diagnostic tests currently available in clinical practice. We will focus on techniques which may be used to support a diagnosis of MPM from cytological specimens and other less invasive modalities, where histological samples cannot be obtained or where results may be non-diagnostic.

2. Pleural Fluid (PF) Cytology

Diagnostic thoracentesis is the primary means of obtaining PF for evaluation and is an essential step in the initial investigation of a unilateral pleural effusion [19]. Diagnostic cytology on PF can spare the patient more invasive investigations to obtain a tissue biopsy, reducing the risk of procedural complication with both cost and time saving in addition. However, the diagnostic yield of MPM from conventional PF cytology alone is highly variable, with sensitivity ranging from 16% to 73% [1]. In one study of 921 patients with an undiagnosed unilateral pleural effusion, fluid cytology was diagnostic in only 9 of 148 (6%) participants with MPM [20].

Several factors contribute to the wide range of sensitivities quoted. Whilst epithelioid cancers can shed malignant cells into pleural effusion fluid, this is rare in sarcomatoid subtypes. Cytological diagnosis is usually limited, therefore, to the epithelioid subtype. Heavy bloodstaining or rich inflammatory cell infiltrate may additionally reduce cellular yield in effusion specimens. Concentration techniques such as cell block and cytospin preparations can overcome these problems and enhance detection of malignant cells. Cell blocks can also provide a substrate on which adjunctive tests, including immunocytochemical and molecular techniques, can be applied. [8,21,22]

Cytologist experience is another important consideration, with cytopathology being a recognised subspecialty in its own right. For example, morphological appearances of benign reactive mesothelial cells can overlap with malignant cells, complicating diagnosis and demanding meticulous assessment. The volume of PF submitted for analysis may be an additional limitation [1,23], with the British Thoracic Society recommending that 20–40 mL should be sent for evaluation [19].

An important limitation on cytology-based diagnosis is the inability to determine tumour invasion into the lung or chest wall on the basis of PF cytology alone [21,24]. Cytological yield in epithelioid mesothelioma is, however, higher in the presence of visceral pleural invasion. In one study of 75 patients with epithelioid MPM, 37/45 (82%) with positive PF cytology at initial thoracentesis had evidence of visceral pleural invasion at local anaesthetic thoracoscopy (defined as masses, nodules, thickening or mixed appearance) compared with 9/30 (30%) patients having negative cytology, giving an odds ratio for an association between visceral pleural invasion and cytological positivity of 11.87 (95% confidence interval (CI): not stated; $p < 0.001$) [25].

3. PF Immunohistochemistry (IHC) and Molecular Techniques

Initial cytomorphology may be sufficient to confirm the presence of malignant cells in PF after routine staining and, in some cases, may confirm MPM. However, more often, ancillary techniques are required to discriminate benign from malignant mesothelial populations and to differentiate MPM from carcinoma or neoplasms of other origins (for example, melanoma). Recent advances in immunocytochemical and molecular testing have facilitated these diagnostic steps [22,26].

3.1. Discriminating Benign from Malignant Mesothelial Populations

Reactive mesothelial proliferation is a common mimic of MPM (and metastatic carcinoma) and has numerous causes, including infection, pulmonary infarction, trauma, autoimmune disease and drug reactions [27]. Cytomorphological features overlap with MPM and include high cellularity, numerous mitotic figures and cytologic atypia. The inability to evaluate tissue invasion in cytology-based specimens means that reactive mesothelial proliferation is more frequently documented in cytologic specimens than in tissue biopsies [24].

Certain immunocytochemical stains are more likely to be positive in benign mesothelial cell proliferation and other stains in malignant mesothelial proliferation. However, most IHC staining patterns do not reliably differentiate malignant from benign mesothelial proliferation. Desmin, reported previously to favour benign reactive mesothelium, shows positivity in up to 56% of mesotheliomas [28]. Similarly, whilst epithelial membrane antigen (EMA), p53 and insulin-like growth-factor 2 messenger ribonucleic acid (RNA)-binding protein 3 (IMP-3) may support a diagnosis of malignancy, benign reactions can also stain positively for these markers [29]. Whilst positive staining with glucose transporter 1 (GLUT1) may have a higher specificity for malignant cell populations in pleural biopsy specimens [1], cytological studies demonstrate lower specificity, with 9/50 patients with benign reactive mesothelial proliferations demonstrating positive polyclonal GLUT-1 staining in one study [30] and 14/38 participants with benign effusions staining positive in another [31].

Detection of specific mesothelioma-associated genetic mutations can help confirm the presence of malignant cells. Loss of BAP1 can be demonstrated on IHC staining and is highly specific for malignancy, whilst fluorescent in situ hybridisation (FISH) can detect deletion of the *CDKN2A/P16* gene, commonly seen in MPM.

3.1.1. BAP1 Loss

BAP1 is a nuclear ubiquitin hydrolase, which functions as a tumour suppressor, and is encoded by the BAP1 gene. It controls DNA repair, expression of genes related to cell cycle and cell proliferation. It can also induce cell death. Cells with reduced or absent BAP1 are unable to repair damaged DNA and cannot execute apoptosis. BAP1-mutant cells are therefore prone to malignant transformation [10].

Somatic mutation of the BAP1 gene in mesothelioma was first described in 2011, with mutations occurring in approximately 70% of epithelioid mesotheliomas [10]. Germline BAP1 mutation is less common, occurring in approximately 1–2% of MPM, usually in the context of the autosomal dominant BAP1 cancer predisposition syndrome [29,32]. Germline BAP1 loss is associated with earlier onset MPM tumours, as well as other BAP1-related malignancies such as uveal melanoma.

BAP1 loss (defined as absence of nuclear staining when a positive internal control is present on a slide) may occur by mutation, biallelic deletion or deletion/insertion [8] and is most reliably detected by IHC [32]. Cells expressing at least one wild-type copy of BAP1 retain IHC staining. Notably, even in tumours arising from germline BAP1 mutation, non-tumour cells express a single wild-type copy and hence produce a positive IHC response. To show loss of BAP1 immunoreactivity, both copies must be mutated, either by a combination of germline and somatic mutation events, as in BAP1 cancer syndrome, or by two somatic events in sporadic cancers [29].

Loss of BAP1 expression has been repeatedly validated in differentiating MPM from benign mesothelial populations and is now in routine use in many pathology laboratories. A recent meta-analysis identified 12 studies of 1824 patients (1016 with MPM), published between 2015 and 2017. The overall pooled sensitivity of BAP1 loss for malignant mesothelioma was 0.56 (95% CI: 0.50–0.62) and specificity 1.00 (95% CI: 0.95–1.00). The area under curve (AUC) was 0.72, indicating moderate diagnostic accuracy. Notably, all studies were of retrospective design, and only four included more than 100 participants. Heterogeneity was evident, with potential explanations including different cut-off values for BAP1 loss, inclusion of participants with pleural and peritoneal mesothelioma and variation in diagnostic accuracy across mesothelioma histological subtypes. For example, the sensitivity ranged from 0.07 (95% CI: 0.00–0.72) in sarcomatoid MPM to 0.74 (95% CI: 0.66–0.80) in epithelioid [33]. Offering additional explanation for this low diagnostic sensitivity, 30–40% of mesotheliomas have been shown to carry a wild-type BAP1 and therefore stain positively in a similar manner to benign lesions [10].

In a subgroup meta-analysis comparing the diagnostic performance of BAP1 loss in histology and cytology specimens, near identical sensitivity and specificity was observed. However, data from the 5 studies evaluating cytology specimens demonstrated reduced diagnostic accuracy with an AUC of 0.69 [33]. Studies of BAP1 loss in cytology specimens have, to date, been hindered by retrospective design, small sample size and the use of cytology specimens in subgroup analyses. Well-designed research is required to accurately determine the diagnostic potential of BAP1 loss in cytology specimens in order to improve current diagnostic pathways and potentially avoid the need for additional invasive procedures.

As a stand-alone test, BAP1 loss has moderate diagnostic sensitivity with excellent specificity for MPM. BAP1 loss is therefore reliable as a "rule in" for mesothelioma, but pleural malignancy cannot be excluded in its absence. Notably, BAP1 loss is uncommon in sarcomatoid and desmoplastic mesothelioma and is demonstrated in other malignancies including melanoma and renal cell carcinoma [34]. Superior diagnostic accuracy may be achieved in combination with other adjunctive tests.

3.1.2. p16 Fluorescence In Situ Hybridization (FISH)

Homozygous deletion of the 9p21 locus is one of the most common genetic alterations in MPM. Its loss affects a cluster of genes, including p16 (also known as cyclin-dependent kinase inhibitor (CDKN)-2A), CDKN2B and methylthioadenosine phosphorylase (MTAP). p16/CDKN2A is a tumour suppressor gene that is present in all healthy cells. Its normal function results in the cessation of the cell cycle; hence, inactivation results in uncontrolled cell proliferation and tumour development.

Homozygous deletion of P16 can be detected using FISH in both cytological and histological specimens [35]; however, the diagnostic sensitivity for MPM is relatively low at 0.53 (95% CI: 0.35–0.70), despite gene profiling studies demonstrating p16/CDKN2A loss in up to 80% of MPM tumours. In part, the low sensitivity reflects variation in p16 deletion across the different MPM subtypes (90–100% loss in sarcomatoid variant compared with a 70% loss in epithelioid and biphasic), although other alterations that affect the 9p21 locus and cannot be detected by FISH also contribute [1,8,21,23,24,29].

An alternative approach, where histological specimens are available, is the application of IHC staining to determine p16 protein expression in cells, which could represent a more accessible ancillary test to laboratories where FISH cannot be performed [36]. However, the sensitivity to discriminate MPM from reactive mesothelial hyperplasia using p16 IHC in combination with BAP1 loss was 10% lower than those of more traditional FISH techniques in one study [35]. IHC techniques may be employed, in addition, to detect MTAP loss, distinguishing malignant from benign proliferations with a specificity of 100% and a sensitivity of 43% (increased to 79.5% when used in combination with BAP1 IHC) in cell block specimens from pleural effusions [37,38]. IHC for MTAP can also discriminate sarcomatoid MPM from fibrous pleuritis. A more recent multicentre evaluation of MTAP loss by IHC demonstrated a 78% sensitivity and a 96% specificity for CDKN2A homozygous deletion, suggesting it to be a reliable surrogate for CDKN2A FISH [39]; however, the use of MTAP is not yet recommended by international guidelines [1,8,15].

Overall, when used in isolation, both FISH and IHC techniques for p16 deletion are limited by low sensitivity. Consequently, whilst p16 deletion can confirm a suspected diagnosis of malignancy, failure to detect its loss does not exclude a diagnosis of MPM. However, combining testing for p16 loss with IHC for BAP1 loss has been shown to increase diagnostic sensitivity (combined sensitivity 0.76 (95% CI: 0.62–0.88)) [40]. Therefore, if BAP1 is intact or a sarcomatoid mesothelioma is suspected, additional testing with p16 FISH may strengthen diagnostic certainty [21] and help to discriminate benign from malignant mesothelial cell populations (Figure 1).

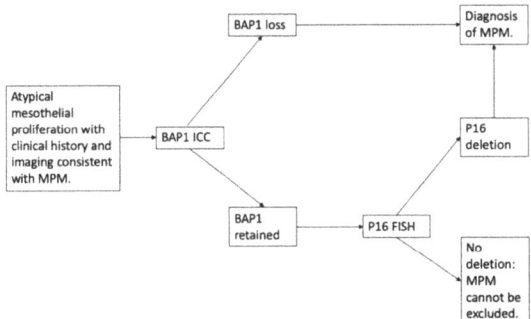

Figure 1. A suggested diagnostic approach where distinction of malignant from benign mesothelial proliferation is unclear on initial fluid cytology. BAP1 loss and p16 deletion support the diagnosis of MPM. MPM, malignant pleural mesothelioma; ICC, immunocytochemistry; FISH, fluorescence in-situ hybridization; BAP1, BRCA 1-associated protein.

3.2. Distinguishing Mesothelioma from Carcinoma

Distinguishing mesothelioma from other causes of malignant pleural effusion is critical in guiding therapeutic strategies and prognosis. Malignancies commonly metastasising to the pleura include lung cancers, breast and gastrointestinal carcinomas. Distinction between epithelioid MPM and carcinomas may be made on morphology and simple histochemical staining alone. As no one marker exhibits a 100% specificity, guidelines recommend a combination of at least two positive mesothelial markers (calretinin, cytokeratin 5/6, Wilms tumour 1 and D2-40) and at least two negative adenocarcinoma IHC markers (thyroid transcription factor 1 (TTF1), carcinoembryonic antigen (CEA) and Ber-EP4) (see Table 1) [1]. Positive markers of other tumour types should be used for differential diagnoses of metastatic carcinomas from other sources, such as hormone receptors in breast and ovarian cancer and PAX8 in renal cell carcinoma [1,15,24].

BAP1 loss may play a role in differentiating mesothelioma from carcinoma, with loss in 46/53 (87%) pleural and peritoneal mesotheliomas compared with 4/204 (2%) (p: <0.001) carcinomas in one study [41]. Further evaluation of the role of BAP1 loss in this context is required, however, before universal adoption is recommended.

3.3. Distinguishing Mesothelioma from Other Malignant Cell Neoplasms

Malignant pleural effusion may be the first presentation of an unknown primary cancer. In this setting, appropriate immunocytochemical panels often enable a precise diagnosis, starting with CK7 and CK20 staining [42]. Other differential diagnoses of MPM depend on histologic category, with epithelioid MPM requiring distinction from carcinomas, sarcomatoid MPM from sarcomas and other spindle cell neoplasms, mixed MPM from other mixed or biphasic tumours such as synovial sarcoma and desmoplastic MPM from fibrous pleuritis. Immunostain selection in this setting would depend on basic morphology [24].

Affirmative markers used in the evaluation of epithelioid MPM are of limited utility in sarcomatoid tumours. More usefully, cytokeratin markers, such as CAM5.2, are important in differentiating sarcomatoid MPM (positive staining) from sarcoma, which is usually keratin-negative [43]. D2-40 (podoplanin) can be used to differentiate sarcomatoid MPM from pulmonary sarcomatoid carcinoma (which also stains positively for TTF1, napsin and p40/p63). Synovial sarcoma can be confirmed by molecular testing for the X; 18 translocation [24].

Table 1. Immunohistochemical markers for differentiating tumour types in malignant pleural effusion [12,24]. Adapted from Bibby et al. [44].

Mesothelial Markers	Adenocarcinoma Markers	Other Markers
Calretinin	TTF1 (lung and thyroid)	Squamous cell lung cancer: p40, p63 and claudin 4
CK 5/6	CEA	Renal cell carcinoma: PAX8, PAX2 and claudin 4
WT1		Pancreas: CA19-9
D2-40	Ber–EP4	Gastrointestinal: CD20 and CDX-2 Gynaecological: PAX-8 and WT1 Prostate: PSA and PSMA Breast: mammaglobin, GCDFP-15, ER, PR and GATA3

Immunocytochemical markers are summarised in Table 1.

4. Diagnostic Biomarkers

Biomarkers present an attractive solution to diagnostic challenges posed by MPM, and consequently, a large number of studies have evaluated potential targets in serum, plasma, PF and exhaled breath. An ideal marker should be obtainable by minimally invasive means and be sufficiently sensitive to detect most cases of MPM, whilst also being highly specific, to avoid false positive results and discriminate individuals with MPM from other pathologies. Protein biomarkers of interest include mesothelin, osteopontin and fibulin-3 [45].

4.1. Mesothelin

Identified in the early 1990s as a surface antigen on ovarian cancer cells, mesothelin is a glycoprotein thought to play a role in cell adhesion and signalling. The mesothelin gene, MSLN, encodes a precursor protein from which membrane-bound mesothelin and a soluble protein megakaryocyte potentiating factor (MPF) are formed. These are commonly referred to as "soluble mesothelin-related peptides" (SMRPs). In normal tissue, mesothelin is only found on mesothelial cells; hence, serum levels of SMRP are low. However, increased concentrations of SMRPs are found in serum samples of patients with ovarian and pancreatic cancers, in addition to mesothelioma. In 2003, Robinson et al. demonstrated that patients with MPM had significantly higher concentrations of serum SMRP than asbestos-exposed healthy controls, non-asbestos-exposed healthy controls and patients with non-mesothelioma malignant or inflammatory pleural disease. They reported a sensitivity of 84% (95% CI: 73–93) and a specificity of 100% (95% CI: 91–100) for MPM. SMRP concentrations were higher in patients with epithelioid tumours and in those with a large tumour bulk (maximum tumour width: >3 cm) [11,46,47]. In contrast, SMRP was less likely to be raised in people with sarcomatoid and biphasic disease; however, small study numbers and non-disclosure of histologic subtype in some studies mean that accurate sensitivity and specificity estimates are difficult to derive for these tumour subtypes [11].

Serum mesothelin has become the most widely studied diagnostic biomarker in MPM, with a meta-analysis in 2014 identifying 28 relevant publications, involving 7550 patients [48]. Pooled sensitivity and specificity estimates were found to be 0.61 and 0.87, respectively, lower than indicated in previous studies. This is mostly accounted for by heterogeneity across the included studies, although publication bias may also play a role. Heterogeneity arose from the use of various ELISA assays, different cut-off values and differences in participant characteristics (i.e., mesothelioma subtypes and choice of control groups). The negative likelihood ratio (NLR) value was 0.43, meaning if participants were serum-SMRP-negative, the probability of having MPM was still moderate at 43%. The authors reported that low sensitivity limited the added value of SMRPs but a positive result may be helpful in confirming MPM, with a positive likelihood ratio of 5.71 [48].

PF mesothelin has been studied as an alternative biomarker, as mesothelin is shed from mesothelioma tumour cells directly into pleural effusion fluid. In 2005, Pass et al. identified that SMRP levels were significantly higher in PF samples from 45 patients with MPM compared to 30 healthy controls [49]. In the first study to assess the clinical utility of PF SMRP, Davies et al. demonstrated levels were 10.9 times greater in patients with MPM compared to benign pleural disease and were highly reproducible [50]. They concluded that the measurement of PF mesothelin contributed valuable additional information to PF cytology alone, especially where initial cytology results were inconclusive. In a meta-analysis by Cui et al., pooled estimates of sensitivity were higher for PF SMRP than serum samples (0.79 compared to 0.61) with PF SMRP specificity remaining robust at 0.85 [48].

Although considered as the current "gold standard" biomarker for MPM in some international guidelines [15], neither serum nor pleural fluid mesothelin is recommended as diagnostic tests in isolation. With low sensitivity, a negative result adds little value and is a frequent finding in non-epithelioid disease. In contrast, a positive result increases the likelihood of mesothelioma; however, false positives are possible in benign inflammatory conditions such as benign asbestos pleural effusion (BAPE) or in the presence of impaired renal function [51]. Consequently, mesothelin testing should be considered as an adjunct in patients with suspicious or inconclusive cytology, who are unsuitable for or decline invasive diagnostic tests with a high pre-test probability of MPM [1,4,8]. Further research into the utility of biomarkers in MPM diagnosis and better understanding of markers of non-epithelioid disease may help to elucidate the role of this test in the diagnostic pathway.

4.2. Other Diagnostic Biomarkers

Osteopontin, a protein mediator of cell matrix interaction, cell signalling and tumour development, has been viewed as a promising biomarker for MPM, but results have been inconsistent. In a meta-analysis of six studies, the overall diagnostic sensitivity and specificity were 0.65 (95% CI: 0.6–7.0) and 0.81 (95% CI: 0.78–0.85), respectively. Notably, the majority of included studies evaluated serum and/or plasma osteopontin from frozen samples with uncertainty regarding the long-term stability of osteopontin in frozen specimens. Degradation of osteopontin during the freezing and defrosting process may explain the low detection rates of this protein in retrospective studies [52]. Similar to mesothelin, the clinical utility of osteopontin is limited by low sensitivity, and further understanding of its added diagnostic value in comparison to other biomarkers is required.

Fibulin 3, an extracellular matrix glycoprotein mediator of cell-to-cell and cell-to-matrix communication, is detectable in blood and PF with a small number of studies reporting varied outcomes on its potential as a biomarker for MPM. Initially promising, with a 97% sensitivity and a 95% specificity to determine MPM from other causes of pleural effusion in one study [53], subsequent analyses have suggested a sensitivity as low as 22% [54]. A questionable diagnostic value was highlighted by one study, with no difference in fibulin 3 levels in pleural effusion samples of patients with MPM and controls. Whilst plasma levels were higher in patients with MPM compared to in controls in a population in Sydney, this was not replicated in a cohort of patients studied in Vienna and the diagnostic accuracy was low (receiver operating curve analyses overall accuracies of 63.2% and 56.2% for correct diagnostic characterisation of MPM in the Sydney and Vienna cohort, respectively). The authors did, however, observe that low pleural effusion fibulin 3 levels were significantly associated with better survival [55]. A meta-analysis of 8 studies demonstrated a pooled diagnostic sensitivity of blood fibulin 3 of 0.87 (95% CI: 0.58–0.97) and a specificity of 0.89 (95% CI: 0.77–0.95) [56]. A subsequent meta-analysis of 7 studies demonstrated a lower overall sensitivity from pooled studies of blood and pleural effusion samples of 0.62 (95% CI: 0.45–0.77) and a specificity of 0.82 (95% CI: 0.73–0.89) [57]. Ultimately the value of fibulin 3 in diagnosing MPM remains unclear, with prospective validation studies ongoing [58].

5. Imaging Techniques

CT with contrast enhancement is the primary imaging modality used for diagnosis and staging of pleural malignancy and can identify the primary tumour, intrathoracic lymphadenopathy and extrathoracic spread [59]. Positive features of malignant pleural disease include circumferential pleural thickening, nodular pleural thickening, parietal pleural thickening of greater than 1 cm and mediastinal pleural involvement [60]. The diagnostic accuracies of CT for detection of pleural malignancy are 68–97% with specificities of 78–89% [1]. CT scanning is widely available and has high clinical utility. However, it has limited soft tissue differentiation, and early malignant disease with minor pleural thickening can be missed. Additionally, subtle invasion of certain structures may be challenging to identify, which has implications for the accuracy of staging. Timing of contrast and reporting of images by non-thoracic radiologists add further variability. Subsequently, 35–46% of patients with pleural malignancy will have a "benign" CT report in routine practice [61].

Differentiating mesothelioma from metastatic pleural malignancy can also be challenging. Parenchymal lung tumours with mediastinal or hilar lymphadenopathy may indicate metastatic pleural disease, whereas the presence of pleural plaques, involvement of the interlobar fissure and absence of lung parenchymal masses favour MPM [1]. It may be particularly difficult to differentiate MPM from pleural metastatic disease, if the tumour presents as a localised pleural or subpleural nodule, a localised anterior mediastinal mass or involves the diaphragmatic pleura with liver invasion, especially in the absence of a pleural effusion [43].

Alternative imaging modalities have been proposed for use in MPM. Positron emission technology (PET)-CT combines high-resolution CT scanning with an injection of a metabolic tracer which accumulates at areas of metabolic activity. Uptake is assessed at regions of interest and reported as standard uptake values (SUV), with a threshold value of 2.0 reliably differentiating between benign and malignant disease [4]. A meta-analysis of 11 PET-CT studies reported a pooled sensitivity of 95% (95% CI: 92–97%) and a specificity of 82% (95% CI: 76–88%) for differentiating malignant from benign disease [62]. False positive results are common, however, particularly in the context of prior talc pleurodesis, active pleural infection, or indolent inflammation such as tuberculous pleuritis. PET-CT cannot distinguish MPM from metastatic pleural disease and, due to poor spatial resolution, has low sensitivity (78%) for extrapleural invasion [61]. Whilst lacking specificity to diagnose MPM routinely, PET-CT may provide functional information on pleural lesions, although it does not appear to be helpful in guiding choice of site for biopsy [63]. It is currently recommended only for staging patients in whom the presence of distant metastatic disease would alter treatment approach [1,8,15].

Magnetic resonance imaging (MRI) offers higher soft tissue contrast than CT, resulting in an increased sensitivity for chest wall and diaphragm invasion, higher contrast with adjacent effusion and higher inter-observer agreement [64]. The contrast enhanced perfusion augments sensitivity in detection of pleural malignancy, even where pleural thickening is minimal [64]. In addition to differentiating malignant from benign pleural disease, diffusion-weighted MRI (DWI-MRI) has distinguished between epithelioid and sarcomatoid MPM with a sensitivity of 60% and a specificity of 94% [1]. At present, the added value of MRI in equivocal or atypical CT scans is unclear, with prospective evaluation required, but, where available, MRI may be considered in difficult diagnostic cases to better delineate invasive disease [1,8,15].

6. Future Directions

The search for novel diagnostic biomarkers is expanding and encompasses multiple branches of medical science. Proteomic analysis has identified new panels of candidate biomarkers [65] with prospective multicentre evaluation of a novel assay ongoing [58]. Gene-expression-based classification has outperformed BAP1 and p16 FISH [40]. Deeper understanding of the genomic and epigenomic factors relevant to MPM may herald new diagnostic techniques that better distinguish MPM from other tumours [66–68]. Circulating plasma micro-RNA [69] and metabolomic profiling [70,71] of PF are other experimental areas of interest.

Whilst these studies may yield new markers which negate the requirement for invasive tissue sampling, all are limited currently to the research setting and are not yet available in clinical practice.

As the range of therapeutic options for MPM expands, the importance of genetic and molecular phenotyping of tumours to enable targeted treatment will increase. Currently, no marker is able to provide this level of personalised tumour phenotyping, so tissue biopsies are likely to remain the diagnostic gold standard for the foreseeable future.

To obtain tissue in patients fit to undergo invasive procedures, a "direct-to-LAT" approach (pathway stratification where selected patients proceed directly to local anaesthetic thoracoscopy (LAT) to obtain pleural biopsies) may be employed in patients where the pre-test probability of MPM is high and the anticipated yield from PF cytology is low [72]. However, a streamlined diagnostic approach is required for more frail patients and those who choose not to undergo pleural biopsy. Research to determine the combined value of the investigations discussed in this article is essential to formalise integrated non-invasive pathways for the diagnosis of MPM.

7. Conclusions

For patients in whom malignant pleural mesothelioma is suspected, tissue diagnosis remains the gold standard and is the only method that can confirm the presence of invasive disease. However, for those unable or unwilling to undergo tissue sampling, the low sensitivity of pleural effusion cytology can be augmented by incorporating ancillary techniques such as immunocytochemical markers to increase reliability [8]. No adjunctive test has a sensitivity and specificity profile to support use in isolation, but findings such as BAP1 loss can provide additional support for a suspected diagnosis if the pre-test probability is high. Where diagnoses remain challenging, even despite use of ancillary techniques, expert radiological review of disease distribution on imaging and occupational history of asbestos exposure are important considerations. Correlation of PF cytology with relevant radiology and supplementary biomarkers can enable an MDT-consensus clinico-radiological-cytological diagnosis to be made, where further invasive tests are not possible or not appropriate [18]. Diagnostic challenges surrounding non-epithelioid MPM are recognised, and there is a critical need for reliable and non-invasive investigative tools in this population.

Author Contributions: Conceptualization, A.D., N.M. and A.B.; writing—original draft preparation, A.D. All authors have read and agreed to the published version of the manuscript.

Funding: This review article received no external funding.

Institutional Review Board Statement: Not applicable.

Informed Consent Statement: Not applicable.

Acknowledgments: The authors would like to thank Richard Daly for reviewing the pathology-based information within the manuscript.

Conflicts of Interest: The authors declare no conflict of interest.

References

1. Woolhouse, I.; Bishop, L.; Darlison, L.; De Fonseka, D.; Edey, A.; Edwards, J.; Faivre-Finn, C.; Fennell, D.A.; Holmes, S.; Kerr, K.M.; et al. British Thoracic Society Guideline for the investigation and management of malignant pleural mesothelioma. *Thorax* **2018**, *73*, i1–i30. [CrossRef]
2. Sekido, Y. Molecular pathogenesis of malignant mesothelioma. *Carcinogenesis* **2013**, *34*, 1413–1419. [CrossRef]
3. Wagner, J.C.; Sleggs, C.A.; Marchand, P. Diffuse pleural mesothelioma and asbestos exposure in the North Western Cape Province. *Br. J. Ind. Med.* **1960**, *17*, 260–271. [CrossRef] [PubMed]
4. Bibby, A.C.; Tsim, S.; Kanellakis, N.; Ball, H.; Talbot, D.C.; Blyth, K.G.; Maskell, N.A.; Psallidas, I. Malignant pleural mesothelioma: An update on investigation, diagnosis and treatment. *Eur. Respir. Rev.* **2016**, *25*, 472–486. [CrossRef] [PubMed]
5. LaDou, J.; Castleman, B.; Frank, A.; Gochfeld, M.; Greenberg, M.; Huff, J.; Joshi, T.K.; Landrigan, P.J.; Lemen, R.; Myers, J.; et al. The Case for a Global Ban on Asbestos. *Environ. Heal Perspect.* **2010**, *118*, 897–901. [CrossRef]
6. Odgerel, C.-O.; Takahashi, K.; Sorahan, T.; Driscoll, T.; Fitzmaurice, C.; Yoko, O.M.; Sawanyawisuth, K.; Furuya, S.; Tanaka, F.; Horie, S.; et al. Estimation of the global burden of mesothelioma deaths from incomplete national mortality data. *Occup. Environ. Med.* **2017**, *74*, 851–858. [CrossRef] [PubMed]
7. Testa, J.R.; Cheung, M.; Pei, J.; Below, J.E.; Tan, Y.; Sementino, E.; Cox, N.J.; Dogan, A.U.; Pass, H.I.; Trusa, S.; et al. P1 mutations predispose to malignant mesothelioma. *Nat. Genet.* **2011**, *43*, 1022–1025. [CrossRef]
8. Scherpereel, A.; Opitz, I.; Berghmans, T.; Psallidas, I.; Glatzer, M.; Rigau, D.; Astoul, P.; Bölükbas, S.; Boyd, J.; Coolen, J.; et al. ERS/ESTS/EACTS/ESTRO guidelines for the management of malignant pleural mesothelioma. *Eur. Respir. J.* **2020**, *55*, 1900953. [CrossRef] [PubMed]
9. Robinson, B.W.S.; Lake, R.A. Advances in Malignant Mesothelioma. *N. Engl. J. Med.* **2005**, *353*, 1591–1603. [CrossRef]
10. Carbone, M.; Adusumilli, P.S.; Alexander, H.R., Jr.; Baas, P.; Bardelli, F.; Bononi, A.; Bueno, R.; Felley-Bosco, E.; Galateau-Salle, F.; Jablons, D.; et al. Mesothelioma: Scientific clues for prevention, diagnosis, and therapy. *CA Cancer J. Clin.* **2019**, *69*, 402–429. [CrossRef]
11. Arnold, D.T.; Maskell, N.A. Biomarkers in mesothelioma. *Ann. Clin. Biochem* **2018**, *55*, 49–58. [CrossRef]
12. Beckett, P.; Edwards, J.; Fennell, D.; Hubbard, R.; Woolhouse, I.; Peake, M. Demographics, management and survival of patients with malignant pleural mesothelioma in the National Lung Cancer Audit in England and Wales. *Lung Cancer* **2015**, *88*, 344–348. [CrossRef] [PubMed]
13. Abo E-Magd, G.H.; Abouissa, A.H.; Abbass, I. Diagnostic yield and safety of medical thoraco-scopic versus CT guided percutaneous tru-cut pleural biopsy. *Eur. Respir. J.* **2019**, *54*, PA3085.

14. Roberts, M.; Neville, E.; Berrisford, R.G.; Antunes, G.; Ali, N.J.; on behalf of the BTS Pleural Disease Guideline Group. Management of a malignant pleural effusion: British Thoracic Society pleural disease guideline 2010. *Thorax* **2010**, *65*, II32–II40. [CrossRef] [PubMed]
15. Kindler, H.L.; Ismaila, N.; Armato, S.G., III; Bueno, R.; Hesdorffer, M.; Jahan, T.; Jones, C.M.; Miettinen, M.; Pass, H.; Rimner, A.; et al. Treatment of Malignant Pleural Mesothelioma: American Society of Clinical Oncology Clinical Practice Guideline. *J. Clin. Oncol* **2018**, *36*, 1343–1373. [CrossRef]
16. Physicians RCo. *National Mesothelioma Audit Report 2020 (for the Audit Period 2016–18)*; National Mesothelioma Audit: London, UK, 2020.
17. Damhuis, R.; Khakwani, A.; De Schutter, H.; Rich, A.; Burgers, J.; Van Meerbeeck, J. Treatment patterns and survival analysis in 9014 patients with malignant pleural mesothelioma from Belgium, the Netherlands and England. *Lung Cancer* **2015**, *89*, 212–217. [CrossRef]
18. Bibby, A.C.; Williams, K.; Smith, S.; Bhatt, N.; A Maskell, N. What is the role of a specialist regional mesothelioma multidisciplinary team meeting? A service evaluation of one tertiary referral centre in the UK. *BMJ Open* **2016**, *6*, e012092. [CrossRef] [PubMed]
19. Hooper, C.; Lee, Y.C.G.; Maskell, N. Investigation of a unilateral pleural effusion in adults: British Thoracic Society pleural disease guideline 2010. *Thorax* **2010**, *65*, ii4-ii17. [CrossRef]
20. Arnold, D.T.; De Fonseka, D.; Perry, S.; Morley, A.; Harvey, J.E.; Medford, A.; Brett, M.; Maskell, N.A. Investigating unilateral pleural effusions: The role of cytology. *Eur. Respir. J.* **2018**, *52*, 1801254. [CrossRef]
21. Porcel, J.M. Biomarkers in the diagnosis of pleural diseases: A 2018 update. *Ther. Adv. Respir. Dis.* **2018**, *12*, 1753466618808660. [CrossRef] [PubMed]
22. Hjerpe, A.; Ascoli, V.; Bedrossian, C.W.M.; Boon, M.E.; Creaney, J.; Davidson, B.; Dejmek, A.; Dobra, K.; Fassina, A.; Field, A.; et al. Guidelines for the Cytopathologic Diagnosis of Epithelioid and Mixed-Type Malignant Mesothelioma: A secondary publication. *Cytopathology* **2015**, *26*, 142–156. [CrossRef] [PubMed]
23. Monaco, S.; Mehrad, M.; Dacic, S. Recent Advances in the Diagnosis of Malignant Mesothelioma: Focus on Approach in Challenging Cases and in Limited Tissue and Cytologic Samples. *Adv. Anat. Pathol.* **2018**, *25*, 24–30. [CrossRef]
24. Husain, A.N.; Colby, T.V.; Ordóñez, N.G.; Allen, T.C.; Attanoos, R.L.; Beasley, M.B.; Butnor, K.J.; Chirieac, L.R.; Churg, A.M.; Dacic, S.; et al. Guidelines for Pathologic Diagnosis of Malignant Mesothelioma 2017 Update of the Consensus Statement From the International Mesothelioma Interest Group. *Arch. Pathol. Lab. Med.* **2018**, *142*, 89–108. [CrossRef] [PubMed]
25. Pinelli, V.; Laroumagne, S.; Sakr, L.; Marchetti, G.P.; Tassi, G.F.; Astoul, P. Pleural Fluid Cytological Yield and Visceral Pleural Invasion in Patients with Epithelioid Malignant Pleural Mesothelioma. *J. Thorac. Oncol.* **2012**, *7*, 595–598. [CrossRef] [PubMed]
26. Chapel, D.B.; Schulte, J.J.; Husain, A.N.; Krausz, T. Application of immunohistochemistry in diagnosis and management of malignant mesothelioma. *Trans. Lung Cancer Res.* **2020**, *9*, S3-S27. [CrossRef] [PubMed]
27. Zeren, E.H.; Demirag, F. Benign and Malignant Mesothelial Proliferation. *Surg. Pathol. Clin.* **2010**, *3*, 83–107. [CrossRef] [PubMed]
28. Attanoos, R.L.; Griffin, A.; Gibbs, A.R. The use of immunohistochemistry in distinguishing reactive from neoplastic mesothelium. A novel use for desmin and comparative evaluation with epithelial membrane antigen, p53, platelet-derived growth factor-receptor, P-glycoprotein and Bcl-2. *Histopathology* **2003**, *43*, 231–238. [CrossRef]
29. Churg, A.; Sheffield, B.S.; Galateau-Salle, F. New Markers for Separating Benign From Malignant Mesothelial Proliferations: Are We There Yet? *Arch. Pathol. Lab. Med.* **2016**, *140*, 318–321. [CrossRef]
30. Ikeda, K.; Tate, G.; Suzuki, T.; Kitamura, T.; Mitsuya, T. Diagnostic usefulness of EMA, IMP3, and GLUT-1 for the immunocytochemical distinction of malignant cells from reactive mesothelial cells in effusion cytology using cytospin preparations. *Diagn. Cytopathol.* **2011**, *39*, 395–401. [CrossRef]
31. Shen, J.; Pinkus, G.S.; Deshpande, V.; Cibas, E.S. Usefulness of EMA, GLUT-1, and XIAP for the cytologic diagnosis of malignant mesothelioma in body cavity fluids. *Am. J. Clin. Pathol.* **2009**, *131*, 516–523. [CrossRef]
32. Pulford, E.; Huilgol, K.; Moffat, D.; Henderson, D.W.; Klebe, S. Malignant Mesothelioma, BAP1 Immunohistochemistry, and VEGFA: Does BAP1 Have Potential for Early Diagnosis and Assessment of Prognosis? *Dis. Markers* **2017**, *2017*, 1–10. [CrossRef]
33. Wang, L.-M.; Shi, Z.-W.; Wang, J.-L.; Lv, Z.; Du, F.-B.; Yang, Q.-B.; Wang, Y. Diagnostic accuracy of BRCA1-associated protein 1 in malignant mesothelioma: A meta-analysis. *Oncotarget* **2017**, *8*, 68863–68872. [CrossRef] [PubMed]
34. Murali, R.; Wiesner, T.; Scolyer, R.A. Tumours associated with BAP1 mutations. *Pathology* **2013**, *45*, 116–126. [CrossRef]
35. Hida, T.; Matsumoto, S.; Hamasaki, M.; Kawahara, K.; Tsujimura, T.; Hiroshima, K.; Kamei, T.; Taguchi, K.; Iwasaki, A.; Oda, Y.; et al. Deletion status of p16 in effusion smear preparation correlates with that of underlying malignant pleural mesothelioma tissue. *Cancer Sci* **2015**, *106*, 1635–1641. [CrossRef] [PubMed]
36. Hida, T.; Hamasaki, M.; Matsumoto, S.; Sato, A.; Tsujimura, T.; Kawahara, K.; Iwasaki, A.; Okamoto, T.; Oda, Y.; Honda, H.; et al. Immunohistochemical detection of MTAP and BAP1 protein loss for mesothelioma diagnosis: Comparison with 9p21 FISH and BAP1 immunohistochemistry. *Lung Cancer* **2017**, *104*, 98–105. [CrossRef]
37. Kinoshita, Y.; Hamasaki, M.; Yoshimura, M.; Matsumoto, S.; Sato, A.; Tsujimura, T.; Ueda, H.; Makihata, S.; Kato, F.; Iwasaki, A.; et al. A combination of MTAP and BAP1 immunohistochemistry is effective for distinguishing sarcomatoid mesothelioma from fibrous pleuritis. *Lung Cancer* **2018**, *125*, 198–204. [CrossRef]
38. Kinoshita, Y.; Hida, T.; Hamasaki, M.; Matsumoto, S.; Sato, A.; Tsujimura, T.; Kawahara, K.; Hiroshima, K.; Oda, Y.; Nabeshima, K. A combination of MTAP and BAP1 immunohistochemistry in pleural effusion cytology for the diagnosis of mesothelioma. *Cancer Cytopathol* **2018**, *126*, 54–63. [CrossRef] [PubMed]

39. Chapel, D.B.; Schulte, J.J.; Berg, K.; Churg, A.; Dacic, S.; Fitzpatrick, C.; Galateau-Salle, F.; Hiroshima, K.; Krausz, T.; Le Stang, N.; et al. MTAP immunohistochemistry is an accurate and reproducible surrogate for CDKN2A fluorescence in situ hybridization in diagnosis of malignant pleural mesothelioma. *Mod. Pathol* **2020**, *33*, 245–254. [CrossRef]
40. Ali, G.; Bruno, R.; Poma, A.M.; Proietti, A.; Ricci, S.; Chella, A.; Melfi, F.; Ambrogi, M.C.; Lucchi, M.; Fontanini, G. A gene-expression-based test can outperform bap1 and p16 analyses in the differential diagnosis of pleural mesothelial proliferations. *Oncol. Lett.* **2020**, *19*, 1060–1065. [PubMed]
41. Davidson, B.; Tötsch, M.; Wohlschlaeger, J.; Hager, T.; Pinamonti, M. The diagnostic role of BAP1 in serous effusions. *Hum. Pathol.* **2018**, *79*, 122–126. [CrossRef] [PubMed]
42. Selves, J.; Long-Mira, E.; Mathieu, M.-C.; Rochaix, P.; Ilié, M. Immunohistochemistry for Diagnosis of Metastatic Carcinomas of Unknown Primary Site. *Cancers* **2018**, *10*, 108. [CrossRef] [PubMed]
43. Fels, E.D.R.; Jones, K.D. Diagnosis of Mesothelioma. *Surg. Pathol. Clin.* **2020**, *13*, 73–89. [CrossRef] [PubMed]
44. Bibby, A.C.; Dorn, P.; Psallidas, I.; Porcel, J.M.; Janssen, J.; Froudarakis, M.; Subotic, D.; Astoul, P.; Licht, P.; Schmid, R.; et al. ERS/EACTS statement on the management of malignant pleural effusions. *Eur. J. Cardio-Thoracic Surg.* **2019**, *55*, 116–132. [CrossRef]
45. Ledda, C.; Senia, P.; Rapisarda, V. Biomarkers for Early Diagnosis and Prognosis of Malignant Pleural Mesothelioma: The Quest Goes on. *Cancers* **2018**, *10*, 203. [CrossRef]
46. Robinson, B.W.; Creaney, J.; Lake, R.; Nowak, A.; Musk, A.W.; de Klerk, N.; Winzell, P.; Hellstrom, K.E.; Hellstrom, I. Mesothelin-family proteins and diagnosis of mesothelioma. *Lancet* **2003**, *362*, 1612–1616. [CrossRef]
47. Creaney, J.; Robinson, B.W.S. Malignant Mesothelioma Biomarkers: From Discovery to Use in Clinical Practice for Diagnosis, Monitoring, Screening, and Treatment. *Chest* **2017**, *152*, 143–149. [CrossRef]
48. Cui, A.; Jin, X.-G.; Zhai, K.; Tong, Z.-H.; Shi, H.-Z. Diagnostic values of soluble mesothelin-related peptides for malignant pleural mesothelioma: Updated meta-analysis. *BMJ Open* **2014**, *4*, e004145. [CrossRef]
49. Pass, H.I.; Wolaniuk, D.; Wali, A.; Thiel, R.; Hellstrom, I.; Sardesai, N.Y. Soluble mesothelin related peptides: A potential biomarker for malignant pleural mesothelioma. *J. Clin. Oncol.* **2005**, *23*, 9532. [CrossRef]
50. Davies, H.E.; Sadler, R.S.; Bielsa, S.; Maskell, N.A.; Rahman, N.M.; Davies, R.J.O.; Ferry, B.L.; Lee, Y.C.G. Clinical Impact and Reliability of Pleural Fluid Mesothelin in Undiagnosed Pleural Effusions. *Am. J. Respir. Crit. Care Med.* **2009**, *180*, 437–444. [CrossRef] [PubMed]
51. Hooper, C.E.; Morley, A.J.; Virgo, P.; Harvey, J.E.; Kahan, B.; Maskell, N.A. A prospective trial evaluating the role of mesothelin in undiagnosed pleural effusions. *Eur. Respir. J.* **2013**, *41*, 18–24. [CrossRef]
52. Hu, Z.-D.; Liu, X.-F.; Ding, C.-M.; Hu, C.-J. Diagnostic accuracy of osteopontin for malignant pleural mesothelioma: A systematic review and meta-analysis. *Clin. Chim. Acta* **2014**, *433*, 44–48. [CrossRef]
53. Pass, H.I.; Levin, S.M.; Harbut, M.R.; Melamed, J.; Chiriboga, L.; Donington, J.; Huflejt, M.; Carbone, M.; Chia, D.; Goodglick, L.; et al. Fibulin-3 as a Blood and Effusion Biomarker for Pleural Mesothelioma. *New Engl. J. Med.* **2012**, *367*, 1417–1427. [CrossRef]
54. Creaney, J.; Dick, I.M.; Meniawy, T.; Leong, S.L.; Leon, J.S.; Demelker, Y.; Segal, A.; Musk, A.W.B.; Lee, Y.C.G.; Skates, S.J.; et al. Comparison of fibulin-3 and mesothelin as markers in malignant mesothelioma. *Thorax* **2014**, *69*, 895–902. [CrossRef] [PubMed]
55. Kirschner, M.B.; Pulford, E.; Hoda, M.A.; Rozsas, A.; Griggs, K.; Cheng, Y.Y.; Edelman, J.J.B.; Kao, S.C.; Hyland, R.; Dong, Y.; et al. Fibulin-3 levels in malignant pleural mesothelioma are associated with prognosis but not diagnosis. *Br. J. Cancer* **2015**, *113*, 963–969. [CrossRef]
56. Ren, R.; Yin, P.; Zhang, Y.; Zhou, J.; Zhou, Y.; Xu, R.; Lin, H.; Huang, C. Diagnostic value of fibulin-3 for malignant pleural mesothelioma: A systematic review and meta-analysis. *Oncotarget* **2016**, *7*, 84851–84859. [CrossRef]
57. Pei, D.; Li, Y.; Liu, X.; Yan, S.; Guo, X.; Xu, X.; Guo, X. Diagnostic and prognostic utilities of humoral fibulin-3 in malignant pleural mesothelioma: Evidence from a meta-analysis. *Oncotarget* **2017**, *8*, 13030–13038. [CrossRef]
58. Tsim, S.; Kelly, C.; Alexander, L.; McCormick, C.; Thomson, F.; Woodward, R.; Foster, J.E.; Stobo, D.B.; Paul, J.; Maskell, N.A.; et al. Diagnostic and Prognostic Biomarkers in the Rational Assessment of Mesothelioma (DIAPHRAGM) study: Protocol of a prospective, multicentre, observational study. *BMJ Open* **2016**, *6*, e013324. [CrossRef]
59. Usuda, K.; Iwai, S.; Funasaki, A.; Sekimura, A.; Motono, N.; Matoba, M.; Doai, M.; Yamada, S.; Ueda, Y.; Uramoto, H. Diffusion-Weighted Imaging Can Differentiate between Malignant and Benign Pleural Diseases. *Cancers* **2019**, *11*, 811. [CrossRef] [PubMed]
60. Leung, A.N.; Müller, N.L.; Miller, R.R. CT in differential diagnosis of diffuse pleural disease. *Am. J. Roentgenol.* **1990**, *154*, 487–492. [CrossRef] [PubMed]
61. Blyth, K.G.; Murphy, D. Progress and challenges in Mesothelioma: From bench to bedside. *Respir. Med.* **2018**, *134*, 31–41. [CrossRef]
62. Treglia, G.; Sadeghi, R.; Annunziata, S.; Lococo, F.; Cafarotti, S.; Bertagna, F.; Prior, J.O.; Ceriani, L.; Giovanella, L. Diagnostic accuracy of 18F-FDG-PET and PET/CT in the differential diagnosis between malignant and benign pleural lesions: A systematic review and meta-analysis. *Acad. Radiol.* **2014**, *21*, 11–20. [CrossRef] [PubMed]
63. DeFonseka, D. PET-CT in the Undiagnosed Effusion: Results of the TARGET Study. In Proceedings of the British Thoracic Society Winter Meeting, London, UK, 4–6 December 2019.
64. Tsim, S.; Cowell, G.W.; Kidd, A.; Woodward, R.; Alexander, L.; Kelly, C.; E Foster, J.; Blyth, K.G. A comparison between MRI and CT in the assessment of primary tumour volume in mesothelioma. *Lung Cancer* **2020**, *150*, 12–20. [CrossRef]

65. Lacerenza, S.; Ciregia, F.; Giusti, L.; Bonotti, A.; Greco, V.; Giannaccini, G.; D'Antongiovanni, V.; Fallahi, P.; Pieroni, L.; Cristaudo, A.; et al. Putative Biomarkers for Malignant Pleural Mesothelioma Suggested by Proteomic Analysis of Cell Secretome. *Cancer Genom. Proteom.* **2020**, *17*, 225–236. [CrossRef]
66. Sage, A.P.; Martinez, V.D.; Minatel, B.C.; Pewarchuk, M.E.; Marshall, E.A.; Macaulay, G.M.; Hubaux, R.; Pearson, D.D.; Goodarzi, A.A.; Dellaire, G.; et al. Genomics and Epigenetics of Malignant Mesothelioma. *High Throughput* **2018**, *7*, 20. [CrossRef]
67. Joseph, N.M.; Chen, Y.-Y.; Nasr, A.; Yeh, I.; Talevich, E.; Onodera, C.; Bastian, B.; Rabban, J.T.; Garg, K.; Zaloudek, C.; et al. Genomic profiling of malignant peritoneal mesothelioma reveals recurrent alterations in epigenetic regulatory genes BAP1, SETD2, and DDX3X. *Mod. Pathol.* **2017**, *30*, 246–254. [CrossRef] [PubMed]
68. Cakiroglu, E.; Senturk, S. Genomics and Functional Genomics of Malignant Pleural Mesothelioma. *Int. J. Mol. Sci.* **2020**, *21*, 6342. [CrossRef] [PubMed]
69. Weber, D.G.; Gawrych, K.; Casjens, S.; Brik, A.; Lehnert, M.; Taeger, D.; Pesch, B.; Kollmeier, J.; Bauer, T.T.; Johnen, G.; et al. Circulating miR-132-3p as a Candidate Diagnostic Biomarker for Malignant Mesothelioma. *Dis. Markers* **2017**, *2017*, 9280170. [CrossRef]
70. Zhou, X.-M.; He, C.-C.; Liu, Y.-M.; Zhao, Y.; Zhao, D.; Du, Y.; Zheng, W.-Y.; Li, J.-X. Metabonomic classification and detection of small molecule biomarkers of malignant pleural effusions. *Anal. Bioanal. Chem.* **2012**, *404*, 3123–3133. [CrossRef] [PubMed]
71. Zennaro, L.; Vanzani, P.; Nicolè, L.; Cappellesso, R.; Fassina, A. Metabonomics by proton nuclear magnetic resonance in human pleural effusions: A route to discriminate between benign and malignant pleural effusions and to target small molecules as potential cancer biomarkers. *Cancer Cytopathol.* **2017**, *125*, 341–348. [CrossRef]
72. Tsim, S.; Paterson, S.; Cartwright, D.; Fong, C.J.; Alexander, L.; Kelly, C.; Holme, J.; Evison, M.; Blyth, K.G. Baseline predictors of negative and incomplete pleural cytology in patients with suspected pleural malignancy—Data supporting 'Direct to LAT' in selected groups. *Lung Cancer* **2019**, *133*, 123–129. [CrossRef]

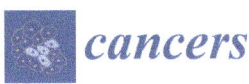 *cancers*

Article

Liquid Biopsies from Pleural Effusions and Plasma from Patients with Malignant Pleural Mesothelioma: A Feasibility Study

Gabriele Moretti [1], Paolo Aretini [2], Francesca Lessi [2], Chiara Maria Mazzanti [2], Guntulu Ak [3,4], Muzaffer Metintaş [3,4], Cecilia Lando [5], Rosa Angela Filiberti [5], Marco Lucchi [6], Alessandra Bonotti [7], Rudy Foddis [8], Alfonso Cristaudo [8], Andrea Bottari [1], Alessandro Apollo [1], Marzia Del Re [9], Romano Danesi [9], Luciano Mutti [10], Federica Gemignani [1,*] and Stefano Landi [1]

1 Department of Biology, Genetic Unit, University of Pisa, via Derna 3, 56126 Pisa, Italy; gabriele.moretti@student.unisi.it (G.M.); a.bottari@studenti.unipi.it (A.B.); alessandro.apollo@humanitasresearch.it (A.A.); stefano.landi@unipi.it (S.L.)
2 Fondazione Pisana per la Scienza, Via Ferruccio Giovannini 13, 56017 San Giuliano Terme, Italy; p.aretini@fpscience.it (P.A.); f.lessi@fpscience.it (F.L.); c.mazzanti@fpscience.it (C.M.M.)
3 Eskisehir Osmangazi University Lung and Pleural Cancers Research and Clinical Center, Eskisehir 26000, Turkey; guntuluak@ogu.edu.tr (G.A.); mmetintas@ogu.edu.tr (M.M.)
4 Department of Chest Diseases, Medical Faculty, Eskisehir Osmangazi University, Eskisehir 26000, Turkey
5 IRCCS Ospedale Policlinico San Martino, Clinical Epidemiology, 16132 Genova, Italy; ceciliafrancesca.lando@hsanmartino.it (C.L.); rosa.filiberti@hsanmartino.it (R.A.F.)
6 Division of Thoracic Surgery, Cardiac-Thoracic and Vascular Department, University Hospital of Pisa, 56124 Pisa, Italy; m.lucchi@med.unipi.it
7 Preventive and Occupational Medicine, University Hospital of Pisa, 56126 Pisa, Italy; abonotti@yahoo.it
8 Department of Translational Research and of New Technologies in Medicine and Surgery, University of Pisa, 56126 Pisa, Italy; rudy.foddis@med.unipi.it (R.F.); alfonso.cristaudo@med.unipi.it (A.C.)
9 Division of Pharmacology, Department of Internal Medicine, University of Pisa, 55, Via Roma, 56126 Pisa, Italy; marzia.delre@ao-pisa.toscana.it (M.D.R.); romano.danesi@unipi.it (R.D.)
10 Sbarro Institute for Cancer Research and Molecular Medicine, Center for Biotechnology, College of Science and Technology, Temple University, Philadelphia, PA 19104, USA; luciano.mutti@temple.edu
* Correspondence: federica.gemignani@unipi.it

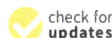

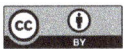

Simple Summary: Patients with malignant pleural mesothelioma (MPM) often have to wait a long time before receiving a diagnosis. To contribute to the research on this neoplasm, we analyzed various samples of tumor biopsy and the relative liquid biopsies from both plasma and pleural fluid. We tested the possibility of obtaining information about the tumor in a quicker and less invasive way compared to the usual solid biopsy. We performed NGS on blood and tumor samples from patients and obtained a list of somatic mutations. With the digital droplet PCR technique, we tested the respective pleural fluids and plasma for the previously found mutations. We discovered that pleural fluid is a good proxy to obtain the mutational landscape of the MPM. We also tracked tumor DNA in plasma, leading to the idea that this could be used in a clinical setting to perform follow-ups of patients and monitor drug responses.

Abstract: Background: Malignant pleural mesothelioma (MPM) is a fatal tumor with a poor prognosis. The recent developments of liquid biopsies could provide novel diagnostic and prognostic tools in oncology. However, there is limited information about the feasibility of this technique for MPMs. Here, we investigate whether cancer-specific DNA sequences can be detected in pleural fluids and plasma of MPM patients as free circulating tumor DNA (ctDNA). Methods: We performed whole-exome sequencing on 14 tumor biopsies from 14 patients, and we analyzed 20 patient-specific somatic mutations with digital droplet PCR (ddPCR) in pleural fluids and plasma, using them as cancer-specific tumor biomarkers. Results: Most of the selected mutations could be detected in pleural fluids (94%) and, noteworthy, in plasma (83%) with the use of ddPCR. Pleural fluids showed similar levels of somatically mutated ctDNA (median = 12.75%, average = 16.3%, standard deviation = 12.3) as those detected in solid biopsies (median = 21.95%; average = 22.21%; standard deviation = 9.57), and their paired difference was weakly statistically significant ($p = 0.048$). On the other hand, the paired difference between solid biopsies and ctDNA from plasma (median = 0.29%, average = 0.89%, standard deviation = 1.40) was highly statistically significant ($p = 2.5 \times 10^{-7}$), corresponding to the important drop of circulating somatically mutated DNA in the bloodstream. However, despite the tiny amount of ctDNA in plasma, varying from 5.57% down to 0.14%, the mutations were detectable at rates similar to those possible for other tumors. Conclusions: We found robust evidence that mutated DNA is spilled from MPMs, mostly into pleural fluids, proving the concept that liquid biopsies are feasible for MPM patients.

Keywords: malignant pleural mesothelioma; liquid biopsies; circulating tumor DNA; plasma; cancer-specific mutations; genomics; cancer biomarkers

1. Introduction

Malignant pleural mesothelioma (MPM) is a fatal cancer that arises from the mesothelial cells of the pleura. Asbestos exposure and the host's predisposing conditions (e.g., inherited mutations within *BAP1* or a chronic inflammatory state of the pleura [1]) play a role in the carcinogenesis of this neoplasm. Fibers are hypothesized to trigger a chronic inflammatory status, inducing a condition known as "frustrated apoptosis" of macrophages [2] and leading to increased production of oxygen reactive species, DNA damage, and cell proliferation, eventually initiating and promoting the malignant process [3,4]. The latency between exposure to asbestos fibers and diagnosis usually takes decades [5], and the first symptoms (which include, but are not limited to, chest pain, breathing difficulties, dyspnea, or increased abdominal volume) are common to other respiratory conditions [6], making a prompt diagnosis very difficult. Widely used imaging methods are not sufficient for the diagnosis of MPM. Thus, to achieve a reliable diagnosis, one needs to perform a biopsy through video-assisted thoracoscopy (VATS) [7,8], although this invasive procedure cannot be routinely used to assess the successive genetic changes.

Liquid biopsies (LBs) represent an innovative approach under development and consist of the analysis of genetic material extracted from body fluids. Events like apoptosis, necroptosis, and cell migration may result in the dispersion of tumor cells or their debris in the fluids surrounding the tumor mass [9]. Therefore, under these circumstances, it is possible to detect circulating tumor cells (CTCs), circulating cell-free tumor DNA (ctDNA), tumor proteins, and tumor-derived extracellular vesicles (tEVs, which include exosomes) in plasma, urine, or other body fluids [9]. Numerous studies have confirmed the possibility of gaining information on many kinds of tumors via blood samples. At first, CTCs were isolated and examined to get more insight into tumor progression and mutational history [10]. CTC phenotypic characterization and count can give hints on the tumor stage and expansion, whereas their DNA can provide information about the tumor mutational landscape [10]. Similarly, ctDNA could also be useful for LBs. In cancer patients, up to 1% of circulating nucleic acids are derived from tumor cells. The ability to isolate and analyze this DNA has made it possible to detect circulating mutations deriving from hepatocellular, breast, lung, and pancreatic carcinoma [11–14]. Evidence suggests the possibility of inferring or confirming the diagnosis of these tumors and performing clinical follow-ups by tracking the mutational load in response to therapies. In specific cases, such as lung adenocarcinoma, the monitoring of mutated ctDNA could provide important information to adjust a personalized therapy based on the use of anti-EGFR drugs [15,16]. On the other hand, other tumors (such as glioblastoma) are not equally capable of spilling ctDNA into the bloodstream [17], and the knowledge, in this regard, on MPM is limited. CtDNA from MPM patients has been analyzed in two previous studies. In 2012, higher DNA integrity was detected in cytologically negative pleural fluids (PFs) from 16 MPM patients (median = 1.2) compared to 23 noncancer patients (median = 0.8). The conclusion is that this biomarker, along with others (e.g., mesothelin), could improve the specificity and sensitivity needed to discriminate MPM from non-MPM patients [18]. More recently, in 2018, 10 MPM patients were analyzed for ctDNA (half of them were treatment-naïve). In this work, tumor biopsies were sequenced, and ctDNA was investigated in plasma samples via digital-droplets PCR (ddPCR). The authors showed that more than half of the treatment-naïve subjects showed positive droplets for mutated ctDNA in their blood samples, demonstrating the presence of tumor-specific mutations in circulating DNA [19]. However, the number of analyzed patients was limited, and not all of them showed mutated ctDNA from MPM in their bloodstream. Furthermore, no other fluids have been analyzed in the attempt to find an alternative approach to increasing the analysis' sensitivity. In order to fill the lack of knowledge on this topic, we analyzed a series of 14 MPM patients and carried out more systematic research on solid tumor biopsies, PF, and plasma withdrawn from the same patient. Thus, we could show that the share of somatically mutated cancer-specific DNA from PFs is similar to that detected in solid biopsies and that the same somatic mutations can also be detected, in tiny amounts, in the plasma of the same patient. Therefore, this feasibility study provides evidence that, in the future, PFs and plasma could constitute a valuable source of information, allowing for the diagnosis, follow-up, and stratification of MPM patients.

2. Materials and Methods

2.1. Patients Cohorts

We analyzed samples from patients diagnosed with MPM from three different hospital centers; we divided them into two groups based on the availability of blood samples.

Group GE consisted of 7 frozen tumor biopsies from San Martino Hospital in Genoa (Italy); each of them was associated with frozen samples of plasma and PF. Biopsies were about 1 mm^3 in size. PF, collected from patients' pleural effusions, and plasma samples were available in different amounts for each subject, ranging from 3 to 6 mL. Patients were diagnosed with MPM at an average age of 71 during the period 2002–2012. All of them were deceased at the moment of this analysis, having a median survival time since diagnosis of 4.6 months, with a minimum of 1 month and a maximum of 33.

Group PT (Pisa and Turkey) consisted of biopsies, frozen whole-blood, and frozen plasma samples from 2 patients (P) from the University Hospital of Cisanello in Pisa (Italy) and 5 patients (T) from Eskişehir Osmangazi University Hospital in Turkey in the period 2017–2019. Patients were diagnosed at a median age of 68. All of them were deceased at the time of the analysis, with a median survival time since diagnosis of 8.9 months and a minimum of 6.4 months and a maximum of 15.5 months. The size of the biopsies was about 1 mm^3, and the volumes of whole blood and plasma were 2 and 1.5 mL, respectively. For patients T, a sample of PF was also available (2 mL). Patients' information is reported in Table S1.

2.2. Sequencing and Filtering

In order to discern somatic from germline mutations, whole-exome sequencing (WES) was carried out on solid biopsies and buffy coats withdrawn from the same patient of Group PT, while specific algorithms and filtering procedures were employed for the patients of Group GE. Genomic DNA was extracted using a PureLink™ Genomic DNA Mini Kit (Thermo Fisher Scientific; Waltham, MA, USA), following manufacturer protocol. This was used for both blood and tumor samples. The final DNA samples' concentration was measured with a Qbit3 (Thermo Fischer Scientific; Waltham, MA, USA). WES was performed on a NextSeq 550 (Illumina; San Diego, CA, USA) and the library was prepared using the kit from the same producer (Nextera DNA Flex Pre-Enrichment Library Prep and Enrichment). Sequencing indexes were also provided by the same manufacturer. Alignment of the resulting FASTA files was performed with Burrows-Wheeler Aligner software [20]. The calling of somatic mutations for the tumor samples was performed with VarScan [21], where paired blood was available; for the remaining cases, GATK tool Mutect2 [22] was used. The resulting single nucleotide variations (SNVs) were annotated using the VEP online tool from the Ensembl portal (http://grch37.ensembl.org/Homo_sapiens/Tools/VEP/ accessed on 16 March 2019).

Since no blood was available for Group GE whereas it was available for the PT group, two alternative filtering procedures, FGE and FPT, were carried out.

FGE was carried out as follows. To maximize the chances of selecting a somatic mutation, we considered those with a ratio of alternative allele reads (i.e., alternative depth, AD) to total reads (i.e., total depth, TD) of 0.25 or lower. This is because such a ratio may originate from mutated tumor cells, whereas a higher ratio could indicate a homozygous or heterozygous mutation present in all the sample's cells, which is less likely somatic. Another parameter of FGE filtering excluded the mutations within noncoding regions. This was done to allow an easier interpretation of the functional consequence of the variation in the context of the carcinogenic progression. The last filter condition required mutations to have an AD greater than 20X and a minor allele frequency (MAF) in the population $\leq 10^{-4}$, according to gnomAD (https://gnomad.broadinstitute.org accessed on 16 March 2019). The former parameter ensures a good NGS quality, while the latter allows us to take into account the negative selection a mutation undergoes in the population, decreasing the possibility of it being germline.

FPT consisted, firstly, in the use of VarScan2, a software based on the statistical analysis of a coverage value for both reference and alternative bases, comparing that found in blood with that of the paired tumor. Then, further filtering was applied using the following criteria: (i) a minor allele frequency (MAF) <1% among Europeans, according to gnomAD, (ii) a read depth $\geq$20X, and (iii) AD = 0 in the blood sample.

From the final list of SNVs obtained with the filtering procedures, up to 5 mutations per patient were selected for further experimental validation. This last choice did not follow a strict criterion but was based on a variety of criteria that included (i) mutations present on a gene already filed for MPM within COSMIC or TCGA databases (https://cancer.sanger.ac.uk/cosmic, https://www.cancer.gov/tcga accessed on 16 March 2019), (ii) the lack of any repeated sequence in the neighboring region of the SNV, and (iii) the lack of paralogues/gene families of the mutated genes.

2.3. Validation and Biostatistical Analysis

SNVs selected following WES were verified in tumor biopsies with an allele-specific oligonucleotide and a real-time quantitative PCR method (ASO–qPCR). For each SNV, the real-time curve obtained with mutation-specific primers was compared with the curve obtained with specific primers designed for the wild-type allele. The results were also compared to the same assay performed on DNA extracted from the whole blood of a healthy subject (reference). This analysis is not quantitative enough to measure the amount of mutated DNA. On the other hand, it is inexpensive and sensitive enough to verify the presence/absence of small amounts of mutated alleles among a plethora of wild-type alleles. Experiments were performed with a CFX96 thermal cycler (Bio-Rad; Hercules, CA, USA) using 5× HOT FIREPol® EvaGreen® qPCR Mix Plus (Solis Biodyne; Tartu, EE, Estonia) and custom oligonucleotides primers (Europhins Genomics, Louxemburg, LU). When ASO–qPCR confirmed the mutation in tumor DNA, we proceeded by using the more sensitive ddPCR for quantification. Thus, for each patient, ddPCR was applied on tumor samples as well as other available fluids.

Circulating DNA was extracted using a QIAamp Circulating Nucleic Acid Kit (Qiagen; Venlo, NL, Netherlands), and the concentrations were measured with a Qbit (Thermo Fisher Scientific; Waltham, MA, USA). DdPCR was used to measure and compare the amount of mutated DNA (using mutation-specific probes) in tumor, blood, PF, and plasma. DNA from a healthy individual and a blank (buffer only) were used as negative controls. We used a QX100 droplet generator to form the reaction droplets and a QX200 droplet reader (Bio-Rad; Hercules, CA, USA) to get the results. The PCR amplification reaction was performed in a T100 thermal cycler from the same manufacturer. For each SNV, we used a pair of TaqMan-like probes, each targeted either to the variant or the common allele, the former being labeled with FAM and the latter with HEX fluorophore. Probes and primers were designed using Bio-Rad's online probes design tool. The reaction mix used was Bio-Rad's ddPCR Supermix for Probes (No dUTP). Differences in the amount of mutated ctDNA from plasma or PF compared to that measured in solid biopsies (as reference) were evaluated with a paired Student's *t*-test analysis, following arcsin transformation for non-normally distributed data, and the nonparametric Wilcoxon signed-rank test.

3. Results

3.1. GE patients, NGS Analysis

For Group GE, NGS analysis yielded an average of 78.67 million reads per tumor, with a mean length of 122 bases. Across all samples, 87.1% of the reads were correctly aligned with the reference, with a mean mapping quality of 59.5 and an average coverage inside the exome regions of 97.7X. After the analysis with the Mutect2 tool, which computed all mismatches in the reads to find mutations, we obtained 97,826 to 123,405 variants, depending on the sample (Table 1). Of those variants, 6.9–10.8% were indels (insertion/deletions) and 89.2–93.1% were SNVs, with an average median coverage of 102X. The values of this parameter fitted a Laplace distribution with a mean of 41.5X.

Then, FGE was optimized to maximize the likelihood of selecting truly somatic mutations. Firstly, variants with the number of AD reads (the ones covering the alternative allele) lower than 25% (arbitrarily chosen), relative to TD (total depth), were positively selected. Between 1065 and 3053 variants passed this step, depending on the sample (Table 1). The second step of selection included only the SNVs within the coding regions (between 593 and 1342). A further step of the FGE procedure was carried out by excluding the variants with less than 20 reads covering the genomic position. Then, among the selected SNVs, those with a MAF $\geq 10^{-4}$ (global, according to gnomAD, arbitrary threshold) were excluded as well. A number of SNVs, between 42 and 184, remained in the final list.

3.2. In GE Patients, Selected Somatic Mutations Were Detected in ctDNA from Plasma and PFs

A total of 25 mutations within 25 genes in 7 subjects were evaluated with ASO–qPCR in tumor biopsies, and 14 were confirmed by this method. The list encompassed *COL1A2*, *BACE2*, *MYBPC1*, *TRPC7*, *ARPP21*, *OR4K2*, *HIST1H2AD*, *OR5AC2*, *SZT2*, *AMPH*, *SPTAN1*, *NLGN1*, *DICER1*, and *FLI1*; most of them had already been reported as somatically mutated in the MPM patients, according to COSMIC or TCGA databases (Table 1). Four SNVs within *BAP1*, *LATS2*, *MUC16*, and *FLG*, the genes most frequently mutated in MPM, together with other 7 mutations in *POTEF*, *RAD50*, *FGFR1*, *UNC79*, *ERBB4*, *CSMD3*, and *CCNL2*, could not be confirmed by ASO–qPCR and were not investigated further with ddPCR.

Table 1. Selected mutations analyzed for Group GE after FGE filtering and relative ASO–qPCR and ddPCR results.

ID	NGS				Selected SNVs				Reads			ddPCR		
	SNV Tot	AD/TD ≤ 0.25	Coding	MAF < 10^{-4} & AD > 20	Gene	Type	ID or Position	MAF [a]	AD/TD	AD (%)	qPCR	% of Variant Allele		
												Tumor	PF	Plasma
696	104,367	1330	797	45	POTEF	S	NM_001099771.2:c.2118T > C	NA	22/112	19.64	No	-	-	-
					COL1A2	S	rs773494330	4.00 × 10^{-6}	23/110	20.91	Yes	0.00	Inhibitor	0.00
1148	106,264	1985	938	122	BACE2	M	rs770736773, COSM5907863	4.00 × 10^{-5}	20/91	21.98	Yes	23.05	Inhibitor	0.16
					BAP1	FS	NM_004656.1:g.52443623del	NA	31/219	14.16	No	-	-	-
					MUC16	M	rs75266616	9.11 × 10^{-5}	22/100	22.00	No	-	-	-
					RAD50	FS	rs7726677708, COSM1143045	2.10 × 10^{-4}	23/197	11.68	No	-	-	-
1725	98,442	1981	920	88	MYBPC1	M	rs752347381	8.00 × 10^{-6}	26/140	18.57	Yes	20.80	23.80	26.55
					TRPC7	M	rs566980923	<10^{-6} [b]	40/256	15.63	Yes	12.50	4.90	0.00
					ARPP21	M	rs1481888266	8.88 × 10^{-6}	22/124	17.74	Yes	16.65	16.00	0.26
					OR4K2	M	rs757533510	4.00 × 10^{-6}	25/98	25.51	Yes	22.40	22.80	24.05
2294	101,976	1810	886	96	FLG	S	rs564106508, COSM5531298	3.60 × 10^{-5}	24/196	12.24	No	-	-	-
					FGFR1	IF	rs138489552	7.20 × 10^{-5}	22/143	15.38	No	-	-	-
					UNC79	M	NM_020818.1:g.94110000C > A	NA	21/99	21.21	No	-	-	-
					HIST1H2AD	M	NM_021065.1:g.26199201G > A	NA	24/217	11.06	Yes	12.05	16.45	0.79
					OR5AC2	S	rs1021819573	2.72 × 10^{-5}	25/163	15.34	Yes	11.10	12.10	5.57
2324	123,405	2852	1178	184	ERBB4	M	NC_000002.12:g.211561993C > T	NA	21/173	12.14	No	-	-	-
					SZT2	M	rs760370909	4.00 × 10^{-6}	27/143	18.88	Yes	0.00	0.00	0.00
2438	97,826	1065	593	42	AMPH	M	COSM1673120 (C > A)	NA [c]	25/171	14.62	Yes	15.10	4.01	0.17
					SPTAN1	M	NM_001130438.3:c.252G > C	NA	28/141	19.86	Yes	21.85	20.20	0.52
					NLGN1	M	COSM4579730 (G > T)	NA [d]	23/104	22.12	Yes	21.95	1.59	0.00
2829	105,292	3053	1342	116	LATS2	S	NM_014572.3:c.1698C > A	NA [e]	22/173	12.72	No	-	-	-
					CSMD3	M	COSM6112252 (G > T)	NA	47/222	21.17	No	-	-	-
					CCNL2	M	NM_030937.3:c.1322747G > T	NA	23/145	15.86	Yes	0.00	0.00	0.00
					DICER1	M	rs775912475	8.00 × 10^{-6}	22/234	9.40	No	-	-	-
					FLI1	M	rs1288594591	4.00 × 10^{-6}	25/156	16.03	Yes	11.88	10.24	0.55

MAF = minor allele frequency; TD = total depth; AD = alternative depth; MA = mutated allele; PF = pleural fluid; S = synonymous; M = missense; FS = frame shift; IF = in frame; SG = stop gain. [a] According to gnomAD (https://gnomad.broadinstitute.org, accessed on 16 March 2019), global frequency. [b] This SNV does not have a frequency in gnomAD (https://gnomad.broadinstitute.org accessed on 16 March 2019). [c] There is a nearby SNP, rs140004238 (G > A), with a global frequency of 3.98 × 10^{-6}, at 7:38516516 (+1bp). [d] There is a SNP, rs134959137 (G > C), with a global frequency of 3.19 × 10^{-5}, at the same genomic position. [e] There is a nearby SNP, rs137701277 (A > G), with a global frequency of 3.98 × 10^{-6}, at 8:113988191 (+2 bp).

The measurements carried out with ddPCR on the 14 confirmed mutations showed that 3 (*COL1A2*-rs773494330, ID = 696; *SZT2*-rs760370909, ID = 2324; *DICER1*-rs775912475, ID = 2829) could not be detected in tumor biopsies with ddPCR, whereas positive results were obtained for 11 mutations found in the biopsies of 7 patients (3 patients were positive for 1 mutation and 4 patients were positive for 2 mutations), as reported in Table 1.

When PFs were analyzed, samples from 6 patients were available. One, ID = 696, could not be analyzed because the amplification failed several times, even after adopting alternative protocols for DNA extraction, suggesting the presence of unknown PCR inhibitors. Thus, only 10 mutations could be compared between tumor biopsies and PFs. Interestingly, for 7 of them, the share of mutated alleles measured in PFs was similar (ranging from 10.24% to 20.20%) to that measured in the respective tumor biopsies. The remaining three mutations showed a reduced amount; however, they were still detectable to a significant extent: *TRPC7*-rs566980923 (ID = 1148), 12.5% in tumor and 4.9% in PF; *AMPH*-COSM1673120 (ID = 2324), 15.1% (tumor) and 4.01% (PF); *NLGN1*-COSM479730 (ID = 2438), 21.95% and 1.59%, respectively (Table 1).

Interestingly, 9 out of 11 mutations of tumor biopsies were also detected in the ctDNA from plasma. Two, *TRPC7*-rs566980923 ID = 1148 and *NLGN1*-COSM479730 ID = 2438, were undetected, and this was in agreement with the low quantity already detected in the respective PF samples. Of the 9 detectable mutations, 2 (*MYBPC1*-rs752347381 ID = 1148 and *OR4K2*-rs757533510 ID = 2294) were likely germline. In fact, for these mutations, the percentage of the alternative allele in PF and plasma was about 25% and of a similar range to that measured in the tumor biopsies. However, as reported in Table 1, the remaining seven mutations were most likely somatic and showed a percentage ranging between 0.16% and 0.79%, whereas their corresponding share within the tumor biopsies ranged between 11.1% and 23.05%. The one showing the highest amount was *OR5AC2*-rs1021819573 (ID = 2294) with a percentage of 5.57 (it was 11.1 in the tumor). Thus, 6 out of 7 patients showed ctDNA in their plasma. Only patient ID = 1148 could not be traced using the selected mutations. Unfortunately, the analysis of the other patient's mutations could not be carried out because of the lack of additional vials of plasma.

3.3. PT Patients, NGS Analysis

NGS analysis on Group PT yielded an average of 80.66 million reads for each subject's tumor sample. The average read length was 98 bases. Across all samples, 70% of the reads were correctly aligned in the exome reference region, with a mapping quality of 54.9 and an average coverage of 72X. After the analysis with the software VarScan2 for each tumor–blood pair, we identified between 102,753 and 130,073 SNVs, of which 1948–3120 were marked as somatic (Table 2). The TD values had a median of 45 and fitted a Laplace distribution with a mean of 50X. The indels were not evaluated in our assays; however, they consisted of a share ranging from 8.89% to 14% of the total variations. FPT consisted of selecting mutations within coding regions, eliciting from 158 to 281 SNVs. Then, SNVs with TD < 20 and a population MAF > 1% (global according to gnomAD) were excluded. The resulting 54–104 SNVs were further filtered by including only mutations with AD = 0 in blood samples, yielding 2 to 42 mutations. Finally, among the available variants filtered for both groups, we selected two mutations per sample for further analyses, as specified in "Materials and Methods" (Tables 1 and 2).

Table 2. Selected mutations analyzed for Group PT after FPT filtering and relative ASO-qPCR and ddPCR results.

							NGS							ddPCR		
							Selected SNVs								% of Variant Allele	
ID	SNV Tot	Somatic [v]	Coding	MAF < 1% & TD > 20	AD = 0 in Blood	Gene	Type	ID or Position	MAF [a]	AD/TD (Blood)	AD/TD (Tumor)	AD (%) (Tumor)	qPCR	Blood	Tumor	PF	Plasma
01T	122,995	2509	158	54	2	JADE1	S	rs775483821	3.99×10^{-6}	0/81	13/53	24.53	Yes	0.00	7.48	12.75	0.20
						SS18	M	NM_001007559.3:c.98A > G	NA	0/44	6/20	30.00	Yes	0.06	0.00	0.10	-
02T	102,753	1948	203	97	22	FLT1	M	NM_002019.4:c.3697C > A	NA	0/125	23/55	41.82	Yes	0.07	32.85	24.85	2.68
						BAP1	SG	COSM4411449(C > T)	NA [b]	0/145	21/96	21.88	Yes	0.00	33.50	22.90	1.39
03T	117,237	2525	281	104	39	DCAF8	M	COSM3319811	NA	0/105	47/129	36.43	Yes	0.00	33.95	36.35	0.58
						PEG10	M	rs368939059 COSM1093296	8.03×10^{-6}	0/78	42/102	41.18	Yes	0.00	35.90	39.70	1.65
04T	130,073	2755	152	75	27	FAM71B	M	rs1404037352	1.6×10^{-5}	0/145	38/138	27.54	Yes	0.00	30.80	9.70	N.A.
						CSMD2	S	rs770364421, COSM5951197	6.60×10^{-5}	0/118	32/117	27.35	Yes	1.45	25.00	8.95	N.A.
05T	126,782	2833	227	81	23	FAT1	M	rs776531396	4.01×10^{-6}	0/150	61/236	25.85	Yes	0.07	23.25	0.00	0.00
						BAP1	SG	rs771713346, COSM6945226	4.00×10^{-6}	0/93	18/75	24.00	Yes	0.00	31.75	36.50	0.14
02P	128,899	3027	266	66	13	VIL1	S	NM_007127.3:c.2070C > T	NA	0/293	29/143	20.28	Yes	0.04	13.20	N.A.	0.29
						OR10A4	M	rs547489107	4.40×10^{-5}	0/137	14/62	22.58	No	-	-	N.A.	-
03P	122,214	3120	239	88	42	NF2	SG	NM_016418.5:c.985A > T	NA	0/155	10/37	27.03	Yes	0.00	15.85	N.A.	0.14
						NLRP6	SG	NM_138329.2:c.403G > T	NA	0/123	30/151	19.87	No	-	-	N.A.	-

MAF = minor allele frequency; TD = total depth; AD = alternative depth; PF = pleural fluid; S = synonymous; M = missense; SG = stop gain. [v] Predicted by VarScan2 tool (DOI:10.1101/gr.129684.111); [a] according to gnomAD (https://gnomad.broadinstitute.org accessed on 16 March 2019), global frequency. [b] There is a SNP, rs770127999 (C > A), with a global frequency of 4.00×10^{-6}, at the same genomic position.

3.4. Selected Mutations for Group PT were also Detected in the ctDNA from Plasma and PF

Fourteen mutations were analyzed with ASO–qPCR in Group PT, and twelve (two for each T patient and one for each P patient) could be confirmed in the tumor biopsies (*OR10A4*-rs547489107 and *NLRP6*-NM_138329.2:c.403G > T were undetected), as reported in Table 2. Thus, we used ddPCR to measure the amount of mutated DNA within the tumor biopsies, and only one mutation (*SS18*-NM_001007559.3:c.98A > G, of subject 01T) could not be detected. Of the remaining 11 mutations in 10 genes (*BAP1* occurred twice), we found that *BAP1*, *NF2*, *FAT1*, *JADE1*, and *FLT1* were already present in the COSMIC and TCGA databases for MPM patients. For eight variants, the percentage of mutated DNA analyzed was of a similar extent to that yielded by NGS, considering an expected 10% error rate. On the other hand, *JADE1*- rs775483821 (ID = 01T) had 7.48% of mutated DNA in ddPCR opposed to 24.53% of the NGS, whereas *BAP1*-COSM4411449(C > T) (ID = 02T) had 33.50% vs. 21.88% and *NF2*- NM_016418.5:c.985A > T (ID = 03P) showed 15.85% vs. 27.03%, respectively. In PF, among the 11 mutations detected in tumor biopsies, 2 (*VIL1*- NM_007127.3:c.2070C > T and *NF2*-NM_016418.5:c.985A > T) could not be analyzed due to the lack of biological specimens of subjects 02P and 03P, whereas 1 (*FAT1*-rs776531396; ID = 05T) was undetectable. The remaining 8 SNVs were detected with percentages compatible with those observed in tumor biopsies, ranging from 12.75% to 39.70%. The only exception was patient 04T, whose mutations (*FAM71B*- rs1404037352 and *CSMD2*-rs770364421) had lower mutated allele relative abundance in PF compared with the tumor sample, namely, 9.7% against 30.80% and 8.95% against 25%, respectively.

The 11 mutations were also investigated in plasma samples. For patient 04T, we could not assay two mutations because of the lack of biological specimens. Of the remaining nine mutations, eight were also detectable in the patients' plasma, whereas *FAT1*- rs776531396 (ID = 05T) was undetectable, in agreement with the lack of detection in his PF. In plasma, the eight mutations could be detected, with percentages ranging from 0.14% to 2.68%. All these results are summarized in Table 2.

Considering both groups of patients and excluding the two mutations highly suspected to be of germline origin and the one not detected in solid biopsy, the percentages of mutated DNA detected in solid biopsies were higher than those detected in ctDNA from PFs: median = 21.95 vs. 12.75 (respectively); average $\pm$ st.dev = 22.21 $\pm$ 9.57 vs. 16.3 $\pm$ 12.3. This difference was statistically significant (p = 0.0237) when analyzed with Student's *t*-test for paired data and not statistically significant when analyzed with nonparametric Wilcoxon's test (p = 0.0648). The difference was much greater when compared to ctDNA from plasma (median = 0.29, average 0.89 $\pm$ 1.40), providing a high statistical significance to the same statistical tests (p = 2.49 $\times$ 10^{-7} and p = 3.2 $\times$ 10^{-4}, respectively).

4. Discussion

In this study, we report a positive feasibility study that in MPM patients, ctDNA is present in PF at high concentrations and cancer-specific DNA can be detected in plasma, although at low percentages. Therefore, we provide evidence that LBs for patients with MPM is feasible, and this could represent a potentially important tool for the diagnosis, therapy, follow-up, and stratification of patients, especially with pleural effusions.

It is noteworthy that we ruled out the possibility of selected germline mutations, either by using stringent filtering procedures or by carrying out WES of the buffy coat, when available. Thus, the present data reinforce and extend the preliminary evidence reported by Hylebos et al. [19], where only 3 out of 10 patients presented ctDNA in plasma samples. In that study, only one mutation was assayed, and no PFs were available. In our study, we started from a selection of 39 total mutations, and 22 could be confirmed in solid biopsies, allowing further investigations in PFs and plasma. Since we considered these SNVs enough for our purposes, we did not pay further attention to the remaining 17 mutations. Likely, they could not be validated because of poor ASO–qPCR probe performance.

In two GE patients, two mutations showed high and similar percentages in tumor, PF, and plasma, strongly suggesting a germline origin. This result was not surprising because, despite the stringent filtering procedure we applied, GE patients' buffy coat was lacking, and WES could not be carried out. However, the remaining 20 were enough for investigating whether MPM patients could carry ctDNA in PF or plasma. With the exception of subjects 696 (PCR could not work for an inhibitor), 02P, and 03P (PFs not available), 16 out of 17 mutations could be detected in PF. The percentages of the mutated allele detected differed by about 7.5%, on average, from those found in the tumor biopsies, a value falling within the intrinsic error of NGS technology (Figure 1). This fact indicates that DNA extracted from PF is a good proxy for its counterpart obtained from the solid tumor. In the future, DNA from PF could be employed instead of the classical solid biopsies to gain insights on the cancer's mutational landscape with much less distress for the patient. Moreover, 15 out of 18 analyzable mutations were also detectable in plasma, with relative abundances varying from 0.14% to 5.57%. Since only a few milliliters of plasma were available from the biobank, we could not analyze a high number of DNA copies in plasma. It is conceivable that the analysis of higher amounts of DNA could have elicited positive results in the three negative cases as well.

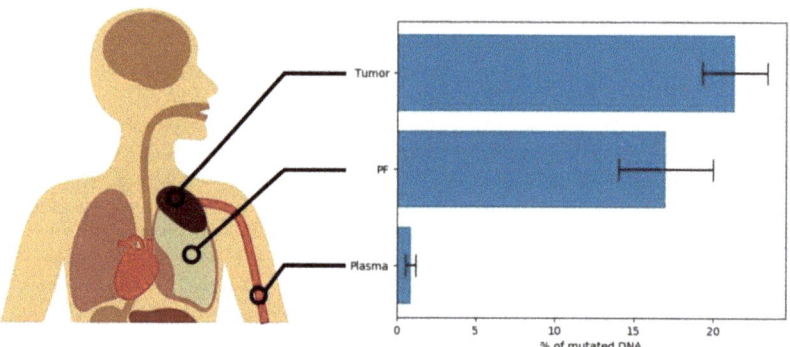

Figure 1. Mean levels of mutated DNA found in the samples from three sources: solid tumor, pleural fluid, and plasma.

The fact that MPM is a locally spreading tumor on the pleural surface could provide a good explanation of the high amount of ctDNA detected in PFs and the low amount detected in plasma. We can hypothesize that the observed interindividual variability of ctDNA levels could be ascribed to the relative amounts of subclones tracked with the picked mutation, the aggressiveness of the subclone carrying the picked mutation, or to the mechanisms involved in the release of tumor DNA.

We foresee that the use of PF or plasma could be very important in the diagnosis process and for a noninvasive clinical follow-up of the patients. An earlier diagnosis could be carried out by integrating the results of ctDNA analysis with currently available biomarkers, such as serum soluble mesothelin levels, and other epigenetic biomarkers under research, such as the expression of the circulating microRNAs miR-16, miR-17, miR-126, miR-486 or CpG methylation at *CDKN2A* or *SFRP* genes [23]. In fact, once the tumor is characterized for its genetic background, specific mutations could be used to monitor the evolution of the disease, allowing early detection of its worsening before any clinical observation. The analysis of cancer-specific mutations through the use of LBs could also allow more accurate monitoring of responses to therapies. With our work, we enlighten the versatility of this method to obtain genetic information on MPM using PF and plasma as starting materials.

One limitation to the present study consisted of the limited clinical information available from the biobanks of the samples G and P. It could be hypothesized that the percentage of mutated copies would be higher in patients presenting the tumors at advanced stages, conceivably with the idea of a higher extent of ctDNA released from largely spread tumors or metastases. At the present time, it is not possible to know whether the mutated DNA could also be detected in LBs from MPM patients with earlier stages of the disease. Future research should be encouraged to approach this task. However, we analyzed whether the amount of mutated DNA could correlate with patients' overall survival (a proxy of the tumor staging), and we could not find any statistically significant correlation. We could hypothesize that this is due to the low statistical power for this type of analysis or to the fact that all MPM patients are diagnosed at late stages. Given the possibility of gathering more clinical and histological data about the tumor, such as cell type, tumor stage, and treatment response, our results may prove even more useful in the clinical field.

5. Conclusions

In summary, this study showed that LBs are feasible in MPM, paving the way for novel tools in the clinical management of these patients. It has been figured out that once the profile of MPM's somatic mutations is fully achieved, the choice of the therapy, its effectiveness, and/or the occurrence of relapses can also be monitored by using PF and plasma as a source of ctDNA.

Supplementary Materials: The following are available online at https://www.mdpi.com/article/10.3390/cancers13102445/s1, Table S1: patients clinical data.

Author Contributions: G.M.: conceptualization, data curation, formal analysis, investigation, methodology, software, validation, writing. C.M.M.: methodology, supervision. P.A.: data curation, methodology, software. F.L.: investigation, methodology. G.A.: data curation, sample collection. M.M.: data curation, sample collection, supervision, writing and editing. C.L.: data curation, sample collection. R.A.F.: data curation, sample collection. M.L.: data curation, sample collection. A.B. (Alessandra Bonotti): data curation, sample collection. R.F.: data curation, sample collection. A.C.: data curation, sample collection. L.M.: writing and editing. A.B. (Andrea Bottari): data curation, formal analysis, investigation, methodology, software, validation. A.A.: data curation, formal analysis, investigation, methodology, software, validation. M.D.R.: validation. R.D.: validation, supervision. F.G.: investigation, project administration, supervision, writing and editing. S.L.: conceptualization, data curation, formal analysis, funding acquisition, investigation, project administration, supervision, visualization, writing and editing. All authors have read and agreed to the published version of the manuscript.

Funding: This research was funded by Fondazione Pisa grant number 153/16.

Institutional Review Board Statement: The study was conducted according to the guidelines of the Declaration of Helsinki and approved by the Institutional Review Boards (or Ethics Committee) of Pi Ge Tu Eskisehir Osmangazy University (protocol code 24.11.2020/22) and Azienda Ospedaliero-Universitaria Pisana (dated 7 February 2013, protocol number 192/53).

Informed Consent Statement: Informed consent was obtained from all subjects involved in the study.

Data Availability Statement: Data is contained within the article or supplementary materia.

Conflicts of Interest: The authors declare there is no conflict of interest. The founding entity had no role in the writing of the manuscript and the performing of the study; in the collection, analyses, or interpretation of data; and in the decision to publish the results.

Abbreviations

AD	number of the reads of the alternative allele (i.e.,: alternative depth)
ASO–qPCR	allele-specific oligonucleotide and real-time quantitative PCR
CTCs	circulating tumor cells
ctDNA	circulating cell-free tumor DNA
ddPCR	digital-droplets PCR
FGE	filtering WES data in GE patients
FPT	filtering of WES data in PT patients
GE	patients from Genova
LB	liquid biopsies
MAF	minor allele frequency
MPM	malignant pleural mesothelioma
NGS	next-generation sequencing
P	patients from Pisa
PFs	pleural fluids
PT	patients from Pisa and Turkey
SNVs	simple nucleotide variants
T	patients from Turkey
TD	total number of reads (i.e., total depth)
tEV	tumor-derived extracellular vesicles
VATS	video-assisted thoracoscopy
WES	whole-exome sequencing.

References

1. Pinato, D.J.; Mauri, F.A.; Ramakrishnan, R.; Wahab, L.; Lloyd, T.; Sharma, R. Inflammation-based prognostic indices in malignant pleural mesothelioma. *J. Thorac. Oncol.* **2012**, *7*, 587–594. [CrossRef] [PubMed]
2. Xue, J.; Patergnani, S.; Giorgi, C.; Suarez, J.; Goto, K.; Bononi, A.; Tanji, M.; Novelli, F.; Pastorino, S.; Xu, R.; et al. Asbestos induces mesothelial cell transformation via HMGB1-driven autophagy. *Proc. Natl. Acad. Sci. USA* **2020**, *117*, 25543–25552. [CrossRef]
3. Carbone, M.; Yang, H. Molecular pathways: Targeting mechanisms of asbestos and erionite carcinogenesis in mesothelioma. *Clin. Cancer Res.* **2012**, *18*, 598–604. [CrossRef]
4. Rehrauer, H.; Wu, L.; Blum, W.; Pecze, L.; Henzi, T.; Serre-Beinier, V.; Aquino, C.; Vrugt, B.; De Perrot, M.; Schwaller, B.; et al. How asbestos drives the tissue towards tumors: YAP activation, macrophage and mesothelial precursor recruitment, RNA editing, and somatic mutations. *Oncogene* **2018**, *37*, 2645–2659. [CrossRef] [PubMed]
5. Marinaccio, A.; Binazzi, A.; Cauzillo, G.; Cavone, D.; Zotti, R.D.; Ferrante, P.; Gennaro, V.; Gorini, G.; Menegozzo, M.; Mensi, C.; et al. Italian Mesothelioma Register (ReNaM) Working Group Analysis of latency time and its determinants in asbestos related malignant mesothelioma cases of the Italian register. *Eur. J. Cancer* **2007**, *43*, 2722–2728. [CrossRef]
6. Carbone, M.; Adusumilli, P.S.; Alexander, H.R., Jr.; Baas, P.; Bardelli, F.; Bononi, A.; Bueno, R.; Felley-Bosco, E.; Galateau-Salle, F.; Jablons, D.; et al. Mesothelioma: Scientific clues for prevention, diagnosis, and therapy. *CA Cancer J. Clin.* **2019**, *69*, 402–429. [CrossRef] [PubMed]
7. Cardinale, L.; Ardissone, F.; Gned, D.; Sverzellati, N.; Piacibello, E.; Veltri, A. Diagnostic Imaging and workup of Malignant Pleural Mesothelioma. *Acta Bio-Medica Atenei Parm.* **2017**, *88*, 134–142.
8. Zhang, W.; Wu, X.; Wu, L.; Zhang, W.; Zhao, X. Advances in the diagnosis, treatment and prognosis of malignant pleural mesothelioma. *Ann. Transl. Med.* **2015**, *3*, 182.
9. Schwarzenbach, H.; Hoon, D.S.B.; Pantel, K. Cell-free nucleic acids as biomarkers in cancer patients. *Nat. Rev. Cancer* **2011**, *11*, 426–437. [CrossRef]
10. Paoletti, C.; Hayes, D.F. Circulating Tumor Cells. In *Novel Biomarkers in the Continuum of Breast Cancer*; Stearns, V., Ed.; Advances in Experimental Medicine and Biology; Springer International Publishing (Switzerland AG): Cham, Switzerland, 2016; Volume 882, pp. 235–258. [CrossRef]
11. Kamyabi, N.; Bernard, V.; Maitra, A. Liquid biopsies in pancreatic cancer. *Expert Rev. Anticancer Ther.* **2019**, *19*, 869–878. [CrossRef]
12. Rolfo, C.; Mack, P.C.; Scagliotti, G.V.; Baas, P.; Barlesi, F.; Bivona, T.G.; Herbst, R.S.; Mok, T.S.; Peled, N.; Pirker, R.; et al. Liquid Biopsy for Advanced Non-Small Cell Lung Cancer (NSCLC): A Statement Paper from the IASLC. *J. Thorac. Oncol.* **2018**, *13*, 1248–1268. [CrossRef]
13. Ye, Q.; Ling, S.; Zheng, S.; Xu, X. Liquid biopsy in hepatocellular carcinoma: Circulating tumor cells and circulating tumor DNA. *Mol. Cancer* **2019**, *18*, 114. [CrossRef] [PubMed]
14. Del Re, M.; Bertolini, I.; Crucitta, S.; Fontanelli, L.; Rofi, E.; De Angelis, C.; Diodati, L.; Cavallero, D.; Gianfilippo, G.; Salvadori, B.; et al. Overexpression of TK1 and CDK9 in plasma-derived exosomes is associated with clinical resistance to CDK4/6 inhibitors in metastatic breast cancer patients. *Breast. Cancer Res. Treat.* **2019**, *178*, 57–62. [CrossRef] [PubMed]

15. Mastoraki, S.; Strati, A.; Tzanikou, E.; Chimonidou, M.; Politaki, E.; Voutsina, A.; Psyrri, A.; Georgoulias, V.; Lianidou, E. ESR1 Methylation: A Liquid Biopsy-Based Epigenetic Assay for the Follow-up of Patients with Metastatic Breast Cancer Receiving Endocrine Treatment. *Clin. Cancer Res.* **2018**, *24*, 1500–1510. [CrossRef]
16. Del Re, M.; Crucitta, S.; Gianfilippo, G.; Passaro, A.; Petrini, I.; Restante, G.; Michelucci, A.; Fogli, S.; de Marinis, F.; Porta, C.; et al. Understanding the Mechanisms of Resistance in EGFR-Positive NSCLC: From Tissue to Liquid Biopsy to Guide Treatment Strategy. *Int. J. Mol. Sci.* **2019**, *20*, 3951. [CrossRef]
17. Saenz-Antoñanzas, A.; Auzmendi-Iriarte, J.; Carrasco-Garcia, E.; Moreno-Cugnon, L.; Ruiz, I.; Villanua, J.; Egaña, L.; Otaegui, D.; Samprón, N.; Matheu, A. Liquid Biopsy in Glioblastoma: Opportunities, Applications and Challenges. *Cancers* **2019**, *11*, 950. [CrossRef]
18. Sriram, K.B.; Relan, V.; Clarke, B.E.; Duhig, E.E.; Windsor, M.N.; Matar, K.S.; Naidoo, R.; Passmore, L.; McCaul, E.; Courtney, D.; et al. Pleural fluid cell-free DNA integrity index to identify cytologically negative malignant pleural effusions including mesotheliomas. *BMC Cancer* **2012**, *12*, 428. [CrossRef]
19. Hylebos, M.; Op de Beeck, K.; Pauwels, P.; Zwaenepoel, K.; van Meerbeeck, J.P.; Van Camp, G. Tumor-specific genetic variants can be detected in circulating cell-free DNA of malignant pleural mesothelioma patients. *Lung Cancer* **2018**, *124*, 19–22. [CrossRef]
20. Li, H.; Durbin, R. Fast and accurate long-read alignment with Burrows-Wheeler transform. *Bioinforma Oxf. Engl.* **2010**, *26*, 589–595. [CrossRef]
21. Koboldt, D.C.; Zhang, Q.; Larson, D.E.; Shen, D.; McLellan, M.D.; Lin, L.; Miller, C.A.; Mardis, E.R.; Ding, L.; Wilson, R.K. VarScan 2: Somatic mutation and copy number alteration discovery in cancer by exome sequencing. *Genome Res.* **2012**, *22*, 568–576. [CrossRef]
22. DePristo, M.A.; Banks, E.; Poplin, R.; Garimella, K.V.; Maguire, J.R.; Hartl, C.; Philippakis, A.A.; Del Angel, G.; Rivas, M.A.; Hanna, M.; et al. A framework for variation discovery and genotyping using next-generation DNA sequencing data. *Nat Genet.* **2011**, *43*, 491–498. [CrossRef] [PubMed]
23. Rozitis, E.; Johnson, B.; Cheng, Y.Y.; Lee, K. The Use of Immunohistochemistry, Fluorescence in situ Hybridization, and Emerging Epigenetic Markers in the Diagnosis of Malignant Pleural Mesothelioma (MPM): A Review. *Front. Oncol.* **2020**, *10*, 1742. [CrossRef]

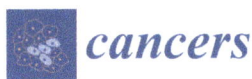

Article

Cross-Species Proteomics Identifies CAPG and SBP1 as Crucial Invasiveness Biomarkers in Rat and Human Malignant Mesothelioma

Joëlle S. Nader [1], Alice Boissard [2], Cécile Henry [2], Isabelle Valo [2], Véronique Verrièle [2], Marc Grégoire [1], Olivier Coqueret [3], Catherine Guette [2] and Daniel L. Pouliquen [3,*]

1. Université de Nantes, Inserm, CRCINA, F-44000 Nantes, France; joelle03nader@gmail.com (J.S.N.); marc.gregoire@inserm.fr (M.G.)
2. Université d'Angers, ICO Cancer Center, Inserm, CRCINA, F-44000 Nantes, France; alice.boissard@ico.unicancer.fr (A.B.); cecile.henry@ico.unicancer.fr (C.H.); isabelle.valo@ico.unicancer.fr (I.V.); Veronique.Verriele@ico.unicancer.fr (V.V.); catherine.guette@ico.unicancer.fr (C.G.)
3. Université d'Angers, Inserm, CRCINA, F-44000 Nantes, France; olivier.coqueret@univ-angers.fr
* Correspondence: daniel.pouliquen@inserm.fr; Tel.: +33-241-352854

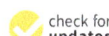

Received: 16 July 2020; Accepted: 23 August 2020; Published: 27 August 2020

Abstract: Malignant mesothelioma (MM) still represents a devastating disease that is often detected too late, while the current effect of therapies on patient outcomes remains unsatisfactory. Invasiveness biomarkers may contribute to improving early diagnosis, prognosis, and treatment for patients, a task that could benefit from the development of high-throughput proteomics. To limit potential sources of bias when identifying such biomarkers, we conducted cross-species proteomic analyzes on three different MM sources. Data were collected firstly from two human MM cell lines, secondly from rat MM tumors of increasing invasiveness grown in immunocompetent rats and human MM tumors grown in immunodeficient mice, and thirdly from paraffin-embedded sections of patient MM tumors of the epithelioid and sarcomatoid subtypes. Our investigations identified three major invasiveness biomarkers common to the three tumor sources, CAPG, FABP4, and LAMB2, and an additional set of 25 candidate biomarkers shared by rat and patient tumors. Comparing the data to proteomic analyzes of preneoplastic and neoplastic rat mesothelial cell lines revealed the additional role of SBP1 in the carcinogenic process. These observations could provide new opportunities to identify highly vulnerable MM patients with poor survival outcomes, thereby improving the success of current and future therapeutic strategies.

Keywords: malignant mesothelioma; biomarkers; proteomics; macrophage-capping protein; fatty acid-binding protein; laminin subunit beta-2; selenium-binding protein 1; carcinogenesis

1. Introduction

The management of malignant mesothelioma (MM) remains a challenge today given its complex biology and aggressiveness, and the absence of specific early symptoms [1]. The effect of current and new therapies on overall survival also remains very modest [2], prompting the need to search for biomarkers that could improve early diagnosis, prognosis, and treatment [3]. Sequential Window Acquisition of all Theoretical Mass Spectra (SWATH-MS) has recently emerged as a promising new tool in cancer proteomics, making it possible to identify biomarkers of increasing stages of invasiveness in MM experimental models, for example [4].

Proteomic analyzes of MM have already provided lists of putative cancer biomarkers, although significant differences are observed between primary and commercial MM cell lines [5], for example, emphasizing the need to use best-suited preclinical cellular models [6]. Moreover, long-established human cell lines [7], some genetically engineered mouse models [8], and subcutaneous xenograft models of human tumors [9,10] often fail to predict drug effects in clinical practice. Therefore, to recapitulate the spectrum of tumor heterogeneity seen in patients, and limit the impact of differences in stromal conditions observed between patient and cancer models, cross-species proteomic analyzes are suggested to improve preclinical evaluation [11].

Remembering the importance of potential sources of bias when identifying biomarkers with potential application in oncology [12,13], to determine which invasiveness biomarkers identified in MM experimental models evolved similarly in human MM, we compared lists of proteins of interest from three biological sources. Data were collected firstly from two MM cell lines, secondly from rat MM tumors grown in syngeneic immunocompetent animals and human MM tumors grown in immunodeficient mice, and thirdly from paraffin-embedded sections of patient MM tumors of the epithelioid and sarcomatoid subtypes. The results identified one main biomarker, CAPG, associated with invasiveness and common to all three categories of tumors and human cell lines. Moreover, two other biomarkers were common to the three tumor sources, while 25 other candidates of interest were shared by rat and patient MM tumors. Finally, comparing these data with proteomic analyzes of a large collection of preneoplastic and neoplastic rat mesothelial cell lines revealed the additional role of SBP1 in the carcinogenic process.

2. Results

2.1. Characterization of Cell Lines and MM Tumors

The four rat MM tumor models shared a sarcomatoid morphology of tumor cells but differed in their infiltrative potential. The M5-T2 tumor is noninvasive, with tumor cell development restricted to the omentum without liver capsular breakthrough (Figure 1A, top left). The F4-T2 tumor is moderately invasive with a regular tumor front (Figure 1A, top right). The F5-T1 and M5-T1 tumors are both characterized by deep infiltration of the liver with irregular tumor fronts, however their respective tumor cells differ in their levels of atypia (Figure 1A, bottom). The highly invasive nature of the M5-T1 tumor is also revealed by necrosis of the liver parenchyma and the presence of apoptotic hepatocytes at the tumor front (Figure 1A, bottom right), associated with the specificities of its proteome [4]. The mean time required for macroscopic tumor development following the injection of $3–5 \times 10^6$ cells i.p. into syngeneic rats also differs among the four models: five weeks for M5-T2, four weeks for F4-T2, and three and a half weeks for F5-T1 and M5-T1.

The tumor rate development of the two models of human MM xenografts grown in NOD SCID mice (mice homozygous for the severe combined immune deficiency spontaneous mutation $Prkdc^{scid}$, characterized by an absence of functional T cells and B cells) also differed markedly, with six weeks for MM34 versus three and a half weeks for MM163. These differences were also confirmed at microscopic level, as MM163 was characterized by tumor cells with heterogeneous nuclei in size and shape, prominent nucleoli, the presence of mitotic figures, and frequent atypia (Figure 1B, right) compared with MM 34 (Figure 1B, left).

The two sarcomatoid MM tumors from patients (SMM-1 and S-MM-2) were characterized by abundant intercellular collagen deposition, the presence of spindle-shaped tumor cells with oval nuclei, considerable heterogeneity in cell dimensions, and frequent atypia (Figure 1C, right column). The two epithelioid MM tumors (EMM-1 and EMM-2) contained tumor cells with abundant eosinophilic cytoplasm, round nuclei, and mild nuclear atypia (Figure 1C, left column).

One of the most frequent genomic alterations found in MM concerned *CDKN2A*, observed in the different histologic types [14]. Analysis of mRNA levels of this gene by qRT PCR in cell lines from the two species has previously revealed a comparable decreased relative expression in human pleural MM cell lines relative to normal mesothelial cells, and in rat MM cell lines relative to preneoplastic mesothelial cell lines [15]. Additionally, *Cdkn2a* relative expression was even more decreased in the three invasive MM cell lines (F4-T2: 2.54; F5-T1: 2.10; and M5-T1: 0.79) relative to the non-invasive M5-T2 cell line (4.97) [15]. The bi-allelic deletion of the *CDKN2A* gene, further confirmed in a list of MM human cell lines including the least invasive MM34 (Meso 34), was found to be strongly associated with overexpression of *IL34* and weakly with mutations of the *NF2* gene (with no association with other genetic alterations in *BAP1*, *LATS2* or *TP53* genes) [16]. MM163 (Meso 163) differed from MM34 by a homozygous deletion of the *IFNB1* gene (located in the same 9p21.3 chromosome region as *CDKN2A*) that encodes IFN-β [17]. A transcriptomic analysis of the group of human MM cell lines sharing the same features as MM163, comparing cells exposed to measles virus with untreated cells, revealed these cells were characterized by a weak IFN-I response, some canonical pathways involved in antigen presentation and cytotoxic T lymphocyte-mediated apoptosis of target cells being particularly hit [17].

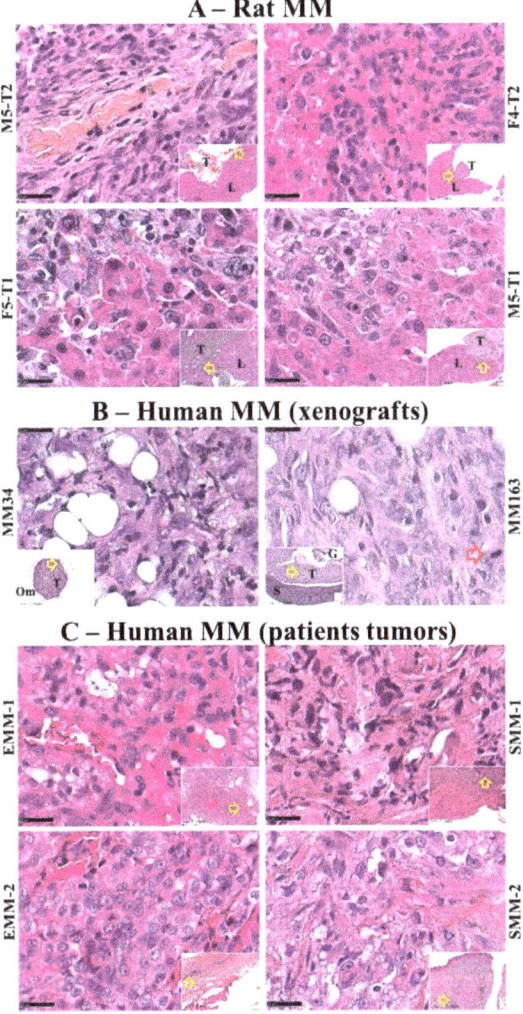

Figure 1. Histological features of the three sources of malignant mesothelioma MM tumors. High magnification views, hematoxylin-phloxine-saffron (HPS) staining (×800, scale bars represent 25 μm), and general views in inserts (×25, scale bars represent 1 mm) with open red arrows indicating the location of magnifications. (**A**) Rat MM tumors of the four experimental models (the names of the corresponding cell lines are indicated on the external side of the photographs). These representative

tumor (T) histological sections included liver tissue (L) and tumor cells exhibiting increasing levels of invasiveness. (**B**) Xenografts of human MM tumors grown in NOD SCID mice, with the corresponding cell line names indicated on the external side of the photographs. (Om) = omentum, (G) = gut, (S) = spleen. The large open arrow shows a mitotic figure. (**C**), Human MM tumors from patients. EMM-1 and EMM-2 (left column) = epithelioid histotype, SMM-1 and SMM-2 (right column) = sarcomatoid histotype.

2.2. Main Biomarkers Sharing the Same Evolution in the Three Sources of MM Tumors

SWATH-MS data on increased MM tumor invasiveness were collected from (1) comparison of the three invasive rat MM tumors (F4-T2, F5-T1, M5-T1) versus the noninvasive one, M5-T2; (2) comparison of Meso 163 xenografts versus Meso 34 human MM tumors grown in immunodeficient mice; and (3) comparison of human MM tumors from patients, sarcomatoid versus epithelioid subtypes. The main findings are summarized in Table 1. The number of proteins with a fold change > 1.5 and statistical p-value < 0.05 estimated by MarkerView was 433, 133, and 191 in each experiment, respectively. Volcano plots for comparisons (1) (2) and (3) are provided in Figure 2A–C, respectively. Comparing these lists, represented by the green, brown, and orange circles, respectively (illustrated in Figure 2D), led us to identify a first pattern of common changes observed in the three experiments and shared by the macrophage-capping protein (encoded by *CAPG*), the fatty acid-binding protein, adipocyte (encoded by *FABP4*), and the laminin subunit beta-2 (encoded by *LAMB2*). These proteins are involved in actin filament finding, lipid transport (fatty acid binding) and extracellular matrix constitution (cell adhesion), respectively. Additional consideration of the comparison of Meso 163 versus Meso 34 human MM cell lines revealed that CAPG was the only biomarker exhibiting similar changes (a strong tendency was also observed for LAMB2), while there were no significant changes for FABP4 (Table 1 and Figure 3). No additional change was observed in the comparison of invasive versus noninvasive rat MM cell lines for the three proteins.

Table 1. Summary of proteomics biomarkers of MM invasiveness and carcinogenesis. Abundance changes: + p < 0.05; - ns (p > 0.09); (+) tendency (0.05 < p < 0.09).

Protein	Rat MM	Patient MM	Human Xenografts	Human MM Cell Lines	Rat MM Carcinogenesis
CAPG	+	+	+	+	+/−
FABP4	+	+	+	−	−
LAMB2	+	+	+	(+)	−
PARP1	+	+	(+)	+	−
NSF	+	+	(+)	+	−
IMDH2	+	+	(+)	+	−
ANXA5	+	+	−	+	−
VAT1	+	+	−	+	+/−
SBP1	+	+	−	+	+
COX2	+	+	−	(+)	−
SC22B	+	+	−	(+)	−
FINC	+	+	−	(+)	+/−
RAB31	+	+	−	−	+
DPYL3	+	+	−	−	−
LRC59	+	+	−	−	−
LTOR1	+	+	−	−	−
TPM3	+	+	−	−	+/−
ERP29	+	+	−	−	−
PRAF3	+	+	−	−	−
IDH3A	+	+	−	−	−
FRIL1	+	+	−	−	−
VATB2	+	+	−	−	−
RS18	+	+	−	−	−
EHD2	+	+	−	−	−
SEPT7	+	+	−	−	−
ALBU	+	+	−	−	−
HBA	+	+	−	−	−
HBB	+	+	−	−	−

A second pattern of common changes was represented by proteins sharing the same differences between rat and human MM but showing no significant changes in human MM xenografts. Three proteins were involved, poly [ADP-ribose] polymerase 1 (encoded by *PARP1*), vesicle-fusing ATPase (encoded by *NSF*), and inosine-5′-monophosphate dehydrogenase (encoded by *IMPDH2*). These proteins are involved in DNA repair, vesicle-mediated transport (Golgi) and de novo synthesis of guanine nucleotides, respectively. This situation confirms that transplantable tumors established subcutaneously in immunodeficient mice are less relevant in terms of stromal/vascular interactions than orthotopic models of tumors in syngeneic animals [6]. However, these limitations were counterbalanced by the observation of tendencies toward an increase in MM163 vs. MM34 xenografts, while significant differences were also found between corresponding human cell lines (Table 1 and Figure 3).

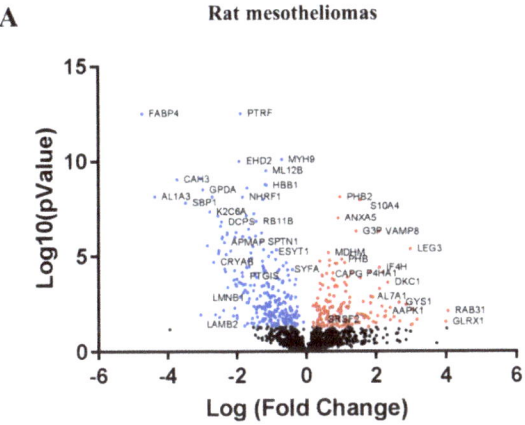

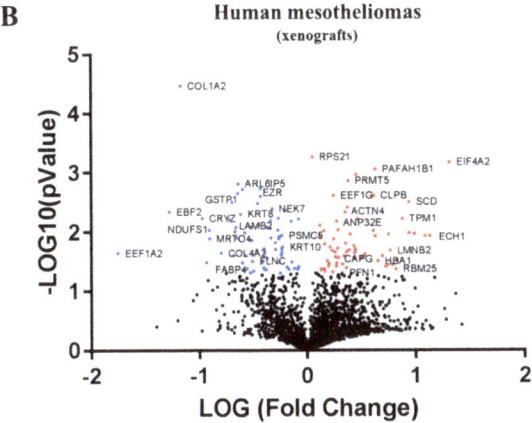

Figure 2. *Cont.*

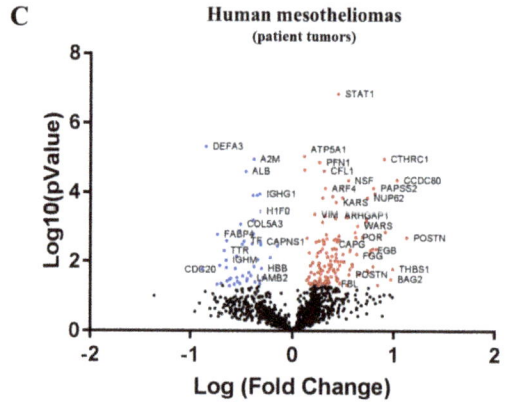

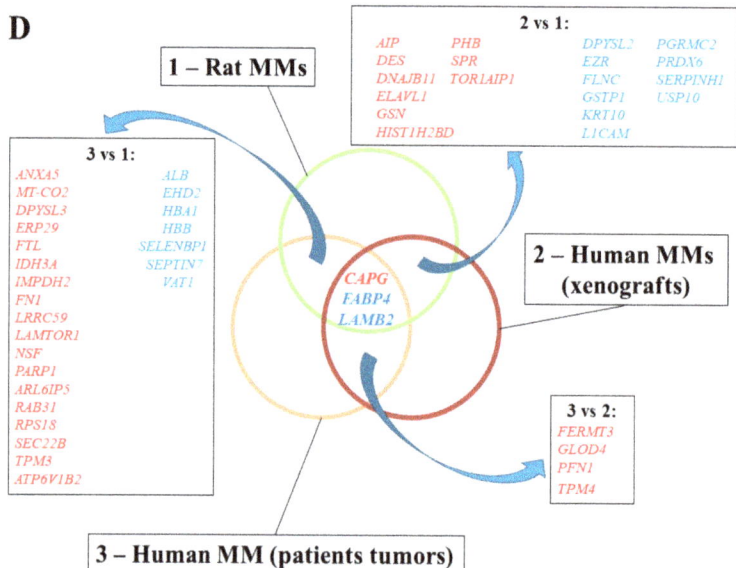

Figure 2. Volcano plots and schematic representation of the comparative proteomic analyzes. (**A**), Volcano plot of the comparison of the three invasive rat MM tumors (F4-T2, F5-T1, and M5-T1) versus the noninvasive one, (M5-T2). (**B**), Volcano plot of the comparison of Meso 163 versus Meso 34 xenografts of human MM tumors grown in immunodeficient mice. (**C**), Volcano plot of the comparison of human MM tumors from patients, sarcomatoid versus epithelioid subtypes. The locations of CAPG (in red), FABP4 and LAMB2 (in blue) are indicated in the three volcano plots. (**D**), Schematic representation of the comparative proteomic analyzes. The three different sources of MM tumors are illustrated by the green (Rat MM), brown (xenografts of human MM grown in NOD SCID mice) and orange (human MM from patient tumor samples) circles. The green circle represents the 433 proteins showing significant changes in abundance ($p < 0.05$) between the three invasive rat MM tumors versus the noninvasive one. The brown circle illustrates the 133 proteins showing significant changes in abundance ($p < 0.05$) between Meso 163 (MM163) and Meso 34 (MM34) xenografts. The orange circle represents the 191 proteins affected by significant changes in abundance ($p < 0.05$) between the two sarcomatoid versus the two epithelioid MM tumors from patients. Genes coding for proteins exhibiting common significant changes are given for *homo sapiens* in italics (increase in red, decrease in blue).

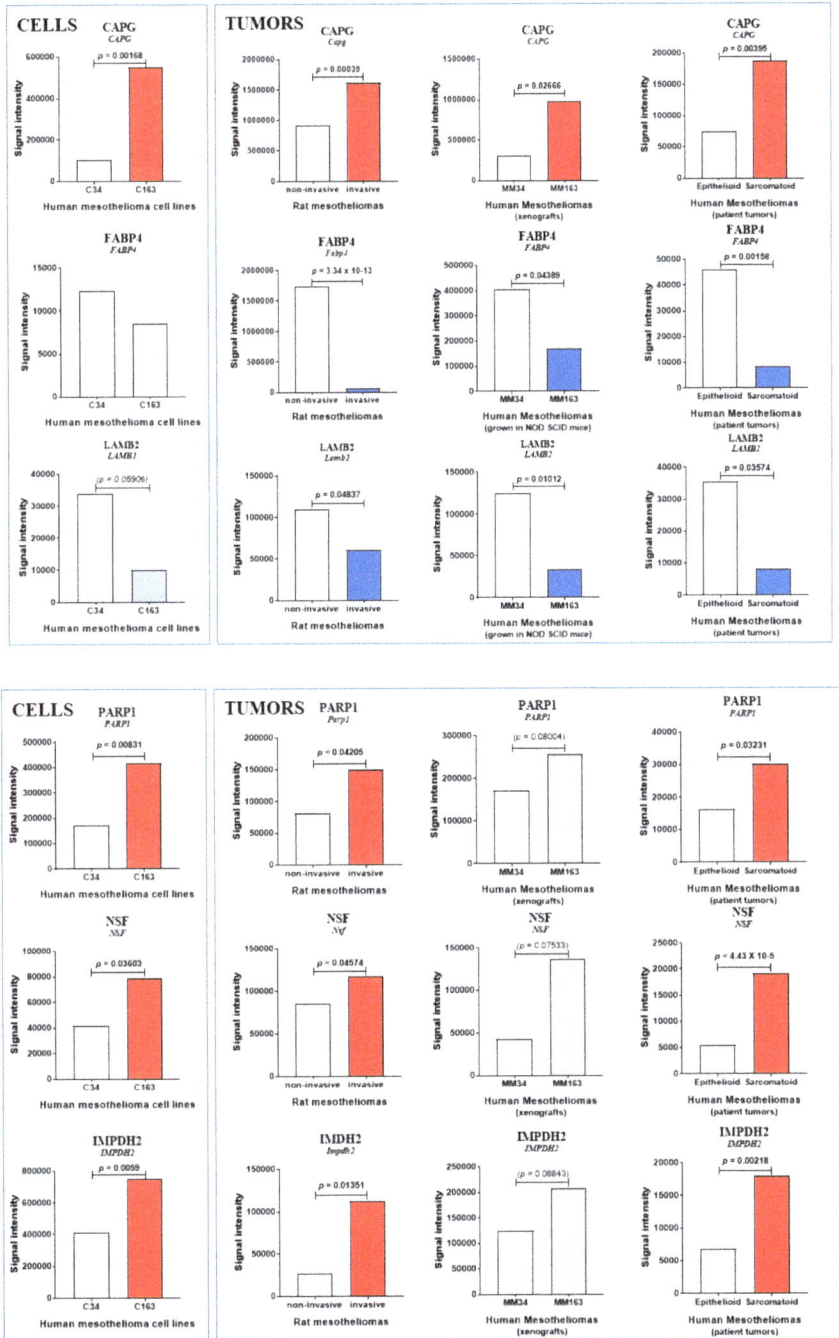

Figure 3. Common biomarkers of MM invasiveness. Proteins showing comparable abundance changes in MM from the three sources and between human mesothelioma cell lines. Increase and decrease are indicated by red and blue bars, respectively (with p values). Blank bars reflect the absence of significant changes ($p > 0.09$), while light red or blue bars indicate tendencies ($0.05 < p < 0.09$).

2.3. Additional Biomarkers of Interest Common to Rat and Human MM

Several additional conclusions were drawn from the common changes in abundance limited to rat and patient MM tumors. Firstly, in the 3 versus 1 comparative analysis (Figure 2D), among the 18 proteins exhibiting a common increase, annexin A5 (encoded by *ANXA5*), involved in the blood coagulation cascade (anticoagulant), was the only one showing the same pattern of changes in human MM cell lines (Figure 4). Moreover, three more proteins revealed the same tendency, cytochrome c oxidase subunit 2 (encoded by *MT-CO2*), vesicle-trafficking protein SC22b (encoded by *SEC22B*), and fibronectin (encoded by *FN1*) (Table 1 and Figure 4). These proteins are involved in electron transport (respiratory chain), vesicle-mediated transport (membrane), and extracellular matrix structural composition (cell adhesion and motility), respectively. Finally, among the seven other proteins exhibiting a decreased abundance, two presented the same pattern, selenium-binding protein 1 (encoded by *SELENBP1*), an oxidoreductase also involved in protein transport, and synaptic vesicle membrane protein VAT-1 homolog (encoded by *VAT1*), which negatively regulates mitochondrial fusion (Table 1 and Figure 4).

The rest of the proteins listed in the 3 versus 1 comparison involved candidate biomarkers for which the difference in abundance between cells was insignificant ($p > 0.090$). By order of magnitude, proteins showing increased abundance with invasiveness included Ras-related protein Rab-31 (encoded by *RAB31*), Ragulator complex protein LAMTOR1 (encoded by *LAMTOR1*), isoform LCRMP-4 of dihydropyrimidinase-related protein 3 (encoded by *DPYSL3*), leucine-rich repeat-containing protein 59 (encoded by *LRRC59*), isoform 2 of tropomyosin alpha-3 chain (encoded by *TPM3*), endoplasmic reticulum resident protein 29 (encoded by *ERP29*), PRA1 family protein 3 (encoded by *ARL6IP5*), ferritin light chain (encoded by *FTL*), isocitrate dehydrogenase [NAD] subunit alpha, mitochondrial (encoded by *IDH3A*), V-type proton ATPase subunit B, brain isoform (encoded by *ATP6V1B2*), and 40S ribosomal protein S18 (encoded by *RPS18*) (Table 1 and Figure 5). Finally, proteins exhibiting a common decrease in both rat and human MM from patients were EH domain-containing protein 2 (encoded by *EHD2*), septin-7 (encoded by *SEPTIN7*), serum albumin (encoded by *ALB*), and two subunits of hemoglobin (encoded by *HBA1* and *HBB*) (Table 1 and Figure 5).

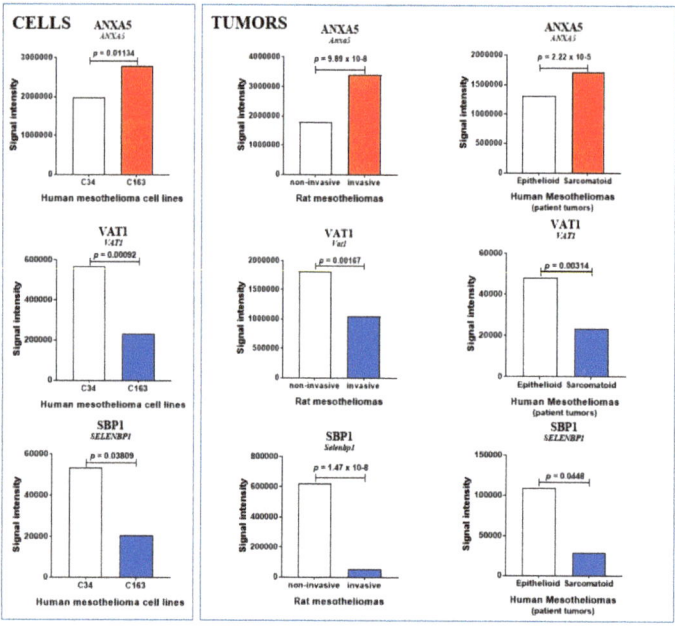

Figure 4. *Cont.*

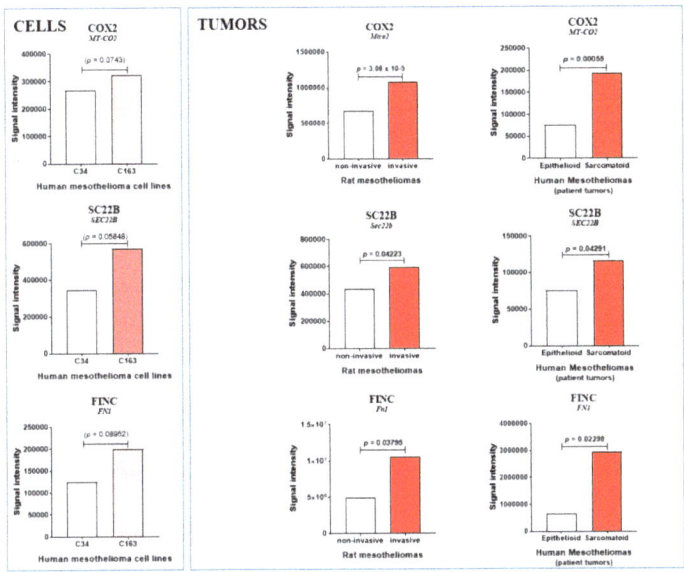

Figure 4. Main invasiveness biomarkers in human vs. rat MM, and cell lines. Proteins showing comparable abundance changes in MM from rat models and patients, and human mesothelioma cell lines. Increase and decrease are indicated by red and blue bars, respectively (with p values). Blank bars reflect the absence of significant changes ($p > 0.09$), while light red bars indicate tendencies ($0.05 < p < 0.09$).

2.4. Candidate Biomarkers Common to Xenografts and Rat or Patient MM

Compared with the previous situation (3 versus 1), the numbers of common proteins found in conditions 2 versus 1, and 3 versus 2, were significantly reduced (Figure 2D). Among these lists, the parallel increase in prohibitin (encoded by *PHB*), and decrease in peroxiredoxin-6 (encoded by *PRDX6*) and ezrin (encoded by *EZR*) have previously been reported to be linked to the acquisition of invasive properties in rat MM models [4]. Moreover, these lists contain several candidate invasiveness biomarkers common to MM and other cancer types and reported in the literature, including gelsolin (encoded by *GSN*), profiling-1 (encoded by *PFN1*), glutathione-S-transferase P (encoded by *GSTP1*), keratin, type I cytoskeletal 10 (encoded by *KRT10*), and serpin H1 (encoded by *SERPINH1*) [13].

2.5. Abundance Changes during Rat MM Carcinogenesis

We next investigated whether some of the 28 candidate biomarkers (the 18 increased and 7 decreased proteins listed in the 3 versus 1 comparison, plus CAPG, FABP4, and LAMB2) common to the rat and human MM (Figure 2D) exhibited additional abundance changes during the carcinogenesis process. For that purpose, we first examined the SWATH-MS proteomic data of the whole biocollection of rat mesothelial cell lines, looking in particular at the list of 674 proteins differentiating preneoplastic cell lines with sarcomatoid versus epithelioid morphology [18]. In a second step, we compared this list to another list of 192 proteins discriminating the two subgroups of preneoplastic cell lines with sarcomatoid morphology PNsarc2 vs. PNsarc1, which differ in their relative expression of *Hif1a* [18]. Finally, comparing the 94 proteins exhibiting significant abundance changes in the two previous situations with the 28 candidate biomarkers described above (see Figure 2D and Sections 2.2 and 2.3), led to six proteins common to the four proteomic analyzes (Figure 6A). The absence of FABP4 in this list (the protein was not detected in cells) suggests a location in the stroma.

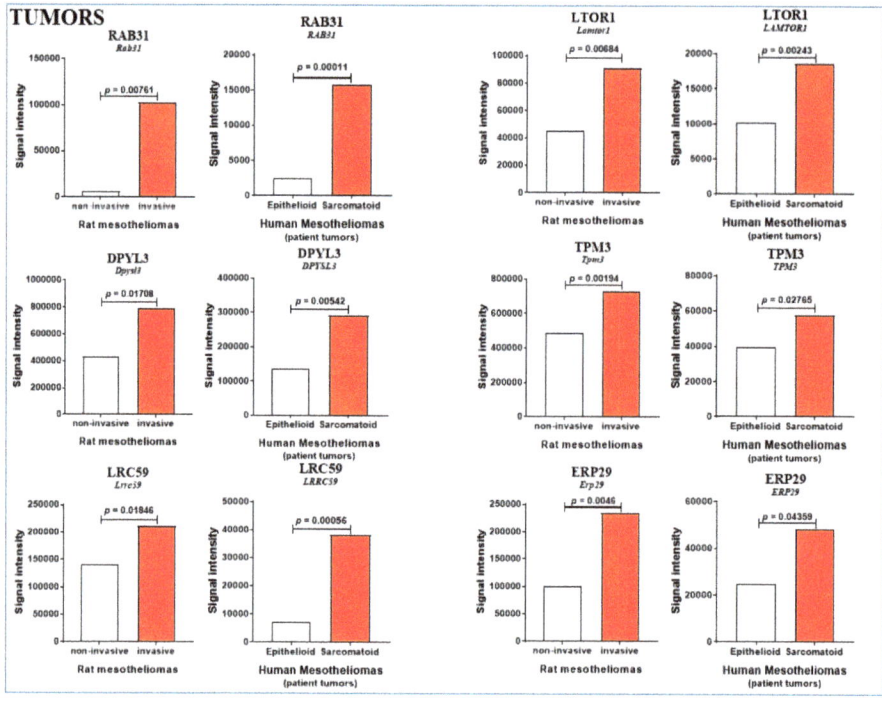
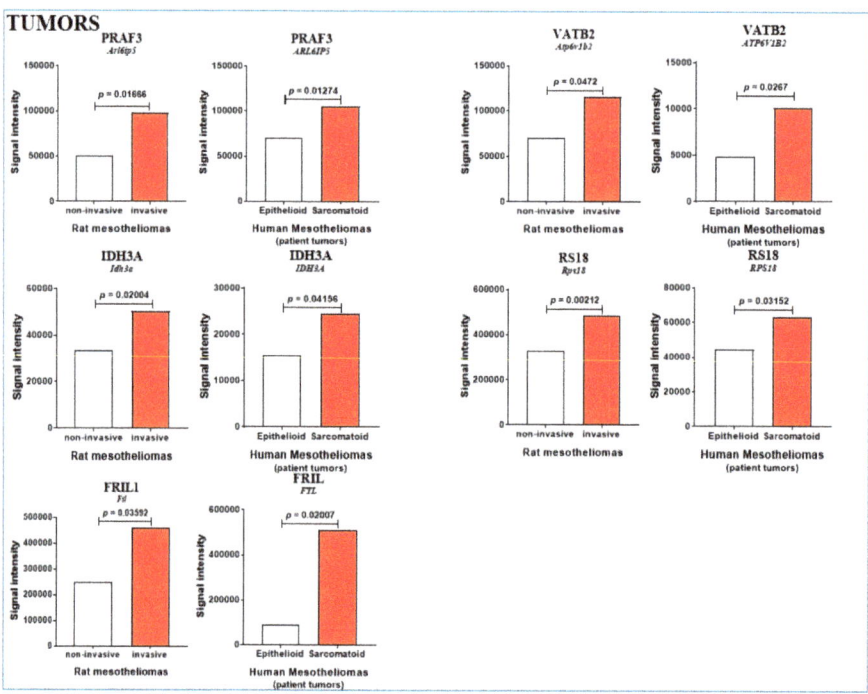

Figure 5. Cont.

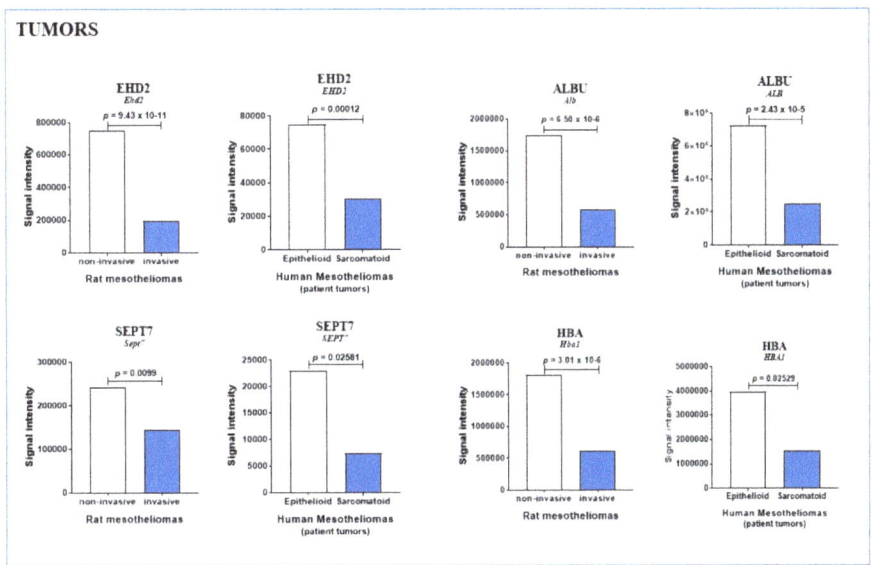

Figure 5. Additional invasiveness biomarkers in MM from patient and rat models. Proteins showing comparable abundance changes only in patient MM vs. rat models. Increase and decrease are indicated by red and blue bars, respectively (with p values). Blank bars reflect the absence of significant changes ($p > 0.09$). For clarity, data on the beta subunit of hemoglobin (encoded by *HBB*) have been excluded as they were similar to those observed for the alpha subunit (encoded by *HBA*).

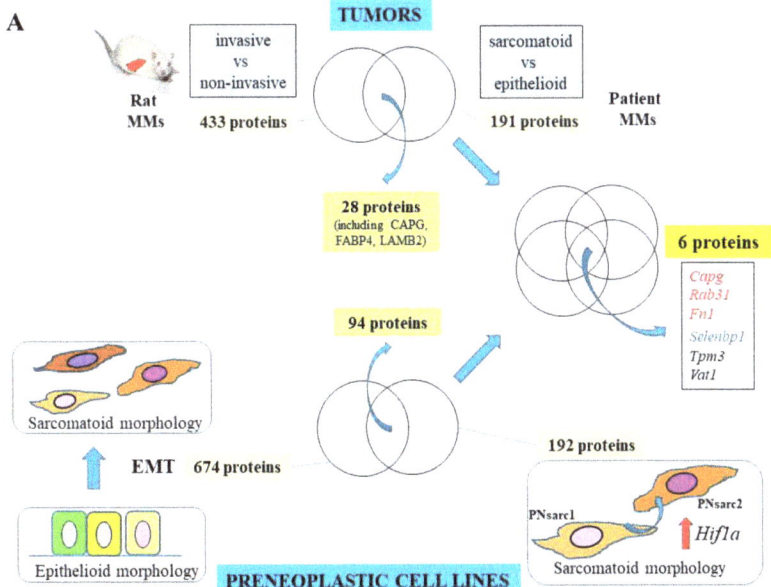

Figure 6. *Cont.*

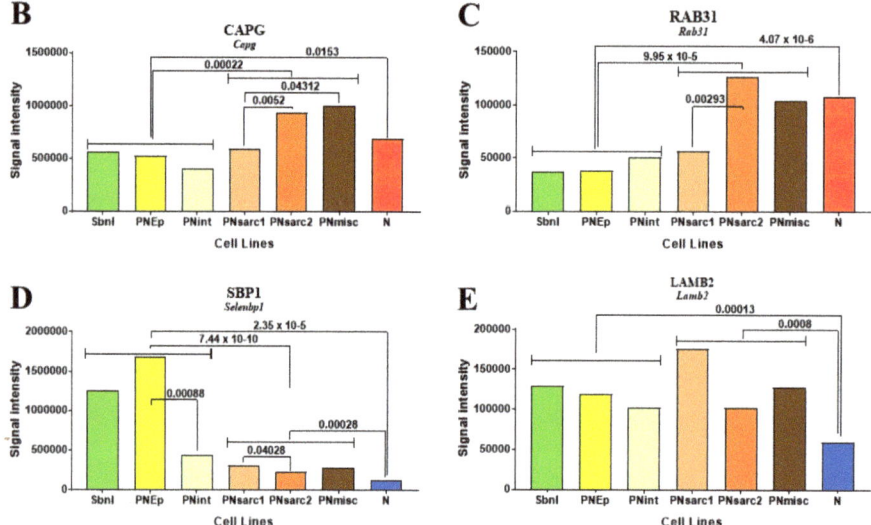

Figure 6. Biomarkers of human vs. rat MM and rat mesothelial cell carcinogenesis. (**A**), Diagram of the methodology used to identify biomarkers showing additional changes during the course of rat mesothelial cell carcinogenesis. For both CAPG (**B**) and RAB31 (**C**), a common rise in abundance was specifically observed in PNsarc2 vs. PNsarc1 and between the whole groups of preneoplastic cell lines with sarcomatoid vs. epithelioid morphology. (**D**), Evolution of abundance changes for SBP1. (**E**), Evolution of abundance changes for LAMB2.

Interestingly, among these six proteins, selenium-binding protein 1 (SBP1, encoded by *Selenbp1*) was the only one exhibiting a continuous decrease from the different subgroups of preneoplastic cell lines with epithelioid morphology to PNsarc1 and PNsarc2, including a final additional decrease in neoplastic cell lines (Table 1 and Figure 6D). Conversely, for CAPG and RAB31, protein abundances in neoplastic cells differed significantly from only one of the two groups of preneoplastic cell lines (Table 1 and Figure 6B,C). For comparison, proteomic data for LAMB2 revealed the absence of significant changes within the different groups and subgroups of preneoplastic cell lines, while there was a dramatic decrease in all neoplastic cell lines (Table 1 and Figure 6E). For fibronectin, the evolution of abundance showed a progressive rise within the first four subgroups of preneoplastic cell lines but as above discrimination with neoplastic cells was incomplete (Table 1 and Figure S1). Finally, for TPM3 and VAT1, no clear evolution was observed within the different groups and subgroups of preneoplastic cells in comparison with neoplastic cells (Table 1 and Figure S1).

3. Discussion

This study investigated the proteomic changes associated with MM invasiveness that were common to experimental and human cell lines or tumor models generated in the F344 rat, human tumor xenografts, and tumor specimens from patients. Our investigations identified three major invasiveness biomarkers not documented so far in integrative molecular studies characterizing MM [14], common to the three tumor sources, CAPG, FABP4, and LAMB2, and an additional set of candidate biomarkers shared by rat and patient tumors. Among these, SBP1 appeared to play an additional crucial role in the carcinogenic process of mesothelial cells.

CAPG, together with ANXA5 and FABP4, was previously found within a group of biomarkers differentiating invasive from noninvasive MM rat tumor models, their abundance being very significantly increased and decreased, respectively [4]. This actin filament end-capping protein was initially reported to be increased in the transformation of human breast cancer cells into a highly metastatic variant [19]. Herein, we confirm that CAPG is also increased in human MM cell lines, human MM tumor models, and patient MM. Interestingly, our observations are consistent with several previous reports showing this protein's overexpression in different cancer types. Its role in promoting the invasiveness of cholangiocarcinoma and hepatocellular carcinoma has been established by Morofuji et al. [20], and Kimura et al. [21], respectively. Its involvement in migration and invasiveness has been documented for ovarian carcinoma by Glaser et al. [22], and for breast cancer by Davalieva et al. [23] and Huang et al. [24]. Its upregulation in clinical high-grade glioblastoma has also been reported by Xing and Zeng [25], while the correlation of its expression level with shorter survival time was demonstrated by Fu et al. [26]. Moreover, the link between its abundance and occurrence of lymph node metastasis has also been documented for three different types of cancer [20,27,28], as well as its association with the prediction of response to treatment [20,29].

FABP4 (also called A-FABP or aP2) is 1 of 10 members of a family of proteins involved in intracellular fatty acid transport and lipid trafficking regulation in cells, which show different tissue-specific expression patterns [30]. Its previously mentioned adipokine function regulating macrophage and adipocyte interactions during inflammation [31] may be consistent with the absence of significant differences observed in our study between mesothelial and MM cell lines. We previously reported that the extent of the decrease was related to increasing invasiveness in rat MM [4]. Interestingly, our observations also agree with the findings of Mathis et al. showing that FABP4 loss was associated with high stage/grade and the presence of metastatic lymph nodes in invasive bladder cancer [32]. Zhong et al. have also demonstrated that similar observations are made in hepatocellular carcinoma, with the protein's overexpression leading to tumor growth inhibition in vivo [33]. A second common protein exhibiting a decreased abundance in all tumor sources was laminin subunit beta-2 (LAMB2). This protein belongs to a family of 16 laminin isoforms, which combine with subunits of collagen IV to build the basement membranes surrounding blood vessels, lymphatics, nerves, and muscle cells. Hewitt et al. initially reported that within carcinomas, vascular basement membrane staining for the subunit beta-2 is clearly weaker relative to normal tissues, probably due to their incomplete maturation [34]. This observation was further confirmed by immunohistochemistry by Mustafa et al. when studying angiogenesis in glioblastoma [35]. The fascinating aspects of their structural diversity have been emphasized by Hohenester and Yurchenco [36], raising crucial questions on the challenge that studying their complex interactions in vivo presents.

The first of an additional subset of common biomarkers of interest, which differed from the previous three by the absence of significant changes in xenografts (only a tendency), was represented by PARP1. The recent development of PARP1 inhibitors for the treatment of cancers presenting compromised HR repair has led to interesting findings on biomarkers associated with their clinical use against MM [37]. Moreover, Gaetani et al. revealed the relationship between PARP1 and miR-126 regulation in the context of asbestos-induced malignancy [38]. Regarding NSF, changes have not yet been documented in the context of cancer invasiveness; however, our data suggest that the increase commonly observed is related to the reassembly pathway of Golgi cisternae at the end of mitosis [39]. Finally, our results are consistent with the recent finding by Kofuji et al. that overexpression of the rate-limiting enzyme for de novo guanine nucleotide biosynthesis, IMDH2, relative to primary glia, promotes glioblastoma tumorigenesis [40]. Among the other biomarkers for which no changes were observed in xenografts, the most significant differences in abundance were found for annexin A5. The potential of the smallest member of the annexin family as a predictive biomarker for tumor development, metastasis, and invasion has already been reviewed [41], with it also being involved in cell membrane repair [42]. Our results are consistent with reports of its overexpression in several other cancer types, including renal cell carcinoma [43], colon cancer [44], and hepatocarcinoma [45,46]. Other highly significant changes mainly involve two proteins, COX2 for increase and VAT1 for decrease. Cytochrome c oxidase dysfunction has already been demonstrated to be related to the Warburg effect in invasive cancers [47]. The involvement of VAT1, a largely uncharacterized enzyme, has also been reported in the regulation of cancer cell motility and its interaction with Talin-1, a key cytoskeletal protein [48].

Two other proteins caught our attention among the second additional subset of common biomarkers of interest, EHD2 and RAB31, characterized by highly significant changes in abundance in both rat and patient MM, but not in human cell lines or in xenografts. The level of the first protein, which belongs to the EHD family associated with plasma membrane, has been reported to be reduced in human esophageal squamous carcinoma in comparison with adjacent normal tissues, linked to increased motility of the tumor cells [49]. Subsequently, a decreased expression was also observed, correlated with histological grade, in an immunohistochemical study of 96 human breast carcinoma samples, leading Shi et al. to suggest that this protein inhibits metastasis by regulating EMT [50]. The second protein, which belongs to the small GTPase family Rab and to the Rab5 subfamily, presents an estrogen receptor-responsive element in its promoter region which can be dysregulated in breast cancer cells, the consequences of this key finding in cancer research having been reviewed by Chua and Tang [51].

Both CAPG and RAB31 shared a similar pattern of changes during the course of rat mesothelial cell carcinogenesis. However, these changes were only observed in the first two subgroups of preneoplastic cell lines with sarcomatoid morphology, suggesting a link to increased *Hifa* expression [18]. The pattern of changes observed for SBP1 markedly contrasted with these situations as decreases in abundance were observed at three main stages of the carcinogenic process. Firstly, the decrease observed between PNep and PNint was concomitant with the first dramatic decrease in the expression of *Cdh1* and *Il10*, and parallel increase in the expression of *Acta 2*, *Tgfb1* [15]. Secondly, the new decrease observed between PNsarc1 and PNsarc2, and continuous decrease from PNep to PNsarc2, confirm the existence of links to both the level of expression of *Hifa* [18] and EMT process [15]. Thirdly, the decrease observed between preneoplastic cell lines with both epithelioid and sarcomatoid morphologies and neoplastic cell lines leads to the conclusion that SBP1 presents additional interest as a biomarker of neoplastic transformation. Finally, the decrease in SBP1 also observed in association with increased invasiveness in human cell lines, rat and patient MM tumors tends to confirm the protein's crucial role. The downregulation of another selenium-containing protein was earlier reported by Apostolou et al., suggesting that selenium could be useful as a chemopreventive agent in individuals at high risk of MM due to asbestos exposure [52]. Interestingly, Rundlöf et al. found differential expression within isoforms of the selenoenzyme thioredoxin reductase 1 (TrxR1) in MM cell lines, with the sarcomatoid phenotype showing the lower total TrxR1 mRNA level [53]. The mechanisms by which dietary selenium may affect MM tumor progression have only been partly explored, mostly in cell lines, pointing to the crucial role of redox metabolism [54]. Although it is well established that low levels of SBP1 are frequently associated with poor clinical outcome [55], the complexity of selenium metabolism has highlighted the fact that among selenocysteine-containing proteins that are members of the glutathione peroxidase family, SBP1 is the only one for which no catalytic function has been assigned [56]. Therefore, many aspects of this research field require further investigation. To give just a few more very recent examples of the protein's importance, Lee et al. have suggested that hepatitis B virus-X-expressing cells, which show markedly decreased *SELENBP1* expression, might be one factor in the development of hepatocellular carcinoma caused by HBV infection [57]. Wang et al. have also reported this protein's novel function in transcriptionally modulating p21 expression through a p53-independent mechanism, with a resulting impact on the G_0/G_1 phase cell cycle arrest in bladder cancer [58].

4. Materials and Methods

4.1. Study Approval

The human studies were conducted according to the ethical guidelines of the Declaration of Helsinki. The paraffin-embedded human MM tumor pieces were prepared from samples of the Tumor Bank of the Reims University Hospital Biological Resource, Collection No. DC-2008-374, declared to the Ministry of Health according to French law, for the use of tissue samples for research. The two human cell lines MM34 (Meso 34) and MM163 (Meso 163) were established from pleural effusions of patients with suspected pleural MM [59], according to the ethics committee approval (Comité de Protection des Personnes Ouest IV-Nantes, dossier n° DC-2011-1399). The animal studies were carried out in agreement with European Union guidelines for the care and use of laboratory animals in research protocols (Agreement #01257.03). All experiments were approved by the ethics committee for animal experiments of the Pays de la Loire Region, France (CEEA.2011.38 and CEEA.2013.7.).

4.2. Rat and Human Cell Lines, and Tumor Samples

The 27 cell lines of the rat biocollection were grown in RPMI 1640 medium, supplemented with 10% heat-inactivated fetal calf serum, 2 mM L-glutamine, 100 U/mL penicillin, and 100 µg/mL streptomycin (all reagents from Gibco Life Technologies Limited, Paisley, UK) at 37 °C in a 5% CO_2 atmosphere. Cells were collected from preconfluent 75 cm^2 flasks and cell pellets of 2×10^6 cells were used for SWATH-MS proteomic analysis after washing in PBS buffer. The four rat neoplastic cell lines (M5-T2, F4-T2, F5-T1, and M5-T1) were injected into syngeneic rats, and tumors collected and fixed as previously described [4]. The two human cell lines Meso 34 and Meso 163 were established from pleural effusions of patients with suspected pleural MM, aseptically collected by thoracocentesis as previously described [56], and cultivated as rat cell lines. Meso 34 and Meso 163 xenografted tumors were collected and fixed after injection of the corresponding cell lines into the peritoneal cavity of two groups of five immunodeficient NOD SCID mice. For patient tumors, four pieces of paraffin-embedded pleural MM tumor pieces collected from four different patients were obtained from the Tumor Bank of the Reims University Hospital Biological Resource. They represented two tumors of the sarcomatoid subtype (S-MM1 and S-MM2) versus two tumors of the epithelioid subtype (E-MM1 and E-MM2).

4.3. SWATH-MS Analysis

The spectral libraries, DDA experiments, peptide identification, and peak extraction of the SWATH data were performed as previously described [4], using either Spectronaut software (v 8.0, Biognosys, Schlieren, Switzerland) or the SWATH micro app embedded in PeakView (v 2.0, AB Sciex Pte. Ltd., Framingham, MA, USA). Sections of the tumors, stained with hematoxylin-phloxine-saffron (HPS), were first examined to select areas of interest, then removed with a scalpel. Five 20 µm thick sections of the samples were used, and the areas of interest collected in a microtube. Samples were deparaffinized, and then cell pellets and dried deparaffinized tumor samples treated as previously described [4]. After centrifugation, salts were removed using OASIS® HLB extraction cartridges (Waters SAS., St Quentin-en-Yvelines, 78, France), and the samples dried under SpeedVac. Peptide concentrations of the samples were determined using the Micro BCA™ protein assay kit (Thermo Fisher Scientific, St Herblain, 44, France).

Five micrograms of each sample were analyzed with a SWATH-MS acquisition method. The method of acquisition, peak extraction of the SWATH data, calibration of the retention time of extracted peptide peaks and quantification followed the procedure already described in [4]. For statistical analysis of the SWATH data set, the peak extraction output data matrix from PeakView was imported into MarkerView (v 2, Sciex, Framingham, MA, USA) for data normalization and relative protein quantification. Proteins with a fold change >1.5 and statistical p-value < 0.05 estimated by MarkerView were declared differentially expressed under different conditions.

5. Conclusions

This study pointed to some proteins of interest that exhibited the same patterns of quantitative changes in different situations, and for which the relationship with tumor invasiveness has already been reported in the literature for other cancer types. Although this study was limited by the small number of samples, an interesting point was the similarity of observations made on malignant mesothelioma cells and tumors from different sources and from two different species. Extending these studies to a larger number of samples would be the logical next step, which may later contribute to improving current therapies for patients with the worst survival outcomes. Another interesting prospect is related to the questions raised by the additional involvement of the selenium-binding protein 1 in the carcinogenic process, a point that would present a good basis for further basic research in cancerology, and probably also for improving early MM diagnosis.

Supplementary Materials: The following are available online at http://www.mdpi.com/2072-6694/12/9/2430/s1, Figure S1: Additional biomarkers of human vs. rat MM and rat mesothelial cell carcinogenesis.

Author Contributions: Conceptualization of experiments (rat experimental cell lines, rat MM tumor models, human MM cell lines, and MM34 and MM163 xenografts in NOD SCID mice), J.S.N. and D.L.P. Preparation of samples from patient tumors and histological examination, I.V. and V.V. Preparation of samples for proteomic analysis, D.L.P., A.B. and C.H. Relative quantification by SWATH-MS acquisition and statistical analysis, validation, C.G. Formal analysis, D.L.P. Funding acquisition, M.G., D.L.P., C.G. and O.C. Original draft preparation, D.L.P. All authors have read and agreed to the published version of the manuscript.

Funding: This study was conducted with the support of the Ligue contre le Cancer (Ligue inter-régionale du Grand-Ouest, comités 16, 29, 44, 72), the Fondation pour la Recherche Médicale (FRM), and the "Comité Féminin 49 Octobre Rose".

Acknowledgments: The authors are indebted to Philippe Birembaut, CHU de Reims, Hôpital Maison Blanche, Laboratoire de Pathologie, F-51092 Reims, France, for his invaluable help in providing human MM tumor samples from patients from the Tumor Bank of the Reims University Hospital Biological Resource, Collection No. DC-2008-374.

Conflicts of Interest: The authors declare no conflict of interest.

References

1. Carbone, M.; Adusumilli, P.S.; Alexander, H.R., Jr.; Baas, P.; Bardelli, F.; Bononi, A.; Bueno, R.; Felley-Bosco, E.; Galateau-Sallé, F.; Jablons, D.; et al. Mesothelioma: Scientific clues for prevention, diagnosis, and therapy. *CA Cancer J. Clin.* **2019**, *69*, 402–429. [CrossRef] [PubMed]
2. Mutti, L.; Peikert, T.; Robinson, B.W.S.; Scherpereel, A.; Tsao, A.S.; de Perrot, M.; Woodard, G.A.; Jablons, D.M.; Wiens, J.; Hirsch, F.R.; et al. Scientific advances and new frontiers in mesothelioma therapeutics. *J. Thorac. Oncol.* **2018**, *13*, 1269–1283. [CrossRef] [PubMed]
3. Panou, V.; Vyberg, M.; Weinreich, U.M.; Meristoudis, C.; Falkmer, U.G.; Røe, O.D. The established and future biomarkers of malignant pleural mesothelioma. *Cancer Treat. Rev.* **2015**, *41*, 486–495. [CrossRef] [PubMed]
4. Nader, J.S.; Abadie, J.; Deshayes, S.; Boissard, A.; Blandin, S.; Blanquart, C.; Boisgerault, N.; Coqueret, O.; Guette, C.; Grégoire, M.; et al. Characterization of increasing stages of invasiveness identifies stromal/cancer cell crosstalk in rat models of mesothelioma. *Oncotarget* **2018**, *9*, 16311–16329. [CrossRef] [PubMed]
5. Chernova, T.; Sun, X.M.; Powley, I.R.; Galavotti, S.; Grosso, S.; Murphy, F.A.; Miles, G.J.; Cresswell, L.; Antonov, A.V.; Bennett, J.; et al. Molecular profiling reveals primary mesothelioma cell lines recapitulate human disease. *Cell Death Differ.* **2016**, *23*, 1152–1164. [CrossRef]
6. Workman, P.; Aboagye, E.O.; Balkwill, F.; Balmain, A.; Bruder, G.; Chaplin, D.J.; Double, J.A.; Everitt, J.; Farningham, D.A.H.; Glennie, M.J.; et al. Guidelines for the welfare and use of animals in cancer research. *Br. J. Cancer* **2010**, *102*, 1555–1577. [CrossRef]
7. Hughes, P.; Marshall, D.; Reid, Y.; Parkes, H.; Gelber, C. The costs of using unauthenticated, over-passaged cell lines: How much more data do we need? *Biotechniques* **2007**, *43*, 577–578. [CrossRef]
8. Olive, K.P.; Tuveson, D.A. The use of targeted mouse models for preclinical testing of novel cancer therapeutics. *Clin. Cancer Res.* **2006**, *12*, 5277–5287. [CrossRef]
9. Kerbel, R.S. Human tumor xenografts as predictive preclinical models for anticancer drug activity in humans: Better than commonly perceived-but they can be improved. *Cancer Biol. Ther.* **2003**, *2*, S134–S139. [CrossRef]
10. Aggarwal, B.B.; Danda, D.; Gupta, S.; Gehlot, P. Models for prevention and treatment of cancer: Problem vs. promises. *Biochem. Pharmacol.* **2009**, *78*, 1083–1094. [CrossRef]
11. Shiozawa, K.; Oyama, R.; Takahashi, M.; Kito, F.; Hattori, E.; Yoshida, A.; Kawai, A.; Ono, M.; Kondo, T. Species-specific quantitative proteomics profiles of sarcoma patient-derived models closely reflect their primary tumors. *Proteom. Clin. Appl.* **2019**, *13*, 1900054. [CrossRef] [PubMed]
12. Henry, N.L.; Hayes, D.F. Cancer biomarkers. *Mol. Oncol.* **2012**, *6*, 140–146. [CrossRef] [PubMed]
13. Pouliquen, D.L.; Boissard, A.; Coqueret, O.; Guette, C. Biomarkers of tumor invasiveness in proteomics (Review). *Int. J. Oncol.* **2020**. [CrossRef] [PubMed]

14. Hmeljak, J.; Sanchez-Vega, F.; Hoadley, K.A.; Shih, J.; Stewart, C.; Heiman, D.; Tarpey, P.; Danilova, L.; Drill, E.; Gibb, E.A.; et al. Integrative molecular characterization of malignant pleural mesothelioma. *Cancer Discov.* **2018**, *8*, 1548–1565. [CrossRef] [PubMed]
15. Roulois, D.; Deshayes, S.; Guilly, M.-N.; Nader, J.S.; Liddell, C.; Robard, M.; Hulin, P.; Ouacher, A.; Le Martelot, V.; Fonteneau, J.-F.; et al. Characterization of preneoplastic and neoplastic rat mesothelial cell lines: The involvement of TETs, DNMTs, and 5-hydroxymethylcytosine. *Oncotarget* **2016**, *7*, 34664–34687. [CrossRef]
16. Blondy, T.; d'Almeida, S.M.; Briolay, T.; Tabiasco, J.; Meiller, C.; Chéné, A.-L.; Cellerin, L.; Deshayes, S.; Delneste, Y.; Fonteneau, J.-F.; et al. Involvement of the M-CSF/IL-34/CSF-1R pathway in malignant pleural mesothelioma. *J. Immunother. Cancer* **2020**, *8*, e000182. [CrossRef]
17. Delaunay, T.; Achard, C.; Boisgerault, N.; Grard, M.; Petithomme, T.; Chatelain, C.; Dutoit, S.; Blanquart, C.; Royer, P.-J.; Minvielle, S.; et al. Frequent homozygous deletions of type I interferon genes in pleural mesothelioma confer sensitivity to oncolytic measles virus. *J. Thor. Oncol.* **2020**, *15*, 827–842. [CrossRef]
18. Nader, J.S.; Guillon, J.; Petit, C.; Boissard, A.; Franconi, F.; Blandin, S.; Lambot, S.; Grégoire, M.; Verrièle, V.; Nawrocki-Raby, B.; et al. S100A4 is a biomarker of tumorigenesis, EMT, invasion, and colonization of host organs in experimental malignant mesothelioma. *Cancers* **2020**, *12*, 939. [CrossRef]
19. Xu, S.-G.; Yan, P.-J.; Shao, Z.-M. Differential proteomic analysis of a highly metastatic variant of human breast cancer cells using two-dimensional differential gel electrophoresis. *J. Cancer Res. Clin. Oncol.* **2010**, *136*, 1545–1556. [CrossRef]
20. Morofuji, N.; Ojima, H.; Onaya, H.; Okusaka, T.; Shimada, K.; Sakamoto, Y.; Esaki, M.; Nara, S.; Kosuge, T.; Asahina, D.; et al. Macrophage-capping protein as a tissue biomarker for prediction of response to gemcitabine treatment and prognosis in cholangiocarcinoma. *J. Proteom.* **2012**, *75*, 1577–1589. [CrossRef]
21. Kimura, K.; Ojima, H.; Kubota, D.; Sakumoto, M.; Nakamura, Y.; Tomonaga, T.; Kosuge, T.; Kondo, T. Proteomic identification of the macrophage-capping protein as a protein contributing to the malignant features of hepatocellular carcinoma. *J. Proteom.* **2013**, *78*, 362–373. [CrossRef] [PubMed]
22. Glaser, J.; Neumann, M.H.D.; Mei, Q.; Betz, B.; Seier, N.; Beyer, I.; Fehm, T.; Neubauer, H.; Niederacher, D.; Fleisch, M.C. Macrophage-capping protein CapG is a putative oncogene involved in migration and invasiveness in ovarian carcinoma. *Biomed. Res. Int.* **2014**, *2014*, 1–8. [CrossRef] [PubMed]
23. Davalieva, K.; Kiprijanovska, S.; Broussard, C.; Petrusevska, G.; Efremov, G.D. Proteomic analysis of infiltrating ductal carcinoma tissues by coupled 2-D DIGE/MS/MS analysis. *Mol. Biol.* **2012**, *46*, 469–480. [CrossRef]
24. Huang, S.; Chi, Y.; Qin, Y.; Wang, Z.; Xiu, B.; Su, Y.; Guo, R.; Guo, L.; Sun, H.; Zheng, C.; et al. CAPG enhances breast cancer metastasis by competing with PRMT5 to modulate STC-1 transcription. *Theranostics* **2018**, *8*, 2549–2564. [CrossRef] [PubMed]
25. Xing, W.; Zeng, C. An integrated transcriptomic and computational analysis for biomarker identification in human glioma. *Tumor Biol.* **2016**, *37*, 7185–7192. [CrossRef]
26. Fu, Q.; Shaya, M.; Li, S.; Kugeluke, Y.; Dilimulati, Y.; Liu, B.; Zhou, Q. Analysis of clinical characteristics of macrophage-capping protein (CAPG) gene expressed in glioma based on TCGA data and clinical experiments. *Oncol. Lett.* **2019**, *18*, 1344–1350. [CrossRef]
27. Ichikawa, H.; Kanda, T.; Kosugi, S.-I.; Kawachi, Y.; Sasaki, H.; Wakai, T.; Kondo, T. Laser microdissection and two-dimensional difference gel electrophoresis reveal the role of a novel macrophage-capping protein in lymph node metastasis in gastric cancer. *J. Proteome Res.* **2013**, *12*, 3780–3791. [CrossRef]
28. Wu, W.; Chen, J.; Ding, Q.; Yang, S.; Wang, J.; Yu, H.; Lin, J. Function of the macrophage-capping protein in colorectal carcinoma. *Oncol. Lett.* **2017**, *14*, 5549–5555. [CrossRef]
29. Westbrook, J.A.; Cairns, D.A.; Peng, J.; Speirs, V.; Hanby, A.M.; Holen, I.; Wood, S.L.; Ottewell, P.D.; Marshall, H.; Banks, R.E.; et al. CAPG and GIPC1: Breast cancer biomarkers for bone metastasis development and treatment. *J. Natl. Cancer Inst.* **2016**, *108*, djv360. [CrossRef]
30. Guaita-Esteruelas, S.; Guma, J.; Masana, L.; Borràs, J. The peritumoural adipose tissue microenvironment and cancer. The roles of fatty acid binding protein 4 and fatty acid binding protein 5. *Mol. Cell. Endocrinol.* **2018**, *462*, 107–118. [CrossRef]
31. Thumser, A.E.; Moore, J.B.; Plant, N.J. Fatty acid binding proteins: Tissue-specific functions in health and disease. *Curr. Opin. Clin. Nutr. Metab. Care* **2014**, *17*, 124–129. [CrossRef] [PubMed]

32. Mathis, C.; Lascombe, I.; Monnien, F.; Bittard, H.; Kleinclauss, F.; Bedgedjian, I.; Fauconnet, S.; Valmary-Degano, S. Down-regulation of A-FABP predicts non-muscle invasive bladder cancer progression: Investigation with a long-term clinical follow-up. *BMC Cancer* **2018**, *18*, 1239. [CrossRef]
33. Zhong, C.-Q.; Zhang, X.-P.; Ma, N.; Zhang, E.-B.; Li, J.J.; Jiang, Y.-B.; Gao, Y.-Z.; Yuan, Y.-M.; Lan, S.-Q.; Xie, D.; et al. FABP4 suppresses proliferation and invasion of hepatocellular carcinoma cells and predicts a poor prognosis for hepatocellular carcinoma. *Cancer Med.* **2018**, *7*, 2629–2640. [CrossRef] [PubMed]
34. Hewitt, R.E.; Powe, D.G.; Morrell, K.; Bailey, E.; Leach, I.H.; Ellis, I.O.; Turner, D.R. Laminin and collagen IV subunit distribution in normal and neoplastic tissues of colorectum and breast. *Br. J. Cancer* **1997**, *75*, 221–229. [CrossRef] [PubMed]
35. Mustafa, D.A.M.; Dekker, L.J.; Stingl, C.; Kremer, A.; Stoop, M.; Sillevis Smitt, P.A.E.; Kros, J.M.; Luider, T.M. A proteome comparison between physiological angiogenesis and angiogenesis in glioblastoma. *Mol. Cell. Proteom.* **2012**, *11*. [CrossRef] [PubMed]
36. Hohenester, E.; Yurchenco, P.D. Laminins in basement membrane assembly. *Cell Adhes. Migr.* **2013**, *7*, 56–63. [CrossRef]
37. Morra, F.; Merolla, F.; D'Abbiero, D.; Ilardi, G.; Campione, S.; Monaco, R.; Guggino, G.; Ambrosio, F.; Staibano, S.; Cerrato, A.; et al. Analysis of CCDC6 as a novel biomarker for the clinical use of PARP1 inhibitors in malignant pleural mesothelioma. *Lung Cancer* **2019**, *135*, 56–65. [CrossRef]
38. Gaetani, S.; Monaco, F.; Alessandrini, F.; Tagliabracci, A.; Sabbatini, A.; Bracci, M.; Valentino, M.; Neuzil, J.; Amati, M.; Santarelli, L.; et al. Mechanism of miR-222 and miR-126 regulation and its role in asbestos-induced malignancy. *Int. J. Biochem. Cell Biol.* **2020**, *121*, 105700. [CrossRef]
39. Rabouille, C.; Kondo, H.; Newman, R.; Hui, N.; Freemont, P.; Warren, G. Syntaxin 5 is a common component of the NSF-and p97-mediated reassembly pathways of Golgi cisternae from mitotic Golgi fragments in vitro. *Cell* **1998**, *92*, 603–610. [CrossRef]
40. Kofuji, S.; Hirayama, A.; Eberhardt, A.O.; Kawaguchi, R.; Sugiura, Y.; Sampetrean, O.; Ikeda, Y.; Warren, M.; Sakamoto, N.; Kitahara, S.; et al. IMP dehydrogenase-2 drives aberrant nucleolar activity and promotes tumorigenesis in glioblastoma. *Nat. Cell Biol.* **2019**, *21*, 1003–1014. [CrossRef]
41. Peng, B.; Guo, C.; Guan, H.; Liu, S.; Sun, M.-Z. Annexin A5 as a potential marker in tumors. *Clin. Chim. Acta* **2014**, *427*, 42–48. [CrossRef] [PubMed]
42. Bouter, A.; Carmeille, R.; Gounou, C.; Bouvet, F.; Degrelle, S.A.; Evain-Brion, D.; Brisson, A.R. Review: Annexin-A5 and cell membrane repair. *Placenta* **2015**, *36*, S43–S49. [CrossRef] [PubMed]
43. Tang, J.; Qin, Z.; Han, P.; Wang, W.; Yang, C.; Xu, Z.; Li, R.; Liu, B.; Qin, C.; Wang, Z.; et al. High annexin A5 expression promotes tumor progression and poor prognosis in renal cell carcinoma. *Int. J. Oncol.* **2017**, *50*, 1839–1847. [CrossRef] [PubMed]
44. Sun, C.-B.; Zhao, A.-Y.; Ji, S.; Han, X.-Q.; Sun, Z.-C.; Wang, M.-C.; Zheng, F.-C. Expression of annexin A5 in serum and tumor tissue of patients with colon cancer and its clinical significance. *World J. Gastroenterol.* **2017**, *23*, 7168–7173. [CrossRef]
45. Sun, X.; Wei, B.; Liu, S.; Guo, C.; Wu, N.; Liu, Q.; Sun, M.-Z. Anxa5 mediates the in vitro malignant behaviours of murine hepatocarcinoma Hca-F cells with high lymph node metastasis potential preferentially via ERK2/p-ERK2/c-Jun/p-c-Jun(Ser73) and E-cadherin. *Biomed. Pharmacother.* **2016**, *84*, 645–654. [CrossRef]
46. Sun, X.; Liu, S.; Wang, J.; Wei, B.; Guo, C.; Chen, C.; Sun, M.-Z. Annexin A5 regulates hepatocarcinoma malignancy via CRKI/II-DOCK180-RAC1 integrin and MEK-ERK pathways. *Cell Death Dis.* **2018**, *9*, 637. [CrossRef]
47. Srinivasan, S.; Guha, M.; Dong, D.W.; Whelan, K.A.; Ruthel, G.; Uchikado, Y.; Natsugoe, S.; Nakagawa, H.; Avadhani, N.G. Disruption of cytochrome c oxidase function induces Warburg effect and metabolic reprogramming. *Oncogene* **2016**, *35*, 1585–1595. [CrossRef]
48. Gleissner, C.M.-L.; Pyka, C.L.; Heydenreuter, W.; Gronauer, T.F.; Atzberger, C.; Korotkov, V.S.; Cheng, W.; Hacker, S.M.; Vollmar, A.M.; Braig, S.; et al. Neocarzilin A is a potent inhibitor of cancer cell motility targeting VAT-1 controlled pathways. *ACS Cent. Sci.* **2019**, *5*, 1170–1178. [CrossRef]
49. Li, M.; Yang, X.; Zhang, J.; Shi, H.; Hang, Q.; Huang, X.; Liu, G.; Zhu, J.; He, S.; Wang, H. Effects of EHD2 interference on migration of esophageal squamous cell carcinoma. *Med. Oncol.* **2013**, *30*, 396. [CrossRef]
50. Shi, Y.; Liu, X.; Sun, Y.; Wu, D.; Qiu, A.; Cheng, H.; Wu, C.; Wang, X. Decreased expression and prognostic role of EHD2 in human breast carcinoma with E-cadherin. *J. Mol. Histol.* **2015**, *46*, 221–231. [CrossRef]

51. Chua, C.E.L.; Tang, B.L. The role of the small GTPase Rab31 in cancer. *J. Cell. Mol. Med.* **2015**, *19*, 1–10. [CrossRef] [PubMed]
52. Apostolou, S.; Klein, J.O.; Mitsuuchi, Y.; Shetler, J.N.; Poulikakos, P.I.; Jhanwar, S.C.; Kruger, W.D.; Testa, J.R. Growth inhibition and induction of apoptosis in mesothelioma cells by selenium and dependence on selenoprotein *SEP15* genotype. *Oncogene* **2014**, *23*, 5032–5040. [CrossRef] [PubMed]
53. Rundlöf, A.-K.; Fernandes, A.P.; Selenius, M.; Babic, M.; Shariatgorji, M.; Nilsonne, G.; Ilag, L.L.; Dobra, K.; Björnsted, M. Quantification of alternative mRNA species and identification of thioredoxin reductase 1 isoforms in human tumor cells. *Differentiation* **2007**, *75*, 123–132. [CrossRef] [PubMed]
54. Rose, A.H.; Bertino, P.; Hoffmann, F.W.; Gaudino, G.; Carbone, M.; Hoffmann, P.R. Increasing dietary selenium elevates reducing capacity and ERK activation associated with accelerated progression of select mesotheliomas tumors. *Am. J. Pathol.* **2014**, *184*, 1041–1049. [CrossRef] [PubMed]
55. Elhodaky, M.; Diamond, A.M. Selenium-binding protein 1 in human health and disease. *Int. J. Mol. Sci.* **2018**, *19*, 3437. [CrossRef]
56. Diamond, A.M. The subcellular location of selenoproteins and the impact on their function. *Nutrients* **2015**, *7*, 3938–3948. [CrossRef]
57. Lee, Y.-M.; Kim, S.; Park, R.-Y.; Kim, Y.-S. Hepatitis B virus-X downregulates expression of selenium binding protein 1. *Viruses* **2020**, *12*, 565. [CrossRef]
58. Wang, Y.; Zhu, W.; Chen, X.; Wei, G.; Jiang, G.; Zhang, G. Selenium-binding protein 1 transcriptionally activates p21 expression via p53-independent mechanism and its frequent reduction associates with poor prognosis in bladder cancer. *J. Transl. Med.* **2020**, *18*, 17. [CrossRef]
59. Blanquart, C.; Gueugnon, F.; Nguyen, J.M.; Roulois, D.; Cellerin, L.; Sagan, C.; Perigaud, C.; Scherpereel, A.; Grégoire, M. CCL2, Galectin-3, and SMRP combination improves the diagnosis of mesothelioma in pleural effusions. *J. Thorac. Oncol.* **2012**, *7*, 883–889. [CrossRef]

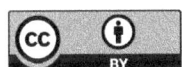

© 2020 by the authors. Licensee MDPI, Basel, Switzerland. This article is an open access article distributed under the terms and conditions of the Creative Commons Attribution (CC BY) license (http://creativecommons.org/licenses/by/4.0/).

Article

Malignant Pleural Mesothelioma Interactome with 364 Novel Protein-Protein Interactions

Kalyani B. Karunakaran [1], Naveena Yanamala [2], Gregory Boyce [2], Michael J. Becich [3] and Madhavi K. Ganapathiraju [3,4,*]

1. Supercomputer Education and Research Centre, Indian Institute of Science, Bangalore 560012, India; kalyanik@iisc.ac.in
2. Exposure Assessment Branch, National Institute of Occupational Safety and Health, Center for Disease Control, Morgantown, WV 26506, USA; yanamala.naveena@gmail.com (N.Y.); omu0@cdc.gov (G.B.)
3. Department of Biomedical Informatics, School of Medicine, University of Pittsburgh, Pittsburgh, PA 15206, USA; becich@pitt.edu
4. Intelligent Systems Program, School of Computing and Information, University of Pittsburgh, Pittsburgh, PA 15213, USA
* Correspondence: madhavi@pitt.edu

Simple Summary: Internal organs like the heart and lungs, and body cavities like the thoracic and abdominal cavities, are covered by a thin, slippery layer called the mesothelium. Malignant pleural mesothelioma (MPM) is an aggressive cancer of the lining of the lung, where genetics and asbestos exposure play a role. It is not diagnosable until it becomes invasive, offering only a short survival time to the patient. To help understand the role of the genes that relate to this disease most of which are poorly understood, we constructed the 'MPM interactome', including in it the protein-protein interactions that we predicted computationally and those that are previously known in the literature. Five novel protein-protein interactions (PPIs) were tested and validated experimentally. 85.65% of the interactome is supported by genetic variant, transcriptomic, and proteomic evidence. Comparative transcriptome analysis revealed 5 repurposable drugs targeting the interactome proteins. We make the interactome available on a freely accessible web application, Wiki-MPM.

Abstract: Malignant pleural mesothelioma (MPM) is an aggressive cancer affecting the outer lining of the lung, with a median survival of less than one year. We constructed an 'MPM interactome' with over 300 computationally predicted protein-protein interactions (PPIs) and over 2400 known PPIs of 62 literature-curated genes whose activity affects MPM. Known PPIs of the 62 MPM associated genes were derived from Biological General Repository for Interaction Datasets (BioGRID) and Human Protein Reference Database (HPRD). Novel PPIs were predicted by applying the HiPPIP algorithm, which computes features of protein pairs such as cellular localization, molecular function, biological process membership, genomic location of the gene, and gene expression in microarray experiments, and classifies the pairwise features as interacting or non-interacting based on a random forest model. We validated five novel predicted PPIs experimentally. The interactome is significantly enriched with genes differentially ex-pressed in MPM tumors compared with normal pleura and with other thoracic tumors, genes whose high expression has been correlated with unfavorable prognosis in lung cancer, genes differentially expressed on crocidolite exposure, and exosome-derived proteins identified from malignant mesothelioma cell lines. 28 of the interactors of MPM proteins are targets of 147 U.S. Food and Drug Administration (FDA)-approved drugs. By comparing disease-associated versus drug-induced differential expression profiles, we identified five potentially repurposable drugs, namely cabazitaxel, primaquine, pyrimethamine, trimethoprim and gliclazide. Preclinical studies may be con-ducted in vitro to validate these computational results. Interactome analysis of disease-associated genes is a powerful approach with high translational impact. It shows how MPM-associated genes identified by various high throughput studies are functionally linked, leading to clinically translatable results such as repurposed drugs. The PPIs are made available on a webserver with interactive user interface, visualization and advanced search capabilities.

Keywords: malignant mesothelioma; protein-protein interactions; systems biology; network analysis; drug repurposing

1. Introduction

Internal organs such as heart and lung, and body cavities such as thoracic and abdominal cavities, are covered by a thin slippery layer of cells called the "mesothelium". This protective layer prevents organ adhesion and plays a number of important roles in inflammation and tissue repair [1]. The mesothelia that line the heart, lung and abdominal cavity are called pericardium, pleura and peritoneum, respectively. Mesothelioma is the cancer that originates from this lining (described in detail in a recent review article [2]). Most types of mesothelioma metastasize to different locations in the body [3]. Pleural mesotheliomas account for ~90% of malignant mesotheliomas and have a short median survival, of less than 1 year [4].

Malignant pleural mesothelioma (MPM) is associated with exposure to asbestos; it has a long latency period after exposure and is conclusively diagnosable only after reaching the invasive phase [3]. It tends to cluster in families and occurs only in a small fraction of the population exposed to asbestos, suggesting the involvement of a genetic component [5]. These factors necessitate expeditious discovery of genetic predispositions, molecular mechanisms and therapeutics for the disease.

The molecular mechanisms of disease are often revealed by the protein-protein interactions (PPIs) of disease-associated genes. For example, the involvement of transcriptional deregulation in MPM pathogenesis was identified through mutations detected in *BAP1* and its interactions with proteins such as *HCF1*, *ASXL1*, *ASXL2*, *ANKRD1*, *FOXK1* and *FOXK2* [6]. PPI of *BAP1* with *BRCA1* was central to understanding the role of *BAP1* in growth-control pathways and cancer; *BAP1* was suggested to play a role in *BRCA1* stabilization [7,8]. Studies on *BAP1* and *BRCA1* later led to clinical trials of the drug vinorelbine as a second line therapy for MPM patients, and the drug was shown to have rare or moderate effects in MPM patients [9,10]. *BAP1* expression was shown to be necessary for vinorelbine activity; 40% of MPM patients in a study showed low *BRCA1* expression and vinorelbine resistance [11–13]. Further, 60% of the disease-associated missense mutations perturb PPIs in human genetic disorders [14].

Despite their importance, only about 10–15% of expected PPIs in the human protein interactome are currently known; for nearly half of the human proteins, not even a single PPI is currently known [15]. Due to the sheer number of PPIs remaining to be discovered in the human interactome, it becomes imperative that biological discovery be accelerated by computational and high-throughput biotechnological methods. We developed a computational model, called HiPPIP (high-precision protein-protein interaction prediction) that is deemed accurate by computational evaluations and experimental validations of 18 predicted PPIs, where all the tested pairs were shown to be true PPIs ([16,17] and current work, and other unpublished works). HiPPIP computes features of protein pairs such as cellular localization, molecular function, biological process membership, genomic location of the gene, and gene expression in microarray experiments, and classifies the pairwise features as interacting or non-interacting based on a random forest model [16]. Though each of the features by itself is not an indicator of an interaction, a machine learning model was able to use the combined features to make predictions with high precision. The threshold of HiPPIP to classify a protein-pair as "a PPI" was set high in such a way that it yields very high-precision predictions, even if low recall. Novel PPIs predicted using this model are making translational impact. For example, they highlighted the role of cilia and mitochondria in congenital heart disease [18,19], that oligoadenylate synthetase-like protein (*OASL*) activates host response during viral infections through RIG-I signaling via its PPI with retinoic acid-inducible gene I (*RIG-I*) [17], and led to the identification of drugs potentially repurposable for schizophrenia [20], one of which is currently under clinical trials.

In this work, we studied MPM-associated genes and their PPIs assembled with HiPPIP and analyzed the MPM interactome to draw translatable results. We demonstrate the various ways in which systems-level analysis of this interactome could lead to biologically insightful and clinically translatable results. We made the interactome available to the cancer biology research community on a webserver with comprehensive annotations, so as to accelerate biomedical research on MPM.

2. Results

We collected 62 MPM-associated genes from the Ingenuity Pathway Analysis (IPA) suite, which will be referred to as 'MPM genes' here; these genes have been reported to affect MPM through gene expression changes or genetic variants, or by being targeted by drugs clinically active against MPM (see details in Data File S1) [21]. Previously known PPIs of the 62 MPM genes were collected from Human Protein Reference Database (HPRD), version 9 [22] and Biological General Repository for Interaction Datasets (BioGRID) version 4.3.194 [23]. Novel (hitherto unknown) PPIs were predicted with HiPPIP, a computational model. We discovered 364 novel PPIs of MPM genes (Table 1), which are deemed highly accurate according to prior evaluation of the HiPPIP model including experimental validations [16]. The MPM interactome thus assembled has 2459 known PPIs and 364 novel PPIs among the 62 MPM-associated genes and 1911 interactors (Figure 1 and Data File S2). Nearly half of the MPM genes had 10 or less known PPIs each, and about 130 novel PPIs have been predicted for these (Figure 2). HiPPIP predicted 920 PPIs of which 556 PPIs were previously known, leaving 364 PPIs to be considered as novel PPIs of the MPM genes. There were an additional 1903 PPIs that are known and not predicted by HiPPIP. This is as expected because the HiPPIP prediction threshold has been fixed to achieve *high precision* by compromising *recall*, which is required for adoption into biology; in other words, it is set to predict only a few PPIs out of the hundreds of thousands of unknown PPIs, but those that are predicted will be highly accurate. It has to be noted that neither PPI prediction nor high throughput PPI screening can be performed with high-precision *and* high-recall. Co-immunoprecipitation (Co-IP) based methods show high-precision and extremely-low recall (detecting only one PPI at a time), whereas multi-screen high-quality yeast 2-hybrid methods show high-precision with low recall (detecting a few tens of thousands of PPIs). Thus, HiPPIP is on par with other methods in terms of precision and the number of new PPIs detected. 18 novel PPIs predicted by HiPPIP were validated to be true (validations have been reported in [16,17], the current work and other unpublished works); the experiments were carried out by diverse research labs.

Table 1. Novel Interactors of each of the malignant pleural mesothelioma (MPM) Genes: Number of known (K) and computationally predicted novel (N) protein-protein interactions (PPIs) and lists the novel interactors. Bold genes in the 4th column are Novel Interactors that were experimentally validated in the current study.

Gene	K	N	Novel Interactors
ATP1B1	21	7	HCRTR1, SERPINC1, TM4SF1, PRRX1, CD84, CREG1, THOC1
ATIC	5	5	MAP3K7, CPS1, KIAA1524, VWC2L, DES
ATXN1	287	5	CNOT6L, XPO7, C7, PITX3, RPL19
BAP1	27	2	PLN, **PARP3**
CDKN2A	168	5	NFX1, DNAI1, GLIPR2, SIT1, CA9
CTLA4	17	10	PLCL1, DCTD, SKP1, GLP1R, AOX1, CD28, ATP5G3, CLK1, BCS1L, CDC26

Table 1. Cont.

Gene	K	N	Novel Interactors
DHFR	10	7	RHOQ, SCZD1, TOMM7, EXOC4, DTYMK, COPS8, CRHBP
FGFR1	67	7	ZFYVE1, NRG1, TPMT, OR51B4, SHB, PPP2CB, EIF4EBP1
FGFR2	46	8	PTPRE, OAT, PLXNA1, SEC23IP, MDM2, MGMT, PLSCR1, ELK4
FGFR3	43	6	GRK4, GMPS, STK32B, IDUA, IRF2BPL, ADD1
FLT1	25	8	MIPEP, RASSF9, HMGB1, FLT3, LATS2, ALOX5AP, ARL2BP, CDK8
FLT3	17	8	FMO1, SNRPA1, PNPLA3, NFIB, GPR12, SHC1, FLT1, CDK8
FLT4	16	4	NKX2-5, HNRNPH1, GRIA1, PNPLA8
FOXO3	27	4	GPR6, HDAC2, PRDM13, SIM1
GART	4	5	TIAM1, NMI, TMPRSS15, JUN, IFNAR1
GIPR	2	0	None
HLA-DQA1	9	6	HLA-DQA2, KLHDC3, TAL2, NXF1, BRD2, HLA-DPB1
HSP90AA1	158	6	IGHA2, MED28, PHLDA2, TCIRG1, IGHD, USP13
HSP90AB1	59	10	SLC25A27, PENK, ZFP36L2, MTX2, TPSAB1, PROS1, GPRC5B, CCR7, GNPDA1, CETN3
HSP90B1	36	2	MMP17, EPB41L4B
IL4R	23	5	RBBP6, NPIPB5, SLC20A1, ERN2, HDGFRP3
KAZN	12	6	KIF1B, NPPA, CELA2A, CELA2B, CTRC, FBLIM1
KDR	60	8	UTP3, SRP72, SHOX2, KIT, **ALB**, CACNA1S, CHIC2, GSTA2
KRT5	25	10	SORD, KRT6A, NADSYN1, SAP18, KRT7, TARBP2, KRT6B, KRT4, DCTN1, GPD1
KRT72	19	8	SP7, KRT78, KRT80, LARP4, MYL6B, KRT74, BCDIN3D, GRASP
LCK	143	5	NCDN, ZSCAN20, YBX1, CITED4, CAMK1D
LY6E	6	8	PIP, GLI4, HSF1, AKR1B1, EIF3H, JRK, GML, GPAA1
LYN	125	12	NEK7, SGK3, PDCD4, TRPA1, TERF1, PNMA2, IL7, CLCF1, AGXT, ARFGEF1, CRH, KLHL41
NTRK2	34	3	NXNL2, KCNS1, CDK20
PDCD1	2	3	COPS8, MCL1, OR6B3
PDGFRA	64	4	SPOCK1, RAPGEF1, **ALB**, CD244
PDGFRB	76	8	PLAUR, TUFM, CDX1, CHRM3, FAXDC2, ITK, CDK14, MITF
PDPN	2	5	PRDM2, PRMT1, ZBTB48, CELA2B, LHX1
POLE	12	7	SCARB1, RAN, VSIG4, ULK1, EIF2B1, MMP17, NOS1
POLE2	19	6	SAV1, PYGL, NID2, PARK7, DRD3, ATOH1
POLE3	7	7	TNC, TRIM32, EIF4G2, ASTN2, GSN, CST3, ALAD
POLE4	7	4	REG3G, SGOL1, EVA1A, B4GALT4
PRR5	5	3	WNT7B, TTC38, SCUBE1

Table 1. Cont.

Gene	K	N	Novel Interactors
RRM1	10	12	SLC22A18AS, SIRPA, SLC22A18, STIM1, SPINK1, ZFPM2, SH2D3A, PSMD13, RNH1, NUP98, CUZD1, RGS4
RRM2	9	10	TAF1B, ST3GAL3, NPBWR2, LPIN1, GCG, MGAT4A, BARX1, ASAP2, ITSN2, LAPTM4A
SP1	146	5	HNRNPA1, REG1A, RAPGEF3, GRIN1, ENDOU
SRC	300	9	ZNF687, ENPP7, FMR1, PI3, PTPRT, CUL4B, DPYD, BARD1, PLTP
TARP	1	4	TBX20, GGCT, IL6, CPVL
TBCE	2	3	SERTAD3, EIF2B2, PRDM2
TTF1	6	3	AMPH, DFNB31, QRFP
TUBA1A	63	3	TUBA1C, AMHR2, ACVR1B
TUBA1C	63	8	PRKAG1, SHMT2, AMHR2, SCAF11, ACVR1B, AQP5, KMT2D, TUBA1A
TUBA3C	12	3	XPO4, EIF3FP2, PARP4
TUBA3D	1	6	TUBA3E, WTH3DI, CCDC74B, FAM168B, LOC151121, IMP4
TUBA4A	51	14	WNT6, ETV6, ATP5G3, CAPN2, CXCR1, SLC11A1, CDK5R2, ALPP, IL1RL1, NUPR1, HPCA, SKP1, DPYSL2, STK16
TUBA8	7	2	POTEH, CCT8L2
TUBB1	1	2	C20orf85, SLMO2
TUBB2A	27	0	None
TUBB3	34	6	PRDM7, SLC7A5, PIEZO1, MVD, TRAPPC2L, TCF25
TUBB4A	10	7	UQCR11, APC2, ABCA7, PLIN3, KDM4B, SBNO2, HMG20B
TUBB4B	19	4	TSC1, NELFB, C9orf9, PTPRE
TUBD1	1	6	TMED1, PTRH2, TRPV1, GJB3, EPX, RFX5
TUBE1	0	6	DPAGT1, NUDC, RPS20, CDC40, GOPC, C6orf203
TUBG1	28	6	WNT3, PHB, RND2, CTRL, SGCA, RARA
TUBG2	3	3	NBR2, IKZF3, CLMP
TYMS	3	9	YES1, TAF3, ITGAM, NDUFV2, EPB41L3, SMCHD1, OCRL, THOC1, NAPG
WT1	64	8	FJX1, PEX3, CAPRIN1, PAX6, BST2, B3GNT3, CALML5, HIPK3

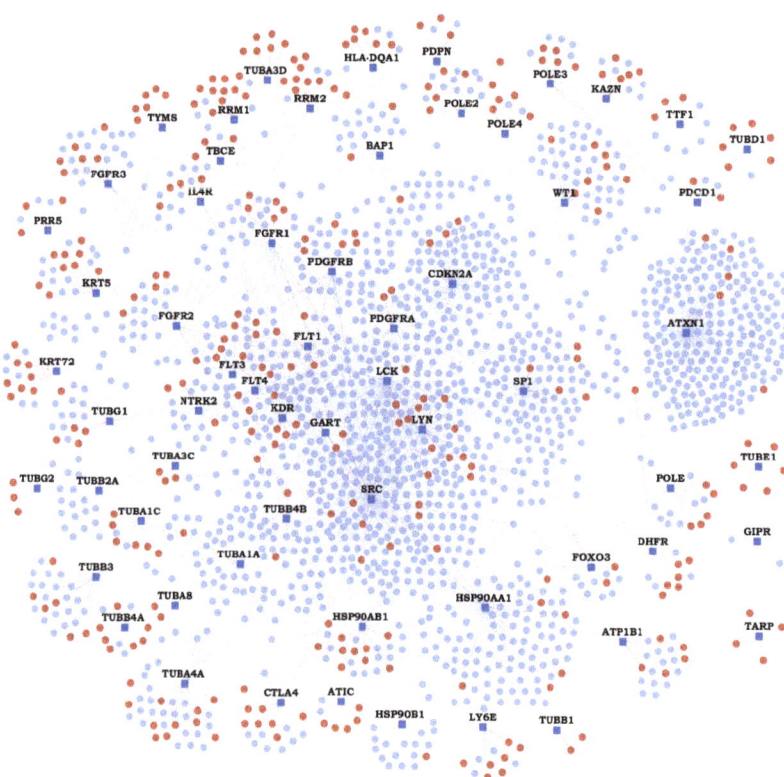

Figure 1. Malignant pleural mesothelioma (MPM) Protein-Protein Interactome: Network view of the MPM interactome is shown as a graph, where genes are shown as nodes and protein-protein interactions (PPIs) as edges connecting the nodes. MPM-associated genes are shown as dark blue square-shaped nodes, novel interactors and known interactors as red and light blue colored circular nodes respectively. Red edges are the novel interactions, whereas blue edges are known interactions.

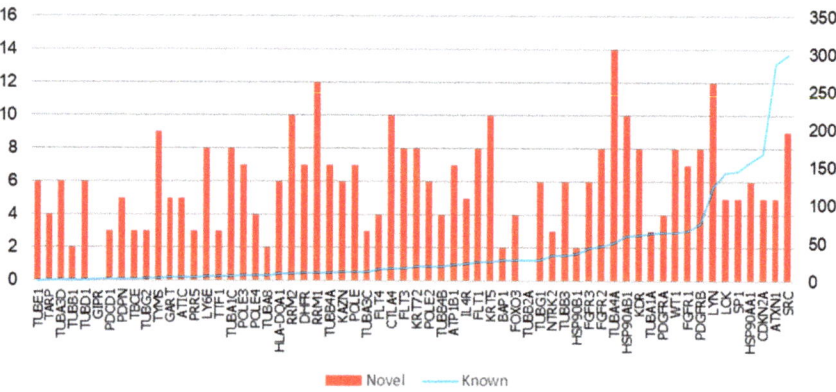

Figure 2. Number of protein-protein interactions (PPIs) in the malignant pleural mesothelioma (MPM) Interactome: The 62 MPM genes are shown along the X-axis, arranged in ascending order of their number of known PPIs. Blue line, right-side axis: Number of known PPIs is shown. Red bars, left-side axis: Number of novel PPIs.

2.1. Experimental Validation of Selected Protein-Protein Interactions (PPIs)

We carried out experimental validations of five predicted PPIs chosen for their biological relevance and proximity to MPM genes, namely, *BAP1-PARP3*, *KDR-ALB*, *PDGFRA-ALB*, *CUTA-HMGB1* and *CUTA-CLPS*. They were validated using protein pull-down followed by protein identification using mass spectrometry (Table S1) or size-based protein detection assay (Figure 3). Each bait protein was also paired with a random prey protein serving as control (specifically, *BAP1*-phospholambin, *ALB-FGFR2* and *CUTA-FGFR2*). All predicted PPIs were validated to be true, while control pairs tested negative. In addition to these five, another PPI from the MPM interactome, namely *HMGB1-FLT1* was validated in our prior work through co-immunoprecipitation [16]. Three novel PPIs, namely *HLA-DQA1— HLA-DQB1*, *FGFR2—FGF2* and *CDKN2A—CDKN2B*, that we reported in the preprint of this work [24], have since been reported as known PPIs in a recent version of BioGRID (downloaded February 2021); these three are treated as known PPIs in the remaining description.

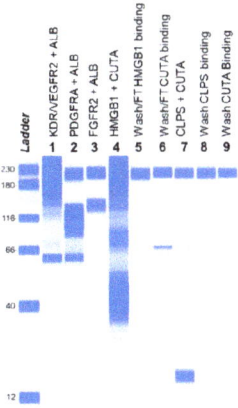

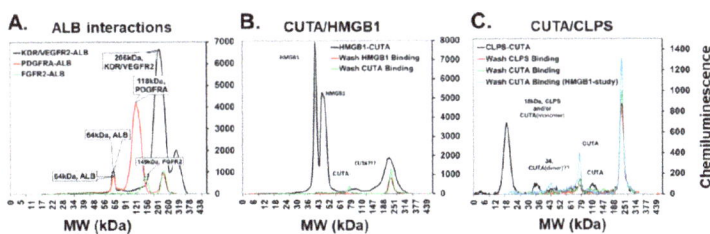

Figure 3. Validation of predicted *ALB* interactions and *CUTA* interactions using Wes™ Simple Western total protein detection assay: Pseudo-gel or virtual-blot like image of the validated interactions of *ALB* (lanes 1–2) and *CUTA* (lanes 4, 7) along with negative control (lane 3). In addition to the final pull-down samples, wash and/or flow through after binding 'bait' and 'prey' proteins for the *CUTA* interactions are also shown (lanes 5, 6, 8 and 9). The electro-pherogram image of Simple Western results using Total protein size-based assay. (**A**) *ALB* interactions with true positives *KDR/VEGFR2*, *PDGFRA* and false positive *FGFR2*. (**B**) *CUTA* interactions with *HMGB1*. (**C**) *CUTA* interactions with *CLPS*. An overlay of the electro-pherogram of the wash from *HMGB1* after *CUTA* binding is also shown in (**C**) for comparison.

2.2. Functional Interactions of Malignant Pleural Mesothelioma (MPM) Genes with Predicted Novel Interactors

We used ReactomeFIViz [25], a Cytoscape plugin, to extract known functional interactions between MPM-associated genes and their novel interactors. Seven novel PPIs had such functional interactions, namely (MPM genes are shown in bold), **PDGFRB**-RAPGEF1 ('part of the same complex', 'bound by the same set of ligands'), **SP1**→HNRNPA1 ('expression regulation'), **HLA-DQA1**→HLA-DPB1, HLA-DQA2→**HLA-DQA1** ('part of the same complex', 'catalysis'), **CTLA4**-CD28, **PDGFRB**-PLAUR ('bound by the same set of ligands') and **FGFR2**-MDM2 ('ubiquitination').

2.3. Web Server

We made the MPM interactome available on a webserver called *Wiki-MPM* (http://severus.dbmi.pitt.edu/wiki-MPM). It has advanced-search capabilities, and presents comprehensive annotations, namely Gene Ontology, diseases, drugs and pathways, of the two proteins of each PPI side-by-side. Here, a user can query for results such as "PPIs where one protein is involved in mesothelioma and the other is involved in immunity", and then see the results with the functional details of the two proteins side-by-side. The PPIs and their annotations also get indexed in major search engines like Google and Bing; thus a user searching for '*KDR* and response to starvation' would find the PPIs *KDR-CAV1* and *KDR-ALB*, where the interactors are each involved in 'response to starvation'. Querying by biomedical associations is a unique feature which we developed in Wiki-Pi that presents known interactions of all human proteins [26]. Wiki-MPM is a specialized version for disseminating the MPM interactome with its novel PPIs, visualizations and browse features. The novel PPIs have a potential to accelerate biomedical discovery in mesothelioma and making them available on this web server brings them to the biologists in an easily-discoverable and usable manner. Wiki-MPM will be integrated into the National Mesothelioma Virtual Bank [27,28], and will be available to the mesothelioma research community as part of our translational support of cancer research.

2.4. Pathway Analysis

We compiled the list of pathways that any of the proteins of MPM interactome are associated with, using Ingenuity Pathway Analysis suite [29]. Top 30 pathways by statistical significance of association are shown in Figure 4A. A number of pathways such as *NF-κB signaling*, *PI3/AKT signaling*, *VEGF signaling* and *natural killer cell signaling*, are highly relevant to mesothelioma etiology. They are found to be connected to MPM genes through novel PPIs that were previously unknown. For example, the PI3K/AKT signaling pathway regulating the cell cycle is aberrantly active in MPM, and the mesothelioma gene *FGFR1* is connected to this pathway via its novel predicted PPIs with *EIF4EBP1* and *PRP2CB* (Figure 4B) [30]. Statistical significance of association to the interactome, and various MPM genes and novel interactors belonging to these pathways are shown in Table 2 and Data File S3. A cancer biologist may utilize the Supplementary Data (Data Files S2 and S3) to study novel PPIs that connect MPM genes to a pathway that they are interested in studying.

Table 2. Pathways that are relevant to the pathophysiology and genetics of malignant pleural mesothelioma: Pathway analysis revealed that molecular mechanisms underlying various types of cancers, axonal guidance signaling, PI3/AKT signaling, VEGF signaling, natural killer cell signaling and inflammation signaling pathways may be pertinent to the development of MPM. A list of all the associated pathways is shown in Data File S3.

Pathway	p-Value	MPM Genes	Novel Interactors
Glucocorticoid Receptor Signaling	6.13×10^{-56}	KRT72, HSP90B1, FGFR3, HSP90AB1, FGFR1, KRT5, FOXO3, FGFR2, HSP90AA1	KRT74, HMGB1, PRKAG1, IL6, KRT6B, KRT78, KRT80, KRT7, KRT4, TAF3, NPPA, MAP3K7, KRT6A
Molecular Mechanisms of Cancer	5.01×10^{-53}	CDKN2A, SRC, FGFR3, FGFR1, FGFR2	CDK14, CDK20, CDKN2B, PRKAG1, WNT7B, RND2, WNT6, CDK8, RHOQ, RAPGEF3, MAP3K7, WNT3
NF-κB Signaling	1.26×10^{-39}	FGFR1, LCK, FLT1, KDR, PDGFRA, FGFR2, NTRK2, FGFR3, PDGFRB, FLT4	MAP3K7
Small Cell Lung Cancer Signaling	2.00×10^{-37}	FGFR1, FGFR2, FGFR3	CDKN2B
Axonal Guidance Signaling	2.51×10^{-37}	TUBB1, TUBA1A, TUBA4A, TUBA8, TUBB2A, NTRK2, FGFR3, FGFR1, TUBB3, TUBG1, TUBA1C, TUBB4B, FGFR2, TUBB4A	MYL6B, DPYSL2, PRKAG1, PLCL1, WNT7B, WNT6, PLXNA1, TUBA3E, WNT3
PI3K/AKT Signaling	1.58×10^{-36}	HSP90B1, FOXO3, HSP90AA1, HSP90AB1	OCRL, PPP2CB, MCL1, EIF4EBP1
VEGF Signaling	3.98×10^{-36}	FGFR1, FLT1, SRC, KDR, FOXO3, FGFR2, FGFR3, FLT4	EIF2B1, EIF2B2
Role of Macrophages, Fibroblasts and Endothelial Cells in Rheumatoid Arthritis	6.31×10^{-36}	SRC, FGFR3, FGFR1, FGFR2	IL1RL1, IL6, PLCL1, WNT7B, IL7, WNT6, CALML5, MAP3K7, WNT3, APC2
Natural Killer Cell Signaling	6.31×10^{-32}	FGFR1, LCK, FGFR2, FGFR3	OCRL, CD244
Actin Cytoskeleton Signaling	1.58×10^{-30}	FGFR1, FGFR2, FGFR3	MYL6B, GSN, APC2
eNOS Signaling	3.16×10^{-30}	FGFR1, FLT1, KDR, HSP90B1, FGFR2, HSP90AA1, FGFR3, FLT4, HSP90AB1	PRKAG1, CALML5, AQP5, CHRM3
Neuroinflammation Signaling Pathway	3.98×10^{-30}	FGFR1, HLA-DQA1, FGFR2, FGFR3	HMGB1, HLA-DQB1, ACVR1B, IL6, GRIN1, GRIA1
Gap Junction Signaling	1.00×10^{-29}	FGFR1, TUBB3, TUBG1, TUBB1, TUBA1C, TUBA1A, SRC, TUBB4B, TUBA4A, FGFR2, TUBA8, TUBB2A, FGFR3, SP1, TUBB4A	GJB3, PRKAG1, TUBA3E, PLCL1, GRIA1
Integrin Signaling	1.58×10^{-28}	FGFR1, SRC, FGFR2, FGFR3	GSN, ITGAM, RHOQ, CAPN2, RND2
IL-6 Signaling	1.58×10^{-28}	FGFR1, FGFR2, FGFR3	IL1RL1, MCL1, IL6, MAP3K7

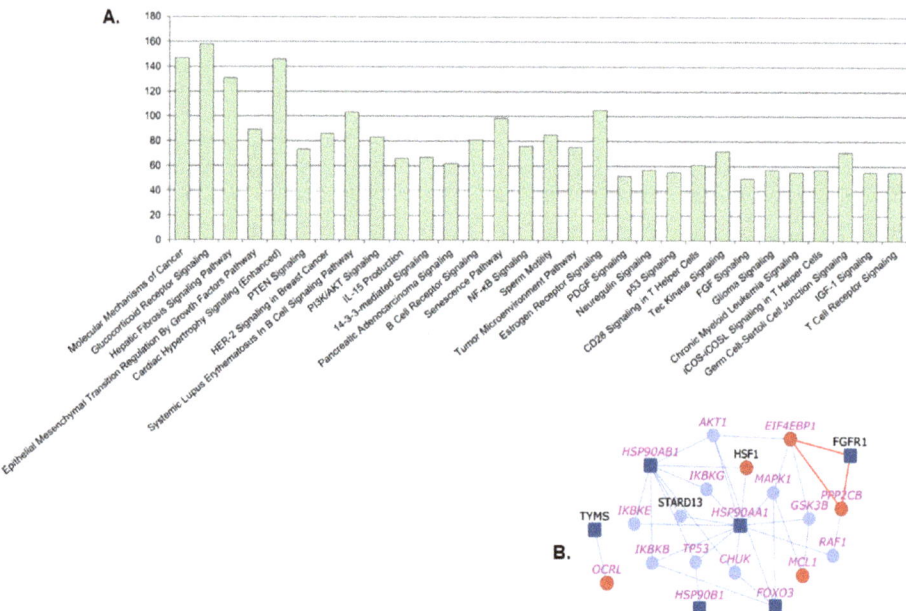

Figure 4. Pathways associated with malignant pleural mesothelioma (MPM) interactome: (**A**) Number of genes from MPM interactome associated with various pathways are shown. Top 30 pathways based on significance of association with the interactome are shown. (**B**) PI3K/AKT Signaling Pathway: Dark blue nodes are MPM genes, light blue nodes are known interactors and red nodes are novel interactors. Nodes with purple labels are genes involved in the PI3K/AKT signaling pathway.

2.5. Potentially Repurposable Drugs

We previously identified drugs potentially repurposable for schizophrenia through interactome analysis, and one of them is currently in clinical trials (ClinicalTrials.gov Identifier: NCT03794076) and another clinical trial has been funded and is yet to start [20]. Following this methodology, we constructed the MPM drug-protein interactome that shows the drugs that target any protein in the MPM interactome. This analysis has been carried out on an earlier version of BioGRID (3.4.159), which had fewer known PPIs, as reported in the preprint version of the paper [24], and has not been recomputed with the latest version of BioGRID unlike the other analyses presented here. There are 513 unique drugs that target 206 of these proteins (of which 28 are novel interactors that are targeted by 147 drugs) (Figure 5 and Data File S4). We adopted the established approach of comparing drug-induced versus disease-associated differential expression using the BaseSpace correlation software (previously called NextBio) [31,32], to identify five drugs that could be potentially repurposable for MPM (Table 3; the table also shows corresponding information for two known MPM drugs). These are: *cabazitaxel*, used in the treatment of refractory prostate cancer; *primaquine* and *pyrimethamine*, two anti-parasitic drugs; *trimethoprim*, an antibiotic; and *gliclazide*, an anti-diabetic drug (See Appendix A, titled 'Repurposable Drugs for Treatment of Malignant Pleural Mesothelioma'). The drugs were selected based on whether they induced a differential expression (DE) in genes that showed a negative correlation with lung cancer associated DE, and affected genes of high DE in MPM tumors/cell lines (GSE51024 [33] and GSE2549 [34]), or underwent prior clinical testing in lung cancer. Lung cancers share common pathways with mesothelioma initiated on asbestos exposure. Therefore, drugs targeting lung cancers can potentially be used in MPM [35]. Table 3 shows pharmacokinetic details of the drugs as reported in Drug Bank [36].

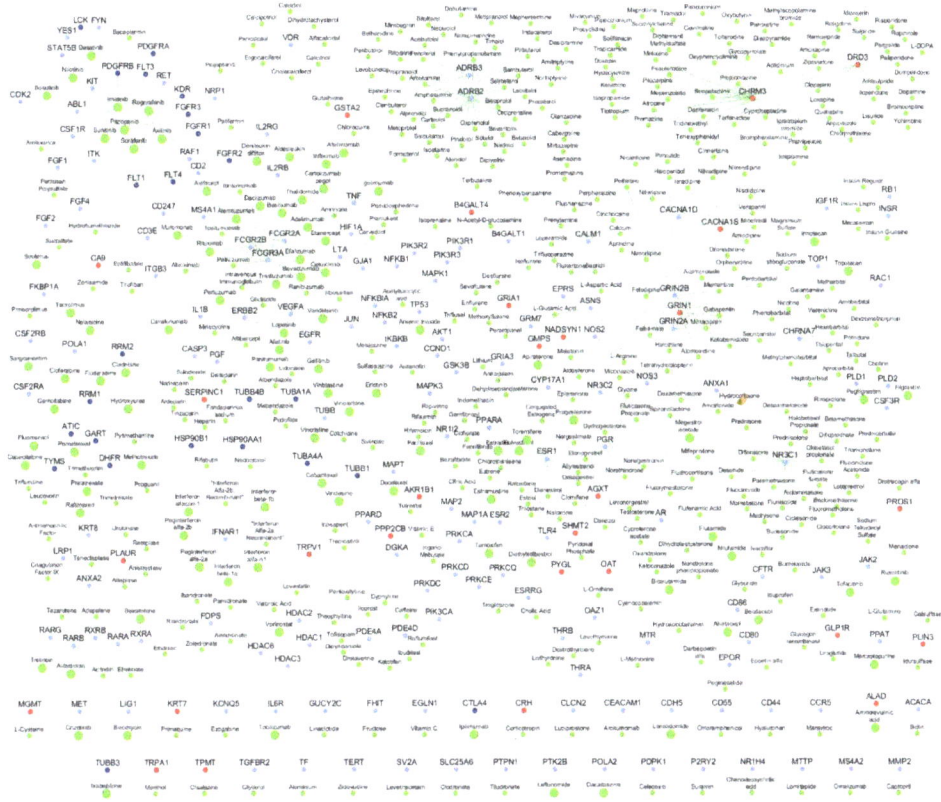

Figure 5. Malignant pleural mesothelioma (MPM) Drug-Protein Interactome: The network shows the drugs (green color nodes) that target the proteins in the MPM interactome. Larger green nodes correspond to drugs that target the anatomic category 'antineoplastic and immunomodulating agents'. The color legend for genes (proteins) is as shown in Figure 1, with MPM genes in dark blue, their known interactors in light blue and novel interactors in red.

Table 3. Pharmacokinetic details of known mesothelioma drugs and the drugs that are presented as candidates for repurposing. Known mesothelioma drugs are shown in bold italics. Score corresponds to scaled correlation score with lung cancer expression studies from BaseSpace (NextBio) analysis.

Drug Name & Score	Original Therapeutic Purpose(s)	Delivery	Half-Life	Toxicity	Targets
Pemetrexed negative 79	Chemotherapeutic drug for pleural mesothelioma and non-small cell lung cancer	Powder for solution; Intravenous	3.5 h	Data not available	ATIC, DHFR, GART, TYMS
Mitomycin negative 64	Chemotherapeutic drug for breast, bladder, esophageal, stomach, pancreas, mesothelioma, lung and liver cancers	Injection, powder or lyophilized for solution; Intravenous	8–48 min	Nausea and vomiting	-
Cabazitaxel negative 79	Anti-neoplastic agent in hormone-refractory metastatic prostate cancer	Solution; Intravenous	Rapid initial-phase of 4 min, intermediate-phase of 2 h and prolonged terminal-phase of 95 h	Neutropenia, hypersensitivity reactions, gastrointestinal symptoms, renal failure	TUBB1, TUBA4A
Pyrimethamine negative 83	Anti-parasitic agent in toxoplasmosis and acute malaria	Tablet; Oral	4 days	Data not available	DHFR

Table 3. Cont.

Drug Name & Score	Original Therapeutic Purpose(s)	Delivery	Half-Life	Toxicity	Targets
Trimethoprim negative 63	Anti-bacterial agent/antibiotic in urinary tract, respiratory tract and middle-ear infections and traveler's diarrhea	Tablet/solution; Oral	8 to 11 h	Oral toxicity in mice at LD50 = 4850 mg/kg	DHFR, TYMS
Primaquine negative 71	Anti-malarial agent	Tablet; Oral	3.7 to 7.4 h	Data not available	KRT7
Gliclazide negative 56	Anti-diabetic/hypoglycemic medication in type 2 diabetes mellitus	Tablet; Oral	10.4 h	Oral toxicity in mice at LD50 = 3000 mg/kg, accumulation in people with severe hepatic and/or renal dysfunction, side-effects of hypoglycemia including dizziness, lack of energy, drowsiness, headache and sweating	VEGFA

Although in each case, there would be some genes that are differentially expressed in the same direction for both the drug and the disorder (for e.g., both the drug and the disease cause some genes to overexpress), the overall effect on the entire transcriptome has an anti-correlation. A correlation score is generated based on the strength of the overlap between the drug and the disease datasets. Statistical criteria such as correction for multiple hypothesis testing are applied and the correlated datasets are then ranked by statistical significance. A numerical score of 100 is assigned to the most significant result, and the scores of the other results are normalized with respect to this top-ranked result. We excluded drugs with unacceptable toxicity (e.g., minocycline) or unsuitable pharmacokinetics. The final list comprised 15 drugs, out of which 10 have already been tested against mesothelioma in clinical trials/animal models, and several of them were found to display clinical activity [37–53] (Table S2). Gemcitabine and pemetrexed are being used as first-line therapy for mesothelioma, in combination with cisplatin [45,53]. Ipilimumab has been identified to be a potential second-line or third-line therapy in combination with nivolumab [47]. Ixabepilone stabilizes cancer progression for up to 28 months [49]. Zoledronate, which showed modest activity in MPM, induced apoptosis and S-phase arrest in human mesothelioma cells and inhibited tumor growth in an orthotopic animal model [54,55]. Sirolimus/cisplatin increased cell death and decreased cell proliferation in MPM cell lines [56]. α-Tocopheryl succinate increased the survival of orthotopic animal models of malignant peritoneal mesothelioma [57]. Pre-clinical testing of vitamin E and its analogs are in progress [58,59].

Primaquine targets KRT7, a novel interactor of KRT5, whose high expression has been correlated with tumour aggressiveness and drug resistance in malignant mesothelioma [60–62]. Primaquine may be re-purposed for MPM treatment at least as an adjunctive drug with pemetrexed, the drug currently used for first-line therapy. Primaquine enhanced the sensitivity of the multi-drug resistant cell line KBV20C to cancer drugs [63]. Gliclazide is an anti-diabetic drug inhibiting VEGFA [64], a known interactor of KDR, and is significantly upregulated in MPM tumour (Log_2FC = 1.83, p-value = 0.0018). Glicazide inhibits VEGF-mediated neovascularization [64]. High levels of VEGF have been correlated with both asbestos exposure in MPM and advanced cancer [65,66]. Glibenclamide, a drug with a similar mechanism of action as that of glicazide, increases caspase activity in MPM cell lines and primary cultures, leading to apoptosis mediated by TRAIL (TNF-related apoptosis inducing ligand) [67].

Eliminating those drugs which are being/have already been tested in mesothelioma with varying results, we arrived at a list of five potentially repurposable drugs in the descending order of negative correlation scores: pyrimethamine, cabazitaxel, primaquine, trimethoprim and gliclazide (Table 3). Cabazitaxel targets the MPM genes, TUBB1 and

TUBA4A, and was effective in treating non-small cell lung cancer (NSCLC) that was resistant to docetaxel, a drug that targets *TUBB1* along with other known interactors of MPM genes [37]. Pyrimethamine and trimethoprim target the MPM gene *TYMS* involved in folate metabolism, which was found to be differentially expressed in MPM tumors (GSE51024 [33]) ($\log_2 FC = 1.82$, p-value = 4.10×10^{-17}). MPM tumors have been shown to be responsive to anti-folates [68].

2.6. Analysis with Other High-Throughput Data

This section describes the overlap of the MPM interactome with various types of MPM-related biological evidence. 1690 (85.65%) proteins in the interactome were supported by genetic variant, transcriptomic, and proteomic evidence, and are listed in Data File S5. Table 4 shows 48 novel interactors that had three or more pieces of biological evidence.

Table 4. Novel interactors in the malignant pleural mesothelioma (MPM) interactome with biological evidences related to MPM. The table shows the following data in columns labeled A to F. (A) 48 novel interactors of MPM associated genes that have been linked to four or more biological evidences related to MPM, namely, **B1**: high or medium gene expression in lungs, **B2**: differential gene expression in MPM tumor versus other thoracic tumors, **B3**: differential gene expression in MPM tumor versus normal adjacent pleural tissue, **B4**: differential gene expression in MPM tumors of epithelioid, biphasic and sarcomatoid types, **B5**: differential gene methylation in MPM, **B6**: gene expression correlated with unfavorable lung cancer prognosis, **B7**: differential gene expression on exposure to asbestos or asbestos-like particles, **C**: isolation as exosome-derived proteins from malignant mesothelioma cell lines, **D**: differential protein abundance levels in epithelioid and sarcomatoid types of malignant mesothelioma, and **E**: genetic variants in MPM. Last column, **F**, gives the total number of sources of evidences for each gene. The complete list of biological evidence for all the genes in the interactome can be found in Data File S5.

A	B							C	D	E	F
Novel Interactor	Differential Gene Expression							Exosome-Derived Proteins	Differential Protein Levels	Genetic Variants	Total
	B1	B2	B3	B4	B5	B6	B7				
CAPRIN1	✓	✓	✓	✓				✓		✓	6
RAN	✓	✓	✓	✓				✓	✓		6
TNC	✓	✓			✓		✓	✓		✓	6
CUL4B	✓	✓	✓	✓				✓			5
GMPS	✓	✓	✓	✓						✓	5
IL6	✓	✓		✓	✓			✓			5
MGMT	✓	✓	✓		✓					✓	5
NFIB	✓		✓	✓		✓				✓	5
NUDC	✓	✓		✓				✓		✓	5
PLAUR	✓	✓		✓	✓	✓					5
PLIN3	✓	✓		✓		✓		✓			5
PLXNA1	✓	✓	✓	✓				✓			5
PRMT1	✓		✓					✓	✓	✓	5
RNH1	✓	✓		✓				✓	✓		5
SCARB1	✓	✓		✓		✓		✓			5
SLC7A5	✓		✓	✓		✓		✓			5
SMCHD1	✓		✓	✓				✓		✓	5
ASAP2	✓	✓		✓				✓			4
B4GALT4	✓	✓		✓		✓					4
CAPN2	✓	✓		✓		✓					4
CDC40	✓		✓	✓		✓					4
DTYMK	✓	✓	✓	✓							4
EIF3H	✓		✓					✓		✓	4
EPB41L3	✓	✓		✓						✓	4

Table 4. Cont.

A	B							C	D	E	F
Novel Interactor	Differential Gene Expression							Exosome-Derived Proteins	Differential Protein Levels	Genetic Variants	Total
	B1	B2	B3	B4	B5	B6	B7				
EXOC4	✓	✓		✓				✓			4
GNPDA1	✓	✓		✓				✓			4
HNRNPA1	✓			✓			✓	✓			4
HNRNPH1	✓		✓	✓				✓			4
LARP4	✓		✓	✓			✓				4
MGAT4A	✓	✓					✓			✓	4
MITF	✓	✓	✓	✓							4
NDUFV2	✓	✓							✓	✓	4
OAT	✓	✓			✓			✓			4
PHB	✓	✓	✓					✓			4
PHLDA2	✓	✓			✓			✓			4
PLCL1		✓	✓	✓						✓	4
PRKAG1	✓	✓						✓		✓	4
PROS1	✓	✓		✓				✓			4
PTRH2		✓		✓			✓			✓	4
PYGL	✓	✓		✓				✓			4
RBBP6	✓		✓	✓						✓	4
SEC23IP	✓	✓	✓	✓							4
SGK3		✓	✓	✓						✓	4
SHMT2	✓	✓	✓	✓							4
SLC20A1	✓	✓		✓						✓	4
TCIRG1	✓	✓		✓				✓			4
XPO4				✓		✓		✓		✓	4
YBX1	✓	✓	✓					✓			4

We compiled the list of genes harboring MPM-associated genetic variants from Bueno et al. [5], and compared this list with all the genes in the MPM interactome (i.e., MPM-associated genes, their known and novel interactors) to identify overlaps. 275 genes in the MPM interactome harbored either germline mutations, or somatic single nucleotide variants (SNVs) or indels (insertions or deletions) (Figure 6, Table 4 and Data File S5) associated with MPM tumors. Of these 275 genes, 37 were novel interactors of MPM genes. *MGMT* carried germline mutations while the following carried somatic mutations: *ASTN2, BARX1, BRD2, CALML5, CAPRIN1, CLK1, CPS1, DPYD, EIF3H, EPB41L3, GMPS, GPR12, ITGAM, KIAA1524, KMT2D, KRT4, MGAT4A, NBR2, NDUFV2, NFIB, NFX1, NUDC, PLCL1, PRDM2, PRKAG1, PRMT1, PTPRT, PTRH2, RBBP6, SGK3, SLC20A1, SMCHD1, SPOCK1, TMPRSS15, TNC* and *XPO4*. Fourteen of these interact with MPM genes that also harbored a genetic variant (MPM genes are shown in bold): **CDKN2A**-*NFX1*, **FLT1**-*LATS2*, **TUBA3C**-*XPO4*, **PDGFRA**-*SPOCK1*, **TYMS**-*SMCHD1*, **TYMS**-*EPB41L3*, **GART**-*TMPRSS15*, **TYMS**-*NDUFV2*, **TYMS**-*ITGAM*, **RRM2**-*BARX1*, **RRM2**-*MGAT4A* and **ATIC**-*CPS1*, **ATIC**-*KIAA1524* and **POLE**-*NOS1*.

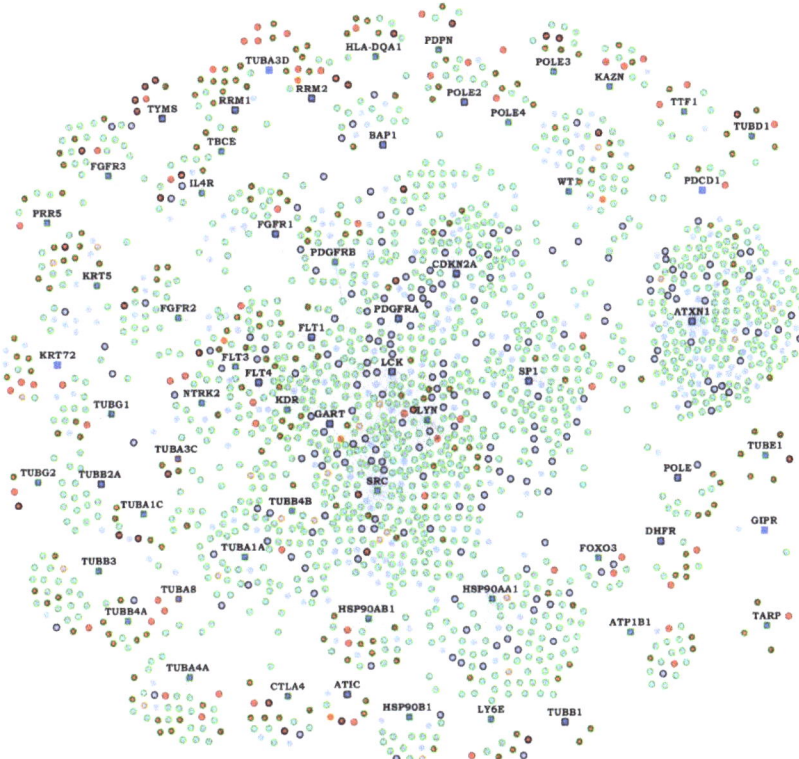

Figure 6. Genes with biological evidences in the malignant pleural mesothelioma (MPM) Protein-Protein Interactome: On the interactome network shown in Figure 1, various biological evidences of relation to malignant pleural mesothelioma (MPM) are shown as node border colors. Genes with variants associated with MPM have orange borders, genes with MPM/lung cancer/asbestos exposure-associated gene/protein expression changes have light green-colored borders and genes with black border have both genetic variants and gene/protein expression changes associated with them. The gene expression-associated features include differential expression in MPM tumors versus normal adjacent pleura, MPM tumors versus other thoracic tumors, differential gene methylation (affecting gene expression) in MPM tumors, gene expression correlated with unfavorable lung cancer prognosis, differential gene expression on exposure to asbestos or asbestos-like particles and high/medium expression in normal lungs. The protein expression-associated features include isolation as exosome-derived proteins from malignant mesothelioma cell lines and differential protein abundance levels in epithelioid and sarcomatoid types of malignant mesothelioma. The complete list of genes in the interactome and their corresponding evidence can be found in Data File S5.

We collected the methylation profile of pleural mesothelioma [69], and found 8 novel interactors to be hypomethylated in pleural mesothelioma versus non-tumor pleural tissue, namely, *ACVR1B*, *IL6*, *MGMT*, *NRG1*, *OAT*, *PHLDA2*, *PLAUR* and *TNC* (Table S3). Some of them have little or no expression in lung tissue but are overexpressed in MPM. *PLAUR* is a prognostic biomarker of MPM [70]. Similarly, *FGFR1* and its novel interactor *NRG1* had elevated mRNA expression in H2722 mesothelioma cell lines and in MPM tissue, both contributing to increased cell growth under tumorigenic conditions [71,72]. *TNC*, involved in invasive growth, is a prognostic biomarker overexpressed in MPM, having low expression in normal lung tissues [73,74]. Thus, these novel interactors, which are not normally expressed in lung tissue, may be hypomethylated in MPM leading to their overexpression, contributing to MPM etiology.

Three hundred and ninety three (393) genes in the MPM interactome were also differentially expressed in mesothelioma tumors versus normal pleural tissue adjacent to tumor (GSE12345 [75]) (p-value of overlap = 9.525 × 10^{-19}, odds ratio = 1.51). 52 out of the 314 novel interactors in the interactome were differentially expressed in this dataset (p-value = 0.046, odds ratio = 1.26). 938 genes, including 132 novel interactors, in the interactome were found to be differentially expressed in MPM tumors of epithelioid, biphasic and sarcomatoid types versus paired normal tissues (GSE51024 [33]) (p-value of overlap = 1.415 × 10^{-18}, odds ratio = 1.24). Genes with fold-change >2 or <$\frac{1}{2}$ were considered as overexpressed and underexpressed, respectively, at a p-value < 0.05. Similarly, 744 genes in the MPM interactome were differentially expressed in MPM tumors versus other thoracic cancers such as thymoma and thyroid cancer (GSE42977 [76]) (p-value = 3.04 × 10^{-41}, odds ratio = 1.53). 112 out of the 314 novel interactors in the interactome were differentially expressed in this dataset (p-value = 7.77 × 10^{-6}, odds ratio = 1.45). This shows that the MPM interactome is enriched with genes whose expression helps in distinguishing MPM from other thoracic tumors and also with genes differentially expressed in mesothelioma tumors versus normal pleural tissue (Figure 6 and Data File S5). From RNA-seq data in GTEx, we found that 1311 genes, including 189 novel interactors, in the interactome have high/medium expression in normal lung tissue (median transcripts-per-million (TPM) > 9) (Figure 6 and Data File S5) [77].

A recent study had examined the gene expression profiles from the lungs of mice exposed to asbestos fibers (crocidolite and tremolite), an asbestiform fiber (erionite) and a mineral fiber (wollastonite) [78]. Crocidolite, tremolite and erionite are capable of inducing lung cancer and mesothelioma in humans and animal models [78]. On the other hand, wollastonite is a low pathogenicity fiber that shows no association with the incidence of lung cancer and mesothelioma in humans, or carcinogenesis in animal models [79]. The MPM interactome showed significant enrichment with all the 4 fibers (Figure 6 and Data File S5). The highest statistical significance was shown for the human orthologs of the mouse genes that were differentially expressed upon crocidolite exposure (199 genes, p-value = 1.16 × 10^{-18}, odds ratio = 1.88). This was followed by tremolite (47 genes, p-value = 2.445 × 10^{-5}, odds ratio = 1.87), wollastonite (16 genes, p-value = 0.0037, odds ratio = 2.09) and erionite (10 genes, p-value = 0.025, odds ratio = 2.01). Altogether, 245 genes in the interactome, including 29 novel interactors, have transcriptomic evidence with respect to exposure to asbestos or asbestos-like fibers. These novel interactors are: *ALB*, *B4GALT4*, *CAPN2*, *CDC40*, *DES*, *FMO1*, *FMR1*, *GML*, *GRIA1*, *HMG20B*, *HNRNPA1*, *ITSN2*, *LARP4*, *LPIN1*, *MGAT4A*, *NEK7*, *NFIB*, *NRG1*, *OCRL*, *PAX6*, *PDCD4*, *PITX3*, *PTRH2*, *REG3G*, *TAF1B*, *THOC1*, *TMED1*, *TNC* and *XPO4*.

From data in Pathology Atlas, we found that high expression of 73 genes, including that of 10 novel interactors, in the interactome has been positively correlated with unfavorable prognosis for lung cancer (p-value = 1.72 × 10^{-9}, odds ratio = 2.05) [80]. These novel interactors are: *SPOCK1*, *SLC7A5*, *SCARB1*, *PLIN3*, *PLAUR*, *PIEZO1*, *KRT6A*, *GJB3*, *B3GNT3* and *ARL2BP*. We predicted *ARL2BP* to interact with *FLT1*, a VEGF receptor expressed in MPM cells. VEGF level in MPM patients is a biomarker for unfavorable prognosis, and lung cancer tumors expressing *FLT1* have been associated with poor prognosis [81,82].

Exosomes are extracellular vesicles secreted into the tumor microenvironment. They facilitate immunoregulation and metastasis by shuttling cellular cargo and directing intercellular communication. In a proteomic profiling study, 2176 proteins were identified in exosomes of at least one of the four human malignant mesothelioma cell lines (JO38, JU77, OLD1612 and LO68) [83]. 324 proteins in the MPM interactome appeared among these exosome-derived proteins (p-value = 8.86 × 10^{-10}, odds ratio = 1.36), out of which 47 were novel interactors. Six hundred and thirty one (631) exosome-derived proteins were identified in all four malignant mesothelioma cell lines. Out of these, 127 occurred in the MPM interactome (p-value = 4.54 × 10^{-12}, odds ratio = 1.84), out of which 15 were novel interactors (*PRKAG1*, *HNRNPA1*, *HNRNPH1*, *SORD*, *RNH1*, *RAN*, *PYGL*, *SLC7A5*, *RPS20*, *PARP4*, *YBX1*, *DCTN1*, *TUFM*, *EXOC4* and *GNPDA1*). In the following novel PPIs, both proteins involved in the interaction appeared among exosome-derived proteins (MPM gene in the interaction is shown in bold): *TUBB3*-SLC7A5, *HSP90AB1*-PROS1, *HSP90AB1*-GNPDA1, *TUBB4A*-PLIN3, *LYN*-ARFGEF1, *HSP90AA1*-PHLDA2, *HSP90AA1*-TCIRG1, *TUBG1*-PHB, *GART*-NMI, *SRC*-CUL4B and *ATIC*-CPS1.

We computed the overlap of the interactome with 142 proteins that showed significant differences in abundance levels between epithelioid and sarcomatoid types of diffuse malignant mesothelioma [84]. In that study, a Fourier transform infrared (FTIR) imaging approach was employed to identify pathologic regions from diffuse malignant mesothelioma tissue samples [84]. These pathologic regions were then harvested using laser capture microdissection for proteomic analysis. 32 proteins in the interactome were more abundant in either epithelioid or sarcomatoid subtypes (p-value = 5.16×10^{-5}, odds ratio = 2.06), including six novel interactors (p-value = 0.038, odds ratio = 2.43). The novel interactors *KRT78*, *NDUFV2*, *PRMT1*, *RAN* and *RNH1*—predicted to interact with the MPM genes *KRT72*, *TYMS*, *PDPN*, *POLE* and *RRM1*, respectively—had higher abundance in epithelioid samples, whereas *IGHA2*—predicted to interact with *HSP90AA1*—had higher abundance in sarcomatoid samples. The predicted interactions of these protein biomarkers with MPM-associated genes provide a mechanistic basis for experimental dissection of their ability to act as factors differentiating epithelioid tumors from sarcomatoid tumors (and vice versa).

3. Discussion

Currently, mesothelioma biologists only study a handful of genes, such as *BAP1*, *CDKN2A* and *NF2*. To shed light onto the other MPM-associated genes, whose functions remain poorly characterized, we assembled the 'MPM interactome' with ~2400 previously known PPIs and 364 computationally predicted PPIs (five of which have been validated in this work), which along with their biological annotations are being made available to researchers. We demonstrate the power of interactome-scale analyses to generate biologically insightful and clinically translatable results. The interactome has highly significant overlaps with MPM-associated genetic variants, genes differentially expressed or methylated in MPM or upon asbestos exposure, genes whose expression has been correlated with lung cancer prognosis, and with exosome-derived proteins in malignant mesothelioma cell lines. The interactome was enriched in cancer-related pathways. We extended the MPM interactome to include the drugs that target any of its proteins and analyzed it to identify a shortlist of 5 drugs that can potentially be repurposed for MPM—an example of a clinically translatable result.

We validated in vitro five novel PPIs in the interactome, namely, *BAP1*-PARP3, *ALB*-KDR, *ALB*-PDGFRA, *CUTA*-HMGB1 and *CUTA*-CLPS. Literature evidence shows that these PPIs may be viable candidates for further experimentation in MPM cell lines or animal models. We hypothesize that the *BAP1*-PARP3 interaction may enhance cancer growth in MPM. *BAP1* is a tumor suppressor protein playing a role in cell cycle progression, repair of DNA breaks, chromatin remodeling, and gene expression regulation; variants in *BAP1* have been implicated in hereditary and sporadic mesothelioma [85]. *PARP3* is involved in DNA repair, regulation of apoptosis, and maintenance of genomic stability and telomere integrity [86]. Interaction of *BAP1* with *BRCA1* has been shown to inhibit breast cancer growth [7]. In the absence of *BRCA1* activity or with a perturbation in its interaction with *BAP1*, cancerous growth is enhanced [87]. Loss of *BRCA1* protein expression has been noted in MPM [12]. In this scenario, it is possible that the novel interaction of *BAP1* with *PARP3* in cancerous cells may be promoting cancerous growth, possibly through regulation of DNA repair and apoptosis. *BAP1* and *PARP3* were found to be moderately overexpressed in sarcomatoid MPM tumors compared with normal pleural tissue ($\log_2$FC = 0.575, p-value = 0.028, and $\log_2$FC = 0.695, p-value = 0.0212, respectively) (GSE42977 [76]). Perturbation of the interaction of *BAP1* with *PARP3*, using *PARP3* inhibitors, may then suppress cancerous growth, at least in sarcomatoid MPM. Several studies and clinical trials [87], have shown that PARP inhibitors influence cancers in which mutations in *BRCA1* or *BRCA2* are observed, which led us to assume that the cancerous growth-inhibiting interaction of *BAP1* with *BRCA1* may already be perturbed in this case, and that PARP inhibitors may actually be blocking the novel interaction of *BAP1* with *PARP3* which enhances cancer growth. It has been pointed out that upon inhibiting PARP activity, cancerous cells that lack *BRCA1* or *BRCA2* activity may undergo cell cycle arrest and apoptosis, possibly due to an accumulation of chromatid aberrations and an inability to perform DNA repair in the absence of BRCA [7,87]. Thus, we suspect that the novel interaction of *BAP1* and *PARP3* may also be perturbed by PARP inhibitors, leading to inhibition of cancer growth.

Low levels of *ALB* have been correlated with poor prognosis in MPM patients [88]. The two MPM genes, *KDR* and *PDGFRA*, that *ALB* is predicted to interact with, are members of the PI3K/AKT pathway which has been shown to be aberrantly active in mesothelioma [89]. High expression of *CUTA* has been correlated with favorable prognosis in lung cancer (Pathology Atlas). It was found to be overexpressed in MPM tumors versus normal pleura ($\log_2 FC = 0.871$, p-value = 0.0039) (GSE2549 [34]). *CLPS* inhibits metastasis of the melanoma cell line, B16F10, to lungs by blocking the signaling pathway involving β1 integrin, *FAK* and paxillin [90]. *CLPS* has a novel interaction with *NEDD9*, which has been shown to mediate β1 integrin signaling and promote metastasis of non-small lung cancer cells [91]. *CD26*, a cancer stem cell marker of malignant mesothelioma, has been shown to associate with the integrin α5β1 (or *ITGA5*, a novel interactor of the MPM gene, *FGFR2*) and promote cell migration and invasion in mesothelioma cells [91]. Another cancer stem cell marker of malignant mesothelioma, *CD9*, inhibits this metastatic effect mediated by *CD26*. Depletion of *CD26* and *CD9* was shown to respectively lead to decreased and increased expression of *NEDD9* and *FAK* in mesothelioma cells lines, hinting at the involvement of *NEDD9* in mesothelioma tumor invasiveness [91]. *NEDD9* has a known interaction with *LYN*, an MPM gene, shown to play a negative role in the regulation of integrin signaling in neutrophils [92]. *CUTA* has a novel interaction with *HMGB1*, which has been shown to activate the integrin αMβ2 (or *ITGAM*, a novel interactor of the MPM gene, *TYMS*) and the cell adhesion and migratory function of neutrophils mediated by αMβ2 [93]. *HMGB1* also has a novel interaction with the MPM gene, *FLT1*, shown to be involved in the migration of multiple myeloma cells by associating with β1 integrin, and mediating PKC activation [94].

A recent bioinformatics study identified the genes differentially expressed in epithelioid MPM tissues versus normal pleural tissues (GSE42977 [76]), and extracted the known PPIs interconnecting these genes from the STRING database [95]. They identified 10 hub genes from this network and shortlisted 31 drugs targeting the proteins in the network based on scores from the Drug-Gene Interaction Database (DGIdb). The DGIdb score takes into account the literature evidence for a particular drug-protein interaction, the number of proteins in the network that interact with the given drug, and the ratio of the average number of known protein interactors for all drugs compared to the number of known protein interactors for the given drug. *CDK1*, which is one of the hub genes identified in their study, is a known interactor of three MPM-associated genes, namely, *LYN*, *SP1* and *RRM2*, and we showed that it has association to MPM in three omics datasets: high expression correlated with unfavorable lung cancer prognosis, differential expression in MPM tumors versus adjacent pleural tissue, and isolation as an exosome-derived protein in malignant mesothelioma cell lines. Our work overall presents a more comprehensive study in terms of a larger number of MPM genes analyzed, which were compiled from multiple sources by IPA, and analysis of a larger number of MPM associated omics data sets, and presents transcriptomic-driven shortlisting of repurposable drugs for which additional evidence is presented from clinical trial data, literature, and differential expression of target genes in MPM datasets.

Our study provides an integrative and mechanistic framework for functional translation of mesothelioma-related multi-omics data. The novelty of our work stems from two key factors: (a) we present computationally predicted PPIs of high precision, which link MPM-related genes from disparate genetic-variant / transcriptomic/proteomic studies in hitherto unknown ways within the functional landscape of the interactome, and (b) the richly annotated MPM interactome is made available on a webserver to facilitate analysis by biologists and computational systems biologists. Our approach has some limitations. The drug-associated expression profiles analyzed in this study were induced in a diverse set of cell lines rather than in mesothelioma cell lines. The effect of the proposed drugs should be examined in MPM cell lines or animal models. We reported the overlap of mouse genes differentially expressed upon asbestos exposure [78] with corresponding human orthologs in the interactome. Mouse models have been routinely used to study pathologic changes associated with asbestos exposure, including gene expression, and these findings have been extrapolated to human diseases such as mesothelioma [96–99]. Nevertheless, our results should be interpreted with caution. It is not possible to draw direct transcriptomic/proteomic/phenotypic equivalences between mice and humans, unless these levels are comprehensively characterized in both the species, and a clear equivalence of factors defining a condition such as asbestos exposure is demonstrated in both the species [100]. Next, it is beyond the scope of our expertise to validate the large number of computationally predicted PPIs in a tissue or cell line of interest. However, we demonstrated the validity of computational predictions on a small number of PPIs on purified proteins with appropriate controls. The computational model has also been validated through additional experiments previously; some of the novel PPIs predicted previously by our method have translated into results of biomedical significance [17–19].

4. Methods

4.1. Data Collection

A search using the keyword "malignant pleural mesothelioma" on IPA (Ingenuity Pathway Analysis) retrieved genes causally related to the disease. IPA retrieves genes from the Ingenuity Knowledge Base which has ~5 million experimental findings expert-curated from biomedical literature or incorporated from other databases [29].

4.2. High-Precision Protein-Protein Interaction Prediction (HiPPIP) Model

PPIs were predicted by computing features of protein pairs, namely, cellular localization, molecular function and biological process membership, genomic location of the gene, gene expression from microarray experiments, protein domains and tissue membership of proteins, as described in Thahir et al. [101], and developing a random forest model to classify the pairwise features as interacting or non-interacting. A random forest with 30 trees was trained using the feature offering maximum information gain out of four random features to split each node; minimum number of samples in each leaf node was set to be 10. The random forest outputs a continuous valued score in the range of [0,1]. The threshold to assign a final label was varied over the range of the score for positive class (i.e., 0 to 1) to find the precision and recall combinations that are observed.

4.3. Evaluation of PPI Prediction Model

Evaluations on a held-out test data showed a precision of 97.5% and a recall of 5% at a threshold of 0.75 on the output score. Next, we created ranked lists for each of the hub genes (i.e., genes that had >50 known PPIs), where we considered all pairs that received a score >0.5 to be novel interactions. The predicted interactions of each of the hub genes are arranged in descending order of the prediction score, and precision versus recall is computed by varying the threshold of predicted score from 1 to 0. Next, by scanning these ranked lists from top to bottom, the number of true positives versus false positives was computed.

4.4. Novel PPIs in the MPM Interactome

Each MPM gene, say Z, is paired with each of the other human genes ($G_1, G_2 \ldots G_N$), and each pair is evaluated with the HiPPIP model. The predicted interactions of each of the MPM genes (namely, the pairs whose score is >0.5) were extracted. These PPIs, combined with the previously known PPIs of MPM genes collectively form the 'MPM interactome'. Interactome figures were created using Cytoscape [102].

Note that 0.5 is the threshold chosen not because it is the midpoint between the two classes, but because the evaluations with hub proteins showed that the pairs that received a score >0.5 are highly confident to be interacting pairs. This was further validated through experiments for a few novel PPIs above this score.

4.5. Previously Known PPIs in the MPM Interactome

Previously known PPIs of the 62 MPM genes were collected from Human Protein Reference Database (HPRD) version 9 [22] and Biological General Repository for Interaction Datasets (BioGRID) version 4.3.194 [23]. The data behind our web-server will be updated once in a year with recent versions of BioGRID, and if novel PPIs are shown validated by such updates to known PPIs, the information will be posted on the web-server.

4.6. In Vitro Pull-Down Assays

An initial screening to find physical interactions was performed using an in vitro pull-down assay for some of the predicted novel PPIs. This technique utilizes a His/biotin tag-fused protein immobilized on an affinity column as the bait protein and a passing-through solution containing the 'prey' protein that binds to the 'bait' protein. The subsequent elution will pull down both the target (prey) and tagged-protein (bait) for further analysis by immunoblotting to confirm the predicted interactions. The pull-down assays were conducted using the Pull-Down PolyHis Protein:Protein Interaction Kit (Pierce™, Rockford, IL, USA) according to the manufacturer's instructions.

4.7. Protein Identification Methods

Peptide sequencing experiments were performed using an EASY-nLC 1000 coupled to a Q Exactive Orbitrap Mass Spectrometer (Thermo Scientific, San Jose, CA, USA) operating in positive ion mode. An EasySpray C18 column (2 μm particle size, 75 μm diameter by 15 cm length) was loaded with 500 ng of protein digest in 22 μL of solvent A (water, 0.1% formic acid) at a pressure of 800 bar. Separations were performed using a linear gradient ramping from 5% solvent B (75% acetonitrile, 25% water, 0.1% formic acid) to 30% solvent B over 120 min, flowing at 300 nL/min.

The mass spectrometer was operated in data-dependent acquisition mode. Precursor scans were acquired at 70,000 resolution over 300–1750 m/z mass range (3e6 AGC target, 20 ms maximum injection time). Tandem MS spectra were acquired using HCD of the top 10 most abundant precursor ions at 17,500 resolution (NCE 28, 1e5 AGC target, 60 ms maximum injection time, 2.0 m/z isolation window). Charge states 1, 6–8 and higher were excluded for fragmentation and dynamic exclusion was set to 20.0 s.

Mass spectra were searched for peptide identifications using Proteome Discoverer 2.1 (Thermo Scientific, Waltham, MA, USA) using the Sequest HT and MSAmanda algorithms, peptide spectral matches were validated using Percolator (target FDR 1%). Initial searches were performed against the complete UniProt database (downloaded 19 March 2018). Peptide matches were restricted to 10 ppm MS1 tolerance, 20 mmu MS2 tolerance, and 2 missed tryptic cleavages. Fixed modifications were limited to cysteine carbamidomethylation, and dynamic modifications were methionine oxidation and protein N-terminal acetylation. Peptide and protein grouping and results validation was performed using Scaffold 4.8.4 (Proteome Software, Portland, OR, USA) along with the X! Tandem algorithm against the previously described database. Proteins were filtered using a 99% FDR threshold.

4.8. Ingenuity Pathway Analysis

Pathway associations of genes in the MPM interactome were computed using Ingenuity Pathway Analysis (IPA). Statistical significance of the overlaps between genes in the MPM interactome and pathways in the Ingenuity Knowledge Base (IKB) was computed with Fisher's exact test based on hypergeometric distribution. In this method, p-value is computed from the probability of k successes in n draws (without replacement) from a finite population of size N containing exactly k objects with an interesting feature, where N = total number of genes associated with pathways in IKB, K = number of genes associated with a particular pathway in IKB, n = number of genes in the MPM interactome and k = K ∩ n. This value was further adjusted for multiple hypothesis correction using the Benjamini-Hochberg procedure.

4.9. Analysis of Differential Gene Expression in Pleural Mesothelioma Tumors and Lungs of Asbestos-Exposed Mice Versus Normal Tissue in Lungs

The overlap of the MPM interactome with genes differentially expressed in pleural mesothelioma tumors compared with normal pleural tissue adjacent to mesothelioma was computed using the dataset GSE12345 [75]. Genes differentially expressed in the lungs of mice exposed to crocidolite and erionite fibers were obtained from the dataset GSE100900 [78]. Genes with fold change >2 or $\frac{1}{2}$ were considered as significantly overexpressed and underexpressed respectively at p-value < 0.05.

4.10. Analysis of DNA Methylation in MPM Tumors

The dataset GSE16559 [69] was used to analyze the methylation profile of pleural mesotheliomas. In this study, genes found to be differentially methylated in mesothelioma were identified from a set of 773 cancer-related genes associated with 1413 autosomal CpG loci. Methylation values (M-values) were computed as $M = \log2 (\beta (1-\beta))$ for both control (non-tumor pleural tissue) and test (pleural mesothelioma) cases, where β is the ratio of methylated probe intensity and overall intensity. Difference between M-values of test and control cases was then computed, and genes with M-value > 1 and M-value < 1 were considered to be hypermethylated and hypomethylated respectively at p-value < 0.05.

4.11. Correlating Expression of MPM Genes with Lung Cancer Prognosis

Data for correlation of gene expression and fraction of patient population surviving after treatment for lung cancer was taken from the Pathology Atlas [80]. Genes with log-rank p-value < 0.001 were considered to be prognostic. Unfavorable prognosis indicates positive correlation of high gene expression with reduced patient survival.

4.12. Identification of Repurposable Drugs in the MPM Drug-Protein Interactome

Negative correlation between lung cancer and drugs were studied using the BaseSpace correlation software, which uses a non-parametric rank-based approach to compute the extent of enrichment of a particular set of genes (or 'bioset') in another set of genes [31]. Readers may refer to Appendix A, titled 'Repurposable Drugs for Treatment of Malignant Pleural Mesothelioma (MPM)' for more details on the methodology used to identify repurposable drugs.

5. Conclusions

Biomedical discovery in the field of MPM research has to be accelerated to fuel clinically translatable results due to an urgent need to diagnose MPM preemptively, prevent its post-treatment recurrence, and curb its predicted increase in incidence in western and economically emerging nations [103]. In this study, we presented the MPM interactome as a valuable resource for mesothelioma biologists. We demonstrated its biological validity through comparison with MPM-related multi-omics data, which served to contextualize the novel PPIs within the mesothelioma landscape. Making novel MPM PPIs available freely on a webserver will catalyze investigations into these by cancer biologists and may lead to biologically or clinically translatable results. The MPM interactome with disease-associated proteins and their interacting partners will help biologists, bioinformaticians and clinicians to piece together an integrated view on how MPM-associated genes from various studies are functionally linked. Biological insights from this 'systems-level' view will help generate testable hypotheses and clinically translatable results. Future work will focus on expanding this interactome by including interactions from additional PPI repositories, other mesothelioma types and mesothelioma datasets.

Supplementary Materials: The following are available online at https://www.mdpi.com/article/10.3390/cancers13071660/s1: Table S1: Identification of protein interactors using liquid chromatography–mass spectrometry (LC-MS), Table S2: Overlaps between drugs tested in NSCLC and drugs occurring in the MPM drug-protein interactome, that were negatively correlated with lung cancer expression studies, Table S3: Some novel interactors which are hypomethylated and their MPM genes, Data File S1: List of MPM genes and their corresponding biological evidences extracted from IPA suite, Data File S2: List of genes from the MPM interactome with their labels (MPM genes, known interactors and novel interactors), Data File S3: List of all the pathways associated with at least one of the MPM genes, Data File S4: List of all the drugs that target any of the genes from the MPM interactome, and Data File S5: Master table of all biological evidences (genetic variant, transcriptomic and proteomic evidence) for each of the MPM interactome genes discussed in the paper.

Author Contributions: In sequence of work: M.K.G. conceptualized and supervised the study and carried out interactome construction and analysis of pathway and drug associations. K.B.K. carried out studies of the overlap of the interactome with various high-throughput data, literature-based evidence gathering, and identification of repurposable drugs. Experimental validations were carried out by N.Y. and G.B. Written description of methods of experimental validation were provided by N.Y. and G.B. Manuscript has been written by K.B.K. and edited by M.K.G., M.J.B. provided consultation and valuable feedback on the manuscript. Manuscript has been read and approved by all authors. All authors have read and agreed to the published version of the manuscript.

Funding: This work has been funded by U24OH009077 (Becich) from the Center for Disease Control (CDC), National Institute of Occupational Safety and Health (NIOSH) and R01MH094564 (Ganapathiraju) from National Institute of Mental Health (NIMH), of National Institutes of Health (NIH), USA. The content is solely the responsibility of the authors and does not necessarily represent the official views of the CDC, NIOSH or NIMH, NIH, USA.

Institutional Review Board Statement: Not applicable.

Informed Consent Statement: Not applicable.

Data Availability Statement: On journal website and at http://severus.dbmi.pitt.edu/wiki-MPM.

Acknowledgments: We thank David Boone (Department of Biomedical Informatics), J. Richard Chaillet (Office of Research Health Sciences) and Adrian Lee (Department of Pharmacology and Chemical Biology) of University of Pittsburgh for detailed and valuable feedback on the manuscript. We thank the team of National Mesothelioma Virtual Bank, particularly Waqas Amin and Jonathan Silverstein (University of Pittsburgh), Harvey Pass (New York University Langone Medical Center) and Carmelo Gaudioso (Roswell Park Comprehensive Cancer Center) for valuable discussions. M.K.G. and K.B.K. thank N. Balakrishnan (Indian Institute of Science) for valuable technical feedback. M.K.G thanks Sai Supreetha Varanasi for system administration assistance in hosting the website.

Conflicts of Interest: The authors declare no conflict of interest.

Appendix A Repurposable Drugs for Treatment of Malignant Pleural Mesothelioma (MPM)

We present here five drugs (*cabazitaxel*, *pyrimethamine*, *trimethoprim*, *primaquine* and *glicazide*) that could potentially be repurposed for the treatment of malignant pleural mesothelioma (MPM). These drugs were shortlisted through three types of analysis: (A) considering those that were already tested in non-small cell lung cancer (NSCLC), (B) gene expression analysis of drugs that target MPM genes or novel interactors in the MPM interactome, or (C) gene expression analysis of drugs that target known interactors in the malignant pleural mesothelioma (MPM) interactome. Drugs were selected based on whether they were already tested against lung cancer in clinical trials and/or showed overall negative correlation with lung cancer expression studies, because both mesothelioma and lung cancers have been shown to share common pathways that are initiated on exposure to asbestos fibres in mesothelial cells and lung epithelial cells respectively [35].

Another criterion used was whether the genes targeted by the drugs showed high differential expression in MPM tumours/cell lines. The details of these methods and observations are presented below.

Appendix A.1 Repurposable Drugs Already Tested in Non-Small Cell Lung Cancer

Nine overlapping drugs were found between drugs tested in NSCLC and drugs occurring in the MPM drug-protein interactome, that were negatively correlated with lung cancer expression studies, namely, cabazitaxel, dasatinib, docetaxel, gemcitabine, ipilimumab, ixabepilone, minocycline, pazopanib and pemetrexed. Minocycline was eliminated due to its toxicity. All of the remaining eight drugs were found to be effective in treatment of NSCLC (Table S2). Out of these eight drugs, cabazitaxel was the only drug that was not tested for treatment of mesothelioma. The fact that the other seven drugs were already tested against mesothelioma in clinical trials demonstrates the validity of our approach. It was interesting to note that drugs that targeted known interactors in addition to some MPM genes were found to have either no effect or limited clinical activity in mesothelioma, for e.g., dasatinib, docetaxel and pazopanib. On the other hand, drugs that targeted only MPM genes were found to be effective in treatment of mesothelioma or were capable of preventing disease progression, for e.g., gemcitabine, ipilimumab, ixabepilone and pemetrexed. This raises the suspicion that drugs that do not act on "off-target" genes (known interactors, in this case) may be more effective. In this respect, cabazitaxel, which targets the MPM genes *TUBB1* and *TUBA4A*, may be a suitable candidate for mesothelioma. Cabazitaxel was found to be effective in treatment of NSCLC resistant to docetaxel, a drug that targets *TUBB1* and other known interactors [37].

Appendix A.2 Repurposable Drugs Targeting MPM Genes and Novel Interactors

The MPM genes that were most differentially expressed with high significance in MPM tumors (GSE51024 [33]) were *TYMS* ($\log_2 FC = 1.82$, p-value $= 4.10 \times 10^{-17}$) and *DHFR* ($\log_2 FC = 0.89$, p-value $= 1.20 \times 10^{-14}$), and the drugs that target these genes (also having negative correlation with lung cancer expression) were pyrimethamine and trimethoprim. The first line drug currently used to treat mesothelioma is premetrexed, which targets proteins in the folate metabolic pathway, namely, *DHFR*, *TYMS* and *GART* [104]. Since MPM tumors have been shown to be responsive to anti-folates [68], both pyrimethamine (which targets only *DHFR*) and trimethoprim (which targets both *DHFR* and *TYMS*), seem to be interesting candidates. Pyrimethamine, an anti-parasitic drug commonly used to treat toxoplasmosis and cystoisosporiasis, has shown anti-tumor activity in metastatic melanoma cells and in murine models of breast cancer [105,106]. Trimethoprim, an antibacterial drug commonly used in the treatment of urinary bladder and respiratory tract infections, is also used to treat bacterial infections in cancer patients [107,108].

Keratin proteins form important components of the cell cytoskeleton, called intermediate filaments, in epithelial cells, and are commonly used as diagnostic markers in cancer [60]. In addition to their role as cancer markers, their involvement in cellular functions such as cell motility, proliferation, cell polarity, protein synthesis, membrane trafficking and most importantly, tumour invasion and metastasis make them attractive as candidates for drug development [60]. *KRT7* is a keratin primarily expressed in mesothelial cells, apart from cells lining ducts and the intestine [60]. In a patient with malignant mesothelioma of the epithelioid type (which spreads to mediastinum and breast), *KRT7* was found to be significantly overexpressed when she developed resistance to pemetrexed/carboplatin, provided as a second line therapy [61]. The cancer cells showed a drastic increase in their immunoreactivity to CK7, the protein encoded by *KRT7* [61]. At the last stage of cancer progression (which was followed by her death), the patient showed dyspnoea (difficulty in breathing), increased tumour volume and pleural fluid [61]. In another case, *KRT7* was found be significantly overexpressed in an aggressive state of MPM, prior to treatment [61]. Two-thirds of malignant mesothelioma cases have been reported to be K7$^+$/K20$^-$ (positive for expression of *KRT7* and negative for expression of *KRT20*) [60]. Expression of

KRT7 in three histological types of mesothelioma, namely, epithelioid, sarcomatid and biphasic, has been used to distinguish them from synovial sarcoma that metastasizes to the lungs and pleura [62]. KRT7 has been identified as marker of circulating tumour cells in lung cancer [109]. KRT7 was also found to be significantly upregulated in MPM tumours ($\log_2 FC$ = 3.80, p-value = 0.0002), and in cell line models of MPM ($\log_2 FC$ = 2.266, p-value = 0.029) (GSE2549 [34]). Positive expression of KRT7 was noted in various types of non-small cell lung cancers, including large cell neuroendocrine carcinoma and lung adenocarcinoma [110,111]. In the MPM interactome, KRT7 was predicted to interact with KRT5, an MPM gene that serves as a marker for malignant mesothelioma, along with vimentin, and is specifically used to distinguish pleural mesothelioma of the epithelioid type from pulmonary adenocarcinoma and non-pulmonary adenocarcinoma metastasizing to pleura [60,112]. KRT7 is a target of primaquine, an-antimalarial agent known to destroy the malarial parasites, *Plasmodium vivax* and *Plasmodium ovale*, inside the liver [113,114]. The exact mechanism of action has not been elucidated for this drug. However, in independent studies, primaquine has been shown to bind to keratin in a concentration-dependent manner, and also mediate strong membrane perturbations in cell membrane models [113,115]. Since high expression of KRT7 has been shown to be related to tumour aggressiveness and drug resistance in malignant mesothelioma, and its high expression was also noted in MPM tumours and cell lines, primaquine may be re-purposed for treatment of MPM at least as an adjunctive drug with pemetrexed, the drug currently used for first line therapy. It is interesting to note that primaquine enhanced the sensitivity of KBV20C cells to cancer drugs, namely, vinblastine, vinorelbine, paclitaxel, docetaxel, vincristine and halaven [63]. KVB20C is a multi-drug resistant cell line derived from oral squamous carcinoma. Primaquine compounds (substituted quinolines) have also been shown to exert anti-tumor activity in breast cancer cells [116].

Appendix A.3 Repurposable Drugs Targeting Known Interactors

Out of the four drugs targeting known interactors in the MPM interactome and showing negative correlation with lung cancer associated gene expression, three drugs were already known to exhibit anti-tumour activity in pre-clinical models of mesothelioma, namely, zoledronate, sirolimus and the vitamin E analog, alpha-tocopheryl succinate, which shows the validity of our approach. Zoledronate, which showed modest activity in MPM, induced apoptosis and S-phase arrest in human mesothelioma cells and inhibited tumor growth in the pleural cavity of an orthotopic animal model [54,55]. Sirolimus/cisplatin increased cell death and decreased cell proliferation in cell lines of MPM [56]. Alpha-tocopheryl succinate increased survival of orthotopic animal models of malignant peritoneal mesothelioma [57]. Zoledronate has demonstrated modest clinical activity in patients with advanced MPM [54]. Sirolimus has not been tested against MPM in clinical trials, but everolimus, a drug derived from sirolimus sharing similar properties with it, has shown only limited clinical activity in MPM, and further testing as a single-agent was not advised based on the results from this study [117]. Both vitamin E and its analog, alpha-tocopheryl succinate have not been tested against MPM in clinical trials. However, testing of vitamin E and its analogs are being carried out in various pre-clinical settings [58,59]. Hence, it was the drug gliclazide that emerged as a potentially repurposable drug, untested against MPM.

Gliclazide, an anti-diabetic drug, inhibits VEGFA, which has been shown to be significantly upregulated ($\log_2 FC$ = 1.83, p-value = 0.0018) in MPM tumour (GSE2549 [34]). This drug inhibits VEGF expression induced by advanced glycation end products in bovine reticular endothelial cells, and VEGF expression induced by ischemia in retinal tissue of mice [64,118]. In the latter case, glicazide also inhibits neovascularization, a process known to be mediated by VEGF. VEGF has been identified as a prognostic marker for MPM. High levels of VEGF have been correlated with both asbestos exposure in MPM, and an advanced stage of the disease [65,66]. It is interesting to note that glibenclamide, a drug whose mechanism of action is similar to that of glicazide, has been shown to increase caspase activity in MPM cell lines and primary cultures, leading to apoptosis mediated by

TNF-related apoptosis inducing ligand (*TRAIL*) [67]. Hence, glicazide may be repurposed to inhibit neovascularization and perhaps enhance apoptosis in MPM.

References

1. Mutsaers, S.E. The mesothelial cell. *Int. J. Biochem. Cell Biol.* **2004**, *36*, 9–16. [CrossRef]
2. Carbone, M.; Adusumilli, P.S.; Alexander, H.R., Jr.; Baas, P.; Bardelli, F.; Bononi, A.; Bueno, R.; Felley-Bosco, E.; Galateau-Salle, F.; Jablons, D.; et al. Mesothelioma: Scientific clues for prevention, diagnosis, and therapy. *CA Cancer J. Clin.* **2019**, *69*, 402–429. [CrossRef] [PubMed]
3. Wang, Z.J.; Reddy, G.P.; Gotway, M.B.; Higgins, C.B.; Jablons, D.M.; Ramaswamy, M.; Hawkins, R.A.; Webb, W.R. Malignant Pleural Mesothelioma: Evaluation with CT, MR Imaging, and PET. *Radiographics* **2004**, *24*, 105–119. [CrossRef] [PubMed]
4. Lang-Lazdunski, L. Malignant pleural mesothelioma: Some progress, but still a long way from cure. *J. Thorac. Dis.* **2018**, *10*, 1172–1177. [CrossRef]
5. Bueno, R.; Stawiski, E.W.; Goldstein, L.D.; Durinck, S.; De Rienzo, A.; Modrusan, Z.; Gnad, F.; Nguyen, T.T.; Jaiswal, B.S.; Chirieac, L.R.; et al. Comprehensive genomic analysis of malignant pleural mesothelioma identifies recurrent mutations, gene fusions and splicing alterations. *Nat. Genet.* **2016**, *48*, 407–416. [CrossRef]
6. Bott, M.; Brevet, M.; Taylor, B.S.; Shimizu, S.; Ito, T.; Wang, L.; Creaney, J.; Lake, R.A.; Zakowski, M.F.; Reva, B.; et al. The nuclear deubiquitinase BAP1 is commonly inactivated by somatic mutations and 3p21.1 losses in malignant pleural mesothelioma. *Nat. Genet.* **2011**, *43*, 668–672. [CrossRef]
7. Jensen, D.E.; Proctor, M.; Marquis, S.T.; Gardner, H.P.; Ha, S.I.; Chodosh, L.A.; Ishov, A.M.; Tommerup, N.; Vissing, H.; Sekido, Y.; et al. BAP1: A novel ubiquitin hydrolase which binds to the BRCA1 RING finger and enhances BRCA1-mediated cell growth suppression. *Oncogene* **1998**, *16*, 1097–1112. [CrossRef] [PubMed]
8. Hakiri, S.; Osada, H.; Ishiguro, F.; Murakami, H.; Murakami-Tonami, Y.; Yokoi, K.; Sekido, Y. Functional differences between wild-type and mutant-type BRCA1-associated protein 1 tumor suppressor against malignant mesothelioma cells. *Cancer Sci.* **2015**, *106*, 990–999. [CrossRef]
9. Zauderer, M.G.; Kass, S.L.; Woo, K.; Sima, C.S.; Ginsberg, M.S.; Krug, L.M. Vinorelbine and gemcitabine as second- or third-line therapy for malignant pleural mesothelioma. *Lung Cancer* **2014**, *84*, 271–274. [CrossRef]
10. Zucali, P.; Perrino, M.; Lorenzi, E.; Ceresoli, G.; De Vincenzo, F.; Simonelli, M.; Gianoncelli, L.; De Sanctis, R.; Giordano, L.; Santoro, A. Vinorelbine in pemetrexed-pretreated patients with malignant pleural mesothelioma. *Lung Cancer* **2014**, *84*, 265–270. [CrossRef]
11. Zauderer, M.G.; Bott, M.; McMillan, R.; Sima, C.S.; Rusch, V.; Krug, L.M.; Ladanyi, M. Clinical characteristics of patients with malignant pleural mesothelioma harboring somatic BAP1 mutations. *J. Thorac. Oncol.* **2013**, *8*, 1430–1433. [CrossRef]
12. Busacca, S.; Sheaff, M.; Arthur, K.; Gray, S.G.; O'Byrne, K.J.; Richard, D.J.; Soltermann, A.; Opitz, I.; Pass, H.; Harkin, D.P.; et al. BRCA1 is an essential mediator of vinorelbine-induced apoptosis in mesothelioma. *J. Pathol.* **2012**, *227*, 200–208. [CrossRef]
13. Toyokawa, G.; Takenoyama, M.; Hirai, F.; Toyozawa, R.; Inamasu, E.; Kojo, M.; Morodomi, Y.; Shiraishi, Y.; Takenaka, T.; Yamaguchi, M.; et al. Gemcitabine and vinorelbine as second-line or beyond treatment in patients with malignant pleural mesothelioma pretreated with platinum plus pemetrexed chemotherapy. *Int. J. Clin. Oncol.* **2013**, *19*, 601–606. [CrossRef]
14. Sahni, N.; Yi, S.; Taipale, M.; Bass, J.I.F.; Coulombe-Huntington, J.; Yang, F.; Peng, J.; Weile, J.; Karras, G.I.; Wang, Y.; et al. Widespread Macromolecular Interaction Perturbations in Human Genetic Disorders. *Cell* **2015**, *161*, 647–660. [CrossRef]
15. Rolland, T.; Taşan, M.; Charloteaux, B.; Pevzner, S.J.; Zhong, Q.; Sahni, N.; Yi, S.; Lemmens, I.; Fontanillo, C.; Mosca, R.; et al. A Proteome-Scale Map of the Human Interactome Network. *Cell* **2014**, *159*, 1212–1226. [CrossRef]
16. Ganapathiraju, M.K.; Thahir, M.; Handen, A.; Sarkar, S.N.; Sweet, R.A.; Nimgaonkar, V.L.; Loscher, C.E.; Bauer, E.M.; Chaparala, S. Schizophrenia interactome with 504 novel protein–protein interactions. *Npj Schizophr.* **2016**, *2*, 16012. [CrossRef]
17. Zhu, J.; Zhang, Y.; Ghosh, A.; Cuevas, R.A.; Forero, A.; Dhar, J.; Ibsen, M.S.; Schmid-Burgk, J.L.; Schmidt, T.; Ganapathiraju, M.K.; et al. Antiviral Activity of Human OASL Protein Is Mediated by Enhancing Signaling of the RIG-I RNA Sensor. *Immunity* **2014**, *40*, 936–948. [CrossRef] [PubMed]
18. Li, Y.; Klena, N.T.; Gabriel, G.C.; Liu, X.; Kim, A.J.; Lemke, K.; Chen, Y.; Chatterjee, B.; Devine, W.; Damerla, R.R.; et al. Global genetic analysis in mice unveils central role for cilia in congenital heart disease. *Nat. Cell Biol.* **2015**, *521*, 520–524. [CrossRef] [PubMed]
19. Liu, X.; Yagi, H.; Saeed, S.; Bais, A.S.; Gabriel, G.C.; Chen, Z.; Peterson, K.; Li, Y.; Schwartz, M.C.; Reynolds, W.T.; et al. The complex genetics of hypoplastic left heart syndrome. *Nat. Genet.* **2017**, *49*, 1152–1159. [CrossRef] [PubMed]
20. Karunakaran, K.B.; Chaparala, S.; Ganapathiraju, M.K. Potentially repurposable drugs for schizophrenia identified from its interactome. *Sci. Rep.* **2019**, *9*, 1–14. [CrossRef] [PubMed]
21. Cedrés, S.; Montero, M.; Martinez, P.; Rodríguez-Freixinós, V.; Torrejon, D.; Gabaldon, A.; Salcedo, M.; Cajal, S.R.Y.; Felip, E. Exploratory analysis of activation of PTEN–PI3K pathway and downstream proteins in malignant pleural mesothelioma (MPM). *Lung Cancer* **2012**, *77*, 192–198. [CrossRef] [PubMed]
22. Prasad, T.S.K.; Goel, R.; Kandasamy, K.; Keerthikumar, S.; Kumar, S.; Mathivanan, S.; Telikicherla, D.; Raju, R.; Shafreen, B.; Venugopal, A.; et al. Human Protein Reference Database—2009 update. *Nucleic Acids Res.* **2008**, *37*, D767–D772. [CrossRef] [PubMed]

23. Stark, C.; Breitkreutz, B.-J.; Reguly, T.; Boucher, L.; Breitkreutz, A.; Tyers, M. BioGRID: A general repository for interaction datasets. *Nucleic Acids Res.* **2006**, *34*, D535–D539. [CrossRef] [PubMed]
24. Karunakaran, K.B.; Yanamala, N.; Boyce, G.; Ganapathiraju, M.K. Mesothelioma Interactome with 367 Novel Protein-Protein Interactions. *bioRxiv* **2018**, 459065. [CrossRef]
25. Wu, G.; Dawson, E.; Duong, A.; Haw, R.; Stein, L. ReactomeFIViz: A Cytoscape app for pathway and network-based data analysis. *F1000Research* **2014**, *3*, 146. [CrossRef]
26. Orii, N.; Ganapathiraju, M.K. Wiki-Pi: A Web-Server of Annotated Human Protein-Protein Interactions to Aid in Discovery of Protein Function. *PLoS ONE* **2012**, *7*, e49029. [CrossRef]
27. Amin, W.; Parwani, A.V.; Melamed, J.; Flores, R.M.; Pennathur, A.; Valdivieso, F.A.; Whelan, N.B.; Landreneau, R.; Luketich, J.D.; Feldman, M.; et al. National Mesothelioma Virtual Bank: A Platform for Collaborative Research and Mesothelioma Biobanking Resource to Support Translational Research. *Lung Cancer Int.* **2013**, *2013*, 1–9. [CrossRef]
28. Amin, W.; Singh, H.; Pople, A.K.; Winters, S.; Dhir, R.; Parwani, A.V.; Becich, M.J. A decade of experience in the development and implementation of tissue banking informatics tools for intra and inter-institutional translational research. *J. Pathol. Inform.* **2010**, *1*, 12. [CrossRef]
29. Krämer, A.; Green, J.; Pollard, J.; Tugendreich, S. Causal analysis approaches in Ingenuity Pathway Analysis. *Bioinformatics* **2014**, *30*, 523–530. [CrossRef]
30. LoPiccolo, J.; Granville, C.A.; Gills, J.J.; Dennis, P.A. Targeting Akt in cancer therapy. *Anti-Cancer Drugs* **2007**, *18*, 861–874. [CrossRef]
31. Kupershmidt, I.; Su, Q.J.; Grewal, A.; Sundaresh, S.; Halperin, I.; Flynn, J.; Shekar, M.; Wang, H.; Park, J.; Cui, W.; et al. Ontology-Based Meta-Analysis of Global Collections of High-Throughput Public Data. *PLoS ONE* **2010**, *5*, e13066. [CrossRef]
32. Chattopadhyay, A.; Ganapathiraju, M.K. Demonstration Study: A Protocol to Combine Online Tools and Databases for Identifying Potentially Repurposable Drugs. *Data* **2017**, *2*, 15. [CrossRef]
33. Suraokar, M.B.; Nunez, M.I.; Diao, L.; Chow, C.W.; Kim, D.; Behrens, C.; Lin, H.; Lee, S.; Raso, G.; Moran, C.; et al. Expression profiling stratifies mesothelioma tumors and signifies deregulation of spindle checkpoint pathway and microtubule network with therapeutic implications. *Ann. Oncol.* **2014**, *25*, 1184–1192. [CrossRef] [PubMed]
34. Gordon, G.J.; Rockwell, G.N.; Jensen, R.V.; Rheinwald, J.G.; Glickman, J.N.; Aronson, J.P.; Pottorf, B.J.; Nitz, M.D.; Richards, W.G.; Sugarbaker, D.J.; et al. Identification of Novel Candidate Oncogenes and Tumor Suppressors in Malignant Pleural Mesothelioma Using Large-Scale Transcriptional Profiling. *Am. J. Pathol.* **2005**, *166*, 1827–1840. [CrossRef]
35. Heintz, N.H.; Janssen-Heininger, Y.M.; Mossman, B.T. Asbestos, lung cancers, and mesotheliomas: From molecular approaches to targeting tumor survival pathways. *Am. J. Respir. Cell Mol. Biol.* **2010**, *42*, 133–139. [CrossRef] [PubMed]
36. Wishart, D.S.; Knox, C.; Guo, A.C.; Cheng, D.; Shrivastava, S.; Tzur, D.; Gautam, B.; Hassanali, M. DrugBank: A knowledgebase for drugs, drug actions and drug targets. *Nuc. Acids Res.* **2008**, *36*, D901–D906. [CrossRef] [PubMed]
37. Kotsakis, A.; Matikas, A.; Koinis, F.; Kentepozidis, N.; Varthalitis, I.I.; Karavassilis, V.; Samantas, E.; Katsaounis, P.; Dermitzaki, E.K.; Hatzidaki, D.; et al. A multicentre phase II trial of cabazitaxel in patients with advanced non-small-cell lung cancer progressing after docetaxel-based chemotherapy. *Br. J. Cancer* **2016**, *115*, 784–788. [CrossRef] [PubMed]
38. Johnson, F.M.; Bekele, B.N.; Feng, L.; Wistuba, I.; Tang, X.M.; Tran, H.T.; Erasmus, J.J.; Hwang, L.-L.; Takebe, N.; Blumenschein, G.R.; et al. Phase II Study of Dasatinib in Patients with Advanced Non–Small-Cell Lung Cancer. *J. Clin. Oncol.* **2010**, *28*, 4609–4615. [CrossRef]
39. Tsao, A.S.; Lin, H.; Carter, B.W.; Lee, J.J.; Rice, D.; Vaporcyan, A.; Swisher, S.; Mehran, R.; Heymach, J.; Nilsson, M.; et al. Biomarker-Integrated Neoadjuvant Dasatinib Trial in Resectable Malignant Pleural Mesothelioma. *J. Thorac. Oncol.* **2018**, *13*, 246–257. [CrossRef]
40. Comer, A.M.; Goa, K.L. Docetaxel. A review of its use in non-small cell lung cancer. *Drugs Aging* **2000**, *17*, 53–80. [CrossRef]
41. Belani, C.P.; Adak, S.; Aisner, S.; Stella, P.J.; Levitan, N.; Johnson, D.H. Docetaxel for malignant mesothelioma: Phase II study of the Eastern Cooperative Oncology Group. *Clin. Lung Cancer* **2004**, *6*, 43–47. [CrossRef]
42. Ralli, M.; Tourkantonis, I.; Makrilia, N.; Gkini, E.; Kotteas, E.; Gkiozos, I.; Katirtzoglou, N.; Syrigos, K. Docetaxel plus gemcitabine as first-line treatment in malignant pleural mesothelioma: A single institution phase II study. *Anticancer Res.* **2009**, *29*, 3441–3444.
43. Tourkantonis, I.; Makrilia, N.; Ralli, M.; Alamara, C.; Nikolaidis, I.; Tsimpoukis, S.; Charpidou, A.; Kotanidou, A.; Syrigos, K. Phase II study of gemcitabine plus docetaxel as second-line treatment in malignant pleural mesothelioma: A single institution study. *Am. J. Clin. Oncol.* **2011**, *34*, 38–42. [CrossRef]
44. Manegold, C. Gemcitabine (Gemzar®) in non-small cell lung cancer. *Expert Rev. Anticancer Ther.* **2004**, *4*, 345–360. [CrossRef]
45. Kindler, H.L.; van Meerbeeck, J.P. The role of gemcitabine in the treatment of malignant mesothelioma. *Semin. Oncol.* **2002**, *29*, 70–76. [CrossRef]
46. Malhotra, J.; Jabbour, S.K.; Aisner, J. Current state of immunotherapy for non-small cell lung cancer. *Transl. Lung Cancer Res.* **2007**, *6*, 196–211. [CrossRef]
47. Scherpereel, A.; Mazieres, J.; Greillier, L.; Dô, P.; Bylicki, O.; Monnet, I.; Corre, R.; Audigier-Valette, C.; Locatelli-Sanchez, M.; Molinier, O. Second-or third-line nivolumab (Nivo) versus nivo plus ipilimumab (Ipi) in malignant pleural mesothelioma (MPM) patients: Results of the IFCT-1501 MAPS2 randomized phase II trial. *Am. Soc. Clin. Oncol.* **2017**, *35*, LBA8507. [CrossRef]

48. Spigel, D.R.; Greco, F.A.; Waterhouse, D.M.; Shipley, D.L.; Zubkus, J.D.; Bury, M.J.; Webb, C.D.; Hart, L.L.; Gian, V.G.; Infante, J.R.; et al. Phase II trial of ixabepilone and carboplatin with or without bevacizumab in patients with previously untreated advanced non-small-cell lung cancer. *Lung Cancer* **2012**, *78*, 70–75. [CrossRef] [PubMed]
49. Puhalla, S.; Brufsky, A. Ixabepilone: A new chemotherapeutic option for refractory metastatic breast cancer. *Biol. Targets Ther.* **2008**, *2*, 505.
50. Altorki, N.; Lane, M.E.; Bauer, T.; Lee, P.C.; Guarino, M.J.; Pass, H.; Felip, E.; Peylan-Ramu, N.; Gurpide, A.; Grannis, F.W.; et al. Phase II Proof-of-Concept Study of Pazopanib Monotherapy in Treatment-Naive Patients with Stage I/II Resectable Non–Small-Cell Lung Cancer. *J. Clin. Oncol.* **2010**, *28*, 3131–3137. [CrossRef] [PubMed]
51. Hiddinga, B.I.; Rolfo, C.; Van Meerbeeck, J.P. Mesothelioma treatment: Are we on target? A review. *J. Adv. Res.* **2015**, *6*, 319–330. [CrossRef]
52. Scagliotti, G.; Parikh, P.; Von Pawel, J.; Biesma, B.; Vansteenkiste, J.; Manegold, C.; Serwatowski, P.; Gatzemeier, U.; Digumarti, R.; Zukin, M.; et al. Phase III Study Comparing Cisplatin Plus Gemcitabine with Cisplatin Plus Pemetrexed in Chemotherapy-Naive Patients with Advanced-Stage Non–Small-Cell Lung Cancer. *J. Clin. Oncol. Off. J. Am. Soc. Clin.* **2008**, *26*, 3543–3551. [CrossRef]
53. Vogelzang, N.J.; Rusthoven, J.J.; Symanowski, J.; Denham, C.; Kaukel, E.; Ruffie, P.; Gatzemeier, U.; Boyer, M.; Emri, S.; Manegold, C.; et al. Phase III Study of Pemetrexed in Combination with Cisplatin Versus Cisplatin Alone in Patients with Malignant Pleural Mesothelioma. *J. Clin. Oncol.* **2003**, *21*, 2636–2644. [CrossRef]
54. Jamil, M.O.; Jerome, M.S.; Miley, D.; Selander, K.S.; Robert, F. A pilot study of zoledronic acid in the treatment of patients with advanced malignant pleural mesothelioma. *Lung Cancer Targets Ther.* **2017**, *8*, 39–44. [CrossRef]
55. Okamoto, S.; Kawamura, K.; Li, Q.; Yamanaka, M.; Yang, S.; Fukamachi, T.; Tada, Y.; Tatsumi, K.; Shimada, H.; Hiroshima, K.; et al. Zoledronic Acid Produces Antitumor Effects on Mesothelioma Through Apoptosis and S-Phase Arrest in p53-Independent and Ras prenylation-Independent Manners. *J. Thorac. Oncol.* **2012**, *7*, 873–882. [CrossRef]
56. Hartman, M.-L.; Esposito, J.M.; Yeap, B.Y.; Sugarbaker, D.J. Combined treatment with cisplatin and sirolimus to enhance cell death in human mesothelioma. *J. Thorac. Cardiovasc. Surg.* **2010**, *139*, 1233–1240. [CrossRef]
57. Tomasetti, M.; Gellert, N.; Procopio, A.; Neuzil, J. A vitamin E analogue suppresses malignant mesothelioma in a preclinical model: A future drug against a fatal neoplastic disease? *Int. J. Cancer* **2004**, *109*, 641–642. [CrossRef] [PubMed]
58. Kovarova, J.; Bajzikova, M.; Vondrusová, M.; Stursa, J.; Goodwin, J.; Nguyen, M.; Zobalova, R.; Pesdar, E.A.; Truksa, J.; Tomasetti, M.; et al. Mitochondrial targeting of α-tocopheryl succinate enhances its anti-mesothelioma efficacy. *Redox Rep.* **2014**, *19*, 16–25. [CrossRef] [PubMed]
59. Sato, A.; Virgona, N.; Sekine, Y.; Yano, T. The evidence to date: A redox-inactive analogue of tocotrienol as a new anti-mesothelioma agent. *J. Rare Dis. Res. Treat.* **2016**, *2*, 38–42.
60. Karantza, V. Keratins in health and cancer: More than mere epithelial cell markers. *Oncogene* **2010**, *30*, 127–138. [CrossRef]
61. Røe, O.D.; Szulkin, A.; Anderssen, E.; Flatberg, A.; Sandeck, H.; Amundsen, T.; Erlandsen, S.E.; Dobra, K.; Sundstrøm, S.H. Molecular resistance fingerprint of pemetrexed and platinum in a long-term survivor of mesothelioma. *PLoS ONE* **2012**, *7*, e40521. [CrossRef] [PubMed]
62. Miettinen, M.; Limon, J.; Niezabitowski, A.; Lasota, J. Calretinin and other mesothelioma markers in synovial sarcoma: Analysis of antigenic similarities and differences with malignant mesothelioma. *Am. J. Surg. Pathol.* **2001**, *25*, 610–617. [CrossRef] [PubMed]
63. Choi, A.-R.; Kim, J.-H.; Woo, Y.H.; Kim, H.S.; Yoon, S. Anti-malarial Drugs Primaquine and Chloroquine Have Different Sensitization Effects with Anti-mitotic Drugs in Resistant Cancer Cells. *Anticancer Res.* **2016**, *36*, 1641–1648. [CrossRef]
64. Kimura, T.; Takagi, H.; Suzuma, K.; Kita, M.; Watanabe, D.; Yoshimura, N. Comparisons between the beneficial effects of different sulphonylurea treatments on ischemia-induced retinal neovascularization. *Free Radic. Biol. Med.* **2007**, *43*, 454–461. [CrossRef]
65. Yasumitsu, A.; Tabata, C.; Tabata, R.; Hirayama, N.; Murakami, A.; Yamada, S.; Terada, T.; Iida, S.; Tamura, K.; Fukuoka, K.; et al. Clinical Significance of Serum Vascular Endothelial Growth Factor in Malignant Pleural Mesothelioma. *J. Thorac. Oncol.* **2010**, *5*, 479–483. [CrossRef]
66. Hirayama, N.; Tabata, C.; Tabata, R.; Maeda, R.; Yasumitsu, A.; Yamada, S.; Kuribayashi, K.; Fukuoka, K.; Nakano, T. Pleural effusion VEGF levels as a prognostic factor of malignant pleural mesothelioma. *Respir. Med.* **2011**, *105*, 137–142. [CrossRef]
67. Pasello, G.; Urso, L.; Conte, P.; Favaretto, A. Effects of Sulfonylureas on Tumor Growth: A Review of the Literature. *Oncologist* **2013**, *18*, 1118–1125. [CrossRef]
68. Krug, L.M.; Heelan, R.T.; Kris, M.G.; Venkatraman, E.; Sirotnak, F.M. Phase II Trial of Pralatrexate (10-Propargyl-10-deazaaminopterin, PDX) in Patients with Unresectable Malignant Pleural Mesothelioma. *J. Thorac. Oncol.* **2007**, *2*, 317–320. [CrossRef] [PubMed]
69. Christensen, B.C.; Marsit, C.J.; Houseman, E.A.; Godleski, J.J.; Longacker, J.L.; Zheng, S.; Yeh, R.-F.; Wrensch, M.R.; Wiemels, J.L.; Karagas, M.R.; et al. Differentiation of Lung Adenocarcinoma, Pleural Mesothelioma, and Nonmalignant Pulmonary Tissues Using DNA Methylation Profiles. *Cancer Res.* **2009**, *69*, 6315–6321. [CrossRef]
70. Wang, S.; Jiang, L.; Han, Y.; Chew, S.H.; Ohara, Y.; Akatsuka, S.; Weng, L.; Kawaguchi, K.; Fukui, T.; Sekido, Y.; et al. Urokinase-type plasminogen activator receptor promotes proliferation and invasion with reduced cisplatin sensitivity in malignant mesothelioma. *Oncotarget* **2016**, *7*, 69565–69578. [CrossRef] [PubMed]
71. Marek, L.A.; Hinz, T.K.; Von Mässenhausen, A.; Olszewski, K.A.; Kleczko, E.K.; Boehm, D.; Weiser-Evans, M.C.; Nemenoff, R.A.; Hoffmann, H.; Warth, A.; et al. Nonamplified FGFR1 Is a Growth Driver in Malignant Pleural Mesothelioma. *Mol. Cancer Res.* **2014**, *12*, 1460–1469. [CrossRef]

72. Wilson, T.R.; Lee, D.Y.; Berry, L.; Shames, D.S.; Settleman, J. Neuregulin-1-Mediated Autocrine Signaling Underlies Sensitivity to HER2 Kinase Inhibitors in a Subset of Human Cancers. *Cancer Cell* **2011**, *20*, 158–172. [CrossRef] [PubMed]
73. Kaarteenaho-Wiik, R.; Soini, Y.; Pöllänen, R.; Pääkkö, P.; Kinnula, V. Over-expression of tenascin-C in malignant pleural mesothelioma. *Histopathology* **2003**, *42*, 280–291. [CrossRef] [PubMed]
74. Lin, C.-C.; Chen, L.-C.; Tseng, V.S.; Yan, J.-J.; Lai, W.-W.; Su, W.-P.; Huang, C.-Y.F. Malignant pleural effusion cells show aberrant glucose metabolism gene expression. *Eur. Respir. J.* **2010**, *37*, 1453–1465. [CrossRef] [PubMed]
75. Crispi, S.; Calogero, R.A.; Santini, M.; Mellone, P.; Vincenzi, B.; Citro, G.; Vicidomini, G.; Fasano, S.; Meccariello, R.; Cobellis, G.; et al. Global Gene Expression Profiling of Human Pleural Mesotheliomas: Identification of Matrix Metalloproteinase 14 (MMP-14) as Potential Tumour Target. *PLoS ONE* **2009**, *4*, e7016. [CrossRef]
76. De Rienzo, A.; Richards, W.G.; Yeap, B.Y.; Coleman, M.H.; Sugarbaker, P.E.; Chirieac, L.R.; Wang, Y.E.; Quackenbush, J.; Jensen, R.V.; Bueno, R. Sequential Binary Gene Ratio Tests Define a Novel Molecular Diagnostic Strategy for Malignant Pleural Mesothelioma. *Clin. Cancer Res.* **2013**, *19*, 2493–2502. [CrossRef]
77. Consortium, G. The Genotype-Tissue Expression (GTEx) pilot analysis: Multitissue gene regulation in humans. *Science* **2015**, *348*, 648–660. [CrossRef] [PubMed]
78. Yanamala, N.; Kisin, E.R.; Gutkin, D.W.; Shurin, M.R.; Harper, M.; Shvedova, A.A. Characterization of pulmonary responses in mice to asbestos/asbestiform fibers using gene expression profiles. *J. Toxicol. Environ. Health Part A* **2017**, *81*, 60–79. [CrossRef] [PubMed]
79. Maxim, L.D.; McConnell, E.E. A Review of the Toxicology and Epidemiology of Wollastonite. *Inhal. Toxicol.* **2005**, *17*, 451–466. [CrossRef]
80. Uhlén, M.; Zhang, C.; Lee, S.; Sjöstedt, E.; Fagerberg, L.; Bidkhori, G.; Benfeitas, R.; Arif, M.; Liu, Z.; Edfors, F.; et al. A pathology atlas of the human cancer transcriptome. *Science* **2017**, *357*, eaan2507. [CrossRef]
81. Strizzi, L.; Catalano, A.; Vianale, G.; Orecchia, S.; Casalini, A.; Tassi, G.; Puntoni, R.; Mutti, L.; Procopio, A. Vascular endothelial growth factor is an autocrine growth factor in human malignant mesothelioma. *J. Pathol.* **2001**, *193*, 468–475. [CrossRef]
82. Seto, T.; Higashiyama, M.; Funai, H.; Imamura, F.; Uematsu, K.; Seki, N.; Eguchi, K.; Yamanaka, T.; Ichinose, Y. Prognostic value of expression of vascular endothelial growth factor and its flt-1 and KDR receptors in stage I non-small-cell lung cancer. *Lung Cancer* **2006**, *53*, 91–96. [CrossRef] [PubMed]
83. Greening, D.W.; Ji, H.; Chen, M.; Robinson, B.W.S.; Dick, I.M.; Creaney, J.; Simpson, R.J. Secreted primary human malignant mesothelioma exosome signature reflects oncogenic cargo. *Sci. Rep.* **2016**, *6*, 32643. [CrossRef]
84. Großerueschkamp, F.; Bracht, T.; Diehl, H.C.; Kuepper, C.; Ahrens, M.; Kallenbach-Thieltges, A.; Mosig, A.; Eisenacher, M.; Marcus, K.; Behrens, T.; et al. Spatial and molecular resolution of diffuse malignant mesothelioma heterogeneity by integrating label-free FTIR imaging, laser capture microdissection and proteomics. *Sci. Rep.* **2017**, *7*, srep44829. [CrossRef]
85. Cigognetti, M.; Lonardi, S.; Fisogni, S.; Balzarini, P.; Pellegrini, V.; Tironi, A.; Bercich, L.; Bugatti, M.; De Rossi, G.; Murer, B.; et al. BAP1 (BRCA1-associated protein 1) is a highly specific marker for differentiating mesothelioma from reactive mesothelial proliferations. *Mod. Pathol.* **2015**, *28*, 1043–1057. [CrossRef]
86. Lupo, B.; Trusolino, L. Inhibition of poly(ADP-ribosyl)ation in cancer: Old and new paradigms revisited. *Biochim. Biophys. Acta (BBA) Bioenerg.* **2014**, *1846*, 201–215. [CrossRef]
87. Nasu, M. *Identification of bap1 as a Predisposing Gene for Malignant Mesothelioma*; University of Hawaii: Manoa, HI, USA, 2012.
88. Yao, Z.-H.; Tian, G.-Y.; Yang, S.-X.; Wan, Y.-Y.; Kang, Y.-M.; Liu, Q.-H.; Yao, F.; Lin, D.-J. Serum albumin as a significant prognostic factor in patients with malignant pleural mesothelioma. *Tumor Biol.* **2014**, *35*, 6839–6845. [CrossRef] [PubMed]
89. Iacono, M.L.; Monica, V.; Righi, L.; Grosso, F.; Libener, R.; Vatrano, S.; Bironzo, P.; Novello, S.; Musmeci, L.; Volante, M.; et al. Targeted Next-Generation Sequencing of Cancer Genes in Advanced Stage Malignant Pleural Mesothelioma: A Retrospective Study. *J. Thorac. Oncol.* **2015**, *10*, 492–499. [CrossRef]
90. Liu, Y.; Zou, X.; Sun, G.; Bao, Y. Codonopsis lanceolata polysaccharide CLPS inhibits melanoma metastasis via regulating integrin signaling. *Int. J. Biol. Macromol.* **2017**, *103*, 435–440. [CrossRef] [PubMed]
91. Okamoto, T.; Iwata, S.; Yamazaki, H.; Hatano, R.; Komiya, E.; Dang, N.H.; Ohnuma, K.; Morimoto, C. CD9 Negatively Regulates CD26 Expression and Inhibits CD26-Mediated Enhancement of Invasive Potential of Malignant Mesothelioma Cells. *PLoS ONE* **2014**, *9*, e86671. [CrossRef] [PubMed]
92. Pereira, S.; Lowell, C. The Lyn Tyrosine Kinase Negatively Regulates Neutrophil Integrin Signaling. *J. Immunol.* **2003**, *171*, 1319–1327. [CrossRef] [PubMed]
93. Orlova, V.V.; Choi, E.Y.; Xie, C.; Chavakis, E.; Bierhaus, A.; Ihanus, E.; Ballantyne, C.M.; Gahmberg, C.G.; Bianchi, M.E.; Nawroth, P.P.; et al. A novel pathway of HMGB1-mediated inflammatory cell recruitment that requires Mac-1-integrin. *EMBO J.* **2007**, *26*, 1129–1139. [CrossRef] [PubMed]
94. Podar, K.; Tai, Y.-T.; Lin, B.K.; Narsimhan, R.P.; Sattler, M.; Kijima, T.; Salgia, R.; Gupta, D.; Chauhan, D.; Anderson, K.C. Vascular Endothelial Growth Factor-induced Migration of Multiple Myeloma Cells Is Associated with β1 Integrin and Phosphatidylinositol 3-Kinase-dependent PKCα Activation. *J. Biol. Chem.* **2002**, *277*, 7875–7881. [CrossRef] [PubMed]
95. Zhang, X.; Yang, L.; Chen, W.; Kong, M. Identification of Potential Hub Genes and Therapeutic Drugs in Malignant Pleural Mesothelioma by Integrated Bioinformatics Analysis. *Oncol. Res. Treat.* **2020**, *43*, 656–671. [CrossRef]

96. Cheresh, P.; Morales-Nebreda, L.; Kim, S.-J.; Yeldandi, A.; Williams, D.B.; Cheng, Y.; Mutlu, G.M.; Budinger, G.R.S.; Ridge, K.; Schumacker, P.T.; et al. Asbestos-Induced Pulmonary Fibrosis Is Augmented in 8-Oxoguanine DNA Glycosylase Knockout Mice. *Am. J. Respir. Cell Mol. Biol.* **2015**, *52*, 25–36. [CrossRef] [PubMed]
97. Bozelka, B.; Sestini, P.; Gaumer, H.; Hammad, Y.; Heather, C.; Salvaggio, J. A murine model of asbestosis. *Am. J. Pathol.* **1983**, *112*, 326.
98. Rehrauer, H.; Wu, L.; Blum, W.; Pecze, L.; Henzi, T.; Serre-Beinier, V.; Aquino, C.; Vrugt, B.; De Perrot, M.; Schwaller, B.; et al. How asbestos drives the tissue towards tumors: YAP activation, macrophage and mesothelial precursor recruitment, RNA editing, and somatic mutations. *Oncogene* **2018**, *37*, 2645–2659. [CrossRef] [PubMed]
99. Altomare, D.A.; Vaslet, C.A.; Skele, K.L.; De Rienzo, A.; Devarajan, K.; Jhanwar, S.C.; McClatchey, A.I.; Kane, A.B.; Testa, J.R. A Mouse Model Recapitulating Molecular Features of Human Mesothelioma. *Cancer Res.* **2005**, *65*, 8090–8095. [CrossRef] [PubMed]
100. Breschi, A.; Gingeras, T.R.; Guigó, A.B.R. Comparative transcriptomics in human and mouse. *Nat. Rev. Genet.* **2017**, *18*, 425–440. [CrossRef]
101. Thahir, M.; Sharma, T.; Ganapathiraju, M.K. An efficient heuristic method for active feature acquisition and its application to protein-protein interaction prediction. *BMC Proc.* **2012**, *6*, S2. [CrossRef]
102. Shannon, P.; Markiel, A.; Ozier, O.; Baliga, N.S.; Wang, J.T.; Ramage, D.; Amin, N.; Schwikowski, B.; Ideker, T. Cytoscape: A Software Environment for Integrated Models of Biomolecular Interaction Networks. *Genome Res.* **2013**, *13*, 2498–2504. [CrossRef] [PubMed]
103. Tagawa, M.; Tada, Y.; Shimada, H.; Hiroshima, K. Gene therapy for malignant mesothelioma: Current prospects and challenges. *Cancer Gene Ther.* **2013**, *20*, 150–156. [CrossRef] [PubMed]
104. Shimizu, T.; Nakanishi, Y.; Nakagawa, Y.; Tsujino, I.; Takahashi, N.; Nemoto, N.; Hashimoto, S. Association between expression of thymidylate synthase, dihydrofolate reductase, and glycinamide ribonucleotide formyltransferase and efficacy of pemetrexed in advanced non-small cell lung cancer. *Anticancer Res.* **2012**, *32*, 4589–4596. [PubMed]
105. Giammarioli, A.M.; Maselli, A.; Casagrande, A.; Gambardella, L.; Gallina, A.; Spada, M.; Giovannetti, A.; Proietti, E.; Malorni, W.; Pierdominici, M. Pyrimethamine Induces Apoptosis of Melanoma Cells via a Caspase and Cathepsin Double-Edged Mechanism. *Cancer Res.* **2008**, *68*, 5291–5300. [CrossRef] [PubMed]
106. Khan, M.W.; Saadalla, A.; Ewida, A.H.; Al-Katranji, K.; Al-Saoudi, G.; Giaccone, Z.T.; Gounari, F.; Zhang, M.; Frank, D.A.; Khazaie, K. The STAT3 inhibitor pyrimethamine displays anti-cancer and immune stimulatory effects in murine models of breast cancer. *Cancer Immunol. Immunother.* **2017**, *67*, 13–23. [CrossRef] [PubMed]
107. Grose, W.E.; Bodey, G.P.; Rodriguez, V. Sulfamethoxazole-Trimethoprim for Infections in Cancer Patients. *JAMA* **1977**, *237*, 352–354. [CrossRef]
108. Bodey, G.P.; Grose, W.E.; Keating, M.J. Use of Trimethoprim-Sulfamethoxazole for Treatment of Infections in Patients with Cancer. *Clin. Infect. Dis.* **1982**, *4*, 579–585. [CrossRef]
109. Lu, S.-H.; Tsai, W.-S.; Chang, Y.-C.; Chou, T.-Y.; Pang, S.-T.; Lin, P.-H.; Tsai, C.-M. Identifying cancer origin using circulating tumor cells. *Cancer Biol. Ther.* **2016**, *17*, 430–438. [CrossRef]
110. Nitadori, J.-i.; Ishii, G.; Tsuta, K.; Yokose, T.; Murata, Y.; Kodama, T.; Nagai, K.; Kato, H.; Ochiai, A. Immunohistochemical differential diagnosis between large cell neuroendocrine carcinoma and small cell carcinoma by tissue microarray analysis with a large antibody panel. *Am. J. Clin. Pathol.* **2006**, *125*, 682–692. [CrossRef]
111. Camilo, R.; Capelozzi, V.L.; Siqueira, S.A.C.; Bernardi, F.D.C. Expression of p63, keratin 5/6, keratin 7, and surfactant-A in non–small cell lung carcinomas. *Hum. Pathol.* **2006**, *37*, 542–546. [CrossRef]
112. Ordóñez, N.G. Value of cytokeratin 5/6 immunostaining in distinguishing epithelial mesothelioma of the pleura from lung adenocarcinoma. *Am. J. Surg. Pathol.* **1998**, *22*, 1215–1221. [CrossRef] [PubMed]
113. Heard, C.; Monk, B.; Modley, A. Binding of primaquine to epidermal membranes and keratin. *Int. J. Pharm.* **2003**, *257*, 237–244. [CrossRef]
114. Kimura, T.; Shirakawa, R.; Yaoita, N.; Hayashi, T.; Nagano, K.; Horiuchi, H. The antimalarial drugs chloroquine and primaquine inhibit pyridoxal kinase, an essential enzyme for vitamin B6 production. *FEBS Lett.* **2014**, *588*, 3673–3676. [CrossRef] [PubMed]
115. Basso, L.G.; Rodrigues, R.Z.; Naal, R.M.; Costa-Filho, A.J. Effects of the antimalarial drug primaquine on the dynamic structure of lipid model membranes. *Biochim. Biophys. Acta (BBA) Biomembr.* **2011**, *1808*, 55–64. [CrossRef] [PubMed]
116. Gakhar, G.; Ohira, T.; Battina, S.; Hua, D.H.; Nguyen, T.A. Anti-Tumor Effect of Primaquine Compounds in Human Breast Cancer Cells. In Proceedings of the AACR Annual Meeting, Las Angeles, CA, USA, 14–18 April 2007; American Association for Cancer Research: Philadelphia, PA, USA, 2007.
117. Ou, S.-H.I.; Moon, J.; Garland, L.L.; Mack, P.C.; Testa, J.R.; Tsao, A.S.; Wozniak, A.J.; Gandara, D.R. SWOG S0722: Phase II Study of mTOR Inhibitor Everolimus (RAD001) in Advanced Malignant Pleural Mesothelioma (MPM). *J. Thorac. Oncol.* **2015**, *10*, 387–391. [CrossRef] [PubMed]
118. Mamputu, J.-C.; Renier, G. Advanced glycation end products increase, through a protein kinase C-dependent pathway, vascular endothelial growth factor expression in retinal endothelial cells: Inhibitory effect of gliclazide. *J. Diabetes Complicat.* **2002**, *16*, 284–293. [CrossRef]

Review
Biomarkers for Malignant Pleural Mesothelioma—A Novel View on Inflammation

Melanie Vogl, Anna Rosenmayr, Tomas Bohanes, Axel Scheed, Milos Brndiar, Elisabeth Stubenberger and Bahil Ghanim *

Department of General and Thoracic Surgery, Karl Landsteiner University of Health Sciences, University Hospital Krems, 3500 Krems an der Donau, Austria; melanie.vogl@krems.lknoe.at (M.V.); arosenmayr@gmail.com (A.R.); bohanest@gmail.com (T.B.); axel.scheed@krems.lknoe.at (A.S.); milos.brndiar@krems.lknoe.at (M.B.); elisabeth.stubenberger@krems.lknoe.at (E.S.)
* Correspondence: bahil.ghanim@kl.ac.at; Tel.: +43-2732-9004-4294

Simple Summary: In view of the recent advances in immunoncology, we want to reevaluate and summarize the role of the immune system in malignant pleural mesothelioma (MPM). MPM is an aggressive disease with limited treatment options and devastating prognosis. Exposure to asbestos and chronic inflammation have long been acknowledged as main risk factors. In this review, we summarize the current knowledge about local and systemic inflammation promoting pathogenesis and progression of MPM. We focus on the prognostic and predictive value of infiltrating immune cells within the tumor and its microenvironment as local inflammation on the one hand and systemic inflammatory parameters on the other. We found that suppression of the specific and activation of the unspecific immune system are essential drivers of MPM, resulting in poor patient outcome. Numerous local and systemic inflammatory parameters are promising potential biomarkers for MPM, worth further research.

Abstract: Malignant pleural mesothelioma (MPM) is an aggressive disease with limited treatment response and devastating prognosis. Exposure to asbestos and chronic inflammation are acknowledged as main risk factors. Since immune therapy evolved as a promising novel treatment modality, we want to reevaluate and summarize the role of the inflammatory system in MPM. This review focuses on local tumor associated inflammation on the one hand and systemic inflammatory markers, and their impact on MPM outcome, on the other hand. Identification of new biomarkers helps to select optimal patient tailored therapy, avoid ineffective treatment with its related side effects and consequently improves patient's outcome in this rare disease. Additionally, a better understanding of the tumor promoting and tumor suppressing inflammatory processes, influencing MPM pathogenesis and progression, might also reveal possible new targets for MPM treatment. After reviewing the currently available literature and according to our own research, it is concluded that the suppression of the specific immune system and the activation of its innate counterpart are crucial drivers of MPM aggressiveness translating to poor patient outcome.

Keywords: malignant pleural mesothelioma; inflammation; infiltrating immune cells; prognostic biomarker; predictive biomarker; immune therapy

1. Introduction

Malignant pleural mesothelioma (MPM) is an aggressive neoplasm of mesothelial origin. Patients face a devastating prognosis of 12 months median survival only after diagnosis [1]. Despite recent—and, in part, promising—developments regarding both systemic therapy and cytoreductive surgery, MPM remains a clinical challenge, especially when it comes to treatment allocation [2,3]. Furthermore, the optimal (multimodal) treatment regimens still remain to be defined from the available arsenal of immune therapy, surgery, radiation and systemic treatment [4].

The pathogenesis of MPM was already associated with chronic inflammation, induced by asbestos exposure, sixty years ago by Wagner et al. [5]. Asbestos remains the main risk factor for developing this rare disease with a latency period of up to 40 years from time of exposure to diagnosis [1,6]. When inhaled, the long and thin asbestos fibers penetrate the lung parenchyma and deposit in the pleura, causing irritation and chronic inflammation. Consequently, the activation of surrounding immune cells leads to the secretion of cytokines, formation of reactive oxygen and nitrogen species, tumor necrosis factor α (TNF-α) release and nuclear factor 'kappa-light-chain-enhancer' of activated B-cells (NFκ-B) expression, in the end resulting in the accumulation of DNA damage and thus malignant evolution as reviewed before [6,7].

The activated immune system—especially with regard to its innate blood derived components—proved to be associated with worse patient outcome, late stage of disease, high Ki67 expression and poor treatment response in MPM as shown before by the authors and other research groups [8–13]. Not only for MPM but generally in oncology, the tumor promoting role of the immune system has been increasingly recognized as reflected in the latest version of the hallmarks of cancer by Hanahan and Weinberg [14]. Most recently, the immune system also evolved as a promising treatment target and modern immune therapy revealed as effective treatment modality in many solid tumors including MPM [15–19].

In light of the past and recent insights regarding the role of inflammation in the development and progression of MPM, inflammatory parameters are currently considered promising biomarkers [20]. In this review, we provide an overview about up to date knowledge of local inflammation in MPM and its involved immune cells as well as the tumor induced systemic inflammatory response. Special focus lies on the use of local and systemic inflammatory parameters as biomarkers for prognostic and predictive purposes in hope to facilitate and optimize treatment decisions and highlight new therapeutic targets for the future management of MPM. Predictive biomarkers might help to answer these crucial questions and are therefore desperately needed [21]. Despite the urgent need, to date there are no biomarkers recommended for MPM in daily practice in the current European guidelines since most studies failed to show sufficient reproducibility, sensitivity and specificity to justify the use of any suggested diagnostic biomarker so far. Unfortunately, the same holds true when it comes to prognostic, predictive or follow up biomarkers and thus further research is requested to better personalize treatment for MPM patients [22].

For this review we performed literature research in PubMed including English literature only. The following search terms were used: mesothelioma combined with prognostic and predictive biomarker, inflammation, inflammatory markers, C-reactive protein, fibrinogen, neutrophil to lymphocyte ratio, monocyte to lymphocyte ratio, thrombocyte to lymphocyte ratio, neutrophils, leukocytes, monocytes, albumin, Glasgow prognostic score, IL-6, ferritin, tumor microenvironment, tumor infiltrating lymphocytes, tumor associated macrophages/monocytes, PD-L1 and PD1, CTLA-4, immune therapy, and complement system. Since mesothelioma is a very rare disease and research regarding inflammatory biomarkers is limited, we included all available studies regarding biomarkers and only excluded case reports

Literature from the very early days of mesothelioma research ranging back to Wagner et al. from 1960 were included [5] as well as the most recent MPM literature from the beginning of 2021, resulting in 194 included references.

2. Findings
2.1. The Role of Local Inflammation in MPM

Several studies proved that (pre)malignant cells of various origins induce an inflammatory response with a paradox tumor promoting effect [23]. Local inflammation and immune cell infiltration within the tumor nests as well as the surrounding tumor microenvironment (TME) strongly influence the development and progression of numerous malignant diseases [23,24] including MPM as reviewed by Hendry et al. [25].

On the other hand, the immune system and its cellular components also play a protective role, especially with regard to acquired immunity as Leigh et al. observed already in 1986 correlating high lymphoid infiltration in mesothelioma specimens to a better prognosis [26]. In the past, the role of different infiltrating immune cells within MPM and the stroma has, therefore, become of increasing research interest since the immune system seems to be characterized here by a—not yet fully understood—duality [12]. Our adaptive immune system is protective against cancer development and spread [27], but it is also well documented that the immune system plays a crucial tumor promoting role in eventually all steps of malignant evolution by contributing to carcinogenesis, proliferation, angiogenesis, local infiltration and finally metastatic progression as reviewed by Coussens and Werb [28].

Very heterogenic immune cell infiltration in MPM tumor specimens and its TME has been described [29–33], with most studies reporting a predominant infiltration of tumor-associated macrophages (TAM) and tumor infiltrating lymphocytes (TIL), in particular CD4+ and CD8+ T-lymphocytes as reviewed by Chu et al. [34]. These cells are assumed to be the key players in the tumor associated immunoreaction. However, also rarer detectable myeloid derived suppressor cells (MDSC) [35,36], natural killer (NK) cells [28,31,32] and regulatory T cells (Treg) [29,36,37] have been studied before. These different immune cells infiltrating the tumor tissue but also contributing to the TME will be summarized in the following paragraphs as well as in Table 1 with regard to their role on MPM outcome and treatment response.

Table 1. Potential local inflammatory biomarkers.

Biomarker	Unfavorable	Univariate Value	Multivariate Value	Impact	Design	Number of Patients/Range	References
B-TIL	Low	HR: N.R.	HR: 0.7	Prog	R	217	[37]
CD8+ TIL	Low	HR: N.S.-N.R.	HR: N.S.-0.4	All prog	All R	16–32	[30,31,38,39]
CD8+ TIL	High	HR: N.R.	HR: N.R.	Prog	R	93	[38]
M2/CD8+ TIL	high	HR: N.R.	HR: 1.6	Prog	R	210	[37]
M2/B-TIL	Low	HR: N.R.	HR: 1.6	Prog	R	210	[37]
CD4+ TIL	Low	HR: N.S.-N.R.	HR: N.S.-N.R.	All prog	All R	27–218	[30–32,37,38]
COX-2	High	HR: N.R.-2.9	HR: N.S.-4.6	All prog	R/R/P	29–77	[39–41]
COX-2	Low	HR: N.R.	HR: N.R.	Prog	R	86	[42]
M2	High	HR: N.S.-1.7	HR: N.S.	All prog	All R	4–210	[38,39,43]
M2/TAM	High	HR: N.R.	HR: N.S.	Prog	R	8	[44]
IL-34	High	HR: N.R.	HR: N.R.	Prog	R	74	[45] *
M-CSF	High	HR: N.R.	HR: N.S.	Prog	R	74	[45] *
PD-L1	High	HR: N.S.-N.R	HR: N.S.-2.3	All prog	All R	33–106	[17,30,43,46,47]

TIL tumor infiltrating lymphocyte, M2 macrophage subtype 2, Treg regulatory T cell, FGF fibroblast growth factor, TGF-β transforming growth factor β, COX-2 cyclooxygenase 2, TAM tumor associated macrophages, IL-34 interleukin 34, M-CSF macrophage colony stimulating factor, NK cells natural killer cells, PD-L1 Programmed cell death ligand 1, HR hazard ratio, N.R. not reported, N.S. not significant, Prog prognostic biomarker, Pred predictive biomarker, R retrospective, P prospective.* measured in pleural effusion.

2.2. Tumor Infiltrating Lymphocytes (TIL)

TIL comprise T- and B-lymphocytes that have left the blood stream and infiltrated the tumor itself as well as the tumor stroma. Invading CD4+ T cells and proinflammatory cytokines prime CD8+ T cells to become effector cytotoxic T-lymphocytes (CTL), which then play a key role in eliminating cancer cells as reviewed before [48]. During tumor progression, cancer cells can avoid this effect by overexpression of programmed death ligand 1 (PD-L1) and cytotoxic T-lymphocyte antigen 4 (CTLA-4) (compare corresponding subchapter). Simultaneously, TIL release cytokines, thereby influencing various other immune cells, including the differentiation of TAM towards the immune suppressive type 2 macrophages (M2). This mechanism represents a negative feedback loop to avoid an over activated immune response. However, both aforementioned—in principal protective—immunosuppressive mechanisms (PD-L1/CLA-4 on the intercellular signaling level and type 2 macrophage differentiation on the cellular level) might lead to tumor immune evasion and thus uncontrolled tumor growth and progression [28,49,50].

For MPM, a predominant infiltration of CD8+ and CD4+ T-lymphocytes has been described by various researchers [30–32,51], but also the role of B lymphocytes [29] and Treg [51] is under investigation as described below.

The influence of B lymphocytes, key players in adaptive humoral immunity, is not fully understood and controversial results have been published so far for mesothelioma. Several studies reported low numbers of infiltrating B lymphocytes as reviewed by Minnema-Luiting [29]. Nevertheless, others discovered high CD 20+ B lymphocytes infiltration as well as the ratio CD163+ macrophages/CD20+ B lymphocytes as independent prognostic factors indicating better prognosis [37].

The prognostic value of CD8+ T lymphocytes, likewise part of the adaptive immunity, is better investigated and thus better understood for different MPM patient populations:

A number of studies investigated tumor samples of patients receiving trimodal therapy including cytoreductive surgery. Some reported an independent favorable prognostic value of high levels of CD8+ TIL [31,32], others found the ratio M2 count/CD8+ TIL count independently indicating negative prognosis [37], also suggesting that patients with low M2 and high CD8+ count have better outcomes. One other study found a correlation of local tumor overgrowth and low levels of CD8+ TIL in surgical patients [49] suggesting again an association with worse prognosis when the adapted immune system is underrepresented in the tumor compared to its innate counterpart.

On the contrary, Pasello et al. found high levels of CD8+ TIL in treatment naïve patients correlating not only with poor prognosis and aggressiveness of the tumor, but also a predictive value of high CD8+ TIL count for low response to chemotherapy. However, high levels of CD8 + TIL correlated additionally with high PD-L1 expression, which the authors speculate to be causal for the observed poor prognosis [38].

Additionally, high CD4+ T cell count in the tumor correlated with better outcome. Yamada et al. showed a tendency for better survival if CD4 + TIL and NK levels were high but did not reach level significance [32]. Marcq et al. compared treatment of naïve patients with those pretreated with chemotherapy and found high count of CD4+ TIL in the TME to be an independent positive prognostic marker for both therapy subgroups [30].

Treg, the immunosuppressive subset of CD4+ T cells, physiologically regulates immune tolerance, but also plays a major role in tumor development. Whereas only scarcely present in healthy tissue, a strong infiltration of Treg has been shown for many tumor entities [50] including MPM [51].

First data suggested that Treg and their deactivation via depletion of the surface marker CD25+ influenced survival in a murine model in a positive way [51]. Additionally, it was hypothesized that response to chemotherapy might be influenced by T effector cells and Treg [30].

While only a few studies analyzed the prognostic and predictive potential of Treg count in MPM, others investigated the cytokines responsible for Treg recruitment and activation, such as transforming growth factor (TGF-β) [6,52–54] and cyclooxygenase-2 (COX-2)/prostaglandin E2 (PGE2) [39–42,55,56], which are released by cancer cells directly or indirectly by cancer associated fibroblasts [50].

2.3. Cancer-Associated Fibroblasts (CAF)

CAF are abundantly present in numerous tumor entities and play a key role in the immunosuppressive effect of TME via cross-talk with Treg. High numbers of CAF are hence often associated with tumor promotion and poor prognosis. In turn, Treg stimulate resident fibroblasts to differentiate into CAF, which emphasizes the tight cross-talk between Tregs and CAFs [50].

A number of studies confirmed high numbers of CAF in TME from MPM samples [29]. As mentioned above, the major cytokines mediating CAF and Treg function have been under thorough investigation. Latest studies suggested a correlation between fibroblast growth factor (FGF) overexpression and high numbers of CAF with tumor aggressiveness and worse prognosis; however, the prognostic or predictive value is currently unknown and further research is obligatory [57,58]. Schelch et al. analyzed the role of different FGFs and their receptors in MPM in vitro and in vivo and proved that the FGF axis promotes cell proliferation, epithelial to mesenchymal transition, migration, invasion and clinical tumor aggressiveness. Inhibition of FGF receptor not only showed anti-proliferative effects itself but also a synergism with radiation and cisplatin and might, therefore, serve as a novel therapeutic target in MPM [58–60]. Furthermore, Li et al. also proved that FGF-2—besides platelet derived growth factor (PDGF) and hepatocyte growth factor (HGF)—is expressed by MPM. In addition, this study showed that MPM cell lines stimulate fibroblast motility and growth on the one hand and fibroblasts vice versa stimulate MPM growth and motility by HGF on the other hand, indicating an important cross-talk and tumor promoting symbiosis of CAFs and MPM cells [57].

2.4. Transforming Growth Factor-β (TGF-β)

TGF-β is known as an important inducer of CAFs and thus supporter of the immunosuppressive TME. Besides this tumor promoting characteristic, TGF-β can directly induce proliferation and epithelial to mesenchymal transition. In addition, TGF-β expression was associated with resistance to immune therapy as summarized recently [61]. With regard to MPM, TGF-β and its subtype activin A have been shown to be overexpressed in MPM cells with tumorigenic effects and thus inhibition or silencing was suggested as possible therapeutic target—first clinical results, however, were unsatisfactory with regard to fresolimumab, a TGF-β targeting antibody [6,53,54]. In addition, activin A blood levels were increased in MPM patients when compared to healthy controls and high activin A levels correlated with advanced tumor stage, high tumor volume and histological subtype translating to poor patient survival [54].

2.5. COX-2

Overexpression of COX-2 is detectable in various tumor cells and mostly associated with worse prognosis [62,63]. Nuvoli et al. reviewed the tumor promoting effects of proinflammatory prostaglandins, synthesized by COX-2 in general and for MPM in particular [55]. COX-2 overexpression was also found in MPM specimens [56]. Although some authors described controversial results regarding the prognostic value of COX-2, the majority reports a negative prognostic value of high tumor COX-2 expression [39–42].

In addition, the therapeutic effect of COX-2-inhibitors such as celecoxib has already been studied in other cancer types extensively [63]. However, COX-2 is not a routine target in modern oncology due to controversial results, e.g., for colorectal [64–66] and lung cancer [67,68]. For MPM on the contrary COX-2-inhibitors achieved promising results in vitro [35,57,69,70] and in vivo [36,71]. Unfortunately, neither NSAIDs nor COX-2 inhibitors prevented MPM development in an asbestos exposed risk group and in murine models [69]. The currently ongoing phase III randomized INFINITE trial assesses the effect of systemic celecoxib and chemotherapy combined with intrapleural INF-α (NCT03710876) and might answer the question whether COX-2 is an eligible treatment target in MPM.

2.6. M2 Macrophages

Under normal conditions, macrophages of the subtype M1 are part of the early inflammatory response enhancing the immune reaction while the immunosuppressive M2 macrophages limit a possible inflammatory overreaction [28,49,50]. A large proportion of M2 of total TAM consequently enforces tumor-promoting and immunosuppressive conditions and has been shown to indicate poor survival for different malignancies [70].

Additionally, for MPM specimens, various studies described strong infiltration of macrophages, predominantly of immunosuppressive M2, as prognostic marker [46,50,72]. High count of infiltrating M2 not only correlated significantly with poor prognosis [73] and increased proliferation rate but also reduced response to chemotherapy [74]. Others found no correlation between prognosis and absolute count of TAM or M2 but reported that high percentage of M2 of total TAM correlates significantly with local overgrowth [49] and negative prognosis [44].

In conclusion, current scarce data indicate that tumor infiltrating M2 might have prognostic and predictive potential. Interestingly, there is abundant research on M2 promoting cytokines and their impact on prognosis and treatment response.

Hematopoietic cytokines, including granulocyte macrophage colony stimulating factor (GM-CSF), were shown to be released by MPM cells especially when exposed to inflammatory cytokines but also autonomously [72,75] promoting the release of monocytes to the peripheral blood.

Additionally, cytokines promoting the M2 differentiation, namely IL-34 [45], macrophage colony stimulating factor (M-CSF) [74] and C-C motif chemokine ligand 2 (CCL2) [76,77] have been found to be elevated in tumor specimens or pleural effusion of MPM patients. High pleural levels of IL-34 correlated with worse prognosis [45], as well as high serum M-CSF, the latter also with response to chemotherapy [78]. Furthermore CCL2, a proinflammatory chemokine for monocyte recruitment, has been investigated over the past years. MPM patients showed significant higher serum levels of CCL2 than an asbestos exposed cohort without evidence of disease [79]. Similar results have been published by Gueugnon et al. as well as Blanquart et al. who found significant higher concentrations of CCL2 in pleural effusion of MPM patients compared to benign effusion or metastatic adenocarcinomas [76,77]. CCL2 released by MPM cells directly plays an important role in monocyte recruitment. CCL2 inhibition is also a potential treatment target and currently under investigation [50,78,80].

2.7. Myeloid-Derived Suppressor Cells (MDSCs)

The immune-suppressive MDSC are immature myeloid cells stimulated by tumor-derived cytokines. Abundantly detectable in MPM TME [35,36] they activate tumor-promoting Treg and inhibit tumor-suppressing CD4+ and CD8+ T cells [36]. A negative prognostic potential of MDSC can, therefore, be assumed; however, to our knowledge, no data regarding the prognostic or predictive value is currently available for MPM.

2.8. Natural Killer Cells and Dendritic Cells (DC)

The majority of studies reported low proportion of DC and NK in MPM specimens [28,31,32]. Yamada et al. additionally investigated the prognostic potential of NK infiltration and found no correlation with outcome [32]. Hegmans et al. confirmed a weak infiltration of DC, although they found a strong infiltration by NK. As possible explanation for low DC numbers they suggest the high levels of Interleukin-6 (IL-6) produced by MPM cells, since IL-6 inhibits the differentiation of progenitor cells to DC [51].

Summarizing these findings, DC and NK—both part of the innate immune system—are currently suspected to play a subordinate role in MPM and are, therefore, underrepresented in medical literature when compared to the aforementioned more prominent cellular players in the tumor and its TME.

2.9. Programmed Death Ligand 1 (PD-L1) and Cytotoxic T-Lymphocyte Antigen 4 (CTLA-4)

PD-L1 is expressed on the surface of various tumor cells and has the ability to bind to PD-1 receptors of CD4+ and CD8+ T Cells thus altering proliferation and cytokine production, leading to T cell inactivation and apoptosis of these important cellular players of adaptive immunity. As reviewed before by Zielinski et al. both PD-1/PD-L1 and CTLA-4 act as similar pathways downregulating lymphocyte response and accordingly adaptive immunity [80]. This tumor immune evasion results in progression and poor prognosis of various solid tumors [81]. With regard to thoracic oncology, the PD-L1 axis and its prognostic role were already analyzed in malignant pleural effusion [82] and stage IV lung cancer [83,84]. Furthermore, PD-L1 expression showed also prognostic potential in MPM as summarized in a recent meta-analysis [85].

PD-L1 positivity in MPM tumor cells was reported at heterogeneous levels ranging from 16 to 68% [29,47,86]. According to Marcq et al., PD-L1 and PD-1 are decreased after chemotherapy [30]. However, for peritoneal mesothelioma, controversial effects of chemotherapy on PD-L1 expression were reported [87]. PD-1 expression on TIL was furthermore described as a negative predictive factor for response to chemotherapy [30]. Additionally, PD-L1 was found to correlate with the sarcomatoid and biphasic histology of MPM [86]. Our study group recently showed that tumor PD-L1 expression is not only prognostic in an international cohort suffering from malignant pleural effusion (in part also caused by MPM) but was significantly interacting with CRP, thus suggesting that the prognostic values of both markers influence each other. This observation translated to the poorest survival in the patient group characterized by high CRP in the patient blood and high PD-L1 expression in the corresponding tumor specimen [82]. Inaguma et al. demonstrated the independent prognostic impact of PD-L1 and activated leukocyte cell adhesion molecule (ALCAM, CD166) in MPM. Expression of both led to the shortest overall survival (OS). Additionally, a significant association between PD-L1 and ALCAM was drawn [46]. Similar prognostic results have been shown previously [43,47].

To reverse the tumor promoting effect of a downregulated specific immune system, checkpoint inhibitors like humanized monoclonal antibodies against PD-1 or PD-L1 have been developed. Immune evasion can be stopped to increase tumor defense [16,81]. The therapeutic benefit of targeting PD-1 with pembrolizumab [16] or nivolumab [17], and PD-L1 with avelumab [18], in pre-treated MPM patients with PD-L1 positive tumors was demonstrated.

The aforementioned other—by malignant disease misused—pathway of adapted immunity downregulation, namely CLTA-4 has also been investigated and proved to be an interesting treatment target to reactivate the immune system against MPM progression as reviewed before [88]. More recently, the combination of nivolumab with ipilimumab was approved by the FDA for unresectable MPM as first line therapy according to promising results documented during the CHECKMATE 743 trial, indicating that the combination of PD-1 and CLTA-4 targeting immune therapy is effective in MPM [19].

Finally, soluble PD-L1 (sPD-L1) from the sera of patients before and during immune therapy was suggested as a predictive biomarker, indicating poor treatment response when elevated before and during immune therapy. Additionally, sPD-L1 levels were also correlating to the inflammatory parameters NLR, neutrophil count and CRP, blood parameters that will be described later on in more detail [15]. Most recently, the role of sPD-L1 was also investigated in pleural effusions [89]. Both serum as well as pleural effusion derived PD-L1 status might represent an easily available method for clinical monitoring of the treatment target during immune therapy in the future.

Although there is great hope for a more personalized immune therapy, the exact background of the heterogeneity in PD-L1 expression and in treatment response is not yet fully understood. The interplay of tumor immunology, immunotherapy and somatic mutations is currently intensively researched [87,90–92]. Yang et al. recently reviewed the complex interactions of molecular characteristics of MPM cells and TME with histological subtype and genomic mutations [93] underlining the need for a deeper understanding of the pathobiological processes in MPM in order to optimize personalized biomarker-guided immunotherapy.

The complex interactions of tumor infiltrating immune cells with MPM cells as well as the resulting systemic inflammatory processes—which will be discussed in the next chapter—are also graphically shown in Figure 1.

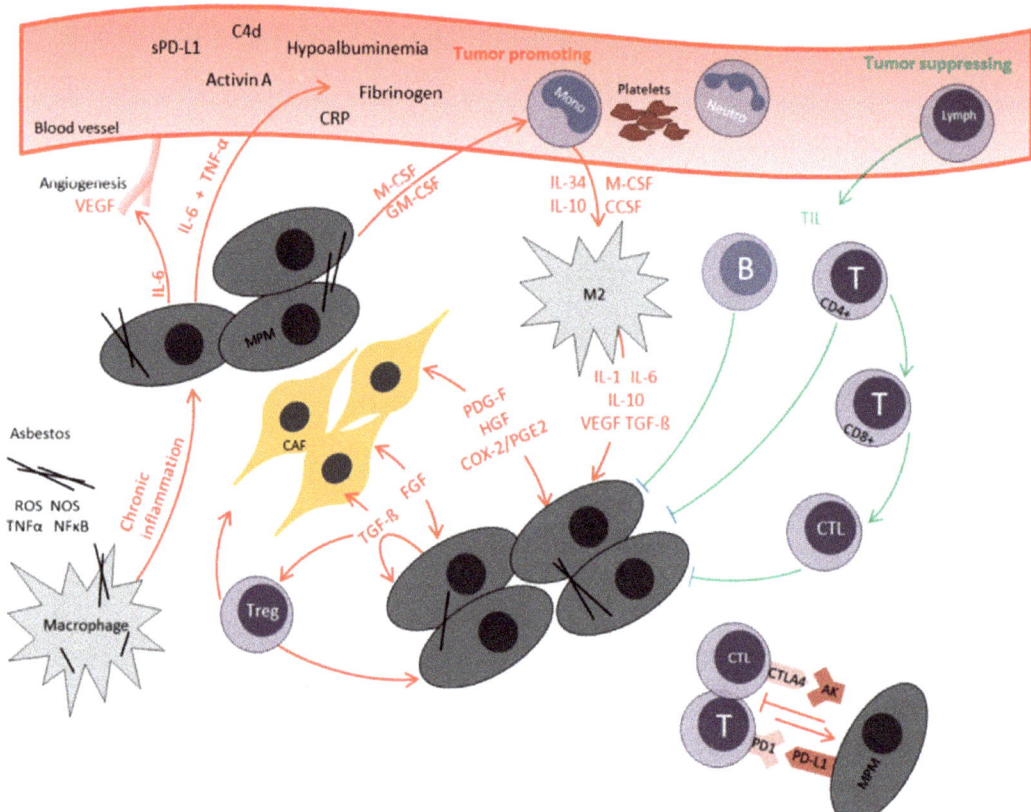

Figure 1. Interaction of local and systemic immune response in malignant pleural mesothelioma. *AB* antibody, *B* B-lymphocyte, *C4d* circulating complement component 4d, *CAF* cancer associated fibroblast, *CCSF* C-C motif chemokine ligand 2, *COX-2* cyclooxygenase-2, *CRP* C-reactive protein, *CTL* cytotoxic T-lymphocyte, *CTLA4* cytotoxic T-Lymphocyte Antigen 4, *FGF* fibroblast growth factor, *GM-CSF* granulocyte macrophage colony stimulating factor, *HGF* hepatocyte growth factor, *IL* interleukin, *Lymph* lymphocyte, *M2* M2-macrophage, *M-CSF* macrophage colony stimulating factor, *Mono* monocyte, *MPM* malignant pleural mesothelioma, NFκB nuclear factor kappa-light-chain-enhancer B, *Neutro* neutrocyte, *PD-1* programmed cell death protein 1, *PD-L1* programmed cell death ligand 1, *PDGF* platelet derived growth factor, *PGE2* prostaglandin E2, RNS reactive nitrogen species, *ROS* reactive oxygen species, *sPD-L1* soluble programmed cell death ligand 1, *T* T-lymphocyte, *TGF-ß* transforming growth factor-ß, *TIL* tumor-infiltrating lymphocyte, *TNF-α* tumor necrosis factor α, *Treg* regulatory T-cell, *VEGF* vascular endothelial growth factor.

In summary, the role of local inflammation and the components of TME in MPM have been investigated by various researchers. We encountered promising data regarding the prognostic potential of the different tumor infiltrating immune cells and also first results for predictive potential of some of these biomarkers. However, most interestingly, we noticed that generally low numbers of specific immune cells as well as high numbers of unspecific immune cells seem to be unfavorable, suggesting a controversial impact of the innate and adaptive immune cells on local tumor progression.

2.10. The Role of Systemic Inflammatory Response in MPM

Systemic inflammation is becoming an increasingly acknowledged factor in the development and progression of different solid tumors, including MPM. Consequently, peripheral blood derived inflammatory markers, which are determined routinely in daily practice for almost all patients, have been extensively examined regarding their applicability as biomarkers in MPM as reviewed before [12].

Since systemic inflammatory parameters can indicate inflammatory and infectious processes in the patient's body as well as malignancy, they are highly unspecific for diagnostic or screening purposes. However, after exclusion of acute inflammation or infection, some of the established and widely available inflammatory markers have been identified as prognostic or predictive markers in various solid tumors [94–99] including MPM [100–102].

As mentioned before, the current European guidelines for MPM management do not recommend any prognostic biomarkers for clinical use [4]. Nevertheless, two prognostic scores have been developed that are widely accepted and well established, namely the EORTC score (European Organization for Research and Treatment of Cancer) [103] and the CALGB score (Cancer and Leukemia Group B) [104]. Both scores have been validated for MPM by different researchers and proved their reproducibility [105–108]. Interestingly, these two scores not only integrate clinical, pathological and epidemiological factors, but also acknowledge systemic inflammation as tumor aggressiveness criteria by including the blood characteristics leukocytosis, thrombocytosis and elevated C-reactive protein (CRP) as negative prognostic factors [103,104]. The following paragraphs discuss the current literature on systemic inflammatory markers in MPM as also summarized in Table 2.

Table 2. Potential Systemic Inflammatory Biomarkers.

Biomarker	Unfavorable	Univariate Value	Multivariate Value	Impact	Design	Number of Patients/Range	Cut-Off Value	References
WBC count	High	HR: N.S.-1.9	HR: N.S.-2.3	All prog	All R	84–363	$8.1–15.6\ 10^9/L / 8.3\ 10^9/L$ *	[102,103,107,109–117]
Lymphocytes	Low	N.S.-N.R.	N.S.	All prog	All R	105–285	$1.27–2.0\ 10^9/L$	[102,114,117]
Monocyte count	High	HR: N.R.-4.0	HR: N.S.-2.7	All prog	All R	105–667	$0.55\ 10^9/L$	[43,102,114]
M-CSF	High	HR: 1.6	HR: N.S	Prog	R	36	1120	[79]
Neutrophil count	High	HR: N.S.-N.R.	HR: N.S.	All prog	All R	105–285	$5.3–5.89\ 10^9/L$	[102,114,117]
Platelet count	High	HR: N.S.-2.1	HR: N.S.-2.1	All prog	All R	84–363	$300–450\ g/L, 400\ 10^9/L$ *	[102,103,107,109–118]
NLR	High	HR: N.S.-2.3	HR: N.S.-2.7	All prog	All R	30–285	3 and 5/5 *	[102–104,109–113,119–121]
NLR normalization after treatment	No			All prog	All R	66–69	Decline to <5	[109,111]
LMR	Low	HR: N.R.	HR: N.S.-1.8	All prog	All R	105–283	2.36–2.74	[102,114,122]
PLR	High	HR: N.R.-1.5	HR: N.S.	All prog	All R	105–285	144–300	[102,03,114]
CRP	High	HR: N.S.-2.8	HR: N.S.-2.7	All prog and [11] pred	All R	115–363	10–50 mg/L/10 mg/L *	[11,102,103,115,116,123]
CAR	High	HR: N.S.-2.6	HR: N.S.-2.1	All prog	All R	100–201	0.58 and 7.5, >0.58 *	[102,104,124]
mGPS	High	HR: N.R.	HR: 2.6	Prog	R	132	1	[103]
Fibrinogen	High	HR: 2.1	HR: 1.8	Prog and pred	R	176	750 mg/dL	[10]
Albumin	Low	HR: N.R.-1.5	HR: N.S.-1.8	All prog	All R	97–278	35–40 g/L, 35 g/L *	[102,103,114,125]
C4d	High	HR: 7.3 high vs. low	HR: 0.3 low vs. high	Prog	R	30	1.5 μg/mL	[8]
Activin A	High	HR: 0.4	HR: 0.4	Prog	R	119	574.0 pg/mL	[55]
sPD-L1	High	HR: N.R.	H.R.: N.S.	Prog	P	40	0.07–1.83 ng/mL measured at 4 timepoints during therapy	[15]

BC white blood cell, M-CSF macrophage colony stimulating factor, NLR neutrophil-to-lymphocyte ratio, LMR lympho-cyte-to-lymphocyte ratio, PLR platelet-to-lymphocyte ratio, IL-6 interleukin 6, CRP C-reactive protein, CAP CRP-to-Albumin ratio, mGPS modified Glasgow prognostic score, C4d Circulating complement component 4d, sPD-L1 soluble programmed cell death ligand 1, HR hazard ratio, N.R. not reported, N.S. not significant, Prog prognostic bi-omarker, Pred predictive biomarker, R retrospective, P prospective, * most frequently used cut-off value.

Leukocytosis, a well-known biomarker of acute inflammation, has been widely investigated as biomarker for MPM and a number of studies reported a negative prognostic value of elevated pretreatment white blood cell count after uni- [103,111,112,116] and multivariate [102,110,115] survival analyses. Absolute lymphocyte count, as sign of an activated specific immune system, was studied by fewer researchers as single biomarker, but an association with poor prognosis and reduced clinical response to chemotherapy has been reported so far [109]. However, the role of lymphocyte count on MPM outcome has been investigated more intensively with regard to different ratios, especially the neutrophil to lymphocyte ratio (NLR) which will be later described more in detail.

Monocyte count on the contrary has been studied more extensively as single prognostic marker in MPM. Burt et al. found an independent negative prognostic value of pretreatment monocytosis for patients undergoing cytoreductive surgery [73] and Zhang et al. and Tanrikulu et al. confirmed these findings for patients receiving different therapies [100,110]. Monocytes, as part of the unspecific immune system, are the procurer cells of tissue specific macrophages [73] including TAM who play an important role in the TME and thus contribute to local immune modulation as mentioned before.

Interestingly, neutrophil count, likewise representing the unspecific immune response, is rarely reported as single blood marker. Few studies describe controversial results, reporting adverse prognostic value of high neutrophil count in univariate analysis [100] or no correlation with prognosis [109,110]. Nevertheless, the neutrophil count compared to the lymphocyte count is more intensively studied when it comes to the NLR.

Thrombocytosis, a known unspecific systemic phenomenon in response to inflammation [126], has long been suggested as independent prognostic factor. Already in 1989, first data suggested an independent negative prognostic value of high platelet count [111], which has been confirmed by others in the following decades [109–111,116,117]. Other studies could not validate the prognostic value at all [112], or found, instead of platelet count, the platelet to lymphocyte ratio (PLR) to be prognostic, as explained more in detail below [102–114].

Next to single blood parameters, special focus has lately been laid on ratios between some blood markers, such as the neutrophil to lymphocyte ratio (NLR), lymphocyte to monocyte ratio (LMR) or platelet to lymphocyte ratio (PLR). These markers are easily accessible and calculated from routine blood cell count and reflect the relation between specific and unspecific systemic immune response.

With increasing knowledge of the role of specific and unspecific immune response in cancer, these ratios have become of rising interest as possible biomarkers in numerous malignancies with promising prognostic potential [94,113–119].

As for other solid tumors [94,113–120], a negative prognostic value of high NLR has been shown for MPM in numerous studies analyzing cohorts of patients receiving different therapy concepts [102,103,112,119,121] including systemic therapy [121]. Furthermore, two studies found in a subgroup analysis that normalization of pretreatment elevated NLR under chemotherapy was predictive for better OS [106,121]. Additionally, for surgical patients undergoing cytoreductive surgery, high NLR was found to correlate with worse prognosis [122].

Low LMR, displaying a domination of unspecific monocytes, has been found to be a negative prognostic marker for numerous malignancies as reviewed by Gu et al. [123]. For MPM, comparable results have been published [102,114,122] showing that low LMR is associated with adverse prognosis in line with the reported negative prognostic value of elevated monocyte count as mentioned before. Of note, Yin et al. published comparable results for peritoneal mesothelioma [124].

Furthermore, high PLR has been studied and reported as a negative prognostic marker for multiple malignancies [119,125,127–129], also including MPM. As already indicated above, of the four named studies with no correlation between platelet count and survival, three, however, did find PLR to be associated with poor prognosis after univariate analyses [102,103,114]. Thus, one might speculate that even if absolute platelet count alone is not prognostic, a relative increase in platelets compared to low lymphocytes might be.

2.11. Acute-Phase Proteins

Already in 1998, Nakano et al. observed significantly elevated serum levels of some acute phase response proteins (APP) and cytokines—namely fibrinogen, IL-6, alpha1-acid glycoprotein and CRP levels—in MPM patients compared to patients with adenocarcinoma of the lung. They also reported significantly higher levels of IL-6 in the pleural fluid of MPM patients and concluded that the pleural IL-6, when entering systemic circulation, enhances the systemic acute phase response (APR) [130].

The APR, as part of the unspecific immune response, is the physiological and biochemical systemic reaction to inflammation, infection, tissue damage due to, for example burn injuries or trauma and malignancies. The process is mediated by proinflammatory cytokines, causing fever, leukocytosis and the release of APP. Gabay et al. provide a detailed list of well-known APP, some of which have been under investigation with regard to applicability as inflammatory biomarkers in MPM—particularly IL-6, CRP, fibrinogen [126].

2.12. Interleukin 6

The proinflammatory cytokine IL-6 is released by various immune cells triggered by IL-1β and TNF, but also produced by tumor cells directly as also proven for MPM with tumor-promoting effects [75,131]. The (patho)physiological functions of IL-6 are reviewed by Hunter in general [132] and by Abdul Rahim et al. for mesothelioma in particular—emphasizing the promoting effect of IL-6 on cell proliferation, angiogenesis via stimulation of VEGF expression, resistance to chemotherapy and physical symptoms negatively influencing wellbeing of the patient [133].

In contrast to other malignancies [134–144] current data does not support the prognostic or predictive value of IL-6 serum concentration for MPM [130]. However, IL-6 levels have been reported to correlate significantly with other markers [130,133] of verified prognostic impact for MPM such as VEGF [145–147], thrombocytosis [107,111,142] and CRP levels [11,116,142]. Adachi et al. found that IL-6 encouraged cell proliferation as autocrine growth factor and the expression of VEGF [148] and accordingly investigated an IL-6 inhibitor as VEGF targeting therapeutic approach in a subsequent study [149].

Antiangiogenic therapeutic approaches have been widely investigated as reviewed recently by Novak et al. [150]. Thus, the clinical use of the VEGF inhibitor bevacizumab is now also regarded as promising improvement of the almost 20 year old standard chemotherapy regimen published by Vogelzang et al. [151] according to the promising results of the MAPS trial [152].

From the current point of view, IL-6 does not seem to be applicable as prognostic or predictive marker for MPM; however, it can be assumed that it plays a major role in promotion of systemic inflammation with release of other proinflammatory cytokines as already suggested two decades ago by Nakano et al. [130].

2.13. C-Reactive Protein (CRP)

CRP, first described in 1930, is one of the earliest discovered and most established acute-phase response proteins [153]. The CRP synthesis in hepatocytes is mainly stimulated by IL-6, IL-1β and tumor necrosis factor α (TNF-α) [126]. Clinical use for inflammation and treatment response is currently well established since elevated CRP levels correlate with the course of chronic and acute infections but also inflammatory (autoimmune) disorders, general tissue injury and various malignancies [154,155]. Lately, elevated serum CRP levels were found to be associated with poor prognosis for multiple tumor entities [82,94,95,97,156–158]. Consequently, this potentially interesting biomarker has also been investigated in MPM. Elevated CRP levels were reported to be associated with shorter survival—regardless of different applied treatment modalities [103,116,123], specifically for patients receiving systemic treatment [112], as well as patients undergoing trimodal therapy including surgery [11]. Some groups even described a level dependent negative prognostic potential of pretreatment CRP serum concentration [112,159].

Furthermore, the predictive potential of CRP for MPM has been explored by the study group of the authors before. It was proven that of patients undergoing aggressive multimodality treatment including cytoreductive surgery only those with normal pretreatment CRP levels benefit from this type of therapy. Thus, patients with normal CRP values before therapy receiving multimodality therapy survived 36 months in median. In contrast to these findings, patients with elevated pretreatment CRP only had 10 months overall survival despite multimodality therapy indicating, that indeed this subgroup of MPM is of distinct treatment responsiveness [11]. Of note, Kao et al. additionally described a correlation between elevated inflammatory markers—specifically elevated CRP and NLR—and advanced clinical symptoms such as fatigue and anorexia in course of an engraved systemic inflammatory response and consequently compromised health-related quality of life [160].

2.14. Fibrinogen

Fibrinogen, a well-known clotting factor, is also an important positive acute phase protein. Its synthesis is increasing significantly when stimulated by proinflammatory cytokines, mainly IL-6 [161]. Fibrinogen as biomarker has been investigated for several diseases including chronic obstructive pulmonary disease and coronary heart disease [161,162]. Additionally, a negative prognostic value of high pretreatment fibrinogen has been found for numerous tumor entities [98,114,163–167]. So far, only the previous study of the authors reported not only a prognostic but also predictive value for pretreatment fibrinogen in MPM. Patients with high fibrinogen plasma levels were shown to have significantly shorter OS. Additionally, of patients receiving trimodal treatment with cytoreductive surgery, those with high pretreatment fibrinogen did not benefit from multimodality treatment [10].

2.15. Albumin—A Negative Acute Phase Protein

Serum albumin not only reflects nutritional status but also inflammatory response as negative acute phase protein mediated by cytokines including IL-6, IL-1β and TNF-α [168]. Hypoalbuminemia has long been acknowledged to impair wound healing and outcome after interventions and surgeries [169–173]. In addition, it was described to indicate short survival in different malignancies [168]. For MPM, hypoalbuminemia has been associated with poor survival for patients receiving different treatment modalities [102,103,114], but also selectively for chemotherapy patients [174] and surgical patients [175].

In a classification and regression tree analysis, Brims et al. found the best survival for patients with no weight loss, a high hemoglobin level and a high serum albumin level [176]. Harris et al. validated these findings for surgical patients undergoing cytoreductive surgery [175].

Hypoalbuminemia and elevated CRP concentration have been integrated in a systemic inflammation based prognostic score, the so-called modified Glasgow Prognostic Score (mGPS). Its prognostic value has also been confirmed for multiple cancer types as reviewed in detail by McMillan [177] and has been acknowledged for mesothelioma in univariate analysis [101].

Furthermore, the prognostic value of elevated CRP/Albumin ratio (CAR), reflecting increased CRP values and decreased albumin concentration as indicator of poor nutritional and activated acute phase response, has been widely explored. Elevated CAR has been shown to predict poor outcome in acute diseases including sepsis [178,179] as well as in various malignant diseases [96,99,180–183]. Takamori et al. investigated CAR for MPM patients and found a high CAR to be independently prognostic [184]. Otoshi et al. confirmed these results for inoperable MPM patients [102] whereas Tanrikulu et al. could not reproduce these results [100].

2.16. Ferritin

The positive APP ferritin is up-regulated under inflammatory or infectious conditions to reduce the iron accessibility of pathogenic organisms [185,186]. For numerous malignancies elevated serum ferritin concentrations have been reported as well, in part with prognostic impact [187]. Healthy human cells, foreign organisms but also cancer cells depend on iron supply for a number of cellular metabolic processes. The role of iron metabolism and its regulation—partially by cells of the TME—have been reviewed excellently by Hsu et al. for cancer in general [187] and by Toyokuni et al. for MPM in particular, especially in context of asbestos-induced oxidative stress [188]. MPM has been associated with elevated ferritin serum levels [189–191], but to our knowledge the prognostic or predictive impact of ferritin has not been investigated so far. However, correlations of ferritin with TAM and modulated lymphocyte function has been suggested [186,187] so in context of the APR as well as the importance of iron metabolism in MPM the study of ferritin as biomarker might reveal interesting new results. Of note, also reduction of iron storage was suggested as possible treatment target after promising preclinical results from a rat model [191,192].

2.17. The Complement System

With regard to the innate immune system and its systemic circulating compartments, the complement component 4d (C4d) was also found to be of prognostic relevance in MPM patients. High plasma C4d levels were associated with high tumor volume, worse response to induction therapy, high acute phase response proteins and shorter survival after multivariate analyses as reported by Klikovits et al. [8]. Furthermore, Agnostinis et al. investigated the role of complement protein C1q in MPM. It was shown that C1q did not activate the classic complement pathway in MPM as one might expect, but instead bound to hyaluronic acid and thereby induced cell adhesion and proliferation of mesothelioma cells. Interestingly, the activation of the classic complement pathway was abandoned by hyaluronic acid [193]. These findings are in line with Klikovits et al., where high C4d (as downstream target of C1q during the classic complement pathway) was not correlating with high C1q [8]. Thus, the activation and exact role of the complement system and its subunits is yet not fully understood and might be of future interest in MPM.

Taken together, many common systemic inflammatory parameters have been studied regarding their prognostic potential for MPM and some additionally for their predictive impact. It is remarkable—compatible with our conclusions on local inflammation—that high unspecific inflammatory markers seem to be adverse whereas high specific inflammatory markers appear to be beneficial reflecting the tumor-promoting influence of the innate immune system and the tumor-suppressing impact of the adaptive immune system, respectively.

3. Conclusions

While preparing the present review and summarizing the established as well as most recent knowledge, it became fairly clear that a large amount of research considering this topic has been performed within the past few decades. Despite the fact that a lot of data is based on retrospective studies—which is most likely explainable by the rare incidence of MPM—high quality research supports the important role of inflammation in MPM. Not only in the setting of pathogenesis, tumor promotion, poor prognosis or treatment response inflammatory processes play a decisive role but inflammation and immune response are also under investigation as promising treatment targets. Most markers and key findings were not only published once but have been validated in the past, thus resulting in several inflammatory related biomarkers characterized by reproducibility and accordingly reliability. Furthermore, comparable results have been documented in other malignancies thus indicating, that some of the above mentioned findings have a universal impact in (immune-) oncology.

In the clinical management of MPM, physicians are confronted with multiple—yet not fully standardized—treatment modalities on the one hand, opposed to poor outcome and treatment resistance on the other hand. Consequently, MPM in general is the ideal candidate for biomarker research especially when it comes to treatment guiding predictive parameters [22].

The immune system plays a key role in MPM, since this rare disease has already been associated with inflammation several decades ago [5]. This theory is supported by many more recent studies summarized in this review. During the past few decades and especially within the last years, it was shown that an upregulated unspecific immune response on the one hand translates to poor outcome. On the one hand, a downregulated specific immune system results in tumor progression, tumor immune evasion and finally poor prognosis, regardless if investigating the inflammatory status in patient blood, pleural effusion, tumor tissue or its associated TME. Thus, the tumor suppressive characteristics of the specific immune system get obvious when the—through MPM suppressed—specific immune response gets reactivated by immune therapy resulting in prolonged survival.

This above-described duality of the immune system in MPM has been analyzed and described before by Linton et al. [12]. However, today we would reply to the question "Inflammation in malignant mesothelioma—friend or foe?" that it is both friend and foe. More precisely, and to simplify the key message from this review, the specific immune system is our friend and its unspecific counterpart the foe which is also reflected in the prognostic value of the corresponding biomarkers—both on a local as well as systemic level.

Further research on the immune system in MPM might help in treating this therapy refractory disease and reveal modern insights in the complex interaction of our immune system with the tumor thus resulting in a better biological understanding, new treatment approaches and finally improved clinical management and patient outcome. There is still need for future studies to gain detailed knowledge about this topic and, thus, we look forward to learning more about the interaction of our immune system with malignant disease in general and MPM in particular.

Author Contributions: All authors contributed to the conceptualization of this review, M.V., B.G. and A.R. conducted the literature research and wrote the manuscript; T.B., A.S., M.B. and E.S. revised the original draft critically; M.V. was responsible for visualization of data in tables and the figure. All authors gave final approval of the version to be published and agreed to be accountable for all aspects of the work in ensuring that questions related to the accuracy or integrity of any part of the work are appropriately investigated and resolved. All authors have read and agreed to the published version of the manuscript.

Funding: This research was funded by Open Access Funding by Karl Landsteiner University of Health Sciences, Krems, Austria.

Informed Consent Statement: Not applicable.

Data Availability Statement: No new data were created or analyzed in this study. Data sharing is not applicable to this article.

Acknowledgments: This work was generously supported by Open Access Publishing Fund of Karl Landsteiner University of Health Sciences, Krems, Austria.

Conflicts of Interest: The authors declare no conflict of interest.

References

1. Robinson, B.W.; Musk, A.W.; Lake, R.A. Malignant mesothelioma. *Lancet (Lond. Engl.)* **2005**, *366*, 397–408. [CrossRef]
2. Ricciardi, S.; Cardillo, G.; Zirafa, C.C.; Carleo, F.; Facciolo, F.; Fontanini, G.; Mutti, L.; Melfi, F. Surgery for malignant pleural mesothelioma: An international guidelines review. *J. Thorac. Dis.* **2018**, *10*, S285–S292. [CrossRef] [PubMed]
3. Ichiki, Y.; Goto, H.; Fukuyama, T.; Nakanishi, K. Should Lung-Sparing Surgery Be the Standard Procedure for Malignant Pleural Mesothelioma? *J. Clin. Med.* **2020**, *9*, 2153. [CrossRef]

4. Opitz, I.; Scherpereel, A.; Berghmans, T.; Psallidas, I.; Glatzer, M.; Rigau, D.; Astoul, P.; Bölükbas, S.; Boyd, J.; Coolen, J.; et al. ERS/ESTS/EACTS/ESTRO guidelines for the management of malignant pleural mesothelioma. *Eur. J. Cardio-Thorac. Surg. Off. J. Eur. Assoc. Cardio-Thorac. Surg.* **2020**, *58*, 1–24. [CrossRef]
5. Wagner, J.C.; Sleggs, C.A.; Marchand, P. Diffuse pleural mesothelioma and asbestos exposure in the North Western Cape Province. *Br. J. Ind. Med.* **1960**, *17*, 260–271. [CrossRef] [PubMed]
6. Bononi, A.; Napolitano, A.; Pass, H.I.; Yang, H.; Carbone, M. Latest developments in our understanding of the pathogenesis of mesothelioma and the design of targeted therapies. *Expert Rev. Respir. Med.* **2015**, *9*, 633–654. [CrossRef]
7. Sekido, Y. Molecular pathogenesis of malignant mesothelioma. *Carcinogenesis* **2013**, *34*, 1413–1419. [CrossRef]
8. Klikovits, T.; Stockhammer, P.; Laszlo, V.; Dong, Y.; Hoda, M.A.; Ghanim, B.; Opitz, I.; Frauenfelder, T.; Nguyen-Kim, T.D.L.; Weder, W.; et al. Circulating complement component 4d (C4d) correlates with tumor volume, chemotherapeutic response and survival in patients with malignant pleural mesothelioma. *Sci. Rep.* **2017**, *7*, 16456. [CrossRef]
9. Ghanim, B.; Klikovits, T.; Hoda, M.A.; Lang, G.; Szirtes, I.; Setinek, U.; Rozsas, A.; Renyi-Vamos, F.; Laszlo, V.; Grusch, M.; et al. Ki67 index is an independent prognostic factor in epithelioid but not in non-epithelioid malignant pleural mesothelioma: A multicenter study. *Br. J. Cancer* **2015**, *112*, 783–792. [CrossRef]
10. Ghanim, B.; Hoda, M.A.; Klikovits, T.; Winter, M.P.; Alimohammadi, A.; Grusch, M.; Dome, B.; Arns, M.; Schenk, P.; Jakopovic, M.; et al. Circulating fibrinogen is a prognostic and predictive biomarker in malignant pleural mesothelioma. *Br. J. Cancer* **2014**, *110*, 984–990. [CrossRef]
11. Ghanim, B.; Hoda, M.A.; Winter, M.P.; Klikovits, T.; Alimohammadi, A.; Hegedus, B.; Dome, B.; Grusch, M.; Arns, M.; Schenk, P.; et al. Pretreatment serum C-reactive protein levels predict benefit from multimodality treatment including radical surgery in malignant pleural mesothelioma: A retrospective multicenter analysis. *Ann. Surg.* **2012**, *256*, 357–362. [CrossRef]
12. Linton, A.; van Zandwijk, N.; Reid, G.; Clarke, S.; Cao, C.; Kao, S. Inflammation in malignant mesothelioma—friend or foe? *Ann. Cardiothorac. Surg.* **2012**, *1*, 516–522. [CrossRef]
13. Opitz, I.; Friess, M.; Kestenholz, P.; Schneiter, D.; Frauenfelder, T.; Nguyen-Kim, T.D.; Seifert, B.; Hoda, M.A.; Klepetko, W.; Stahel, R.A.; et al. A New Prognostic Score Supporting Treatment Allocation for Multimodality Therapy for Malignant Pleural Mesothelioma: A Review of 12 Years' Experience. *J. Thorac. Oncol.* **2015**, *10*, 1634–1641. [CrossRef] [PubMed]
14. Hanahan, D.; Weinberg, R.A. Hallmarks of cancer: The next generation. *Cell* **2011**, *144*, 646–674. [CrossRef] [PubMed]
15. Chiarucci, C.; Cannito, S.; Daffinà, M.G.; Amato, G.; Giacobini, G.; Cutaia, O.; Lofiego, M.F.; Fazio, C.; Giannarelli, D.; Danielli, R.; et al. Circulating Levels of PD-L1 in Mesothelioma Patients from the NIBIT-MESO-1 Study: Correlation with Survival. *Cancers* **2020**, *12*, 361. [CrossRef] [PubMed]
16. Alley, E.W.; Lopez, J.; Santoro, A.; Morosky, A.; Saraf, S.; Piperdi, B.; van Brummelen, E. Clinical safety and activity of pembrolizumab in patients with malignant pleural mesothelioma (KEYNOTE-028): Preliminary results from a non-randomised, open-label, phase 1b trial. *Lancet Oncol.* **2017**, *18*, 623–630. [CrossRef]
17. Quispel-Janssen, J.; van der Noort, V.; de Vries, J.F.; Zimmerman, M.; Lalezari, F.; Thunnissen, E.; Monkhorst, K.; Schouten, R.; Schunselaar, L.; Disselhorst, M.; et al. Programmed Death 1 Blockade With Nivolumab in Patients With Recurrent Malignant Pleural Mesothelioma. *J. Thorac. Oncol.* **2018**, *13*, 1569–1576. [CrossRef]
18. Hassan, R.; Thomas, A.; Nemunaitis, J.J.; Patel, M.R.; Bennouna, J.; Chen, F.L.; Delord, J.P.; Dowlati, A.; Kochuparambil, S.T.; Taylor, M.H.; et al. Efficacy and Safety of Avelumab Treatment in Patients With Advanced Unresectable Mesothelioma: Phase 1b Results From the JAVELIN Solid Tumor Trial. *Jama Oncol.* **2019**, *5*, 351–357. [CrossRef]
19. Wright, K. FDA Approves Nivolumab Plus Ipilimumab for Previously Untreated Unresectable Malignant Pleural Mesothelioma. *Oncology (Williston Park)* **2020**, *34*, 502–503. [CrossRef]
20. Opitz, I.; Furrer, K. Preoperative Identification of Benefit from Surgery for Malignant Pleural Mesothelioma. *Thorac. Surg. Clin.* **2020**, *30*, 435–449. [CrossRef]
21. La Thangue, N.B.; Kerr, D.J. Predictive biomarkers: A paradigm shift towards personalized cancer medicine. *Nat. Rev. Clin. Oncol.* **2011**, *8*, 587–596. [CrossRef]
22. Scherpereel, A.; Opitz, I.; Berghmans, T.; Psallidas, I.; Glatzer, M.; Rigau, D.; Astoul, P.; Bolukbas, S.; Boyd, J.; Coolen, J.; et al. ERS/ESTS/EACTS/ESTRO guidelines for the management of malignant pleural mesothelioma. *Eur Respir J.* **2020**, *55*. [CrossRef]
23. Mantovani, A.; Allavena, P.; Sica, A.; Balkwill, F. Cancer-related inflammation. *Nature* **2008**, *454*, 436–444. [CrossRef]
24. Badalamenti, G.; Fanale, D.; Incorvaia, L.; Barraco, N.; Listì, A.; Maragliano, R.; Vincenzi, B.; Calò, V.; Iovanna, J.L.; Bazan, V.; et al. Role of tumor-infiltrating lymphocytes in patients with solid tumors: Can a drop dig a stone? *Cell. Immunol.* **2019**, *343*, 103753. [CrossRef] [PubMed]
25. Hendry, S.; Salgado, R.; Gevaert, T.; Russell, P.A.; John, T.; Thapa, B.; Christie, M.; van de Vijver, K.; Estrada, M.V.; Gonzalez-Ericsson, P.I.; et al. Assessing Tumor-Infiltrating Lymphocytes in Solid Tumors: A Practical Review for Pathologists and Proposal for a Standardized Method from the International Immuno-Oncology Biomarkers Working Group: Part 2: TILs in Melanoma, Gastrointestinal Tract Carcinomas, Non-Small Cell Lung Carcinoma and Mesothelioma, Endometrial and Ovarian Carcinomas, Squamous Cell Carcinoma of the Head and Neck, Genitourinary Carcinomas, and Primary Brain Tumors. *Adv. Anat. Pathol.* **2017**, *24*, 311–335. [CrossRef] [PubMed]
26. Leigh, R.A.; Webster, I. Lymphocytic infiltration of pleural mesothelioma and its significance for survival. *South. Afr. Med. J. Suid-Afrik. Tydskr. Vir Geneeskd.* **1982**, *61*, 1007–1009.

27. Koebel, C.M.; Vermi, W.; Swann, J.B.; Zerafa, N.; Rodig, S.J.; Old, L.J.; Smyth, M.J.; Schreiber, R.D. Adaptive immunity maintains occult cancer in an equilibrium state. *Nature* **2007**, *450*, 903–907. [CrossRef] [PubMed]
28. Coussens, L.M.; Werb, Z. Inflammation and cancer. *Nature* **2002**, *420*, 860–867. [CrossRef]
29. Minnema-Luiting, J.; Vroman, H.; Aerts, J.; Cornelissen, R. Heterogeneity in Immune Cell Content in Malignant Pleural Mesothelioma. *Int. J. Mol. Sci.* **2018**, *19*, 1041. [CrossRef] [PubMed]
30. Marcq, E.; Siozopoulou, V.; De Waele, J.; van Audenaerde, J.; Zwaenepoel, K.; Santermans, E.; Hens, N.; Pauwels, P.; van Meerbeeck, J.P.; Smits, E.L. Prognostic and predictive aspects of the tumor immune microenvironment and immune checkpoints in malignant pleural mesothelioma. *Oncoimmunology* **2017**, *6*, e1261241. [CrossRef]
31. Anraku, M.; Cunningham, K.S.; Yun, Z.; Tsao, M.S.; Zhang, L.; Keshavjee, S.; Johnston, M.R.; de Perrot, M. Impact of tumor-infiltrating T cells on survival in patients with malignant pleural mesothelioma. *J. Thorac. Cardiovasc. Surg.* **2008**, *135*, 823–829. [CrossRef]
32. Yamada, N.; Oizumi, S.; Kikuchi, E.; Shinagawa, N.; Konishi-Sakakibara, J.; Ishimine, A.; Aoe, K.; Gemba, K.; Kishimoto, T.; Torigoe, T.; et al. CD8+ tumor-infiltrating lymphocytes predict favorable prognosis in malignant pleural mesothelioma after resection. *Cancer Immunol. Immunother. Cii* **2010**, *59*, 1543–1549. [CrossRef]
33. Awad, M.M.; Jones, R.E.; Liu, H.; Lizotte, P.H.; Ivanova, E.V.; Kulkarni, M.; Herter-Sprie, G.S.; Liao, X.; Santos, A.A.; Bittinger, M.A.; et al. Cytotoxic T Cells in PD-L1-Positive Malignant Pleural Mesotheliomas Are Counterbalanced by Distinct Immunosuppressive Factors. *Cancer Immunol. Res.* **2016**, *4*, 1038–1048. [CrossRef] [PubMed]
34. Chu, G.J.; van Zandwijk, N.; Rasko, J.E.J. The Immune Microenvironment in Mesothelioma: Mechanisms of Resistance to Immunotherapy. *Front. Oncol.* **2019**, *9*, 1366. [CrossRef] [PubMed]
35. Yap, T.A.; Aerts, J.G.; Popat, S.; Fennell, D.A. Novel insights into mesothelioma biology and implications for therapy. *Nat. Rev. Cancer* **2017**, *17*, 475–488. [CrossRef]
36. Veltman, J.D.; Lambers, M.E.; van Nimwegen, M.; Hendriks, R.W.; Hoogsteden, H.C.; Aerts, J.G.; Hegmans, J.P. COX-2 inhibition improves immunotherapy and is associated with decreased numbers of myeloid-derived suppressor cells in mesothelioma. Celecoxib influences MDSC function. *BMC Cancer* **2010**, *10*, 464. [CrossRef]
37. Ujiie, H.; Kadota, K.; Nitadori, J.I.; Aerts, J.G.; Woo, K.M.; Sima, C.S.; Travis, W.D.; Jones, D.R.; Krug, L.M.; Adusumilli, P.S. The tumoral and stromal immune microenvironment in malignant pleural mesothelioma: A comprehensive analysis reveals prognostic immune markers. *Oncoimmunology* **2015**, *4*, e1009285. [CrossRef] [PubMed]
38. Pasello, G.; Zago, G.; Lunardi, F.; Urso, L.; Kern, I.; Vlacic, G.; Grosso, F.; Mencoboni, M.; Ceresoli, G.L.; Schiavon, M.; et al. Malignant pleural mesothelioma immune microenvironment and checkpoint expression: Correlation with clinical-pathological features and intratumor heterogeneity over time. *Ann. Oncol. Off. J. Eur. Soc. Med. Oncol.* **2018**, *29*, 1258–1265. [CrossRef] [PubMed]
39. Baldi, A.; Santini, D.; Vasaturo, F.; Santini, M.; Vicidomini, G.; Di Marino, M.P.; Esposito, V.; Groeger, A.M.; Liuzzi, G.; Vincenzi, B.; et al. Prognostic significance of cyclooxygenase-2 (COX-2) and expression of cell cycle inhibitors p21 and p27 in human pleural malignant mesothelioma. *Thorax* **2004**, *59*, 428–433. [CrossRef] [PubMed]
40. Mineo, T.C.; Ambrogi, V.; Cufari, M.E.; Pompeo, E. May cyclooxygenase-2 (COX-2), p21 and p27 expression affect prognosis and therapeutic strategy of patients with malignant pleural mesothelioma? *Eur. J. Cardio-Thorac. Surg. Off. J. Eur. Assoc. Cardio-Thorac. Surg.* **2010**, *38*, 245–252. [CrossRef]
41. Edwards, J.G.; Faux, S.P.; Plummer, S.M.; Abrams, K.R.; Walker, R.A.; Waller, D.A.; O'Byrne, K.J. Cyclooxygenase-2 expression is a novel prognostic factor in malignant mesothelioma. *Clin. Cancer Res. Off. J. Am. Assoc. Cancer Res.* **2002**, *8*, 1857–1862.
42. O'Kane, S.L.; Cawkwell, L.; Campbell, A.; Lind, M.J. Cyclooxygenase-2 expression predicts survival in malignant pleural mesothelioma. *Eur. J. Cancer (Oxf. Engl. 1990)* **2005**, *41*, 1645–1648. [CrossRef]
43. Cedrés, S.; Ponce-Aix, S.; Zugazagoitia, J.; Sansano, I.; Enguita, A.; Navarro-Mendivil, A.; Martinez-Marti, A.; Martinez, P.; Felip, E. Analysis of expression of programmed cell death 1 ligand 1 (PD-L1) in malignant pleural mesothelioma (MPM). *PLoS ONE* **2015**, *10*, e0121071. [CrossRef] [PubMed]
44. Cornelissen, R.; Lievense, L.A.; Maat, A.P.; Hendriks, R.W.; Hoogsteden, H.C.; Bogers, A.J.; Hegmans, J.P.; Aerts, J.G. Ratio of intratumoral macrophage phenotypes is a prognostic factor in epithelioid malignant pleural mesothelioma. *PLoS ONE* **2014**, *9*, e106742. [CrossRef] [PubMed]
45. Blondy, T.; d'Almeida, S.M.; Briolay, T.; Tabiasco, J.; Meiller, C.; Chéné, A.L.; Cellerin, L.; Deshayes, S.; Delneste, Y.; Fonteneau, J.F.; et al. Involvement of the M-CSF/IL-34/CSF-1R pathway in malignant pleural mesothelioma. *J. Immunother. Cancer* **2020**, *8*. [CrossRef]
46. Inaguma, S.; Lasota, J.; Wang, Z.; Czapiewski, P.; Langfort, R.; Rys, J.; Szpor, J.; Waloszczyk, P.; Okoń, K.; Biernat, W.; et al. Expression of ALCAM (CD166) and PD-L1 (CD274) independently predicts shorter survival in malignant pleural mesothelioma. *Hum. Pathol.* **2018**, *71*, 1–7. [CrossRef] [PubMed]
47. Mansfield, A.S.; Roden, A.C.; Peikert, T.; Sheinin, Y.M.; Harrington, S.M.; Krco, C.J.; Dong, H.; Kwon, E.D. B7-H1 expression in malignant pleural mesothelioma is associated with sarcomatoid histology and poor prognosis. *J. Thorac. Oncol. Off. Publ. Int. Assoc. Study Lung Cancer* **2014**, *9*, 1036–1040. [CrossRef] [PubMed]
48. Farhood, B.; Najafi, M.; Mortezaee, K. CD8(+) cytotoxic T lymphocytes in cancer immunotherapy: A review. *J. Cell. Physiol.* **2019**, *234*, 8509–8521. [CrossRef]

49. Cornelissen, R.; Lievense, L.A.; Robertus, J.L.; Hendriks, R.W.; Hoogsteden, H.C.; Hegmans, J.P.; Aerts, J.G. Intratumoral macrophage phenotype and CD8+ T lymphocytes as potential tools to predict local tumor outgrowth at the intervention site in malignant pleural mesothelioma. *Lung Cancer (Amst. Neth.)* **2015**, *88*, 332–337. [CrossRef]
50. Najafi, M.; Farhood, B.; Mortezaee, K. Contribution of regulatory T cells to cancer: A review. *J. Cell. Physiol.* **2019**, *234*, 7983–7993. [CrossRef]
51. Hegmans, J.P.; Hemmes, A.; Hammad, H.; Boon, L.; Hoogsteden, H.C.; Lambrecht, B.N. Mesothelioma environment comprises cytokines and T-regulatory cells that suppress immune responses. *Eur. Respir. J.* **2006**, *27*, 1086–1095. [CrossRef]
52. Fitzpatrick, D.R.; Bielefeldt-Ohmann, H.; Himbeck, R.P.; Jarnicki, A.G.; Marzo, A.L.; Robinson, B.W. Transforming growth factor-beta: Antisense RNA-mediated inhibition affects anchorage-independent growth, tumorigenicity and tumor-infiltrating T-cells in malignant mesothelioma. *Growth Factors (ChurSwitz.)* **1994**, *11*, 29–44. [CrossRef]
53. Hoda, M.A.; Münzker, J.; Ghanim, B.; Schelch, K.; Klikovits, T.; Laszlo, V.; Sahin, E.; Bedeir, A.; Lackner, A.; Dome, B.; et al. Suppression of activin A signals inhibits growth of malignant pleural mesothelioma cells. *Br. J. Cancer* **2012**, *107*, 1978–1986. [CrossRef]
54. Hoda, M.A.; Dong, Y.; Rozsas, A.; Klikovits, T.; Laszlo, V.; Ghanim, B.; Stockhammer, P.; Ozsvar, J.; Jakopovic, M.; Samarzija, M.; et al. Circulating activin A is a novel prognostic biomarker in malignant pleural mesothelioma—A multi-institutional study. *Eur. J. Cancer (Oxf. Engl. 1990)* **2016**, *63*, 64–73. [CrossRef] [PubMed]
55. Nuvoli, B.; Galati, R. Cyclooxygenase-2, epidermal growth factor receptor, and aromatase signaling in inflammation and mesothelioma. *Mol. Cancer Ther.* **2013**, *12*, 844–852. [CrossRef]
56. Marrogi, A.; Pass, H.I.; Khan, M.; Metheny-Barlow, L.J.; Harris, C.C.; Gerwin, B.I. Human mesothelioma samples overexpress both cyclooxygenase-2 (COX-2) and inducible nitric oxide synthase (NOS2): In vitro antiproliferative effects of a COX-2 inhibitor. *Cancer Res.* **2000**, *60*, 3696–3700.
57. Li, Q.; Wang, W.; Yamada, T.; Matsumoto, K.; Sakai, K.; Bando, Y.; Uehara, H.; Nishioka, Y.; Sone, S.; Iwakiri, S.; et al. Pleural mesothelioma instigates tumor-associated fibroblasts to promote progression via a malignant cytokine network. *Am. J. Pathol.* **2011**, *179*, 1483–1493. [CrossRef] [PubMed]
58. Schelch, K.; Hoda, M.A.; Klikovits, T.; Münzker, J.; Ghanim, B.; Wagner, C.; Garay, T.; Laszlo, V.; Setinek, U.; Dome, B.; et al. Fibroblast growth factor receptor inhibition is active against mesothelioma and synergizes with radio- and chemotherapy. *Am. J. Respir. Crit. Care Med.* **2014**, *190*, 763–772. [CrossRef] [PubMed]
59. Schelch, K.; Wagner, C.; Hager, S.; Pirker, C.; Siess, K.; Lang, E.; Lin, R.; Kirschner, M.B.; Mohr, T.; Brcic, L.; et al. FGF2 and EGF induce epithelial-mesenchymal transition in malignant pleural mesothelioma cells via a MAPKinase/MMP1 signal. *Carcinogenesis* **2018**, *39*, 534–545. [CrossRef]
60. Vlacic, G.; Hoda, M.A.; Klikovits, T.; Sinn, K.; Gschwandtner, E.; Mohorcic, K.; Schelch, K.; Pirker, C.; Peter-Vorosmarty, B.; Brankovic, J.; et al. Expression of FGFR1-4 in Malignant Pleural Mesothelioma Tissue and Corresponding Cell Lines and its Relationship to Patient Survival and FGFR Inhibitor Sensitivity. *Cells* **2019**, *8*, 1091. [CrossRef] [PubMed]
61. Ghahremanifard, P.; Chanda, A.; Bonni, S.; Bose, P. TGF-beta Mediated Immune Evasion in Cancer-Spotlight on Cancer-Associated Fibroblasts. *Cancers* **2020**, *12*, 3650. [CrossRef]
62. Hashemi Goradel, N.; Najafi, M.; Salehi, E.; Farhood, B.; Mortezaee, K. Cyclooxygenase-2 in cancer: A review. *J. Cell. Physiol.* **2019**, *234*, 5683–5699. [CrossRef] [PubMed]
63. Tołoczko-Iwaniuk, N.; Dziemiańczyk-Pakieła, D.; Nowaszewska, B.K.; Celińska-Janowicz, K.; Miltyk, W. Celecoxib in Cancer Therapy and Prevention—Review. *Curr. Drug Targets* **2019**, *20*, 302–315. [CrossRef]
64. Zhou, X.; Wang, X.; Zhao, Y.; Yi, C. The role of celecoxib for colorectal cancer treatment: A systematic review. *Transl. Cancer Res.* **2018**, *7*, 1527–1536. [CrossRef]
65. Van Cutsem, E.; Cervantes, A.; Adam, R.; Sobrero, A.; Van Krieken, J.H.; Aderka, D.; Aranda Aguilar, E.; Bardelli, A.; Benson, A.; Bodoky, G.; et al. ESMO consensus guidelines for the management of patients with metastatic colorectal cancer. *Ann. Oncol. Off. J. Eur. Soc. Med. Oncol.* **2016**, *27*, 1386–1422. [CrossRef] [PubMed]
66. Chen, E.Y.; Blanke, C.D.; Haller, D.G.; Benson, A.B.; Dragovich, T.; Lenz, H.J.; Robles, C.; Li, H.; Mori, M.; Mattek, N.; et al. A Phase II Study of Celecoxib with Irinotecan, 5-Fluorouracil, and Leucovorin in Patients With Previously Untreated Advanced or Metastatic Colorectal Cancer. *Am. J. Clin. Oncol.* **2018**, *41*, 1193–1198. [CrossRef] [PubMed]
67. Zhang, W.; Yi, L.; Shen, J.; Zhang, H.; Luo, P.; Zhang, J. Comparison of the benefits of celecoxib combined with anticancer therapy in advanced non-small cell lung cancer: A meta-analysis. *J. Cancer* **2020**, *11*, 1816–1827. [CrossRef]
68. Yi, L.; Zhang, W.; Zhang, H.; Shen, J.; Zou, J.; Luo, P.; Zhang, J. Systematic review and meta-analysis of the benefit of celecoxib in treating advanced non-small-cell lung cancer. *Drug Des. Dev. Ther.* **2018**, *12*, 2455–2466. [CrossRef]
69. Robinson, C.; Alfonso, H.; Woo, S.; Olsen, N.; Bill Musk, A.W.; Robinson, B.W.; Nowak, A.K.; Lake, R.A. Effect of NSAIDS and COX-2 inhibitors on the incidence and severity of asbestos-induced malignant mesothelioma: Evidence from an animal model and a human cohort. *Lung Cancer (Amst. Neth.)* **2014**, *86*, 29–34. [CrossRef]
70. López-Janeiro, Á.; Padilla-Ansala, C.; de Andrea, C.E.; Hardisson, D.; Melero, I. Prognostic value of macrophage polarization markers in epithelial neoplasms and melanoma. A systematic review and meta-analysis. *Mod. Pathol. Off. J. United States Can. Acad. Pathol. Inc.* **2020**, *33*, 1458–1465. [CrossRef]

71. Catalano, A.; Graciotti, L.; Rinaldi, L.; Raffaelli, G.; Rodilossi, S.; Betta, P.; Gianni, W.; Amoroso, S.; Procopio, A. Preclinical evaluation of the nonsteroidal anti-inflammatory agent celecoxib on malignant mesothelioma chemoprevention. *Int. J. Cancer* **2004**, *109*, 322–328. [CrossRef] [PubMed]
72. Demetri, G.D.; Zenzie, B.W.; Rheinwald, J.G.; Griffin, J.D. Expression of colony-stimulating factor genes by normal human mesothelial cells and human malignant mesothelioma cells lines in vitro. *Blood* **1989**, *74*, 940–946. [CrossRef] [PubMed]
73. Burt, B.M.; Rodig, S.J.; Tilleman, T.R.; Elbardissi, A.W.; Bueno, R.; Sugarbaker, D.J. Circulating and tumor-infiltrating myeloid cells predict survival in human pleural mesothelioma. *Cancer* **2011**, *117*, 5234–5244. [CrossRef]
74. Chéné, A.L.; d'Almeida, S.; Blondy, T.; Tabiasco, J.; Deshayes, S.; Fonteneau, J.F.; Cellerin, L.; Delneste, Y.; Grégoire, M.; Blanquart, C. Pleural Effusions from Patients with Mesothelioma Induce Recruitment of Monocytes and Their Differentiation into M2 Macrophages. *J. Thorac. Oncol. Off. Publ. Int. Assoc. Study Lung Cancer* **2016**, *11*, 1765–1773. [CrossRef] [PubMed]
75. Schmitter, D.; Lauber, B.; Fagg, B.; Stahel, R.A. Hematopoietic growth factors secreted by seven human pleural mesothelioma cell lines: Interleukin-6 production as a common feature. *Int. J. Cancer* **1992**, *51*, 296–301. [CrossRef] [PubMed]
76. Gueugnon, F.; Leclercq, S.; Blanquart, C.; Sagan, C.; Cellerin, L.; Padieu, M.; Perigaud, C.; Scherpereel, A.; Gregoire, M. Identification of novel markers for the diagnosis of malignant pleural mesothelioma. *Am. J. Pathol.* **2011**, *178*, 1033–1042. [CrossRef] [PubMed]
77. Blanquart, C.; Gueugnon, F.; Nguyen, J.M.; Roulois, D.; Cellerin, L.; Sagan, C.; Perigaud, C.; Scherpereel, A.; Gregoire, M. CCL2, galectin-3, and SMRP combination improves the diagnosis of mesothelioma in pleural effusions. *J. Thorac. Oncol. Off. Publ. Int. Assoc. Study Lung Cancer* **2012**, *7*, 883–889. [CrossRef]
78. Dudek, A.Z.; Pang, H.; Kratzke, R.A.; Otterson, G.A.; Hodgson, L.; Vokes, E.E.; Kindler, H.L. Phase II study of dasatinib in patients with previously treated malignant mesothelioma (cancer and leukemia group B 30601): A brief report. *J. Thorac. Oncol. Off. Publ. Int. Assoc. Study Lung Cancer* **2012**, *7*, 755–759. [CrossRef]
79. Kishimoto, T.; Fujimoto, N.; Ebara, T.; Omori, T.; Oguri, T.; Niimi, A.; Yokoyama, T.; Kato, M.; Usami, I.; Nishio, M.; et al. Serum levels of the chemokine CCL2 are elevated in malignant pleural mesothelioma patients. *Bmc Cancer* **2019**, *19*, 1204. [CrossRef]
80. Zielinski, C.; Knapp, S.; Mascaux, C.; Hirsch, F. Rationale for targeting the immune system through checkpoint molecule blockade in the treatment of non-small-cell lung cancer. *Ann. Oncol* **2013**, *24*, 1170–1179. [CrossRef]
81. Xiang, X.; Yu, P.C.; Long, D.; Liao, X.L.; Zhang, S.; You, X.M.; Zhong, J.H.; Li, L.Q. Prognostic value of PD -L1 expression in patients with primary solid tumors. *Oncotarget* **2018**, *9*, 5058–5072. [CrossRef]
82. Ghanim, B.; Rosenmayr, A.; Stockhammer, P.; Vogl, M.; Celik, A.; Bas, A.; Kurul, I.C.; Akyurek, N.; Varga, A.; Plönes, T.; et al. Tumour cell PD-L1 expression is prognostic in patients with malignant pleural effusion: The impact of C-reactive protein and immune-checkpoint inhibition. *Sci. Rep.* **2020**, *10*, 5784. [CrossRef]
83. Ettinger, D.S.; Wood, D.E.; Aggarwal, C.; Aisner, D.L.; Akerley, W.; Bauman, J.R.; Bharat, A.; Bruno, D.S.; Chang, J.Y.; Chirieac, L.R.; et al. NCCN Guidelines Insights: Non-Small Cell Lung Cancer, Version 1.2020. *J. Natl. Compr. Cancer Netw.* **2019**, *17*, 1464–1472. [CrossRef]
84. Low, J.L.; Walsh, R.J.; Ang, Y.; Chan, G.; Soo, R.A. The evolving immuno-oncology landscape in advanced lung cancer: First-line treatment of non-small cell lung cancer. *Adv. Med. Oncol.* **2019**, *11*, 1758835919870360. [CrossRef]
85. Jin, L.; Gu, W.; Li, X.; Xie, L.; Wang, L.; Chen, Z. PD-L1 and prognosis in patients with malignant pleural mesothelioma: A meta-analysis and bioinformatics study. *Adv. Med. Oncol.* **2020**, *12*, 1758835920962362. [CrossRef]
86. Brosseau, S.; Danel, C.; Scherpereel, A.; Mazières, J.; Lantuejoul, S.; Margery, J.; Greillier, L.; Audigier-Valette, C.; Gounant, V.; Antoine, M.; et al. Shorter Survival in Malignant Pleural Mesothelioma Patients With High PD-L1 Expression Associated With Sarcomatoid or Biphasic Histology Subtype: A Series of 214 Cases From the Bio-MAPS Cohort. *Clin. Lung Cancer* **2019**, *20*, e564–e575. [CrossRef] [PubMed]
87. White, M.G.; Schulte, J.J.; Xue, L.; Berger, Y.; Schuitevoerder, D.; Vining, C.C.; Kindler, H.L.; Husain, A.; Turaga, K.K.; Eng, O.S. Heterogeneity in PD-L1 expression in malignant peritoneal mesothelioma with systemic or intraperitoneal chemotherapy. *Br. J. Cancer* **2020**. [CrossRef] [PubMed]
88. de Gooijer, C.J.; Borm, F.J.; Scherpereel, A.; Baas, P. Immunotherapy in Malignant Pleural Mesothelioma. *Front. Oncol.* **2020**, *10*, 187. [CrossRef] [PubMed]
89. Carosio, R.; Fontana, V.; Mastracci, L.; Ferro, P.; Grillo, F.; Banelli, B.; Canessa, P.A.; Dessanti, P.; Vigani, A.; Morabito, A.; et al. Characterization of soluble PD-L1 in pleural effusions of mesothelioma patients: Potential implications in the immune response and prognosis. *J. Cancer Res. Clin. Oncol.* **2021**, *147*, 459–468. [CrossRef] [PubMed]
90. Yang, H.; Hall, S.R.R.; Sun, B.; Yao, F. Comment on "Heterogeneity in PD-L1 expression in malignant peritoneal mesothelioma with systemic or intraperitoneal chemotherapy". *Br. J. Cancer* **2020**. [CrossRef] [PubMed]
91. Kiyotani, K.; Park, J.H.; Inoue, H.; Husain, A.; Olugbile, S.; Zewde, M.; Nakamura, Y.; Vigneswaran, W.T. Integrated analysis of somatic mutations and immune microenvironment in malignant pleural mesothelioma. *Oncoimmunology* **2017**, *6*, e1278330. [CrossRef] [PubMed]
92. Yang, H.; Xu, D.; Yang, Z.; Yao, F.; Zhao, H.; Schmid, R.A.; Peng, R.W. Systematic Analysis of Aberrant Biochemical Networks and Potential Drug Vulnerabilities Induced by Tumor Suppressor Loss in Malignant Pleural Mesothelioma. *Cancers* **2020**, *12*, 2310. [CrossRef] [PubMed]
93. Yang, H.; Xu, D.; Schmid, R.A.; Peng, R.W. Biomarker-guided targeted and immunotherapies in malignant pleural mesothelioma. *Ther. Adv. Med. Oncol.* **2020**, *12*, 1758835920971421. [CrossRef]

94. Semeniuk-Wojtaś, A.; Lubas, A.; Stec, R.; Syryło, T.; Niemczyk, S.; Szczylik, C. Neutrophil-to-lymphocyte Ratio, Platelet-to-lymphocyte Ratio, and C-reactive Protein as New and Simple Prognostic Factors in Patients With Metastatic Renal Cell Cancer Treated With Tyrosine Kinase Inhibitors: A Systemic Review and Meta-analysis. *Clin. Genitourin. Cancer* **2018**, *16*, e685–e693. [CrossRef] [PubMed]
95. O'Dowd, C.; McRae, L.A.; McMillan, D.C.; Kirk, A.; Milroy, R. Elevated preoperative C-reactive protein predicts poor cancer specific survival in patients undergoing resection for non-small cell lung cancer. *J. Thorac. Oncol. Off. Publ. Int. Assoc. Study Lung Cancer* **2010**, *5*, 988–992. [CrossRef]
96. Liu, Y.; Chen, S.; Zheng, C.; Ding, M.; Zhang, L.; Wang, L.; Xie, M.; Zhou, J. The prognostic value of the preoperative c-reactive protein/albumin ratio in ovarian cancer. *BMC Cancer* **2017**, *17*, 285. [CrossRef] [PubMed]
97. Liu, Z.Q.; Chu, L.; Fang, J.M.; Zhang, X.; Zhao, H.X.; Chen, Y.J.; Xu, Q. Prognostic role of C-reactive protein in prostate cancer: A systematic review and meta-analysis. *Asian J. Androl.* **2014**, *16*, 467–471. [CrossRef]
98. Lin, Y.; Liu, Z.; Qiu, Y.; Zhang, J.; Wu, H.; Liang, R.; Chen, G.; Qin, G.; Li, Y.; Zou, D. Clinical significance of plasma D-dimer and fibrinogen in digestive cancer: A systematic review and meta-analysis. *Eur. J. Surg. Oncol. J. Eur. Soc. Surg. Oncol. Br. Assoc. Surg. Oncol.* **2018**, *44*, 1494–1503. [CrossRef]
99. Liu, Z.; Shi, H.; Chen, L. Prognostic role of pre-treatment C-reactive protein/albumin ratio in esophageal cancer: A meta-analysis. *BMC Cancer* **2019**, *19*, 1161. [CrossRef]
100. Tanrikulu, A.C.; Abakay, A.; Komek, H.; Abakay, O. Prognostic value of the lymphocyte-to-monocyte ratio and other inflammatory markers in malignant pleural mesothelioma. *Environ. Health Prev. Med.* **2016**, *21*, 304–311. [CrossRef]
101. Pinato, D.J.; Mauri, F.A.; Ramakrishnan, R.; Wahab, L.; Lloyd, T.; Sharma, R. Inflammation-based prognostic indices in malignant pleural mesothelioma. *J. Thorac. Oncol. Off. Publ. Int. Assoc. Study Lung Cancer* **2012**, *7*, 587–594. [CrossRef]
102. Otoshi, T.; Kataoka, Y.; Kaku, S.; Iki, R.; Hirabayashi, M. Prognostic Impact of Inflammation-related Biomarkers on Overall Survival of Patients with Inoperable Malignant Pleural Mesothelioma. *Vivo (Athens Greece)* **2018**, *32*, 445–450. [CrossRef]
103. Curran, D.; Sahmoud, T.; Therasse, P.; van Meerbeeck, J.; Postmus, P.E.; Giaccone, G. Prognostic factors in patients with pleural mesothelioma: The European Organization for Research and Treatment of Cancer experience. *J. Clin. Oncol. Off. J. Am. Soc. Clin. Oncol.* **1998**, *16*, 145–152. [CrossRef]
104. Herndon, J.E.; Green, M.R.; Chahinian, A.P.; Corson, J.M.; Suzuki, Y.; Vogelzang, N.J. Factors predictive of survival among 337 patients with mesothelioma treated between 1984 and 1994 by the Cancer and Leukemia Group B. *Chest* **1998**, *113*, 723–731. [CrossRef] [PubMed]
105. Fennell, D.A.; Parmar, A.; Shamash, J.; Evans, M.T.; Sheaff, M.T.; Sylvester, R.; Dhaliwal, K.; Gower, N.; Steele, J.; Rudd, R. Statistical validation of the EORTC prognostic model for malignant pleural mesothelioma based on three consecutive phase II trials. *J. Clin. Oncol. Off. J. Am. Soc. Clin. Oncol.* **2005**, *23*, 184–189. [CrossRef] [PubMed]
106. Meniawy, T.M.; Creaney, J.; Lake, R.A.; Nowak, A.K. Existing models, but not neutrophil-to-lymphocyte ratio, are prognostic in malignant mesothelioma. *Br. J. Cancer* **2013**, *109*, 1813–1820. [CrossRef] [PubMed]
107. Edwards, J.G.; Abrams, K.R.; Leverment, J.N.; Spyt, T.J.; Waller, D.A.; O'Byrne, K.J. Prognostic factors for malignant mesothelioma in 142 patients: Validation of CALGB and EORTC prognostic scoring systems. *Thorax* **2000**, *55*, 731–735. [CrossRef]
108. Sandri, A.; Guerrera, F.; Roffinella, M.; Olivetti, S.; Costardi, L.; Oliaro, A.; Filosso, P.L.; Lausi, P.O.; Ruffini, E. Validation of EORTC and CALGB prognostic models in surgical patients submitted to diagnostic, palliative or curative surgery for malignant pleural mesothelioma. *J. Thorac. Dis.* **2016**, *8*, 2121–2127. [CrossRef]
109. Billé, A.; Krug, L.M.; Woo, K.M.; Rusch, V.W.; Zauderer, M.G. Contemporary Analysis of Prognostic Factors in Patients with Unresectable Malignant Pleural Mesothelioma. *J. Thorac. Oncol. Off. Publ. Int. Assoc. Study Lung Cancer* **2016**, *11*, 249–255. [CrossRef]
110. Zhang, A.; Cao, S.; Jin, S.; Cao, J.; Shen, J.; Pan, B.; Zhu, R.; Yu, Y. Elevated aspartate aminotransferase and monocyte counts predict unfavorable prognosis in patients with malignant pleural mesothelioma. *Neoplasma* **2017**, *64*, 114–122. [CrossRef]
111. Ruffie, P.; Feld, R.; Minkin, S.; Cormier, Y.; Boutan-Laroze, A.; Ginsberg, R.; Ayoub, J.; Shepherd, F.A.; Evans, W.K.; Figueredo, A.; et al. Diffuse malignant mesothelioma of the pleura in Ontario and Quebec: A retrospective study of 332 patients. *J. Clin. Oncol. Off. J. Am. Soc. Clin. Oncol.* **1989**, *7*, 1157–1168. [CrossRef] [PubMed]
112. Baud, M.; Strano, S.; Dechartres, A.; Jouni, R.; Triponez, F.; Chouaid, C.; Forgez, P.; Damotte, D.; Roche, N.; Régnard, J.F.; et al. Outcome and prognostic factors of pleural mesothelioma after surgical diagnosis and/or pleurodesis. *J. Thorac. Cardiovasc. Surg.* **2013**, *145*, 1305–1311. [CrossRef] [PubMed]
113. Bowen, R.C.; Little, N.A.B.; Harmer, J.R.; Ma, J.; Mirabelli, L.G.; Roller, K.D.; Breivik, A.M.; Signor, E.; Miller, A.B.; Khong, H.T. Neutrophil-to-lymphocyte ratio as prognostic indicator in gastrointestinal cancers: A systematic review and meta-analysis. *Oncotarget* **2017**, *8*, 32171–32189. [CrossRef] [PubMed]
114. Janik, S.; Raunegger, T.; Hacker, P.; Ghanim, B.; Einwallner, E.; Müllauer, L.; Schiefer, A.I.; Moser, J.; Klepetko, W.; Ankersmit, H.J.; et al. Prognostic and diagnostic impact of fibrinogen, neutrophil-to-lymphocyte ratio, and platelet-to-lymphocyte ratio on thymic epithelial tumors outcome. *Oncotarget* **2018**, *9*, 21861–21875. [CrossRef] [PubMed]
115. Ethier, J.L.; Desautels, D.; Templeton, A.; Shah, P.S.; Amir, E. Prognostic role of neutrophil-to-lymphocyte ratio in breast cancer: A systematic review and meta-analysis. *Breast Cancer Res. Bcr* **2017**, *19*, 2. [CrossRef] [PubMed]
116. Haram, A.; Boland, M.R.; Kelly, M.E.; Bolger, J.C.; Waldron, R.M.; Kerin, M.J. The prognostic value of neutrophil-to-lymphocyte ratio in colorectal cancer: A systematic review. *J. Surg. Oncol.* **2017**, *115*, 470–479. [CrossRef]

117. Diem, S.; Schmid, S.; Krapf, M.; Flatz, L.; Born, D.; Jochum, W.; Templeton, A.J.; Früh, M. Neutrophil-to-Lymphocyte ratio (NLR) and Platelet-to-Lymphocyte ratio (PLR) as prognostic markers in patients with non-small cell lung cancer (NSCLC) treated with nivolumab. *Lung Cancer (Amst. Neth.)* **2017**, *111*, 176–181. [CrossRef]
118. Kiriu, T.; Yamamoto, M.; Nagano, T.; Hazama, D.; Sekiya, R.; Katsurada, M.; Tamura, D.; Tachihara, M.; Kobayashi, K.; Nishimura, Y. The time-series behavior of neutrophil-to-lymphocyte ratio is useful as a predictive marker in non-small cell lung cancer. *PLoS ONE* **2018**, *13*, e0193018. [CrossRef]
119. Yodying, H.; Matsuda, A.; Miyashita, M.; Matsumoto, S.; Sakurazawa, N.; Yamada, M.; Uchida, E. Prognostic Significance of Neutrophil-to-Lymphocyte Ratio and Platelet-to-Lymphocyte Ratio in Oncologic Outcomes of Esophageal Cancer: A Systematic Review and Meta-analysis. *Ann. Surg. Oncol.* **2016**, *23*, 646–654. [CrossRef]
120. Ghanim, B.; Schweiger, T.; Jedamzik, J.; Glueck, O.; Glogner, C.; Lang, G.; Klepetko, W.; Hoetzenecker, K. Elevated inflammatory parameters and inflammation scores are associated with poor prognosis in patients undergoing pulmonary metastasectomy for colorectal cancer. *Interact. Cardiovasc. Thorac. Surg.* **2015**, *21*, 616–623. [CrossRef]
121. Kao, S.C.; Pavlakis, N.; Harvie, R.; Vardy, J.L.; Boyer, M.J.; van Zandwijk, N.; Clarke, S.J. High blood neutrophil-to-lymphocyte ratio is an indicator of poor prognosis in malignant mesothelioma patients undergoing systemic therapy. *Clin. Cancer Res. Off. J. Am. Assoc. Cancer Res.* **2010**, *16*, 5805–5813. [CrossRef]
122. Kao, S.C.; Klebe, S.; Henderson, D.W.; Reid, G.; Chatfield, M.; Armstrong, N.J.; Yan, T.D.; Vardy, J.; Clarke, S.; van Zandwijk, N.; et al. Low calretinin expression and high neutrophil-to-lymphocyte ratio are poor prognostic factors in patients with malignant mesothelioma undergoing extrapleural pneumonectomy. *J. Thorac. Oncol. Off. Publ. Int. Assoc. Study Lung Cancer* **2011**, *6*, 1923–1929. [CrossRef]
123. Gu, L.; Li, H.; Chen, L.; Ma, X.; Li, X.; Gao, Y.; Zhang, Y.; Xie, Y.; Zhang, X. Prognostic role of lymphocyte to monocyte ratio for patients with cancer: Evidence from a systematic review and meta-analysis. *Oncotarget* **2016**, *7*, 31926–31942. [CrossRef]
124. Yin, W.; Zheng, G.; Su, S.; Liang, Y. The Value of COX-2, NF-κB, and Blood Routine Indexes in the Prognosis of Malignant Peritoneal Mesothelioma. *Oncol. Res. Treat.* **2019**, *42*, 334–341. [CrossRef]
125. Li, B.; Zhou, P.; Liu, Y.; Wei, H.; Yang, X.; Chen, T.; Xiao, J. Platelet-to-lymphocyte ratio in advanced Cancer: Review and meta-analysis. *Clin. Chim. Acta Int. J. Clin. Chem.* **2018**, *483*, 48–56. [CrossRef] [PubMed]
126. Gabay, C.; Kushner, I. Acute-phase proteins and other systemic responses to inflammation. *N. Engl. J. Med.* **1999**, *340*, 448–454. [CrossRef] [PubMed]
127. Chen, N.; Li, W.; Huang, K.; Yang, W.; Huang, L.; Cong, T.; Li, Q.; Qiu, M. Increased platelet-lymphocyte ratio closely relates to inferior clinical features and worse long-term survival in both resected and metastatic colorectal cancer: An updated systematic review and meta-analysis of 24 studies. *Oncotarget* **2017**, *8*, 32356–32369. [CrossRef]
128. Zhou, Y.; Cheng, S.; Fathy, A.H.; Qian, H.; Zhao, Y. Prognostic value of platelet-to-lymphocyte ratio in pancreatic cancer: A comprehensive meta-analysis of 17 cohort studies. *Oncotargets Ther.* **2018**, *11*, 1899–1908. [CrossRef] [PubMed]
129. Zhang, H.; Gao, L.; Zhang, B.; Zhang, L.; Wang, C. Prognostic value of platelet to lymphocyte ratio in non-small cell lung cancer: A systematic review and meta-analysis. *Sci. Rep.* **2016**, *6*, 22618. [CrossRef] [PubMed]
130. Nakano, T.; Chahinian, A.P.; Shinjo, M.; Tonomura, A.; Miyake, M.; Togawa, N.; Ninomiya, K.; Higashino, K. Interleukin 6 and its relationship to clinical parameters in patients with malignant pleural mesothelioma. *Br. J. Cancer* **1998**, *77*, 907–912. [CrossRef]
131. Monti, G.; Jaurand, M.C.; Monnet, I.; Chretien, P.; Saint-Etienne, L.; Zeng, L.; Portier, A.; Devillier, P.; Galanaud, P.; Bignon, J.; et al. Intrapleural production of interleukin 6 during mesothelioma and its modulation by gamma-interferon treatment. *Cancer Res.* **1994**, *54*, 4419–4423.
132. Hunter, C.A.; Jones, S.A. IL-6 as a keystone cytokine in health and disease. *Nat. Immunol.* **2015**, *16*, 448–457. [CrossRef] [PubMed]
133. Abdul Rahim, S.N.; Ho, G.Y.; Coward, J.I. The role of interleukin-6 in malignant mesothelioma. *Transl. Lung Cancer Res.* **2015**, *4*, 55–66. [CrossRef] [PubMed]
134. Scambia, G.; Testa, U.; Benedetti Panici, P.; Foti, E.; Martucci, R.; Gadducci, A.; Perillo, A.; Facchini, V.; Peschle, C.; Mancuso, S. Prognostic significance of interleukin 6 serum levels in patients with ovarian cancer. *Br. J. Cancer* **1995**, *71*, 354–356. [CrossRef] [PubMed]
135. Bachelot, T.; Ray-Coquard, I.; Menetrier-Caux, C.; Rastkha, M.; Duc, A.; Blay, J.Y. Prognostic value of serum levels of interleukin 6 and of serum and plasma levels of vascular endothelial growth factor in hormone-refractory metastatic breast cancer patients. *Br. J. Cancer* **2003**, *88*, 1721–1726. [CrossRef]
136. Vainer, N.; Dehlendorff, C.; Johansen, J.S. Systematic literature review of IL-6 as a biomarker or treatment target in patients with gastric, bile duct, pancreatic and colorectal cancer. *Oncotarget* **2018**, *9*, 29820–29841. [CrossRef]
137. Hao, W.; Zhu, Y.; Zhou, H. Prognostic value of interleukin-6 and interleukin-8 in laryngeal squamous cell cancer. *Med. Oncol. (Northwood Lond. Engl.)* **2013**, *30*, 333. [CrossRef]
138. Chang, C.H.; Hsiao, C.F.; Yeh, Y.M.; Chang, G.C.; Tsai, Y.H.; Chen, Y.M.; Huang, M.S.; Chen, H.L.; Li, Y.J.; Yang, P.C.; et al. Circulating interleukin-6 level is a prognostic marker for survival in advanced nonsmall cell lung cancer patients treated with chemotherapy. *Int. J. Cancer* **2013**, *132*, 1977–1985. [CrossRef]
139. Ujiie, H.; Tomida, M.; Akiyama, H.; Nakajima, Y.; Okada, D.; Yoshino, N.; Takiguchi, Y.; Tanzawa, H. Serum hepatocyte growth factor and interleukin-6 are effective prognostic markers for non-small cell lung cancer. *Anticancer Res.* **2012**, *32*, 3251–3258.

140. Jia, Y.; Li, X.; Zhao, C.; Jiang, T.; Zhao, S.; Zhang, L.; Liu, X.; Shi, J.; Qiao, M.; Luo, J.; et al. Impact of serum vascular endothelial growth factor and interleukin-6 on treatment response to epidermal growth factor receptor tyrosine kinase inhibitors in patients with non-small-cell lung cancer. *Lung Cancer (Amst. Neth.)* **2018**, *125*, 22–28. [CrossRef]
141. Kallio, J.; Hämäläinen, M.; Luukkaala, T.; Moilanen, E.; Tammela, T.L.; Kellokumpu-Lehtinen, P.L. Resistin and interleukin 6 as predictive factors for recurrence and long-term prognosis in renal cell cancer. *Urol. Oncol.* **2017**, *35*, 544.e525–544.e531. [CrossRef]
142. Kang, D.H.; Park, C.K.; Chung, C.; Oh, I.J.; Kim, Y.C.; Park, D.; Kim, J.; Kwon, G.C.; Kwon, I.; Sun, P.; et al. Baseline Serum Interleukin-6 Levels Predict the Response of Patients with Advanced Non-small Cell Lung Cancer to PD-1/PD-L1 Inhibitors. *Immune Netw.* **2020**, *20*, e27. [CrossRef]
143. Pilskog, M.; Nilsen, G.H.; Beisland, C.; Straume, O. Elevated plasma interleukin 6 predicts poor response in patients treated with sunitinib for metastatic clear cell renal cell carcinoma. *Cancer Treat. Res. Commun.* **2019**, *19*, 100127. [CrossRef]
144. Chen, M.F.; Chen, P.T.; Lu, M.S.; Lin, P.Y.; Chen, W.C.; Lee, K.D. IL-6 expression predicts treatment response and outcome in squamous cell carcinoma of the esophagus. *Mol. Cancer* **2013**, *12*, 26. [CrossRef]
145. Kao, S.C.; Harvie, R.; Paturi, F.; Taylor, R.; Davey, R.; Abraham, R.; Clarke, S.; Marx, G.; Cullen, M.; Kerestes, Z.; et al. The predictive role of serum VEGF in an advanced malignant mesothelioma patient cohort treated with thalidomide alone or combined with cisplatin/gemcitabine. *Lung Cancer (Amst. Neth.)* **2012**, *75*, 248–254. [CrossRef] [PubMed]
146. Edwards, J.G.; Cox, G.; Andi, A.; Jones, J.L.; Walker, R.A.; Waller, D.A.; O'Byrne, K.J. Angiogenesis is an independent prognostic factor in malignant mesothelioma. *Br. J. Cancer* **2001**, *85*, 863–868. [CrossRef] [PubMed]
147. Strizzi, L.; Catalano, A.; Vianale, G.; Orecchia, S.; Casalini, A.; Tassi, G.; Puntoni, R.; Mutti, L.; Procopio, A. Vascular endothelial growth factor is an autocrine growth factor in human malignant mesothelioma. *J. Pathol.* **2001**, *193*, 468–475. [CrossRef] [PubMed]
148. Adachi, Y.; Aoki, C.; Yoshio-Hoshino, N.; Takayama, K.; Curiel, D.T.; Nishimoto, N. Interleukin-6 induces both cell growth and VEGF production in malignant mesotheliomas. *Int. J. Cancer* **2006**, *119*, 1303–1311. [CrossRef] [PubMed]
149. Adachi, Y.; Yoshio-Hoshino, N.; Aoki, C.; Nishimoto, N. VEGF targeting in mesotheliomas using an interleukin-6 signal inhibitor based on adenovirus gene delivery. *Anticancer Res.* **2010**, *30*, 1947–1952.
150. Nowak, A.K.; Brosseau, S.; Cook, A.; Zalcman, G. Antiangiogeneic Strategies in Mesothelioma. *Front. Oncol.* **2020**, *10*, 126. [CrossRef]
151. Vogelzang, N.J.; Rusthoven, J.J.; Symanowski, J.; Denham, C.; Kaukel, E.; Ruffie, P.; Gatzemeier, U.; Boyer, M.; Emri, S.; Manegold, C.; et al. Phase III study of pemetrexed in combination with cisplatin versus cisplatin alone in patients with malignant pleural mesothelioma. *J. Clin. Oncol. Off. J. Am. Soc. Clin. Oncol.* **2003**, *21*, 2636–2644. [CrossRef] [PubMed]
152. Zalcman, G.; Mazieres, J.; Margery, J.; Greillier, L.; Audigier-Valette, C.; Moro-Sibilot, D.; Molinier, O.; Corre, R.; Monnet, I.; Gounant, V.; et al. Bevacizumab for newly diagnosed pleural mesothelioma in the Mesothelioma Avastin Cisplatin Pemetrexed Study (MAPS): A randomised, controlled, open-label, phase 3 trial. *Lancet* **2016**, *387*, 1405–1414. [CrossRef]
153. Tillett, W.S.; Francis, T. Serological Reactions in Pneumonia with a Non-Protein Somatic Fraction of Pneumococcus. *J. Exp. Med.* **1930**, *52*, 561–571. [CrossRef] [PubMed]
154. Pepys, M.B.; Hirschfield, G.M. C-reactive protein: A critical update. *J. Clin. Investig.* **2003**, *111*, 1805–1812. [CrossRef]
155. Black, S.; Kushner, I.; Samols, D. C-reactive Protein. *J. Biol. Chem.* **2004**, *279*, 48487–48490. [CrossRef]
156. Ibuki, Y.; Hamai, Y.; Hihara, J.; Emi, M.; Taomoto, J.; Furukawa, T.; Yamakita, I.; Kurokawa, T.; Okada, M. Role of Postoperative C-Reactive Protein Levels in Predicting Prognosis After Surgical Treatment of Esophageal Cancer. *World J. Surg.* **2017**, *41*, 1558–1565. [CrossRef]
157. Yu, Q.; Yu, X.F.; Zhang, S.D.; Wang, H.H.; Wang, H.Y.; Teng, L.S. Prognostic role of C-reactive protein in gastric cancer: A meta-analysis. *Asian Pac. J. Cancer Prev. APJCP* **2013**, *14*, 5735–5740. [CrossRef]
158. Janik, S.; Bekos, C.; Hacker, P.; Raunegger, T.; Ghanim, B.; Einwallner, E.; Beer, L.; Klepetko, W.; Müllauer, L.; Ankersmit, H.J.; et al. Elevated CRP levels predict poor outcome and tumor recurrence in patients with thymic epithelial tumors: A pro- and retrospective analysis. *Oncotarget* **2017**, *8*, 47090–47102. [CrossRef]
159. Nojiri, S.; Gemba, K.; Aoe, K.; Kato, K.; Yamaguchi, T.; Sato, T.; Kubota, K.; Kishimoto, T. Survival and prognostic factors in malignant pleural mesothelioma: A retrospective study of 314 patients in the west part of Japan. *Jpn. J. Clin. Oncol.* **2011**, *41*, 32–39. [CrossRef]
160. Kao, S.C.; Vardy, J.; Harvie, R.; Chatfield, M.; van Zandwijk, N.; Clarke, S.; Pavlakis, N. Health-related quality of life and inflammatory markers in malignant pleural mesothelioma. *Supportive Care Cancer Off. J. Multinatl. Assoc. Supportive Care Cancer* **2013**, *21*, 697–705. [CrossRef]
161. Duvoix, A.; Dickens, J.; Haq, I.; Mannino, D.; Miller, B.; Tal-Singer, R.; Lomas, D.A. Blood fibrinogen as a biomarker of chronic obstructive pulmonary disease. *Thorax* **2013**, *68*, 670–676. [CrossRef] [PubMed]
162. Rosenson, R.S.; Koenig, W. Utility of inflammatory markers in the management of coronary artery disease. *Am. J. Cardiol.* **2003**, *92*, 10i–18i. [CrossRef]
163. Zhang, Y.; Cao, J.; Deng, Y.; Huang, Y.; Li, R.; Lin, G.; Dong, M.; Huang, Z. Pretreatment plasma fibrinogen level as a prognostic biomarker for patients with lung cancer. *Clinics (Sao Paulo Braz.)* **2020**, *75*, e993. [CrossRef] [PubMed]
164. Li, M.; Wu, Y.; Zhang, J.; Huang, L.; Wu, X.; Yuan, Y. Prognostic value of pretreatment plasma fibrinogen in patients with colorectal cancer: A systematic review and meta-analysis. *Medicine* **2019**, *98*, e16974. [CrossRef] [PubMed]
165. Cheng, F.; Zeng, C.; Zeng, L.; Chen, Y. Clinicopathological and prognostic value of preoperative plasma fibrinogen in gastric cancer patients: A meta-analysis. *Medicine* **2019**, *98*, e17310. [CrossRef]

166. Perisanidis, C.; Psyrri, A.; Cohen, E.E.; Engelmann, J.; Heinze, G.; Perisanidis, B.; Stift, A.; Filipits, M.; Kornek, G.; Nkenke, E. Prognostic role of pretreatment plasma fibrinogen in patients with solid tumors: A systematic review and meta-analysis. *Cancer Treat. Rev.* **2015**, *41*, 960–970. [CrossRef]
167. Seebacher, V.; Polterauer, S.; Grimm, C.; Husslein, H.; Leipold, H.; Hefler-Frischmuth, K.; Tempfer, C.; Reinthaller, A.; Hefler, L. The prognostic value of plasma fibrinogen levels in patients with endometrial cancer: A multi-centre trial. *Br. J. Cancer* **2010**, *102*, 952–956. [CrossRef]
168. Gupta, D.; Lis, C.G. Pretreatment serum albumin as a predictor of cancer survival: A systematic review of the epidemiological literature. *Nutr. J.* **2010**, *9*, 69. [CrossRef]
169. Cross, M.B.; Yi, P.H.; Thomas, C.F.; Garcia, J.; Della Valle, C.J. Evaluation of malnutrition in orthopaedic surgery. *J. Am. Acad. Orthop. Surg.* **2014**, *22*, 193–199. [CrossRef] [PubMed]
170. Hsieh, W.C.; Aboud, A.; Henry, B.M.; Omara, M.; Lindner, J.; Pirk, J. Serum albumin in patients undergoing transcatheter aortic valve replacement: A meta-analysis. *Rev. Cardiovasc. Med.* **2019**, *20*, 161–169. [CrossRef] [PubMed]
171. Karas, P.L.; Goh, S.L.; Dhital, K. Is low serum albumin associated with postoperative complications in patients undergoing cardiac surgery? *Interact. Cardiovasc. Thorac. Surg.* **2015**, *21*, 777–786. [CrossRef] [PubMed]
172. Salvetti, D.J.; Tempel, Z.J.; Goldschmidt, E.; Colwell, N.A.; Angriman, F.; Panczykowski, D.M.; Agarwal, N.; Kanter, A.S.; Okonkwo, D.O. Low preoperative serum prealbumin levels and the postoperative surgical site infection risk in elective spine surgery: A consecutive series. *J. Neurosurg. Spine* **2018**, *29*, 549–552. [CrossRef] [PubMed]
173. Loftus, T.J.; Brown, M.P.; Slish, J.H.; Rosenthal, M.D. Serum Levels of Prealbumin and Albumin for Preoperative Risk Stratification. *Nutr. Clin. Pract. Off. Publ. Am. Soc. Parenter. Enter. Nutr.* **2019**, *34*, 340–348. [CrossRef] [PubMed]
174. Yao, Z.H.; Tian, G.Y.; Yang, S.X.; Wan, Y.Y.; Kang, Y.M.; Liu, Q.H.; Yao, F.; Lin, D.J. Serum albumin as a significant prognostic factor in patients with malignant pleural mesothelioma. *Tumour Biol. J. Int. Soc. Oncodev. Biol. Med.* **2014**, *35*, 6839–6845. [CrossRef] [PubMed]
175. Harris, E.J.A.; Kao, S.; McCaughan, B.; Nakano, T.; Kondo, N.; Hyland, R.; Nowak, A.K.; de Klerk, N.H.; Brims, F.J.H. Prediction modelling using routine clinical parameters to stratify survival in Malignant Pleural Mesothelioma patients undergoing cytoreductive surgery. *J. Thorac. Oncol. Off. Publ. Int. Assoc. Study Lung Cancer* **2019**, *14*, 288–293. [CrossRef] [PubMed]
176. Brims, F.J.; Meniawy, T.M.; Duffus, I.; de Fonseka, D.; Segal, A.; Creaney, J.; Maskell, N.; Lake, R.A.; de Klerk, N.; Nowak, A.K. A Novel Clinical Prediction Model for Prognosis in Malignant Pleural Mesothelioma Using Decision Tree Analysis. *J. Thorac. Oncol. Off. Publ. Int. Assoc. Study Lung Cancer* **2016**, *11*, 573–582. [CrossRef]
177. McMillan, D.C. The systemic inflammation-based Glasgow Prognostic Score: A decade of experience in patients with cancer. *Cancer Treat. Rev.* **2013**, *39*, 534–540. [CrossRef]
178. Fairclough, E.; Cairns, E.; Hamilton, J.; Kelly, C. Evaluation of a modified early warning system for acute medical admissions and comparison with C-reactive protein/albumin ratio as a predictor of patient outcome. *Clin. Med. (Lond. Engl.)* **2009**, *9*, 30–33. [CrossRef] [PubMed]
179. Ranzani, O.T.; Zampieri, F.G.; Forte, D.N.; Azevedo, L.C.; Park, M. C-reactive protein/albumin ratio predicts 90-day mortality of septic patients. *PLoS ONE* **2013**, *8*, e59321. [CrossRef] [PubMed]
180. Kudou, K.; Saeki, H.; Nakashima, Y.; Kamori, T.; Kawazoe, T.; Haruta, Y.; Fujimoto, Y.; Matsuoka, H.; Sasaki, S.; Jogo, T.; et al. C-reactive protein/albumin ratio is a poor prognostic factor of esophagogastric junction and upper gastric cancer. *J. Gastroenterol. Hepatol.* **2019**, *34*, 355–363. [CrossRef]
181. Xie, Q.; Wang, L.; Zheng, S. Prognostic and Clinicopathological Significance of C-Reactive Protein to Albumin Ratio in Patients With Pancreatic Cancer: A Meta-Analysis. *Dose-Response A Publ. Int. Hormesis Soc.* **2020**, *18*, 1559325820931290. [CrossRef]
182. Deng, T.B.; Zhang, J.; Zhou, Y.Z.; Li, W.M. The prognostic value of C-reactive protein to albumin ratio in patients with lung cancer. *Medicine* **2018**, *97*, e13505. [CrossRef]
183. Wang, F.; Li, P.; Li, F.S. Prognostic role of C-reactive protein to albumin ratio in colorectal cancer: A meta analysis. *Medicine* **2019**, *98*, e16064. [CrossRef]
184. Takamori, S.; Toyokawa, G.; Shimokawa, M.; Kinoshita, F.; Kozuma, Y.; Matsubara, T.; Haratake, N.; Akamine, T.; Hirai, F.; Seto, T.; et al. The C-Reactive Protein/Albumin Ratio is a Novel Significant Prognostic Factor in Patients with Malignant Pleural Mesothelioma: A Retrospective Multi-institutional Study. *Ann. Surg. Oncol.* **2018**, *25*, 1555–1563. [CrossRef] [PubMed]
185. Thachil, J. The beneficial effect of acute phase increase in serum ferritin. *Eur. J. Intern. Med.* **2016**, *35*, e16–e17. [CrossRef] [PubMed]
186. Kernan, K.F.; Carcillo, J.A. Hyperferritinemia and inflammation. *Int. Immunol.* **2017**, *29*, 401–409. [CrossRef] [PubMed]
187. Hsu, M.Y.; Mina, E.; Roetto, A.; Porporato, P.E. Iron: An Essential Element of Cancer Metabolism. *Cells* **2020**, *9*, 2591. [CrossRef]
188. Toyokuni, S. Iron addiction with ferroptosis-resistance in asbestos-induced mesothelial carcinogenesis: Toward the era of mesothelioma prevention. *Free Radic. Biol. Med.* **2019**, *133*, 206–215. [CrossRef]
189. Döngel, İ.; Akbaş, A.; Benli, İ.; Bayram, M. Comparison of serum biochemical markers in patients with mesothelioma and pleural plaques versus healthy individuals exposed to environmental asbestos. *Turk. Gogus Kalp Damar Cerrahisi Derg.* **2019**, *27*, 374–380. [CrossRef]
190. Sezgi, C.; Taylan, M.; Sen, H.S.; Evliyaoğlu, O.; Kaya, H.; Abakay, O.; Abakay, A.; Tanrıkulu, A.C.; Senyiğit, A. Oxidative status and acute phase reactants in patients with environmental asbestos exposure and mesothelioma. *Sci. World J.* **2014**, *2014*, 902748. [CrossRef] [PubMed]

191. Jiang, L.; Akatsuka, S.; Nagai, H.; Chew, S.H.; Ohara, H.; Okazaki, Y.; Yamashita, Y.; Yoshikawa, Y.; Yasui, H.; Ikuta, K.; et al. Iron overload signature in chrysotile-induced malignant mesothelioma. *J. Pathol.* **2012**, *228*, 366–377. [CrossRef] [PubMed]
192. Ohara, Y.; Chew, S.H.; Shibata, T.; Okazaki, Y.; Yamashita, K.; Toyokuni, S. Phlebotomy as a preventive measure for crocidolite-induced mesothelioma in male rats. *Cancer Sci.* **2018**, *109*, 330–339. [CrossRef] [PubMed]
193. Agostinis, C.; Vidergar, R.; Belmonte, B.; Mangogna, A.; Amadio, L.; Geri, P.; Borelli, V.; Zanconati, F.; Tedesco, F.; Confalonieri, M.; et al. Complement Protein C1q Binds to Hyaluronic Acid in the Malignant Pleural Mesothelioma Microenvironment and Promotes Tumor Growth. *Front. Immunol.* **2017**, *8*, 1559. [CrossRef] [PubMed]

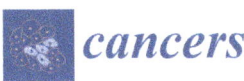

Review

Pathological Characterization of Tumor Immune Microenvironment (TIME) in Malignant Pleural Mesothelioma

Francesca Napoli [1], Angela Listì [2], Vanessa Zambelli [1], Gianluca Witel [3], Paolo Bironzo [1,2], Mauro Papotti [1,4], Marco Volante [1], Giorgio Scagliotti [1,2,†] and Luisella Righi [1,*,†]

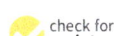

1. Department of Oncology, University of Turin, 10043 Orbassano, Italy; francesca.napoli@unito.it (F.N.); vanessa.zambelli@unito.it (V.Z.); paolo.bironzo@unito.it (P.B.); mauro.papotti@unito.it (M.P.); marco.volante@unito.it (M.V.); giorgio.scagliotti@unito.it (G.S.)
2. Thoracic Oncology Unit, San Luigi Hospital, 10043 Orbassano, Italy; alisti@live.it
3. Department of Medical Sciences, University of Turin, City of Health and Science, 10126 Torino, Italy; gianlucarobert.witel@unito.it
4. Pathology Unit, City of Health and Science, 10126 Torino, Italy
* Correspondence: luisella.righi@unito.it
† These are co-last authors.

Simple Summary: Tumor immune microenvironment is an important structural component of malignant pleural mesothelioma that contributes to disease growth support and progression. Its study and pathological characterization are important tools to find new biomarkers for advanced therapeutic strategies.

Abstract: Malignant pleural mesothelioma (MPM) is a rare and highly aggressive disease that arises from pleural mesothelial cells, characterized by a median survival of approximately 13–15 months after diagnosis. The primary cause of this disease is asbestos exposure and the main issues associated with it are late diagnosis and lack of effective therapies. Asbestos-induced cellular damage is associated with the generation of an inflammatory microenvironment that influences and supports tumor growth, possibly in association with patients' genetic predisposition and tumor genomic profile. The chronic inflammatory response to asbestos fibers leads to a unique tumor immune microenvironment (TIME) composed of a heterogeneous mixture of stromal, endothelial, and immune cells, and relative composition and interaction among them is suggested to bear prognostic and therapeutic implications. TIME in MPM is known to be constituted by immunosuppressive cells, such as type 2 tumor-associated macrophages and T regulatory lymphocytes, plus the expression of several immunosuppressive factors, such as tumor-associated PD-L1. Several studies in recent years have contributed to achieve a greater understanding of the pathogenetic mechanisms in tumor development and pathobiology of TIME, that opens the way to new therapeutic strategies. The study of TIME is fundamental in identifying appropriate prognostic and predictive tissue biomarkers. In the present review, we summarize the current knowledge about the pathological characterization of TIME in MPM.

Keywords: mesothelioma; tumor microenvironment; tumor-associated macrophages; dendritic cells; immunohistochemistry

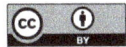

1. Introduction

Malignant pleural mesothelioma (MPM) is a rare and highly aggressive disease arising from pleural mesothelial cells. The recognized risk factors of MPM are asbestos, radiation exposure, genetic mutations, and the exposition to Simian Virus 40, but asbestos is certainly the most relevant and most well-known cause [1]. The overall prognosis of advanced stage MPM is poor, with a median survival of less than 15 months [2]. MPM consists of three histological variants: epithelioid (~60% of mesotheliomas), sarcomatoid, characterized by spindle cell morphology (~20% of mesotheliomas), and biphasic, which presents both epithelioid and sarcomatoid features (~20% of mesotheliomas) [3]. Diagnosis of MPM relies on an integration of clinical, radiological, and pathological findings, with histological examination being the mainstay for diagnosis and prognostication [4,5]. Since MPM is diagnosed in advanced stage in the majority of cases, the standard of care consists in systemic chemotherapy. However, the standard combination of cisplatin and pemetrexed chemotherapy agents [6] prolongs the median survival time by approximately 3 months only [7]. In the last years, genetic studies on MPM reported a low prevalence of oncogene driver mutations and low tumor mutational burden, but frequent copy-number losses and recurrent somatic mutations in oncosuppressor genes such as BAP1, NF2, and CDKN2A [8–13]. Unfortunately, no targeted therapies exploiting these alterations have emerged.

The etiopathogenetic evolution of MPM is mostly due to the generation of a tumor immune microenvironment (TIME) as a consequence of asbestos-induced damage, that may support tumor growth, possibly in association to genetic predisposition [14,15]. Over time, chronic inflammation determines an increased production of free radicals and reactive oxygen species by inflammatory cells and/or an alteration of immunocompetent cells, resulting in a reduction of tumor immunity [16].

The unique role of TIME in MPM development and progression still needs an accurate characterization in terms of infiltrating cell types, expression of co-inhibitory molecules, and activation of immune pathways (e.g., INFγ). As histological examination remains the gold standard in the diagnosis of MPM, the characterization of TIME could be crucial to visualize all cellular components and achieve a better understanding of the disease. Despite the different biological and clinical features between pleural and peritoneal mesothelioma [17], the presence of tertiary lymphoid structures (TLS) as a component of the host immune response was highlighted in epithelioid peritoneal mesothelioma (EMPM), as well. However, no association between TLS-EMPM and different oncological outcomes was found, thus suggesting that TLS would reflect an indirect mechanism of therapy resistance to drugs in EMPM as in its pleural counterpart [18].

Given the role of TIME in MPM, the use of immune checkpoint inhibition treatment has the rationale to provide new potential therapeutic opportunities. Indeed, the combination of monoclonal antibodies directed against programmed cell death protein 1 (PD-1) and cytotoxic T-lymphocyte-associated protein 4 (CTLA-4) recently showed its superiority over platinum-pemetrexed chemotherapy in a phase 3 trial [19]. Notably, a greater benefit was observed in biphasic/sarcomatoid MPM. Moreover, single-agent anti-PD-1 therapy demonstrated to significantly increase survival as compared to best supportive care in platinum pre-treated patients [20].

Another novel potential treatment in MPM is cell therapy. Clinical trials using CAR-T cells in MPM have shown that this potential therapy is relatively safe, but efficacy remains modest, likely due to the strong immunosuppressive conditions in MPM microenvironment [21,22]. Furthermore, preclinical studies are ongoing in a bimodal treatment approach consisting of dendritic cell (DC) vaccination to prime tumor-specific T cells, a strategy to reprogram the desmoplastic microenvironment in mesothelioma and pancreatic cancer [23].

The most adequate tissue specimens for MPM pathological characterization derive from video-assisted thoracoscopic (VATS) biopsies or pleurectomies, which are the recommended samples for complete histological diagnosis [2,3,7]. The availability of large amounts of tissue allows both the definition of histological tumor features and immune cells' spatial distribution on routine hematoxylin-eosin slide. On these specimens, the cheapest and fastest tool used for pathological characterization studies is immunohistochemistry (IHC), that allows to visualize both tumor cells and microenvironment components, according to their immunophenotype and biomarker expression (Figure 1). Despite its advantages, a limitation of chromogen-based IHC analysis is the impossibility of using more than one or two markers per slide. Novel and innovative multiplex immunophenotyping techniques are in development to deeply analyze as a whole both the spatial distribution and immunophenotypic interaction of each single cell subtype [24–26].

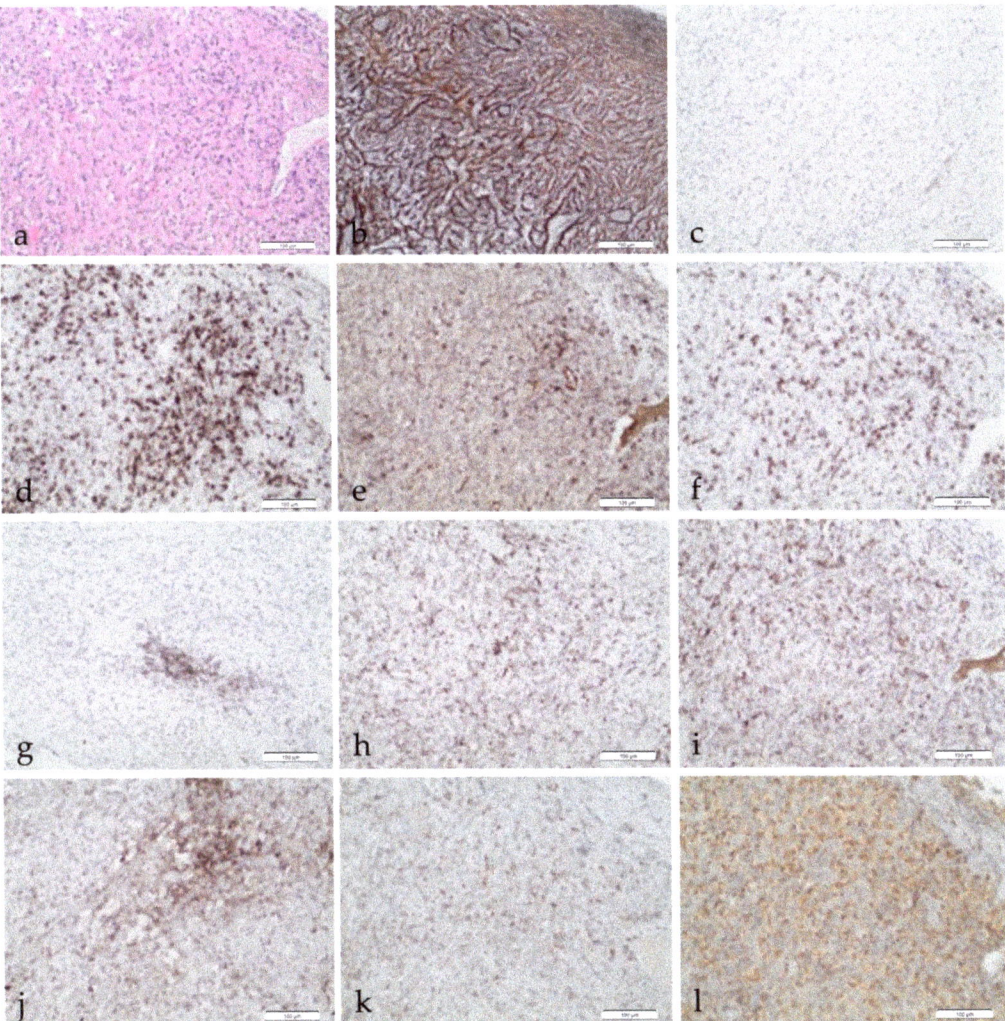

Figure 1. Pathological characterization of TIME in MPM. Histological appearance of MPM, epithelioid type (**a**), Ematoxilin & eosin (100×); reticulin stain showing connective tissue around neoplastic cells (**b**), (100×); SMA IHC stain showing scattered fibrocytes (**c**), (100×); CD3 IHC stain highlighting T lymphocytes (**d**), (100×); CD4 IHC stain showing scattered T cells (**e**), (100×); CD8 IHC stain showing moderate T lymphocyte infiltrate (**f**), (100×); CD20 IHC stain showing a small aggregate of B lymphocytes (**g**), (100×); CD68 IHC stain showing diffuse macrophage infiltration (**h**), (100×); CD163 IHC stain showing activated TAMs (**i**), (100×); PD-L1 IHC stain showing small aggregates of positive tumor cells (**j**), (100×); VISTA IHC stain showing moderate expression in immune cells (**k**), (100×); STING IHC stain showing diffuse immune cell positivity (**l**), (100×). Notes: TIME: tumor immune microenvironment; MPM: malignant pleural mesothelioma; SMA: smooth muscle actin; IHC: immunohistochemistry; PD-L1: programmed death ligand 1; VISTA: V-domain Ig-containing suppressor of T-cell activation; STING: STimulator of Interferon Genes.

Given the need to explore TIME in its components and constituents, in this review, we summarize the current data on TIME pathological characterization and biomarker identification in MPM.

2. The Tumor Immune Microenvironment

TIME is a complex and heterogeneous mixture of stromal, endothelial, and immune cells admixed in a connective matrix and its composition differs among individuals and histological types. In fact, studies suggest that TIME profoundly differs between epithelioid and non-epithelioid pleural mesotheliomas: the former typically have an immune-activated TIME with greater proportion of plasmacytoid dendritic cells (DC), CD20+ B cells, CD4+ helper T cells, and exhausted CD8+ tumor-infiltrating lymphocytes (TILs), whereas non-epithelioid mesotheliomas have a TIME with a larger proportion of macrophages, regulatory T cells, mesothelioma stem cells, and neutrophils [27].

In past years, the prognostic and predictive role of TIME in MPM was investigated mainly on small and heterogeneous series, with no conclusive data due to difficulties in MPM microenvironment characterization [28,29]. Moreover, qualitative and quantitative changes in tumor/stroma ratio may produce a dramatic rewiring in the MPM-infiltrating immune cell subsets [30].

Increasing evidence suggests that analysis of gene expression or copy numbers in cancer samples helps to understand immune cell infiltration into the tumor ME. Yoshihara et al., by means of transcription profiling, have developed the ESTIMATE algorithm (Estimation of STromal and Immune cells in MAlignant Tumor tissues using Expression data) to analyze the stromal and immune infiltration associated to tumor cellularity in cancer samples [31]. Using gene expression data, a 'stromal signature', that describes the presence of stroma in tumor tissue, and an 'immune signature', that represents the infiltration of immune cells, were identified. Recently, the ESTIMATE algorithm was applied to MPM samples and the involvement of 14 immune/stromal-related genes was found to have significant prognostic potential. In silico analyses revealed that all these genes are involved in immune responses and may predict the survival of patients with MPM, playing also a role as biomarkers of the sensitivity to immunotherapy [32].

Additionally, Lee and coworkers, using mass spectrometry and comprehensive analysis of intra-tumoral immune system, described a distinct immunogenic TIME signature which was associated with favorable OS and response to checkpoint blockade [33]. The importance of understanding TIME of different MPM histotypes in relation to hypofractionated radiation therapy response was recently demonstrated as well [27].

2.1. Extracellular Matrix and Stroma Components

In MPM, the intra-tumoral stroma is not merely a scaffold but also promotes tumor growth, invasion, and protection from an anti-tumor immune response.

Several studies reported that many genes involved in extracellular matrix (ECM) production and remodeling are upregulated in MPM, especially in the biphasic [34] and sarcomatoid [35] variants. Furthermore, increased expression of these ECM-related genes is associated with "immune desert" tumor regions, characterized by a poor lymphocytic infiltrate, suggesting that MPM-altered stroma might act as a barrier to the immune response [36]. Very recent studies that analyze public mRNA-sequencing datasets through bioinformatic analyses have identified several differentially expressed genes (DEGs) in MPM. In these studies, genes specifically associated to the ECM component, structural constituents, organization, and receptor interaction were found overexpressed. These genes resulted in being involved in different protein–protein interaction (PPI) networks, gene ontology (GO), biological processes (BC), and molecular functions [37,38], and were also validated in MPM cell line models [39].

ECM components such as collagen, laminin, fibronectin, and integrins can be produced by mesothelioma cells that can also promote, under the influence of various growth factors, the synthesis of matrix metalloproteases (MMP), favoring ECM remodeling and tumor cell invasion [40].

In vitro studies demonstrated that different histotypes are characterized by specific ECM profiles, and that these differences determine a varying ability of MPM cells to spread and migrate towards ECM substrates [41,42]. In particular, characterization of cell culture conditions showed that 3D growth of malignant cells was enhanced in the presence of their own ECM, while invasion was stimulated by fibronectin in epithelioid and biphasic MPM histotypes, while homologous cell-derived ECM stimulated invasion in the most aggressive (sarcomatoid) form of MPM.

Furthermore, inhibition of collagen production delays MPM tumor growth [43]. Morphometric and immunohistochemical analysis of tumor collagen V (Col V), along with the quantitative inverse relationship between Col V and CD8+ T lymphocytes, demonstrated that high levels of Col V and low CD8+ T lymphocytes confer an immune-privileged TIME for tumor invasion and poor patients' prognosis [44,45].

The architecture of connective tissue in MPM per se, highlighted by silver-based reticulin staining (Figure 1b), has been recently proposed to distinguish the transitional variant of MPM, showing intermediate features between epithelioid and sarcomatoid histotypes, and bearing a specific prognosis [46]; in fact, a delicate reticulin pattern around single cells is indicative of this transitional type, as compared to a rough pattern banding individual cells in the sarcomatoid, and a large cluster pattern in the epithelioid type [47].

Cancer-Associated Fibroblasts (CAFs)

Tumor stroma is mostly composed by both fibrocytes with small spindle-shaped nuclei, derived from macrophages or dendritic cells, and activated fibroblasts (or cancer-associated fibroblasts, CAFs) that are identified by alpha smooth muscle actin (SMA) (Figure 1c) [48,49].

In recent years, fibroblast growth factor receptor (FGFR) signaling has been recognized as increasingly important, both in cancer pathogenesis and as a potential therapeutic target [50]. There are strong preclinical data suggesting that FGF is important in MPM as well. In MPM cell lines, FGFR1 and FGFR2 are co-expressed and their expression is strongly associated with sensitivity to FGFR-active tyrosine kinase inhibitors [51]. Inhibiting FGF autocrine signaling using an FGF-ligand trap reduces proliferation in MPM cell lines and reduces tumor growth in xenografts [52]. Unfortunately, the phase II clinical trial with a FGFR 1–3 inhibitor did not demonstrate efficacy in patients with MPM, who had progressed after first-line treatment with platinum-based chemotherapy [53].

CAFs have been shown to exert pro-tumorigenic effects by secreting several growth factors that promote cancer cell proliferation and invasion [54]. Literature data reported that TGFβ, IL-6, and CCL2, synthetized by CAFs [55], were detected in pleural effusions of MPM patients, where they seem to contribute to the recruitment and differentiation of immunosuppressive cells [56,57].

Our group identified Caveolin 1 (CAV1)-positive CAFs in a subgroup of epithelioid MPM with poorer prognosis [58]. CAV1 acts as a multifunctional scaffolding protein with multiple binding partners and is associated with cell surface caveolae in the regulation of lipid raft domains, but it is also involved in cancer growth and progression, modulating tissue responses through architectural regulation of the microenvironment. Recently, caveolae and their components emerged as integrators of different cell functions, mechano-transduction, and ECM–cell interactions [59]. Furthermore, in vitro studies on quantitative proteomic profiling revealed that CAV1 is required for exosomal sorting of ECM protein cargo subsets and for fibroblast-derived exosomes to efficiently deposit ECM and promote tumor invasion of breast cancer cells [60].

Furthermore, connective tissue growth factor (CTGF), a pro-tumorigenic CAF marker [49], is more expressed in sarcomatoid than in epithelioid MPM [61], and it is produced by both MPM cells and fibroblasts, and promotes the invasion of MPM cells in vitro [62]. Ohara's group has demonstrated that a CTGF-specific monoclonal antibody (FG-3019, pamrevlumab) could inhibit mesothelioma cell growth in vitro [63]. Based on these data, it was suggested that the use of FG-3019, currently under clinical trials for idiopathic pulmonary fibrosis [64] and pancreatic ductal adenocarcinoma [65], could be a therapeutic option for MPM. This is supported by preclinical data including a strong in vivo cancer growth inhibition observed in melanoma and pancreatic cancer with the use of the same anti-CTGF monoclonal antibody [66,67].

2.2. Inflammatory Cellular Component of TIME

2.2.1. Tumor-Associated Macrophages

Macrophages are specialized phagocytic cells that play a dual role in cancer depending on their differentiation. Tumor-associated macrophages (TAMs) derive from circulating monocytic precursors and are the major component of MPM TIME (Figure 1h,i). They are divided into two classes: classically activated (M1) macrophages, which have pro-inflammatory, tissue destructive, and anti-tumor activity, and alternatively activated (M2) macrophages, which have pro-tumorigenic properties [68]. M2 macrophages are the ones mostly present in MPM and their differentiation is regulated by interleukins, such as IL-4, IL-13, and IL-10, produced by tumor-infiltrating lymphocytes (TILs) [69].

Asbestos phagocytosis by macrophages triggers the formation of the inflammasome complex and promotes secretion of IL-1β [70,71]. Additionally, IL-1β/IL-1 receptor (IL-1R) signaling was reported to contribute to the oncogenesis of asbestos-induced mesothelioma [72]. These studies highlight the important role of the inflammasome in MPM development. The phagocytosed asbestos fibers remain undegraded and induce apoptosis of macrophages [73]. Undegraded asbestos fibers then undergo phagocytosis by nearby macrophages. Thus, asbestos is not completely removed and constitutively activates the inflammasome in macrophages. Moreover, it was reported that high mobility group box 1 (HMGB1) protein is abundantly secreted by MPM cells and serum levels of HMGB1 are associated with poor prognosis in MPM patients [74,75]. HMGB1 is one of the damage-associated molecular pattern proteins and promotes pro-IL-1β production functioning as an agonist of Toll-like receptor 4 (TLR4) [76]. Both HMGB1 derived from MPM cells and asbestos-activated inflammasome in TAMs induce IL-1β production, resulting in enhanced aggressiveness of MPM [77].

The tissue localization of M2 macrophages has been investigated in different immunohistochemical studies. Marcq and coworkers demonstrated that the number of stromal CD68+ macrophages found in MPM specimens was positively correlated to the number of stromal Tregs, suggesting a direct action of macrophages on stimulating and recruiting CD4+ immunosuppressive cells [78]. Burt et al. found that the absolute number of CD68+ macrophages was associated with worse prognosis in non-epithelioid MPM [79]. Finally, Cornelissen and coworkers reported that patients who develop recurrence after radiation treatment have a higher M2/total TAM ratio and lower CD8+ cell count at diagnosis, compared to patients who did not develop this outgrowth [80].

2.2.2. T Cells and Natural Killer Cells

The CD3+ T-lymphocytes are the second most common immune cell type in MPM (Figure 1d–f) TIME and constitute, on average, 20–42% of the immune cell infiltrate [68,81]. T helper CD4+ cells play an important role in the generation of T cell-mediated antitumor response via activation of antigen-presenting cells (APCs), which stimulate CD8+ cytotoxic TILs and natural killer (NK) cells. The latter are lymphoid cells of the innate immune system with strong immunostimulatory functions and cytotoxic capacity [82].

A recent study by Alay and coworkers, performing an integrative transcriptome analysis on a publicly available dataset of 516 MPMs, revealed a clinically relevant immune-based classification based on CD4+ T-helper 2 (TH2) and CD8+ cytotoxic T cells, that were found to be consistently associated with better overall survival [83].

CD8+, CD4+, and CD4+/FoxP3+ T-cells are present in the majority of patients [84], but the number of T-reg cells in pleural effusions of MPM patients is lower than in other solid tumors [85], confirming the presence of an immunosuppressive milieu in MPM tumoral mass, rather than in pleural effusion [86]. The positive effect of CD4+ tumor-infiltrating lymphocytes (TILs) on prognosis has been previously suggested for epithelioid [78,87–89], but remains controversial in sarcomatoid MPM [81,88]. On the other hand, low CD8+

and high FoxP3+ TILs counts were shown to correlate with a high risk of both death and recurrence, regardless of the presence of a sarcomatoid component [87–90].

Ujiie and coworkers demonstrated the prognostic role of CD8+ and CD20+ expressing lymphocytes in 230 epithelioid mesothelioma patients [29]. In particular, they found that rather than the single type of infiltrating cells, the combination of high M2-polarized TAMs (CD163+) with low CD8+ T cells, and low M2-polarized TAMs (CD163+) with high CD20+ B cells, were independent markers of worse and better overall survival, respectively. These data were confirmed by Pasello et al., except for the fact that CD8+ T-lymphocytes were found in MPM samples showing aggressive features (sarcomatoid/biphasic histology, higher necrosis, and proliferation index), when associated with higher CD68+ macrophages and PD-L1 expression [90].

In a study by our group, Salaroglio et al. [91] performed a simultaneous comprehensive analysis of the immune infiltrate in pleural fluid and fresh pleural biopsy tissues aiming to identify an immune phenotype with diagnostic and prognostic value in MPM patients. It was confirmed that CD8+ TILs in pleural effusion have no prognostic significance, while intratumor immune infiltrate is more effective in predicting the patient's outcome. The same result was obtained by Chee et al., who state that high proportions of FoxP3+ T cells are associated with a poor prognosis in epithelioid and sarcomatoid tumors [88].

Moreover, Fusco et al. found an increased presence of stromal CD4+ T and CD19+ B lymphocytes with a positive correlation between each other, possibly indicating a positive feedback loop between these two lineages [92].

Our group also characterized TIME in MPM by immunohistochemistry, as a validation step of gene expression profiling. In MPM cases with higher expression of T-cell lineage genes, T-effector genes, and T-regulatory genes, we observed a high expression of CD3+ T-infiltrating lymphocytes, with a similar amount of CD4+ and CD8+ T-cells. On the contrary, high amounts of CD20+ B lymphocytes, with follicular chronic inflammation as a morphological hallmark, were observed in the group that showed higher relative expression of B cell and lower expression of T cell genes [36].

2.2.3. Myeloid-Derived Suppressor Cells

Myeloid-derived suppressor cells (MDSC) are myeloid cells with suppressive activity on innate and adaptive immune cells that have been described to inactivate immune response against the tumor in cancer patients [93]. Based on their surface markers, MDSC can be subdivided in granulocytic MDSC (GR-MDSC), which express granulocytic markers like CD66b and/or CD15, and monocytic MDSC (MO-MDSC), which express the monocytic antigen CD14 [91]. The main mechanisms by which MDSC exert their suppressive activity on other immune cells are the depletion of arginine and tryptophan by expression of effector enzymes arginase I (Arg I), inducible NO-synthase (iNOS), and indolamin-2,3-dioxygenase (IDO), as well as by production of reactive oxygen species (ROS) [93].

In mice, MDSCs are characterized by IL-4 expression [94]. Burt et al. found IL-4R to be highly expressed on the surface of human MPM tumor cells: IL-4R was present in 97% of epithelial and 95% of non-epithelial tumors. Only a scattered and small fraction of stromal cells stained positive for IL-4R, and conversely, IL-4R-positive macrophages were predominantly found in the stroma [95]. Myeloid CD33+ cells were found to represent approximately 42% of CD45+ immune cells: 0.6–31% of these myeloid cells were typed as MDSCs [96].

In their study, Salaroglio et al. reported that GR- and MO-MDSCs abrogated proliferation and cytotoxic activity of autologous TILs and of TILs derived from patients with pleuritis, suggesting an important role of MDSCs in immunosuppression mediation. Moreover, the intratumor-infiltrating MDSCs, but not the MDSCs of pleural fluid, resulted significantly associated with poorer PFS and OS [91].

Furthermore, it was recently reported that MPM TIME is enriched in infiltrating granulocytes, which inhibit T-cell proliferation and activation. Immunohistochemistry and transcriptomic analysis revealed that a majority of MPMs express GM-CSF, and that high GM-CSF expression correlates with clinical progression. Blockade of GM-CSF with neutralizing antibodies or ROS inhibition restores T-cell proliferation, suggesting that targeting GM-CSF could be of therapeutic benefit in MPM patients [97].

2.2.4. Dendritic Cells

Dendritic cells (DCs) are powerful antigen-presenting cells with key roles in the initiation and regulation of immune responses. DCs are unique in their ability to activate naïve T cells and initiate primary immune responses in lymph nodes, and they also play a central role in reactivating memory T-cell responses in the lungs. DC-derived signals regulate both the degree of T-cell activation and the nature of immune response (e.g., T helper (Th) 1, Th2, Th17, B-cell help) [98]. Several DC subpopulations have been defined: DCs are broadly divided into myeloid dendritic cells (mDCs), usually referred to as conventional dendritic cells (cDCs), and plasmacytoid dendritic cells (pDCs). In human lungs, cDCs form dense networks throughout the epithelium of large conducting airways, bronchioles, alveoli, and interstitial space, and they express CD141, CD1c, and the C-type lectin domain family 9 member A (CLEC9A) [99,100]. pDCs are best characterized by their ability to synthesize great amounts of IFN. They are relatively inefficient at presenting antigens to T cells and seem to play an important role in tolerance induction, probably via induction of regulatory T cells. In humans, pDCs are identified by surface markers such as CD303 (a C-type lectin), CD304 or neuropilin-1, Ig-like transcript 7, and IL-3 receptor-α chain [101]. Under normal conditions, activated pDCs exhibit robust IFN-α production and promote both innate and adaptive immune responses. In several cancer models [102], including MPM [103], pDCs demonstrate an impaired response to T activation, decreased or absent IFN-α production, and contribute in establishing an immunosuppressive TIME and a reduced ability to generate effective anti-mesothelioma T cell responses. On the other hand, a comprehensive proteomic analysis on 12 surgically resected MPMs highlighted a correlation between the presence of activated pDCs (CD40+ and CD86+) and tumors having a good TIME signature as well as a favorable response to immune checkpoint therapy [33]. Finally, evidence to date suggests that CD40+ DC activation is a critical and nonredundant mechanism to convert "cold" tumors (i.e., lacking a T cell tumor infiltrate) into "hot" ones (i.e., having a prominent T cell tumor infiltrate), sensitizing them to checkpoint inhibition therapy [104,105].

2.2.5. B Lymphocytes

B lymphocytes contribute to humoral immunity as they can differentiate into antibody-secreting plasma cells. Additionally, B cells can stimulate T cells or serve as APCs. In MPM, B lymphocyte infiltrate is associated with better patient survival [29,90]. Generally, B cell infiltrate in mesothelioma is scant [55,89].

As mentioned above, in our study on immune gene expression profiling in MPM, the subgroup with downregulated T-cell effector and upregulated B-cell genes failed to show correlation with increased expression of genes associated with antigen presentation, thus we concluded that these B cells may be part of the adaptive cytotoxic response [36].

2.3. PD-L1 and Other Immune Checkpoints

The programmed cell death pathway (PD-1/PD-L1) plays a critical role in tumor immune escape control. PD-1 is mainly expressed on activated CD4/CD8 T cells and B cells [96]. PD-L1, the ligand of PD-1, is not only expressed in immune cells, but also in others, including cancer cells, helping immune evasion by interacting with PD-1 on T-cells [106]. The interaction between tumor PD-L1 and PD-1 on T cells results in the inhibition of T cell activation and proliferation, as well as immune evasion by PD-L1-expressing tumors [107].

PD-L1 immunohistochemical expression in tumor tissue has been widely accepted as a predictive biomarker [108], because of its association with increased efficacy of immune checkpoint inhibitors (ICIs) in several malignancies [109]. Immunotherapy based on monoclonal antibodies against PD-1 and PD-L1 has also been tested for MPMs in clinical trials (Figure 1j). Several nonrandomized phase I/II trials, testing single-agent ICI, showed variable antitumor activity (9–29%) and median progression-free survival ranging from 2.8 to 6.2 months [110]. Preliminary results from phase II clinical trials combining inhibitors of cytotoxic T-lymphocyte-associated antigen 4 (CTLA4) and anti-PD1/PD-L1, such as ipilimumab, nivolumab, tremelimumab, or durvalumab, showed promising results but significant toxicity [111]. In those clinical trials, PD-L1 expression showed limited value in predicting benefit from ICIs, and PD-L1 expression analysis currently has no role as a clinical predictive biomarker in MPM. Moreover, the prognostic value of PD-L1 expression in MPM is controversial. In a recent meta-analysis, Jin et al. reported that PD-L1 overexpression significantly correlated with poor overall survival, irrespective of the sample size of the series, treatment method, or PD-L1 cut-off value. Furthermore, overexpression of PD-L1 was associated with sarcomatoid and biphasic histology [112].

The above-mentioned integrative transcriptome analysis of MPM [83] revealed a clinically relevant immune-based classification of the same, identifying three immune groups (IG1–IG3) that represent different immune infiltration patterns and are associated with distinct survival outcomes. The group with the shortest overall survival (IG1) represented more than 50% of cases, whereas the IG3 group, having the best prognosis, accounted for 8.5% of cases only. Interestingly, while most immune checkpoint markers correlated with the different immune groups, CD276 (B7-H3) showed an opposite expression pattern, decreasing from IG1 to IG3. CD276 is a member of the B7 family of immunoregulatory proteins and is overexpressed in several tumor types. It has been shown that CD276 can promote tumor proliferation, angiogenesis, and metastasis, and is associated with shorter survival time in multiple tumor types [113]. A recent study reported a wide immunohistochemical expression of B7-H3 in MPM and demonstrated that PD-L1 and B7-H3 were significantly co-expressed in tumor cells of the non-epithelioid histotype [114]. Similarly, CD44 is the only T-cell exhaustion marker that showed negative correlation with the immune groups [83]. This marker has been associated with metastasis and low survival rates in multiple cancer types [115]. In MPM, CD44 has been shown to promote invasiveness when interacting with hyaluronan [116,117].

V-domain Ig-containing suppressor of T-cell activation (VISTA) is another immune checkpoint that inhibits anti-tumor immune responses (Figure 1k). In a TCGA-based study, VISTA gene expression was reported to be higher in MPM than in all other cancer types. This was particularly observed in the epithelioid subtype and strongly correlated with mesothelin expression [11]. Moreover, VISTA was recently described as a new potential target for mesothelioma immunotherapy. Muller et al. investigated the tissue expression of VISTA and PD-L1 in a large cohort of MPMs. They found frequent expression of VISTA and infrequent expression of PD-L1 (88% and 33% of epithelioid, 90% and 43% of biphasic, and 42% and 75% of sarcomatoid) with favorable and unfavorable survival correlations, respectively [118].

In this context, the expression of STimulator of Interferon Genes (STING) protein is described as having a crucial role in identifying "inflamed" or "hot" tumors that could be successfully treated with immunotherapy (Figure 1l). STING absence implies a tumor environment with no activation of the INFγ pathway, which is a known parameter of response to ICIs [119]. Moreover, it has been reported that targeting DNA damage response promotes anti-tumor immunity through STING-mediated T-cell activation in small-cell lung cancer [120].

3. Angiogenesis

The prognosis of MPM is best explained by a continuous model, which shows specific expression patterns of genes involved in angiogenesis and immune response [121]. Asbestos fibers have a direct effect on mesothelial cells, causing the release, together with inflammatory cytokines, of vascular endothelial growth factor (VEGF), which attracts leukocytes [122]. VEGF signaling is crucial in MPM pathophysiology [123], regulating blood vessel function, inducing tumor cell growth, and suppressing immune activation [124]. VEGF also acts as a powerful mitogen for mesothelial cells themselves. Indeed, MPM cell lines secrete VEGF-A and VEGF-C, as well as expressing both VEGF receptors Flt-1 (VEGF-R1) and KDR (VEGFR-2) [125,126]. Thus, VEGF signaling can induce MPM cell growth in an autocrine fashion. This may explain why mesothelioma cells show striking sensitivity to anti-VEGF agents, in addition to the more canonical role of such agents in inhibiting neo-angiogenesis. Moreover, MPM has been shown to produce the highest levels of VEGF among solid tumors [127].

Other growth factors can also regulate migration, survival, and differentiation of endothelial cells, contributing to neoangiogenesis, such as TGFb, EGF, angiogenin, IL-8, and platelet-derived growth factor (PDGF) [128]. All this evidence provides the rationale for the development of VEGF and angiogenesis inhibitors as a therapeutic strategy in MPM [129].

Although there has been over a decade of intense investigation, there are still no validated biomarkers of angiogenesis able to predict the efficacy of anti-angiogenic agents both in MPM and in other cancers [130]. The complementary LUME-Meso biomarker study has reviewed the plasma levels of 58 angiogenic factors and single-nucleotide polymorphisms (SNPs) in genes for VEGFR1 (FLT1), and VEGFR3 (FLT4) and mesothelin (MSLN), and assessed micro-vessel density via CD31 immunohistochemistry on archival biopsy samples. Although PFS and OS benefits were observed in patients with low plasma endoglin and homozygous VEGFR1/3 genotypes, no biomarkers showed any significant and conclusive association with antiangiogenic efficacy [131].

Recently, Chia and coworkers evaluated VEGF, PDGF, FGFR, and CD31 by immunohistochemistry in tissue microarrays from 329 patients who underwent surgical resection or biopsy for MPM. They found that high CD31 density and high PDGF expression levels were associated with poor prognosis in the epithelioid MPM group [132].

4. Conclusions

TIME is a challenging component with an emerging pathogenic, immunomodulatory, and growth-promoting role in MPM. Given the relatively low mutational burden of MPM, biological events other than genetics may be critical determinants of MPM growth and aggressiveness and could influence cells' immune-escape.

A greater understanding of infiltrating immune cells, their role and function, and the presence of ligand or modulatory marker expression will give a wider and better structured picture of the tumor–immune cell interplay (Figure 2).

A precise pathological and immuno-phenotypical characterization of TIME, in terms of extracellular matrix profiles, subtypes of immune-infiltrating cells, expression of co-inhibitory molecules, and activation of immune pathways could provide important knowledge for translational pathology studies. Practical identification of specific biomarkers that could influence the host immunity has to be performed and would represent a major advance for clinical translation of neoantigen-directed immunotherapies, paving the way to understand how to personalize future therapeutic approaches in MPM patients.

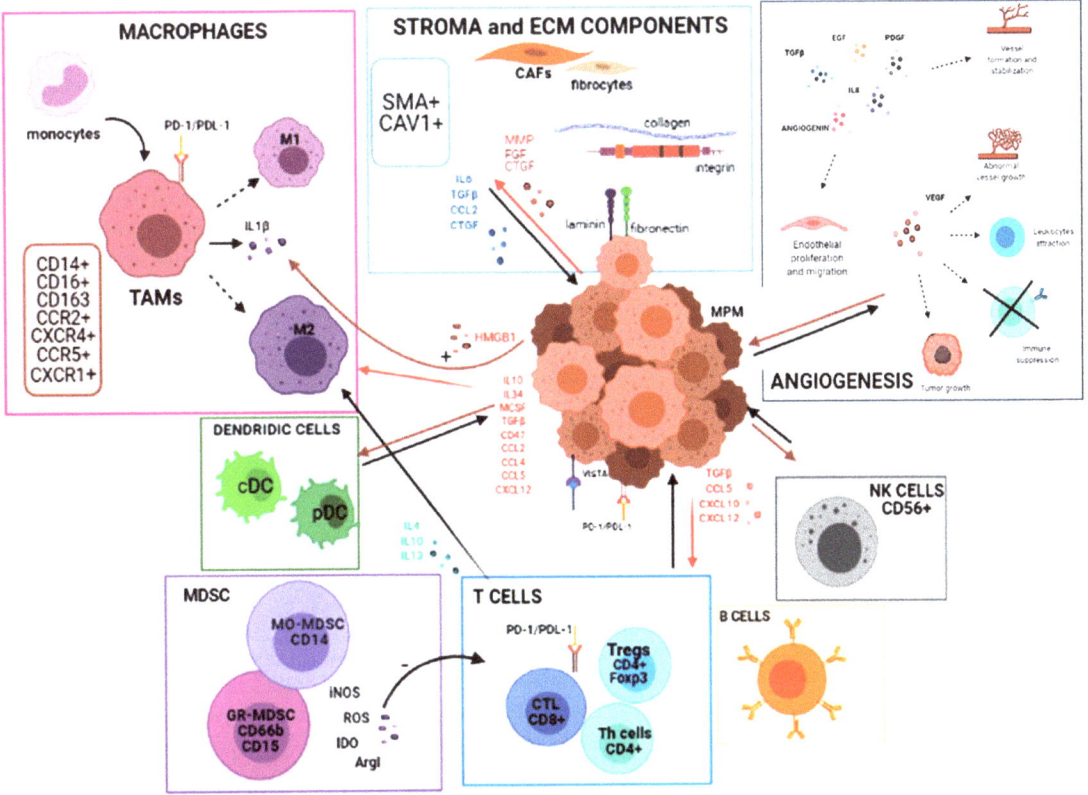

Figure 2. Graphical representation of tumor immune microenvironment interactions in MPM.

Author Contributions: Conceptualization, L.R. and F.N.; methodology, F.N.; software, F.N.; validation, F.N., A.L. and V.Z.; formal analysis, F.N. and G.W.; investigation, F.N.; resources, L.R., M.P., M.V., P.B. and G.S.; data curation, F.N. and L.R.; writing—original draft preparation, F.N.; writing—review and editing, G.W., L.R., M.P., P.B., M.V. and G.S.; visualization, L.R.; supervision, M.V., M.P. and G.S.; project administration, L.R.; funding acquisition, G.S. and P.B. All authors have read and agreed to the published version of the manuscript.

Funding: The research plan has received funding from AIRC under IG 2019-ID. 23760 project—to G.S., and from University of Turin, Ricerca Locale (Ex 60%) Funding 2019, to P.B.

Conflicts of Interest: The authors declare no conflict of interest.

References

1. Yang, H.; Testa, J.R.; Carbone, M. Mesothelioma Epidemiology, Carcinogenesis, and Pathogenesis. *Curr. Treat. Opt. Oncol.* **2008**, *9*, 147–157. [CrossRef]
2. Kindler, H.L.; Ismaila, N.; Armato, S.G.; Bueno, R.; Hesdorffer, M.; Jahan, T.; Jones, C.M.; Miettinen, M.; Pass, H.; Rimner, A.; et al. Treatment of Malignant Pleural Mesothelioma: American Society of Clinical Oncology Clinical Practice Guideline. *JCO* **2018**, *36*, 1343–1373. [CrossRef] [PubMed]
3. Nicholson, A.G.; Sauter, J.L.; Nowak, A.K.; Kindler, H.L.; Gill, R.R.; Remy-Jardin, M.; Armato, S.G.; Fernandez-Cuesta, L.; Bueno, R.; Alcala, N.; et al. EURACAN/IASLC Proposals for Updating the Histologic Classification of Pleural Mesothelioma: Towards a More Multidisciplinary Approach. *J. Thorac. Oncol.* **2020**, *15*, 29–49. [CrossRef]
4. Opitz, I.; Scherpereel, A.; Berghmans, T.; Psallidas, I.; Glatzer, M.; Rigau, D.; Astoul, P.; Bölükbas, S.; Boyd, J.; Coolen, J.; et al. ERS/ESTS/EACTS/ESTRO Guidelines for the Management of Malignant Pleural Mesothelioma. *Eur. J. Cardio Thorac. Surg.* **2020**, *58*, 1–24. [CrossRef] [PubMed]

5. Van Gerwen, M.; Alpert, N.; Wolf, A.; Ohri, N.; Lewis, E.; Rosenzweig, K.E.; Flores, R.; Taioli, E. Prognostic Factors of Survival in Patients with Malignant Pleural Mesothelioma: An Analysis of the National Cancer Database. *Carcinogenesis* **2019**, *40*, 529–536. [CrossRef]
6. Vogelzang, N.J.; Rusthoven, J.J.; Symanowski, J.; Denham, C.; Kaukel, E.; Ruffie, P.; Gatzemeier, U.; Boyer, M.; Emri, S.; Manegold, C.; et al. Phase III Study of Pemetrexed in Combination with Cisplatin versus Cisplatin Alone in Patients with Malignant Pleural Mesothelioma. *J. Clin. Oncol.* **2003**, *21*, 2636–2644. [CrossRef] [PubMed]
7. Baas, P.; Fennell, D.; Kerr, K.M.; Van Schil, P.E.; Haas, R.L.; Peters, S. ESMO Guidelines Committee Malignant Pleural Mesothelioma: ESMO Clinical Practice Guidelines for Diagnosis, Treatment and Follow-Up. *Ann. Oncol.* **2015**, *26* (Suppl. S5), v31–v39. [CrossRef] [PubMed]
8. Bueno, R.; Stawiski, E.W.; Goldstein, L.D.; Durinck, S.; De Rienzo, A.; Modrusan, Z.; Gnad, F.; Nguyen, T.T.; Jaiswal, B.S.; Chirieac, L.R.; et al. Comprehensive Genomic Analysis of Malignant Pleural Mesothelioma Identifies Recurrent Mutations, Gene Fusions and Splicing Alterations. *Nat. Genet.* **2016**, *48*, 407–416. [CrossRef] [PubMed]
9. Cakiroglu, E.; Senturk, S. Genomics and Functional Genomics of Malignant Pleural Mesothelioma. *Int. J. Mol. Sci.* **2020**, *21*, 6342. [CrossRef]
10. Guo, G.; Chmielecki, J.; Goparaju, C.; Heguy, A.; Dolgalev, I.; Carbone, M.; Seepo, S.; Meyerson, M.; Pass, H.I. Whole-Exome Sequencing Reveals Frequent Genetic Alterations in BAP1, NF2, CDKN2A, and CUL1 in Malignant Pleural Mesothelioma. *Cancer Res.* **2015**, *75*, 264–269. [CrossRef]
11. Hmeljak, J.; Sanchez-Vega, F.; Hoadley, K.A.; Shih, J.; Stewart, C.; Heiman, D.; Tarpey, P.; Danilova, L.; Drill, E.; Gibb, E.A.; et al. Integrative Molecular Characterization of Malignant Pleural Mesothelioma. *Cancer Discov.* **2018**, *8*, 1548–1565. [CrossRef]
12. Kang, H.C.; Kim, H.K.; Lee, S.; Mendez, P.; Kim, J.W.; Woodard, G.; Yoon, J.-H.; Jen, K.-Y.; Fang, L.T.; Jones, K.; et al. Whole Exome and Targeted Deep Sequencing Identify Genome-Wide Allelic Loss and Frequent SETDB1 Mutations in Malignant Pleural Mesotheliomas. *Oncotarget* **2016**, *7*, 8321–8331. [CrossRef]
13. Lo Iacono, M.; Monica, V.; Righi, L.; Grosso, F.; Libener, R.; Vatrano, S.; Bironzo, P.; Novello, S.; Musmeci, L.; Volante, M.; et al. Targeted Next-Generation Sequencing of Cancer Genes in Advanced Stage Malignant Pleural Mesothelioma: A Retrospective Study. *J. Thorac. Oncol.* **2015**, *10*, 492–499. [CrossRef]
14. Bott, M.; Brevet, M.; Taylor, B.S.; Shimizu, S.; Ito, T.; Wang, L.; Creaney, J.; Lake, R.A.; Zakowski, M.F.; Reva, B.; et al. The Nuclear Deubiquitinase BAP1 Is Commonly Inactivated by Somatic Mutations and 3p21.1 Losses in Malignant Pleural Mesothelioma. *Nat. Genet.* **2011**, *43*, 668–672. [CrossRef]
15. Testa, J.R.; Cheung, M.; Pei, J.; Below, J.E.; Tan, Y.; Sementino, E.; Cox, N.J.; Dogan, A.U.; Pass, H.I.; Trusa, S.; et al. Germline BAP1 Mutations Predispose to Malignant Mesothelioma. *Nat. Genet.* **2011**, *43*, 1022–1025. [CrossRef]
16. Matsuzaki, H.; Maeda, M.; Lee, S.; Nishimura, Y.; Kumagai-Takei, N.; Hayashi, H.; Yamamoto, S.; Hatayama, T.; Kojima, Y.; Tabata, R.; et al. Asbestos-Induced Cellular and Molecular Alteration of Immunocompetent Cells and Their Relationship with Chronic Inflammation and Carcinogenesis. *J. Biomed. Biotechnol.* **2012**, *2012*, 492608. [CrossRef] [PubMed]
17. Kusamura, S.; Kepenekian, V.; Villeneuve, L.; Lurvink, R.J.; Govaerts, K.; De Hingh, I.H.J.T.; Moran, B.J.; Van der Speeten, K.; Deraco, M.; Glehen, O.; et al. Peritoneal Mesothelioma: PSOGI/EURACAN Clinical Practice Guidelines for Diagnosis, Treatment and Follow-Up. *Eur. J. Surg. Oncol.* **2021**, *47*, 36–59. [CrossRef] [PubMed]
18. Benzerdjeb, N.; Dartigues, P.; Kepenekian, V.; Valmary-Degano, S.; Mery, E.; Avérous, G.; Chevallier, A.; Laverriere, M.-H.; Villa, I.; Harou, O.; et al. Tertiary Lymphoid Structures in Epithelioid Malignant Peritoneal Mesothelioma Are Associated with Neoadjuvant Chemotherapy, but Not with Prognosis. *Virchows Arch.* **2021**. [CrossRef] [PubMed]
19. Baas, P.; Scherpereel, A.; Nowak, A.; Fujimoto, N.; Peters, S.; Tsao, A.; Mansfield, A.; Popat, S.; Jahan, T.; Antonia, S.; et al. ID:2908 First-Line Nivolumab + Ipilimumab vs. Chemotherapy in Unresectable Malignant Pleural Mesothelioma: CheckMate 743. *J. Thorac. Oncol.* **2020**, *15*, e42. [CrossRef]
20. Fennell, D.; Ottensmeier, C.; Califano, R.; Hanna, G.; Ewings, S.; Hill, K.; Wilding, S.; Danson, S.; Nye, M.; Steele, N.; et al. PS01.11 Nivolumab Versus Placebo in Relapsed Malignant Mesothelioma: The CONFIRM Phase 3 Trial. *J. Thorac. Oncol.* **2021**, *16*, S62. [CrossRef]
21. Castelletti, L.; Yeo, D.; van Zandwijk, N.; Rasko, J.E.J. Anti-Mesothelin CAR T Cell Therapy for Malignant Mesothelioma. *Biomark. Res.* **2021**, *9*, 11. [CrossRef] [PubMed]
22. Hiltbrunner, S.; Britschgi, C.; Schuberth, P.; Bankel, L.; Nguyen-Kim, T.D.L.; Gulati, P.; Weder, W.; Opitz, I.; Lauk, O.; Caviezel, C.; et al. Local Delivery of CAR T Cells Targeting Fibroblast Activation Protein Is Safe in Patients with Pleural Mesothelioma: First Report of FAPME, a Phase I Clinical Trial. *Ann. Oncol.* **2021**, *32*, 120–121. [CrossRef] [PubMed]
23. Lau, S.P.; van Montfoort, N.; Kinderman, P.; Lukkes, M.; Klaase, L.; van Nimwegen, M.; van Gulijk, M.; Dumas, J.; Mustafa, D.A.M.; Lievense, S.L.A.; et al. Dendritic Cell Vaccination and CD40-Agonist Combination Therapy Licenses T Cell-Dependent Antitumor Immunity in a Pancreatic Carcinoma Murine Model. *J. Immunother. Cancer* **2020**, *8*, e000772. [CrossRef]
24. Parra, E.R.; Zhai, J.; Tamegnon, A.; Zhou, N.; Pandurengan, R.K.; Barreto, C.; Jiang, M.; Rice, D.C.; Creasy, C.; Vaporciyan, A.A.; et al. Identification of Distinct Immune Landscapes Using an Automated Nine-Color Multiplex Immunofluorescence Staining Panel and Image Analysis in Paraffin Tumor Tissues. *Sci. Rep.* **2021**, *11*, 4530. [CrossRef] [PubMed]
25. Ijsselsteijn, M.E.; van der Breggen, R.; Farina Sarasqueta, A.; Koning, F.; de Miranda, N.F.C.C. A 40-Marker Panel for High Dimensional Characterization of Cancer Immune Microenvironments by Imaging Mass Cytometry. *Front. Immunol.* **2019**, *10*, 2534. [CrossRef] [PubMed]

26. Mungenast, F.; Fernando, A.; Nica, R.; Boghiu, B.; Lungu, B.; Batra, J.; Ecker, R.C. Next-Generation Digital Histopathology of the Tumor Microenvironment. *Genes* **2021**, *12*, 538. [CrossRef]
27. De Perrot, M.; Wu, L.; Cabanero, M.; Perentes, J.Y.; McKee, T.D.; Donahoe, L.; Bradbury, P.; Kohno, M.; Chan, M.-L.; Murakami, J.; et al. Prognostic Influence of Tumor Microenvironment after Hypofractionated Radiation and Surgery for Mesothelioma. *J. Thorac. Cardiovasc. Surg.* **2020**, *159*, 2082–2091.e1. [CrossRef]
28. Suzuki, K.; Kadota, K.; Sima, C.S.; Sadelain, M.; Rusch, V.W.; Travis, W.D.; Adusumilli, P.S. Chronic Inflammation in Tumor Stroma Is an Independent Predictor of Prolonged Survival in Epithelioid Malignant Pleural Mesothelioma Patients. *Cancer Immunol. Immunother.* **2011**, *60*, 1721–1728. [CrossRef]
29. Ujiie, H.; Kadota, K.; Nitadori, J.-I.; Aerts, J.G.; Woo, K.M.; Sima, C.S.; Travis, W.D.; Jones, D.R.; Krug, L.M.; Adusumilli, P.S. The Tumoral and Stromal Immune Microenvironment in Malignant Pleural Mesothelioma: A Comprehensive Analysis Reveals Prognostic Immune Markers. *Oncoimmunology* **2015**, *4*, e1009285. [CrossRef]
30. Lievense, L.A.; Bezemer, K.; Cornelissen, R.; Kaijen-Lambers, M.E.H.; Hegmans, J.P.J.J.; Aerts, J.G.J.V. Precision Immunotherapy; Dynamics in the Cellular Profile of Pleural Effusions in Malignant Mesothelioma Patients. *Lung Cancer* **2017**, *107*, 36–40. [CrossRef] [PubMed]
31. Yoshihara, K.; Shahmoradgoli, M.; Martínez, E.; Vegesna, R.; Kim, H.; Torres-Garcia, W.; Treviño, V.; Shen, H.; Laird, P.W.; Levine, D.A.; et al. Inferring Tumour Purity and Stromal and Immune Cell Admixture from Expression Data. *Nat. Commun.* **2013**, *4*, 2612. [CrossRef] [PubMed]
32. Xu, X.; Cheng, L.; Fan, Y.; Mao, W. Tumor Microenvironment-Associated Immune-Related Genes for the Prognosis of Malignant Pleural Mesothelioma. *Front. Oncol.* **2020**, *10*, 544789. [CrossRef]
33. Lee, H.-S.; Jang, H.-J.; Choi, J.M.; Zhang, J.; de Rosen, V.L.; Wheeler, T.M.; Lee, J.-S.; Tu, T.; Jindra, P.T.; Kerman, R.H.; et al. Comprehensive Immunoproteogenomic Analyses of Malignant Pleural Mesothelioma. *JCI Insight* **2018**, *3*. [CrossRef] [PubMed]
34. Gordon, G.J.; Rockwell, G.N.; Jensen, R.V.; Rheinwald, J.G.; Glickman, J.N.; Aronson, J.P.; Pottorf, B.J.; Nitz, M.D.; Richards, W.G.; Sugarbaker, D.J.; et al. Identification of Novel Candidate Oncogenes and Tumor Suppressors in Malignant Pleural Mesothelioma Using Large-Scale Transcriptional Profiling. *Am. J. Pathol.* **2005**, *166*, 1827–1840. [CrossRef]
35. Blum, Y.; Meiller, C.; Quetel, L.; Elarouci, N.; Ayadi, M.; Tashtanbaeva, D.; Armenoult, L.; Montagne, F.; Tranchant, R.; Renier, A.; et al. Dissecting Heterogeneity in Malignant Pleural Mesothelioma through Histo-Molecular Gradients for Clinical Applications. *Nat. Commun.* **2019**, *10*, 1333. [CrossRef] [PubMed]
36. Patil, N.S.; Righi, L.; Koeppen, H.; Zou, W.; Izzo, S.; Grosso, F.; Libener, R.; Loiacono, M.; Monica, V.; Buttigliero, C.; et al. Molecular and Histopathological Characterization of the Tumor Immune Microenvironment in Advanced Stage of Malignant Pleural Mesothelioma. *J. Thorac. Oncol.* **2018**, *13*, 124–133. [CrossRef]
37. Liu, X.; Qian, K.; Lu, G.; Chen, P.; Zhang, Y. Identification of Genes and Pathways Involved in Malignant Pleural Mesothelioma Using Bioinformatics Methods. *BMC Med. Genom.* **2021**, *14*, 104. [CrossRef]
38. Duan, W.; Wang, K.; Duan, Y.; Chen, X.; Chu, X.; Hu, P.; Xiong, B. Combined Analysis of RNA Sequence and Microarray Data Reveals a Competing Endogenous RNA Network as Novel Prognostic Markers in Malignant Pleural Mesothelioma. *Front. Oncol.* **2021**, *11*, 615234. [CrossRef] [PubMed]
39. Morani, F.; Bisceglia, L.; Rosini, G.; Mutti, L.; Melaiu, O.; Landi, S.; Gemignani, F. Identification of Overexpressed Genes in Malignant Pleural Mesothelioma. *Int. J. Mol. Sci.* **2021**, *22*, 2738. [CrossRef]
40. Liu, Z.; Klominek, J. Regulation of Matrix Metalloprotease Activity in Malignant Mesothelioma Cell Lines by Growth Factors. *Thorax* **2003**, *58*, 198–203. [CrossRef]
41. Scarpa, S.; Giuffrida, A.; Fazi, M.; Coletti, A.; Palumbo, C.; Pass, H.I.; Procopio, A.; Modesti, A. Migration of Mesothelioma Cells Correlates with Histotype-Specific Synthesis of Extracellular Matrix. *Int. J. Mol. Med.* **1999**, *4*, 67–71. [CrossRef]
42. Jagirdar, R.M.; Papazoglou, E.D.; Pitaraki, E.; Kouliou, O.A.; Rouka, E.; Giannakou, L.; Giannopoulos, S.; Sinis, S.I.; Hatzoglou, C.; Gourgoulianis, K.I.; et al. Cell and Extracellular Matrix Interaction Models in Benign Mesothelial and Malignant Pleural Mesothelioma Cells in 2D and 3D In-Vitro. *Clin. Exp. Pharmacol. Physiol.* **2021**, *48*, 543–552. [CrossRef]
43. Abayasiriwardana, K.S.; Wood, M.K.; Prêle, C.M.; Birnie, K.A.; Robinson, B.W.; Laurent, G.J.; McAnulty, R.J.; Mutsaers, S.E. Inhibition of Collagen Production Delays Malignant Mesothelioma Tumor Growth in a Murine Model. *Biochem. Biophys. Res. Commun.* **2019**, *510*, 198–204. [CrossRef]
44. Balancin, M.L.; Teodoro, W.R.; Farhat, C.; de Miranda, T.J.; Assato, A.K.; de Souza Silva, N.A.; Velosa, A.P.; Falzoni, R.; Ab'Saber, A.M.; Roden, A.C.; et al. An Integrative Histopathologic Clustering Model Based on Immuno-Matrix Elements to Predict the Risk of Death in Malignant Mesothelioma. *Cancer Med.* **2020**, *9*, 4836–4849. [CrossRef]
45. Balancin, M.L.; Teodoro, W.R.; Baldavira, C.M.; Prieto, T.G.; Farhat, C.; Velosa, A.P.; da Costa Souza, P.; Yaegashi, L.B.; Ab'Saber, A.M.; Takagaki, T.Y.; et al. Different Histological Patterns of Type-V Collagen Levels Confer a Matrices-Privileged Tissue Microenvironment for Invasion in Malignant Tumors with Prognostic Value. *Pathol. Res. Pract.* **2020**, *216*, 153277. [CrossRef] [PubMed]
46. Galateau Salle, F.; Le Stang, N.; Nicholson, A.G.; Pissaloux, D.; Churg, A.; Klebe, S.; Roggli, V.L.; Tazelaar, H.D.; Vignaud, J.M.; Attanoos, R.; et al. New Insights on Diagnostic Reproducibility of Biphasic Mesotheliomas: A Multi-Institutional Evaluation by the International Mesothelioma Panel From the MESOPATH Reference Center. *J. Thorac. Oncol.* **2018**, *13*, 1189–1203. [CrossRef] [PubMed]

47. Galateau Salle, F.; Le Stang, N.; Tirode, F.; Courtiol, P.; Nicholson, A.G.; Tsao, M.-S.; Tazelaar, H.D.; Churg, A.; Dacic, S.; Roggli, V.; et al. Comprehensive Molecular and Pathologic Evaluation of Transitional Mesothelioma Assisted by Deep Learning Approach: A Multi-Institutional Study of the International Mesothelioma Panel from the MESOPATH Reference Center. *J. Thorac. Oncol.* **2020**, *15*, 1037–1053. [CrossRef] [PubMed]
48. LeBleu, V.S.; Kalluri, R. A Peek into Cancer-Associated Fibroblasts: Origins, Functions and Translational Impact. *Dis. Models Mech.* **2018**, *11*, dmm029447. [CrossRef] [PubMed]
49. Ohara, Y.; Enomoto, A.; Tsuyuki, Y.; Sato, K.; Iida, T.; Kobayashi, H.; Mizutani, Y.; Miyai, Y.; Hara, A.; Mii, S.; et al. Connective Tissue Growth Factor Produced by Cancer-Associated Fibroblasts Correlates with Poor Prognosis in Epithelioid Malignant Pleural Mesothelioma. *Oncol. Rep.* **2020**, *44*, 838–848. [CrossRef]
50. Katoh, M.; Nakagama, H. FGF Receptors: Cancer Biology and Therapeutics. *Med. Res. Rev.* **2014**, *34*, 280–300. [CrossRef]
51. Marek, L.A.; Hinz, T.K.; von Mässenhausen, A.; Olszewski, K.A.; Kleczko, E.K.; Boehm, D.; Weiser-Evans, M.C.; Nemenoff, R.A.; Hoffmann, H.; Warth, A.; et al. Nonamplified FGFR1 Is a Growth Driver in Malignant Pleural Mesothelioma. *Mol. Cancer Res.* **2014**, *12*, 1460–1469. [CrossRef]
52. Blackwell, C.; Sherk, C.; Fricko, M.; Ganji, G.; Barnette, M.; Hoang, B.; Tunstead, J.; Skedzielewski, T.; Alsaid, H.; Jucker, B.M.; et al. Inhibition of FGF/FGFR Autocrine Signaling in Mesothelioma with the FGF Ligand Trap, FP-1039/GSK3052230. *Oncotarget* **2016**, *7*, 39861–39871. [CrossRef] [PubMed]
53. Lam, W.-S.; Creaney, J.; Chen, F.K.; Chin, W.L.; Muruganandan, S.; Arunachalam, S.; Attia, M.S.; Read, C.; Murray, K.; Millward, M.; et al. A Phase II Trial of Single Oral FGF Inhibitor, AZD4547, as Second or Third Line Therapy in Malignant Pleural Mesothelioma. *Lung Cancer* **2020**, *140*, 87–92. [CrossRef] [PubMed]
54. Chen, X.; Song, E. Turning Foes to Friends: Targeting Cancer-Associated Fibroblasts. *Nat. Rev. Drug Discov.* **2019**, *18*, 99–115. [CrossRef]
55. Hegmans, J.P.J.J.; Hemmes, A.; Hammad, H.; Boon, L.; Hoogsteden, H.C.; Lambrecht, B.N. Mesothelioma Environment Comprises Cytokines and T-Regulatory Cells That Suppress Immune Responses. *Eur. Respir. J.* **2006**, *27*, 1086–1095. [CrossRef]
56. Schelch, K.; Hoda, M.A.; Klikovits, T.; Münzker, J.; Ghanim, B.; Wagner, C.; Garay, T.; Laszlo, V.; Setinek, U.; Dome, B.; et al. Fibroblast Growth Factor Receptor Inhibition Is Active against Mesothelioma and Synergizes with Radio- and Chemotherapy. *Am. J. Respir. Crit. Care Med.* **2014**, *190*, 763–772. [CrossRef] [PubMed]
57. Kumar-Singh, S.; Weyler, J.; Martin, M.J.; Vermeulen, P.B.; Van Marck, E. Angiogenic Cytokines in Mesothelioma: A Study of VEGF, FGF-1 and -2, and TGF Beta Expression. *J. Pathol.* **1999**, *189*, 72–78. [CrossRef]
58. Righi, L.; Cavallo, M.C.; Gatti, G.; Monica, V.; Rapa, I.; Busso, S.; Albera, C.; Volante, M.; Scagliotti, G.V.; Papotti, M. Tumor/Stromal Caveolin-1 Expression Patterns in Pleural Mesothelioma Define a Subgroup of the Epithelial Histotype with Poorer Prognosis. *Am. J. Clin. Pathol.* **2014**, *141*, 816–827. [CrossRef]
59. Lolo, F.N.; Jiménez-Jiménez, V.; Sánchez-Álvarez, M.; Del Pozo, M.Á. Tumor-Stroma Biomechanical Crosstalk: A Perspective on the Role of Caveolin-1 in Tumor Progression. *Cancer Metastasis Rev.* **2020**, *39*, 485–503. [CrossRef]
60. Albacete-Albacete, L.; Navarro-Lérida, I.; López, J.A.; Martín-Padura, I.; Astudillo, A.M.; Ferrarini, A.; Van-Der-Heyden, M.; Balsinde, J.; Orend, G.; Vázquez, J.; et al. ECM Deposition Is Driven by Caveolin-1-Dependent Regulation of Exosomal Biogenesis and Cargo Sorting. *J. Cell Biol.* **2020**, *219*, e202006178. [CrossRef]
61. Fujii, M.; Toyoda, T.; Nakanishi, H.; Yatabe, Y.; Sato, A.; Matsudaira, Y.; Ito, H.; Murakami, H.; Kondo, Y.; Kondo, E.; et al. TGF-β Synergizes with Defects in the Hippo Pathway to Stimulate Human Malignant Mesothelioma Growth. *J. Exp. Med.* **2012**, *209*, 479–494. [CrossRef] [PubMed]
62. Jiang, L.; Yamashita, Y.; Chew, S.-H.; Akatsuka, S.; Ukai, S.; Wang, S.; Nagai, H.; Okazaki, Y.; Takahashi, T.; Toyokuni, S. Connective Tissue Growth Factor and β-Catenin Constitute an Autocrine Loop for Activation in Rat Sarcomatoid Mesothelioma. *J. Pathol.* **2014**, *233*, 402–414. [CrossRef]
63. Ohara, Y.; Chew, S.H.; Misawa, N.; Wang, S.; Somiya, D.; Nakamura, K.; Kajiyama, H.; Kikkawa, F.; Tsuyuki, Y.; Jiang, L.; et al. Connective Tissue Growth Factor-Specific Monoclonal Antibody Inhibits Growth of Malignant Mesothelioma in an Orthotopic Mouse Model. *Oncotarget* **2018**, *9*, 18494–18509. [CrossRef]
64. Richeldi, L.; Fernández Pérez, E.R.; Costabel, U.; Albera, C.; Lederer, D.J.; Flaherty, K.R.; Ettinger, N.; Perez, R.; Scholand, M.B.; Goldin, J.; et al. Pamrevlumab, an Anti-Connective Tissue Growth Factor Therapy, for Idiopathic Pulmonary Fibrosis (PRAISE): A Phase 2, Randomised, Double-Blind, Placebo-Controlled Trial. *Lancet Respir. Med.* **2020**, *8*, 25–33. [CrossRef]
65. Picozzi, V.J.; Pipas, J.M.; Koong, A.; Giaccia, A.; Bahary, N.; Krishnamurthi, S.S.; Lopez, C.D.; O'Dwyer, P.J.; Modelska, K.; Poolman, V.; et al. FG-3019, a Human Monoclonal Antibody to CTGF, with Gemcitabine/Erlotinib in Patients with Locally Advanced or Metastatic Pancreatic Ductal Adenocarcinoma. *JCO* **2013**, *31*, 213. [CrossRef]
66. Finger, E.C.; Cheng, C.-F.; Williams, T.R.; Rankin, E.B.; Bedogni, B.; Tachiki, L.; Spong, S.; Giaccia, A.J.; Powell, M.B. CTGF Is a Therapeutic Target for Metastatic Melanoma. *Oncogene* **2014**, *33*, 1093–1100. [CrossRef] [PubMed]
67. Neesse, A.; Frese, K.K.; Bapiro, T.E.; Nakagawa, T.; Sternlicht, M.D.; Seeley, T.W.; Pilarsky, C.; Jodrell, D.I.; Spong, S.M.; Tuveson, D.A. CTGF Antagonism with MAb FG-3019 Enhances Chemotherapy Response without Increasing Drug Delivery in Murine Ductal Pancreas Cancer. *Proc. Natl. Acad. Sci. USA* **2013**, *110*, 12325–12330. [CrossRef]
68. Abbott, D.M.; Bortolotto, C.; Benvenuti, S.; Lancia, A.; Filippi, A.R.; Stella, G.M. Malignant Pleural Mesothelioma: Genetic and Microenviromental Heterogeneity as an Unexpected Reading Frame and Therapeutic Challenge. *Cancers* **2020**, *12*, 1186. [CrossRef]

69. Solinas, G.; Germano, G.; Mantovani, A.; Allavena, P. Tumor-Associated Macrophages (TAM) as Major Players of the Cancer-Related Inflammation. *J. Leukoc. Biol.* **2009**, *86*, 1065–1073. [CrossRef]
70. Carbone, M.; Yang, H. Molecular Pathways: Targeting Mechanisms of Asbestos and Erionite Carcinogenesis in Mesothelioma. *Clin. Cancer Res.* **2012**, *18*, 598–604. [CrossRef]
71. Sayan, M.; Mossman, B.T. The NLRP3 Inflammasome in Pathogenic Particle and Fibre-Associated Lung Inflammation and Diseases. *Part. Fibre Toxicol.* **2016**, *13*, 51. [CrossRef]
72. Kadariya, Y.; Menges, C.W.; Talarchek, J.; Cai, K.Q.; Klein-Szanto, A.J.; Pietrofesa, R.A.; Christofidou-Solomidou, M.; Cheung, M.; Mossman, B.T.; Shukla, A.; et al. Inflammation-Related IL1β/IL1R Signaling Promotes the Development of Asbestos-Induced Malignant Mesothelioma. *Cancer Prev. Res.* **2016**, *9*, 406–414. [CrossRef]
73. Hamilton, R.F.; Iyer, L.L.; Holian, A. Asbestos Induces Apoptosis in Human Alveolar Macrophages. *Am. J. Physiol.* **1996**, *271*, L813–L819. [CrossRef]
74. Jube, S.; Rivera, Z.S.; Bianchi, M.E.; Powers, A.; Wang, E.; Pagano, I.; Pass, H.I.; Gaudino, G.; Carbone, M.; Yang, H. Cancer Cell Secretion of the DAMP Protein HMGB1 Supports Progression in Malignant Mesothelioma. *Cancer Res.* **2012**, *72*, 3290–3301. [CrossRef]
75. Tabata, C.; Shibata, E.; Tabata, R.; Kanemura, S.; Mikami, K.; Nogi, Y.; Masachika, E.; Nishizaki, T.; Nakano, T. Serum HMGB1 as a Prognostic Marker for Malignant Pleural Mesothelioma. *BMC Cancer* **2013**, *13*, 205. [CrossRef]
76. Maroso, M.; Balosso, S.; Ravizza, T.; Liu, J.; Aronica, E.; Iyer, A.M.; Rossetti, C.; Molteni, M.; Casalgrandi, M.; Manfredi, A.A.; et al. Toll-like Receptor 4 and High-Mobility Group Box-1 Are Involved in Ictogenesis and Can Be Targeted to Reduce Seizures. *Nat. Med.* **2010**, *16*, 413–419. [CrossRef] [PubMed]
77. Horio, D.; Minami, T.; Kitai, H.; Ishigaki, H.; Higashiguchi, Y.; Kondo, N.; Hirota, S.; Kitajima, K.; Nakajima, Y.; Koda, Y.; et al. Tumor-Associated Macrophage-Derived Inflammatory Cytokine Enhances Malignant Potential of Malignant Pleural Mesothelioma. *Cancer Sci.* **2020**, *111*, 2895–2906. [CrossRef] [PubMed]
78. Marcq, E.; Siozopoulou, V.; De Waele, J.; van Audenaerde, J.; Zwaenepoel, K.; Santermans, E.; Hens, N.; Pauwels, P.; van Meerbeeck, J.P.; Smits, E.L.J. Prognostic and Predictive Aspects of the Tumor Immune Microenvironment and Immune Checkpoints in Malignant Pleural Mesothelioma. *Oncoimmunology* **2017**, *6*, e1261241. [CrossRef]
79. Burt, B.M.; Rodig, S.J.; Tilleman, T.R.; Elbardissi, A.W.; Bueno, R.; Sugarbaker, D.J. Circulating and Tumor-Infiltrating Myeloid Cells Predict Survival in Human Pleural Mesothelioma. *Cancer* **2011**, *117*, 5234–5244. [CrossRef]
80. Cornelissen, R.; Lievense, L.A.; Robertus, J.-L.; Hendriks, R.W.; Hoogsteden, H.C.; Hegmans, J.P.J.J.; Aerts, J.G.J.V. Intratumoral Macrophage Phenotype and CD8+ T Lymphocytes as Potential Tools to Predict Local Tumor Outgrowth at the Intervention Site in Malignant Pleural Mesothelioma. *Lung Cancer* **2015**, *88*, 332–337. [CrossRef]
81. Chu, G.J.; van Zandwijk, N.; Rasko, J.E.J. The Immune Microenvironment in Mesothelioma: Mechanisms of Resistance to Immunotherapy. *Front. Oncol.* **2019**, *9*, 1366. [CrossRef] [PubMed]
82. Van Acker, H.H.; Capsomidis, A.; Smits, E.L.; Van Tendeloo, V.F. CD56 in the Immune System: More Than a Marker for Cytotoxicity? *Front. Immunol.* **2017**, *8*, 892. [CrossRef]
83. Alay, A.; Cordero, D.; Hijazo-Pechero, S.; Aliagas, E.; Lopez-Doriga, A.; Marín, R.; Palmero, R.; Llatjós, R.; Escobar, I.; Ramos, R.; et al. Integrative Transcriptome Analysis of Malignant Pleural Mesothelioma Reveals a Clinically Relevant Immune-Based Classification. *J. Immunother. Cancer* **2021**, *9*, e001601. [CrossRef]
84. DeLong, P.; Carroll, R.G.; Henry, A.C.; Tanaka, T.; Ahmad, S.; Leibowitz, M.S.; Sterman, D.H.; June, C.H.; Albelda, S.M.; Vonderheide, R.H. Regulatory T Cells and Cytokines in Malignant Pleural Effusions Secondary to Mesothelioma and Carcinoma. *Cancer Biol. Ther.* **2005**, *4*, 342–346. [CrossRef] [PubMed]
85. Thapa, B.; Salcedo, A.; Lin, X.; Walkiewicz, M.; Murone, C.; Ameratunga, M.; Asadi, K.; Deb, S.; Barnett, S.A.; Knight, S.; et al. The Immune Microenvironment, Genome-Wide Copy Number Aberrations, and Survival in Mesothelioma. *J. Thorac. Oncol.* **2017**, *12*, 850–859. [CrossRef] [PubMed]
86. Murthy, P.; Ekeke, C.N.; Russell, K.L.; Butler, S.C.; Wang, Y.; Luketich, J.D.; Soloff, A.C.; Dhupar, R.; Lotze, M.T. Making Cold Malignant Pleural Effusions Hot: Driving Novel Immunotherapies. *OncoImmunology* **2019**, *8*, e1554969. [CrossRef] [PubMed]
87. Yamada, N.; Oizumi, S.; Kikuchi, E.; Shinagawa, N.; Konishi-Sakakibara, J.; Ishimine, A.; Aoe, K.; Gemba, K.; Kishimoto, T.; Torigoe, T.; et al. CD8+ Tumor-Infiltrating Lymphocytes Predict Favorable Prognosis in Malignant Pleural Mesothelioma after Resection. *Cancer Immunol. Immunother.* **2010**, *59*, 1543–1549. [CrossRef]
88. Chee, S.J.; Lopez, M.; Mellows, T.; Gankande, S.; Moutasim, K.A.; Harris, S.; Clarke, J.; Vijayanand, P.; Thomas, G.J.; Ottensmeier, C.H. Evaluating the Effect of Immune Cells on the Outcome of Patients with Mesothelioma. *Br. J. Cancer* **2017**, *117*, 1341–1348. [CrossRef]
89. Anraku, M.; Cunningham, K.S.; Yun, Z.; Tsao, M.-S.; Zhang, L.; Keshavjee, S.; Johnston, M.R.; de Perrot, M. Impact of Tumor-Infiltrating T Cells on Survival in Patients with Malignant Pleural Mesothelioma. *J. Thorac. Cardiovasc. Surg.* **2008**, *135*, 823–829. [CrossRef]
90. Pasello, G.; Zago, G.; Lunardi, F.; Urso, L.; Kern, I.; Vlacic, G.; Grosso, F.; Mencoboni, M.; Ceresoli, G.L.; Schiavon, M.; et al. Malignant Pleural Mesothelioma Immune Microenvironment and Checkpoint Expression: Correlation with Clinical–Pathological Features and Intratumor Heterogeneity over Time. *Ann. Oncol.* **2018**, *29*, 1258–1265. [CrossRef]

91. Salaroglio, I.C.; Kopecka, J.; Napoli, F.; Pradotto, M.; Maletta, F.; Costardi, L.; Gagliasso, M.; Milosevic, V.; Ananthanarayanan, P.; Bironzo, P.; et al. Potential Diagnostic and Prognostic Role of Microenvironment in Malignant Pleural Mesothelioma. *J. Thorac. Oncol.* **2019**, *14*, 1458–1471. [CrossRef] [PubMed]
92. Fusco, N.; Vaira, V.; Righi, I.; Sajjadi, E.; Venetis, K.; Lopez, G.; Cattaneo, M.; Castellani, M.; Rosso, L.; Nosotti, M.; et al. Characterization of the Immune Microenvironment in Malignant Pleural Mesothelioma Reveals Prognostic Subgroups of Patients. *Lung Cancer* **2020**, *150*, 53–61. [CrossRef] [PubMed]
93. Greten, T.F.; Manns, M.P.; Korangy, F. Myeloid Derived Suppressor Cells in Human Diseases. *Int. Immunopharmacol.* **2011**, *11*, 802–807. [CrossRef]
94. Mandruzzato, S.; Solito, S.; Falisi, E.; Francescato, S.; Chiarion-Sileni, V.; Mocellin, S.; Zanon, A.; Rossi, C.R.; Nitti, D.; Bronte, V.; et al. IL4Ralpha+ Myeloid-Derived Suppressor Cell Expansion in Cancer Patients. *J. Immunol.* **2009**, *182*, 6562–6568. [CrossRef]
95. Burt, B.M.; Bader, A.; Winter, D.; Rodig, S.J.; Bueno, R.; Sugarbaker, D.J. Expression of Interleukin-4 Receptor Alpha in Human Pleural Mesothelioma Is Associated with Poor Survival and Promotion of Tumor Inflammation. *Clin. Cancer Res.* **2012**, *18*, 1568–1577. [CrossRef] [PubMed]
96. Minnema-Luiting, J.; Vroman, H.; Aerts, J.; Cornelissen, R. Heterogeneity in Immune Cell Content in Malignant Pleural Mesothelioma. *Int. J. Mol. Sci.* **2018**, *19*, 1041. [CrossRef]
97. Khanna, S.; Graef, S.; Mussai, F.; Thomas, A.; Wali, N.; Yenidunya, B.G.; Yuan, C.; Morrow, B.; Zhang, J.; Korangy, F.; et al. Tumor-Derived GM-CSF Promotes Granulocyte Immunosuppression in Mesothelioma Patients. *Clin. Cancer Res.* **2018**, *24*, 2859–2872. [CrossRef] [PubMed]
98. Upham, J.W.; Xi, Y. Dendritic Cells in Human Lung Disease: Recent Advances. *Chest* **2017**, *151*, 668–673. [CrossRef]
99. Guilliams, M.; Lambrecht, B.N.; Hammad, H. Division of Labor between Lung Dendritic Cells and Macrophages in the Defense against Pulmonary Infections. *Mucosal Immunol.* **2013**, *6*, 464–473. [CrossRef]
100. Kopf, M.; Schneider, C.; Nobs, S.P. The Development and Function of Lung-Resident Macrophages and Dendritic Cells. *Nat. Immunol.* **2015**, *16*, 36–44. [CrossRef]
101. Lynch, J.P.; Mazzone, S.B.; Rogers, M.J.; Arikkatt, J.J.; Loh, Z.; Pritchard, A.L.; Upham, J.W.; Phipps, S. The Plasmacytoid Dendritic Cell: At the Cross-Roads in Asthma. *Eur. Respir. J.* **2014**, *43*, 264–275. [CrossRef] [PubMed]
102. Mitchell, D.; Chintala, S.; Dey, M. Plasmacytoid Dendritic Cell in Immunity and Cancer. *J. Neuroimmunol.* **2018**, *322*, 63–73. [CrossRef] [PubMed]
103. Gardner, J.K.; Mamotte, C.D.S.; Patel, P.; Yeoh, T.L.; Jackaman, C.; Nelson, D.J. Mesothelioma Tumor Cells Modulate Dendritic Cell Lipid Content, Phenotype and Function. *PLoS ONE* **2015**, *10*, e0123563. [CrossRef] [PubMed]
104. Jackaman, C.; Cornwall, S.; Graham, P.T.; Nelson, D.J. CD40-Activated B Cells Contribute to Mesothelioma Tumor Regression. *Immunol. Cell Biol.* **2011**, *89*, 255–267. [CrossRef]
105. Vonderheide, R.H. CD40 Agonist Antibodies in Cancer Immunotherapy. *Annu. Rev. Med.* **2020**, *71*, 47–58. [CrossRef]
106. Hegde, P.S.; Karanikas, V.; Evers, S. The Where, the When, and the How of Immune Monitoring for Cancer Immunotherapies in the Era of Checkpoint Inhibition. *Clin. Cancer Res.* **2016**, *22*, 1865–1874. [CrossRef]
107. Hu, Z.I.; Ghafoor, A.; Sengupta, M.; Hassan, R. Malignant Mesothelioma: Advances in Immune Checkpoint Inhibitor and Mesothelin-Targeted Therapies. *Cancer* **2021**, *127*, 1010–1020. [CrossRef]
108. Paver, E.C.; Cooper, W.A.; Colebatch, A.J.; Ferguson, P.M.; Hill, S.K.; Lum, T.; Shin, J.-S.; O'Toole, S.; Anderson, L.; Scolyer, R.A.; et al. Programmed Death Ligand-1 (PD-L1) as a Predictive Marker for Immunotherapy in Solid Tumours: A Guide to Immunohistochemistry Implementation and Interpretation. *Pathology* **2021**, *53*, 141–156. [CrossRef]
109. Akinleye, A.; Rasool, Z. Immune Checkpoint Inhibitors of PD-L1 as Cancer Therapeutics. *J. Hematol. Oncol.* **2019**, *12*, 92. [CrossRef]
110. McCambridge, A.J.; Napolitano, A.; Mansfield, A.S.; Fennell, D.A.; Sekido, Y.; Nowak, A.K.; Reungwetwattana, T.; Mao, W.; Pass, H.I.; Carbone, M.; et al. Progress in the Management of Malignant Pleural Mesothelioma in 2017. *J. Thorac. Oncol.* **2018**, *13*, 606–623. [CrossRef]
111. Scherpereel, A.; Wallyn, F.; Albelda, S.M.; Munck, C. Novel Therapies for Malignant Pleural Mesothelioma. *Lancet Oncol.* **2018**, *19*, e161–e172. [CrossRef]
112. Jin, L.; Gu, W.; Li, X.; Xie, L.; Wang, L.; Chen, Z. PD-L1 and Prognosis in Patients with Malignant Pleural Mesothelioma: A Meta-Analysis and Bioinformatics Study. *Adv. Med. Oncol.* **2020**, *12*, 1758835920962362. [CrossRef]
113. Seaman, S.; Zhu, Z.; Saha, S.; Zhang, X.M.; Yang, M.Y.; Hilton, M.B.; Morris, K.; Szot, C.; Morris, H.; Swing, D.A.; et al. Eradication of Tumors through Simultaneous Ablation of CD276/B7-H3-Positive Tumor Cells and Tumor Vasculature. *Cancer Cell* **2017**, *31*, 501–515.e8. [CrossRef]
114. Matsumura, E.; Kajino, K.; Abe, M.; Ohtsuji, N.; Saeki, H.; Hlaing, M.T.; Hino, O. Expression Status of PD-L1 and B7-H3 in Mesothelioma. *Pathol. Int.* **2020**, *70*, 999–1008. [CrossRef]
115. Chen, C.; Zhao, S.; Karnad, A.; Freeman, J.W. The Biology and Role of CD44 in Cancer Progression: Therapeutic Implications. *J. Hematol. Oncol.* **2018**, *11*, 64. [CrossRef]
116. Cortes-Dericks, L.; Schmid, R.A. CD44 and Its Ligand Hyaluronan as Potential Biomarkers in Malignant Pleural Mesothelioma: Evidence and Perspectives. *Respir. Res.* **2017**, *18*, 58. [CrossRef] [PubMed]

117. Ohno, Y.; Shingyoku, S.; Miyake, S.; Tanaka, A.; Fudesaka, S.; Shimizu, Y.; Yoshifuji, A.; Yamawaki, Y.; Yoshida, S.; Tanaka, S.; et al. Differential Regulation of the Sphere Formation and Maintenance of Cancer-Initiating Cells of Malignant Mesothelioma via CD44 and ALK4 Signaling Pathways. *Oncogene* **2018**, *37*, 6357–6367. [CrossRef] [PubMed]
118. Muller, S.; Victoria Lai, W.; Adusumilli, P.S.; Desmeules, P.; Frosina, D.; Jungbluth, A.; Ni, A.; Eguchi, T.; Travis, W.D.; Ladanyi, M.; et al. V-Domain Ig-Containing Suppressor of T-Cell Activation (VISTA), a Potentially Targetable Immune Checkpoint Molecule, Is Highly Expressed in Epithelioid Malignant Pleural Mesothelioma. *Mod. Pathol.* **2020**, *33*, 303–311. [CrossRef] [PubMed]
119. Galon, J.; Bruni, D. Approaches to Treat Immune Hot, Altered and Cold Tumours with Combination Immunotherapies. *Nat. Rev. Drug Discov.* **2019**, *18*, 197–218. [CrossRef] [PubMed]
120. Sen, T.; Rodriguez, B.L.; Chen, L.; Corte, C.M.D.; Morikawa, N.; Fujimoto, J.; Cristea, S.; Nguyen, T.; Diao, L.; Li, L.; et al. Targeting DNA Damage Response Promotes Antitumor Immunity through STING-Mediated T-Cell Activation in Small Cell Lung Cancer. *Cancer Discov.* **2019**, *9*, 646–661. [CrossRef] [PubMed]
121. Alcala, N.; Mangiante, L.; Le-Stang, N.; Gustafson, C.E.; Boyault, S.; Damiola, F.; Alcala, K.; Brevet, M.; Thivolet-Bejui, F.; Blanc-Fournier, C.; et al. Redefining Malignant Pleural Mesothelioma Types as a Continuum Uncovers Immune-Vascular Interactions. *EBioMedicine* **2019**, *48*, 191–202. [CrossRef]
122. Sekido, Y. Molecular Pathogenesis of Malignant Mesothelioma. *Carcinogenesis* **2013**, *34*, 1413–1419. [CrossRef] [PubMed]
123. Strizzi, L.; Catalano, A.; Vianale, G.; Orecchia, S.; Casalini, A.; Tassi, G.; Puntoni, R.; Mutti, L.; Procopio, A. Vascular Endothelial Growth Factor Is an Autocrine Growth Factor in Human Malignant Mesothelioma. *J. Pathol.* **2001**, *193*, 468–475. [CrossRef]
124. Ellis, L.M.; Hicklin, D.J. VEGF-Targeted Therapy: Mechanisms of Anti-Tumour Activity. *Nat. Rev. Cancer* **2008**, *8*, 579–591. [CrossRef] [PubMed]
125. König, J.-E.; Tolnay, E.; Wiethege, T.; Müller, K.-M. Expression of Vascular Endothelial Growth Factor in Diffuse Malignant Pleural Mesothelioma. *Virchows Arch.* **1999**, *435*, 8–12. [CrossRef]
126. Ohta, Y.; Shridhar, V.; Bright, R.K.; Kalemkerian, G.P.; Du, W.; Carbone, M.; Watanabe, Y.; Pass, H.I. VEGF and VEGF Type C Play an Important Role in Angiogenesis and Lymphangiogenesis in Human Malignant Mesothelioma Tumours. *Br. J. Cancer* **1999**, *81*, 54–61. [CrossRef] [PubMed]
127. Linder, C.; Linder, S.; Munck-Wikland, E.; Strander, H. Independent Expression of Serum Vascular Endothelial Growth Factor (VEGF) and Basic Fibroblast Growth Factor (BFGF) in Patients with Carcinoma and Sarcoma. *Anticancer Res.* **1998**, *18*, 2063–2068. [PubMed]
128. Antony, V.B.; Hott, J.W.; Godbey, S.W.; Holm, K. Angiogenesis in Mesotheliomas. Role of Mesothelial Cell Derived IL-8. *Chest* **1996**, *109*, 21S–22S. [CrossRef]
129. Nowak, A.K.; Brosseau, S.; Cook, A.; Zalcman, G. Antiangiogeneic Strategies in Mesothelioma. *Front. Oncol.* **2020**, *10*, 126. [CrossRef]
130. De Marinis, F.; Bria, E.; Ciardiello, F.; Crinò, L.; Douillard, J.Y.; Griesinger, F.; Lambrechts, D.; Perol, M.; Ramalingam, S.S.; Smit, E.F.; et al. International Experts Panel Meeting of the Italian Association of Thoracic Oncology on Antiangiogenetic Drugs for Non-Small Cell Lung Cancer: Realities and Hopes. *J. Thorac. Oncol.* **2016**, *11*, 1153–1169. [CrossRef]
131. Nowak, A.; Grosso, F.; Steele, N.; Novello, S.; Popat, S.; Greillier, L.; John, T.; Leighl, N.; Reck, M.; Pavlakis, N.; et al. MA 19.03 Nintedanib + Pemetrexed/Cisplatin in Malignant Pleural Mesothelioma (MPM): Phase II Biomarker Data from the LUME-Meso Study. *J. Thorac. Oncol.* **2017**, *12*, S1884. [CrossRef]
132. Chia, P.L.; Russell, P.; Asadi, K.; Thapa, B.; Gebski, V.; Murone, C.; Walkiewicz, M.; Eriksson, U.; Scott, A.M.; John, T. Analysis of Angiogenic and Stromal Biomarkers in a Large Malignant Mesothelioma Cohort. *Lung Cancer* **2020**, *150*, 1–8. [CrossRef] [PubMed]

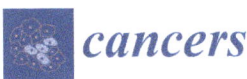

Article

Identification of Redox-Sensitive Transcription Factors as Markers of Malignant Pleural Mesothelioma

Martina Schiavello [1], Elena Gazzano [2,3], Loredana Bergandi [4], Francesca Silvagno [4], Roberta Libener [5], Chiara Riganti [3,4] and Elisabetta Aldieri [3,4,*]

[1] Department of Medical Sciences, University of Torino, 10126 Torino, Italy; martina.schiavello@unito.it
[2] Department of Life Sciences and Systems Biology, University of Torino, 10135 Torino, Italy; elena.gazzano@unito.it
[3] Interdepartmental Center for Studies on Asbestos and Other Toxic Particulates "G. Scansetti", University of Torino, 10126 Torino, Italy; chiara.riganti@unito.it
[4] Department of Oncology, University of Torino, 10126 Torino, Italy; loredana.bergandi@unito.it (L.B.); francesca.silvagno@unito.it (F.S.)
[5] Department of Integrated Activities Research and Innovation, Azienda Ospedaliera SS. Antonio e Biagio e Cesare Arrigo, 15121 Alessandria, Italy; rlibener@ospedale.al.it
* Correspondence: elisabetta.aldieri@unito.it; Tel.: +39-0116705844

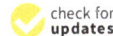

Citation: Schiavello, M.; Gazzano, E.; Bergandi, L.; Silvagno, F.; Libener, R.; Riganti, C.; Aldieri, E. Identification of Redox-Sensitive Transcription Factors as Markers of Malignant Pleural Mesothelioma. *Cancers* **2021**, *13*, 1138. https://doi.org/10.3390/cancers13051138

Academic Editor: Daniel L. Pouliquen

Received: 17 February 2021
Accepted: 3 March 2021
Published: 7 March 2021

Publisher's Note: MDPI stays neutral with regard to jurisdictional claims in published maps and institutional affiliations.

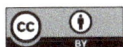

Copyright: © 2021 by the authors. Licensee MDPI, Basel, Switzerland. This article is an open access article distributed under the terms and conditions of the Creative Commons Attribution (CC BY) license (https://creativecommons.org/licenses/by/4.0/).

Simple Summary: Malignant pleural mesothelioma is a lung tumor associated with asbestos exposure, with a poor prognosis, and a difficult pharmacological approach. Asbestos exposure is very toxic for the lungs, which counteract this toxic effect by activating some antioxidant defense proteins. When these proteins are more active that in normal conditions, as in several cancers, these tumors become able to survive and resist to stress or chemotherapy. In our laboratory, we collected cellular samples of mesothelioma and non-transformed mesothelium from Hospital's Biobank and we evaluated these proteins. Our results demonstrated these proteins are upregulated in mesothelioma cells and not in non-transformed mesothelium. This event could be associated to toxic effects evoked by asbestos exposure, highlighting the need in the future to monitor asbestos-exposed people by measuring biomarkers identified, in the attempt to identify them as possible predictive markers and potential pharmacological targets addressed to improve mesothelioma prognosis.

Abstract: Although asbestos has been banned in most countries around the world, malignant pleural mesothelioma (MPM) is a current problem. MPM is an aggressive tumor with a poor prognosis, so it is crucial to identify new markers in the preventive field. Asbestos exposure induces oxidative stress and its carcinogenesis has been linked to a strong oxidative damage, event counteracted by antioxidant systems at the pulmonary level. The present study has been focused on some redox-sensitive transcription factors that regulate cellular antioxidant defense and are overexpressed in many tumors, such as Nrf2 (Nuclear factor erythroid 2-related factor 2), Ref-1 (Redox effector factor 1), and FOXM1 (Forkhead box protein M1). The research was performed in human mesothelial and MPM cells. Our results have clearly demonstrated an overexpression of Nrf2, Ref-1, and FOXM1 in mesothelioma towards mesothelium, and a consequent activation of downstream genes controlled by these factors, which in turn regulates antioxidant defense. This event is mediated by oxidative free radicals produced when mesothelial cells are exposed to asbestos fibers. We observed an increased expression of Nrf2, Ref-1, and FOXM1 towards untreated cells, confirming asbestos as the mediator of oxidative stress evoked at the mesothelium level. These factors can therefore be considered predictive biomarkers of MPM and potential pharmacological targets in the treatment of this aggressive cancer.

Keywords: malignant pleural mesothelioma; mesothelium; oxidative stress; redox-sensitive factors; asbestos; biomarkers

1. Introduction

Exposure to asbestos has been clearly associated to the development of lung diseases, among which the most serious is the Malignant Pleural Mesothelioma (MPM), a tumor that originates from the pleura, with an increased incidence throughout the world due to the long latency period, and the direct correlation between asbestos exposure and MPM development is unequivocal [1]. Histologically, three main subtypes of MPM can be distinguished: epithelioid (60–80%), sarcomatoid (<10%), and biphasic or mixed (10–15%) [2]. Although this is a rather rare neoplasm, the incidence is expected to grow over the next few years with a peak between 2020 and 2030 [3], mainly due to the extensive exposure to asbestos fibers in the past years [3]. Most patients are diagnosed at an advanced stage of the disease [4], and for this reason the MPM needs a timely diagnosis and an improvement in the prognosis.

Numerous studies have been focused on trying to clarify the molecular mechanisms underlying the carcinogenesis induced by asbestos, however, some aspects still need to be defined [5]. It is known that asbestos causes chronic inflammation and induces a strong oxidative damage mediated by an increased production of Reactive Oxygen Species (ROS), free radicals that have been shown to be carcinogenetic mediators, by causing DNA mutations and inducing tumor cell proliferation [6]. Several studies have shown that ROS are important second messengers in mediating the toxicity of asbestos [6], especially at the level of the pulmonary mesothelium [7]. Thus, ROS production can modulate different redox-sensitive signal pathways by different transcription factors, in the attempt to counteract the oxidative damage [8]. Among these, a role in carcinogenesis has been shown to be linked to the following redox-sensitive transcription factors: Nuclear factor erythroid 2—related factor 2 (Nrf2 o NFE2L2)/Kelch-like protein ECH-associated protein 1 (KEAP-1) [9], Apurinic-apyrimidinic endonuclease 1 (APE-1)/Redox effector factor 1 (Ref-1) [10] and Forkhead box protein M1 (FOXM1) [11].

The need of these factors in survival of tumor cells, strongly suggests a fundamental role of their activation in carcinogenesis [9–11]. Cancer cells become able to survive against oxidative stress by activating these factors constitutively in different types of tumors (lung, pancreas, breast) [12–14], with increased aggressiveness and resistance to chemotherapy [15], thus up-regulating pro-survival antioxidant responses.

Nrf2 is a redox-sensitive factor belonging to the subfamily cap'n'collar (CNC), containing seven conserved domains (Neh1-7), the latter being involved in the regulation of its stability and transcriptional activity [16]. The intracellular regulator of Nrf2 is KEAP-1, containing 27 cysteines sensitive to oxidative stress: under basal conditions, KEAP-1 degrades Nrf2 by promoting its ubiquitination via proteasome [17]. It has been shown that cancer cells are able to survive against oxidative stress by activating Nrf2 constitutively, and in this way upregulating the antioxidant response in different types of tumors (lung, pancreas, breast, and endometrium), with increased tumor aggression and resistance to chemotherapy [18,19]. Particularly in lung cancer, inactivating somatic mutations on KEAP-1 cysteine residues have been observed, resulting in constitutive activation of Nrf2 [20]. Elevated levels of ROS, by acting on cysteine residues, cause a conformational change of KEAP-1 with the dissociation of the Nrf2/KEAP-1 complex and consequent nuclear translocation of Nrf2, which in turn activates genes that regulate the antioxidant response, such as Mn-Superoxide Dismutase (SOD2) and catalase (CAT), and upregulating the expression of phase II detoxification (glutathione S-transferase, GST) and antioxidant (heme oxygenase 1, HO-1) enzymes [18,19], thus playing a central role in cellular antioxidant defense [20]. Moreover, ROS increase induces the phosphorylation of Nrf2 at the N-terminal region, resulting in a further detachment from KEAP-1 and translocation of the transcription factor from the cytoplasm into the nucleus [21]. Nrf2 is active against oxidative stress when phosphorylated by different kinases, such as MAPK (Mitogen-activated protein kinase)/Erk (Extracellular signal-regulated kinase), PKC (Protein kinase C), and PI3K (Phosphoinositide 3-kinase) at the level of serine and threonine residues, by breaking the binding with the KEAP-1 inhibitor and thus translocating into the nucleus [21].

APE-1/Ref-1 is a multifunctional enzyme involved, respectively, in DNA repair and cellular redox regulation. The two main activities are encoded by two distinct regions of the protein: N-terminal region controls the redox function and C-terminal region checks the DNA repair [10]. Redox-sensitive factor Ref-1, when activated, induces in turn various transcription factors, among which the Nuclear Factor kappa B (NF-kB), the Activator Protein-1 (AP-1) [10], both involved in redox cellular control, and the Hypoxia-Inducible Factor 1 α (HIF-1α), and modulates some tumor suppressors, such as p53 and PTEN (Phosphatase and tensin homolog) [22]. It is known that DNA oxidative damage accelerates cancer development: ROS has been shown to activate the overexpression of Ref-1 with consequent increase in endonuclease activity [22]. As Nrf2, Ref-1 results to be overexpressed in various types of tumors, with increased resistance to antineoplastic therapies [23]: some studies showed an increased expression of Ref-1 in non-small cell lung cancer (NSCLC) with consequent resistance to cisplatin treatment [23], and in knock-down mice there is a significant improvement against the cytotoxic response to drugs [24].

FOXM1 is a transcription factor of the Forkhead box (FoxO) protein superfamily [25]. Unlike FoxO transcription factors, which are activated in quiescent cells and inhibit cell proliferation, FOXM1 is only expressed in proliferating cells and has critical functions in cell-cycle progression [25,26]. Expression of FOXM1 is induced by increased oncogenic stress requiring ROS, and the upregulated FOXM1 counteracts elevated intracellular ROS levels by stimulating the expression of antioxidant enzyme genes to protect tumor cells from oxidative stress [27], such as those involved in the antioxidant system. It has been demonstrated that elevated FOXM1 downregulates ROS levels by stimulating the expression of ROS scavenger genes, such as *SOD2* and *CAT* [27]. As Nrf2 and Ref-1, FOXM1 is overexpressed in different human cancers [28], particularly in lung cancers, and resulted activated by oncogenic pathways, such as those mediated by the axis Ras/MAPK/Erk [26]: induction of FOXM1 by oncogenic Ras requires ROS increase [27], so stimulating FOXM1 nuclear translocation via MAPK/Erk and thus promoting the transcriptional activity of FOXM1 [29].

In this context, our study has been addressed to clarify the correlation between oxidative stress, asbestos and the development of mesothelioma, going to investigate the involvement of all these factors associated to the antioxidant response at a diagnostic and therapeutic level. However, although there are some evidence in literature that demonstrate the overexpression of Nrf2, Ref-1, and FOXM1 in MPM, a close correlation between the pro-oxidant effects exerted by asbestos and these factors, in association to the development of mesothelioma, has not yet been clearly demonstrated. Actually, speaking of asbestos, it should be noted that asbestos includes six different types of fibers [30], among which the most pathogenic in inducing MPM are the iron-containing fibers crocidolite and amosite [31], in particular the crocidolite asbestos (used in this work) has been demonstrated to be the most carcinogenic asbestos fiber [31]. Recent evidence of activation of Nrf2, caused by exposure to asbestos, is reported in murine peritoneal macrophages, in which the use of Nrf2 inhibitory molecules showed an increased apoptosis of tumor cells [32], while other studies in human mesothelioma cell lines showed the involvement of the antioxidant role of Nrf2 in resistance to chemotherapy [33] or in improving therapeutic approach against MPM [34]. Moreover, a proteomic analysis identified Nrf2 as one of the proteins more expressed on biphasic MPM [35] and experiments in human mesothelioma MSTO-211H cells demonstrated Nrf2 overexpression via ROS induction [36], although not in association with asbestos exposure. Concerning Ref-1, Flaherty et al. [37] demonstrated an increased Ref-1 activity after crocidolite asbestos incubation in human alveolar macrophages, as already previously shown in rat pleural mesothelial cells by Fung et al. [38], but, until now, no clear evidence has been associated to MPM. Finally, in recent literature, the role of FOXM1 in association to MPM, particularly by considering the emerging role of FOXM1 as hallmark in many tumors is emerging [28], has been studied. Cunniff et al. [39,40] demonstrated a link between FOXM1 expression and the mitochondrial oxidant metabolism in mesothelioma cell lines, Mizuno et al. [41] showed a direct regulation of FOXM1 transcription in mesothelioma cells by YAP (Yes-associated protein) oncogenic protein, and Romagnoli et al. [42] identified, by gene expression analysis, FOXM1 as a potential target for novel therapies against mesothelioma. Nevertheless, until now, no link has been shown to correlate FOXM1 overexpression to primary asbestos exposure.

In literature, the characterization of new markers, potentially useful in the diagnosis and therapy of asbestos-related diseases, is becoming increasingly important. In recent years, some molecules such as Mesothelin [5] and BAP1 (BRCA1 associated protein-1) [43] have had special relevance and now are used in MPM diagnosis. Moreover, also the High Mobility Group Box 1 (HMGB1), mediator of pulmonary inflammation, has been detected at high level in the serum of patients exposed to asbestos compared to those not exposed [4,5]. Notably, by examining The Cancer Genome Atlas (TCGA) and Genomic Data Commons (GDC) datasets concerning MPM patients analyzed and eventual Nrf2, Ref-1, and FOXM1 prognostic values, the results showed, out of 87 MPM samples analyzed, that none of the three proposed transcription factors have been analyzed up to now, although in lung cancer they have already been identified and quite associated with a worse prognosis. However, markers as Mesothelin or BAP1 are not able to provide an early diagnosis of MPM. We therefore evaluated the possible involvement of the above mentioned redox-sensitive transcription factors in MPM development in correlation to crocidolite asbestos exposure, analyzing the expression of these factors in human mesothelial and mesothelioma cells, notably the last ones derived from asbestos exposed MPM patients. This is a crucial point aimed to identify these redox-sensitive transcription factors as predictive markers for this aggressive cancer.

2. Results

2.1. Nrf2, Ref-1, and FOXM1 Are Overexpressed in MPM Cells

We evaluated the expression of Nrf2, Ref-1, and FOXM1 in human mesothelial cells (HMC) and MPM cells. Our results showed clearly an increased basal expression of the redox-sensitive transcription factors in all three histological types of MPM, epithelioid (EMM), sarcomatoid (SMM), and biphasic (BMM) forms, towards HMC (Figure 1A,B). As documented in literature, we used NSCLC cells (A549) as positive control of the basal overexpression of these factors in lung tumor cells.

2.2. Nrf2 Phosphorylation in MPM Cells Mediates its Nuclear Translocation

ROS increase induces the phosphorylation of Nrf2 in the N-terminal region [21]. We evaluated the presence of the phosphorylated form of Nrf2 (p-Nrf2) in nuclear extracts of HMC and MPM (EMM, SMM, BMM) cells, and in A549 cell line, used as positive control of basal Nrf2 phosphorylation. As shown in Figure 2A,B, the presence of the phosphorylated form of Nrf2 in all histological types of MPM cells unless the mesothelium demonstrated the activation of Nrf2 via its phosphorylation, as the mechanism which drives and activates Nrf2.

2.3. Increased Antioxidant Target Genes Induced by by Nrf2, Ref-1, and FOXM1 in MPM Cells

Nrf2 activation drives the transcription and induction of some target genes involved in the antioxidant response, some of these already associated to asbestos exposure [44]. We demonstrated an increased expression of SOD2, GST, CAT, and HO-1 proteins in MPM cells towards HMC, as shown in Figure 3A,B.

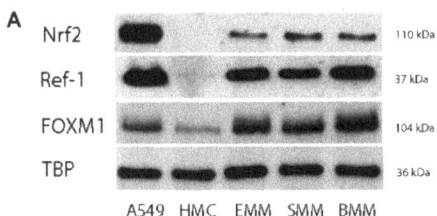

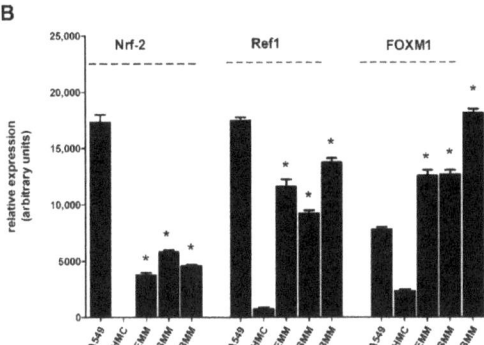

Figure 1. Nrf2, Ref-1, and FOXM1 overexpression in MPM cells. (**A**) Western blot analysis of Nrf2, Ref-1, FOXM1, and TBP proteins on nuclear extracts of HMC, EMM, SMM, BMM, and A549 cells. (**B**) Densitometric analysis of the expression levels of Nrf2 ($n = 3$, * $p < 0.001$), Ref-1 ($n = 3$, * $p < 0.001$) and FOXM1 ($n = 3$, * $p < 0.001$).

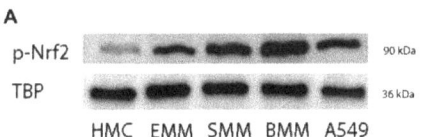

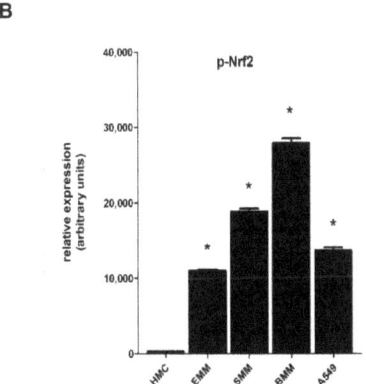

Figure 2. Phospho-Nrf2 overexpression in MPM cells. (**A**) Western Blot analysis of phosphorylated Nrf2 (p-Nrf2) and TBP proteins on nuclear extracts of HMC, EMM, SMM, BMM, and A549 cells. (**B**) Densitometric analysis of the relative expression of p-Nrf2 ($n = 3$, * $p < 0.001$).

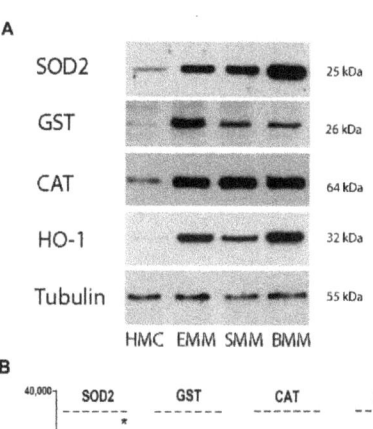
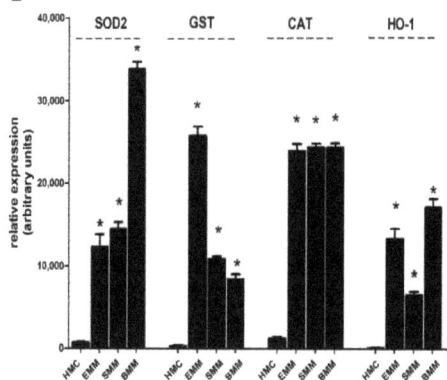

Figure 3. Expression of antioxidant genes induced by Nrf2 and FOXM1 in MPM cells. (**A**) Western Blot of SOD2, GST, CAT, HO-1, and Tubulin proteins in HMC, EMM, SMM, and BMM cells. (**B**) Densitometric analysis of the relative expression of SOD2, GST, CAT, and HO-1 ($n = 3$, * $p < 0.001$).

As Nrf2, also FOXM1 activated the antioxidant proteins SOD2 and CAT in MPM cells towards HMC (Figure 3A,B), so counteracting oxidative stress in tumor cells.

Ref-1, when activated, still controls some target genes involved in the antioxidant response, such as NF-kB. Our results demonstrated an increased nuclear accumulation of p50 active subunit of NF-kB in MPM cells towards HMC (Figure 4A,B). Among Ref-1 related controlled genes, the tumor suppressors p53 and PTEN are crucial in cancer suppression when expressed at nuclear level. So, in our experimental models, both p53 and PTEN are significantly expressed in the cytosol of MPM cells in comparison to HMC (Figure 4C,D), thus both not working as tumor suppressors at nuclear level.

At the same time, we evaluated p53 and PTEN at nuclear level: the results evidentiated a partially not so significative downregulation of PTEN and p53 proteins in MPM cells towards HMC (Figure S1), although both resulted partially decreased in MPM cells.

2.4. Phosphorylation of Erk Mediates Nrf2 Phosphorylation and FOXM1 Overexpression

Nrf2 phosphorylation has been demonstrated to be mediated by different kinases, among which the MAPK/Erk pathway is one of the main involved [21]. Besides, ERK phosphorylation has been widely documented in mesothelial cells exposed to crocidolite asbestos and in MPM cells [45]. Our results show an increased active phosphorylated form of Erk (p-Erk) in all three histological types of MPM cells and not in HMC (Figure 5A,B).

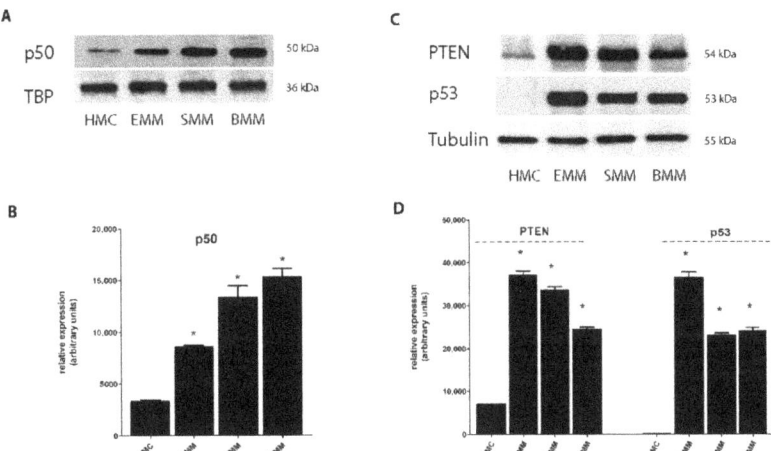

Figure 4. Expression of genes induced by Ref-1 in MPM cells. (**A**) Western Blot of nuclear p50 active subunit of NF-kB and TBP protein in HMC, EMM, SMM, and BMM cells, and (**B**) the relative densitometric analysis ($n = 3$, * $p < 0.001$). (**C**) Western Blot of cytosolic p53, PTEN and Tubulin proteins in HMC, EMM, SMM, and BMM cells, and (**D**) the relative densitometric analysis ($n = 3$, * $p < 0.001$).

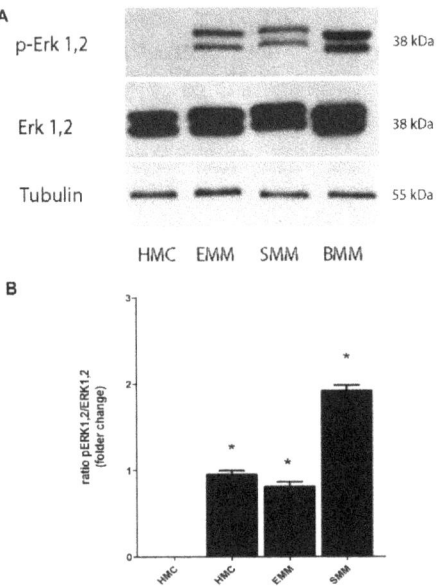

Figure 5. Erk phosphorylation mediates Nrf2 and FOXM1 activation. (**A**) Western Blot of phosho-Erk (p-Erk), Erk (1,2) and Tubulin proteins in HMC, EMM, SMM, and BMM cells. (**B**) Densitometric analysis of the relative expression of p-Erk versus Erk ($n = 3$, * $p < 0.001$).

Several mechanisms have been proposed to explain the activity of FOXM1 in cancer progression, including the activation of this factor by several oncogenic protein and signaling pathways, such as Ras and MAPK/Erk [29]. As for Nrf2, our results demonstrated an overexpression of the p-Erk in MPM cells (Figure 5A,B) and not in mesothelial cells.

2.5. Increased Expression of Nrf2, Ref-1, and FOXM1 after Crocidolite Asbestos Exposure in Mesothelial Cells

Crocidolite asbestos (the most carcinogenic variant of asbestos fibers) exposure, as well known in literature, is strictly associated to the development of cellular oxidative stress, induced both by fibers themselves and generated by pulmonary cells, particularly at the mesothelium level, in response to asbestos exposure [46].

We already demonstrated that in HMC incubated with crocidolite asbestos fibers there is a strong induction of an oxidative stress, via a significant increase in ROS production, event completely reverted by antioxidants co-incubation [47]. In our experimental model, as expected, HMC incubated with crocidolite asbestos showed an increased significant expression of Nrf2, Ref-1 and FOXM1 compared to untreated cells, in a dose dependent manner (Figure 6A,B).

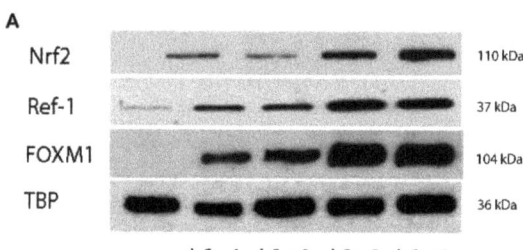

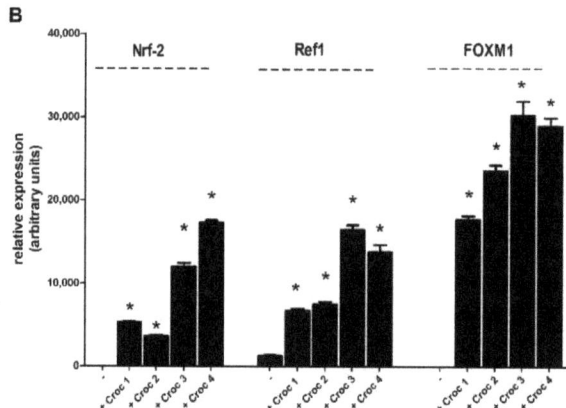

Figure 6. Increased expression of Nrf2, Ref-1 and FOXM1 after crocidolite asbestos exposure. (**A**) Western Blot of nuclear extracts of Nrf2, Ref-1 and FOXM1 from HMC untreated (-) or treated (+) for 24 h with crocidolite (Croc) asbestos (Croc 1: 1 µg/cm^2; Croc 2: 5 µg/cm^2 Croc 3: 10 µg/cm^2; Croc 4: 25 µg/cm^2). (**B**) Densitometric analysis of the relative expression of Nrf2 ($n = 3$, * $p < 0.001$), Ref-1 ($n = 3$, * $p < 0.001$) and FOXM1 ($n = 3$, * $p < 0.001$), respectively.

To confirm our results, we also performed some experiments by incubating HMC with an inert, nonpathogenic monodispersed synthetic amorphous silica, made up of spheres (MSS): results demonstrated clearly that Nrf2, Ref-1 and FOXM1 are overexpressed only when incubated with crocidolite asbestos and not after MSS exposure (Figure S2).

Furthermore, to correlate Nrf2, Ref-1 and FOXM1 overexpression, evoked by asbestos exposure, to MPM development, we measured the basal ROS level in HMC and MPM cells. The results (Figure S3) showed a significant lower level of ROS in MPM cells than in HMC, thus confirming that the hyper-activation of these redox-sensitive transcription factors in MPM is crucial in mediating MPM development and promoting mesothelioma resistance against oxidative stress.

3. Discussion

Malignant mesothelioma is a tumor with a poor prognosis and, to date, the only therapeutic approach remains surgical excision and chemotherapy, although the latter is not so effective, and the survival is low. There is therefore growing interest in identifying more precise and unequivocal methods of investigation and treatment. Above all, the attempt is addressed, on the one hand, to clarify the bio-molecular mechanisms underlying the neoplastic transformation of the mesothelium after asbestos exposure and, on the other hand, to identify new and more specific predictive and diagnostic markers for this aggressive tumor.

Some mechanisms have been clarified with reference to the toxicity of asbestos at the pulmonary level. In particular, both cytotoxicity and genotoxicity have been widely associated with an increased oxidative stress, mediated by the production of ROS, induced by fibers themselves or as a response from the lung to asbestos [48]. Consequently, this increased ROS production at cellular level represents one of the causes underlying the known toxic effects exerted by asbestos in the lung, particularly at mesothelial level, which seek to counteract oxidative stress by inducing antioxidant cellular defense.

In our cellular mesothelial and MPM models, we evaluate three redox-sensitive factors that recently have been demonstrated to be overexpressed in different tumors and strictly involved in antioxidant defense, Nrf2, Ref-1, and FOXM1 [19,22,26]. In comparison to not transformed HMC, Nrf2, Ref-1, and FOXM1 resulted overexpressed in MPM, and this overexpression was confirmed also in NSCLC pulmonary carcinoma (A549 cells). The results obtained clearly show the overexpression of Nrf2, Ref-1, and FOXM1 in all histologic types of MPM cells (epithelioid, sarcomatous, and biphasic) but not in the not transformed mesothelium. Particularly, Nrf2 translocates into the nucleus when phosphorylated by different kinases, such as MAPK/Erk [21]. We have demonstrated clearly the phosphorylation of Erk in MPM cells but not in HMC, thus proposing this molecular mechanism in mediating Nrf2 phosphorylation and activation.

Asbestos fibers exposure induces a strong oxidative stress. Previous results in our lab demonstrated that crocidolite asbestos increased ROS production in HMC, event completely reverted by antioxidants co-incubation [47]. These results have been confirmed in our experimental models, in which HMC cells exposed to crocidolite asbestos showed an increased and significantly activation of Nrf2, Ref-1, and FOXM1, in a dose-dependent manner, in HMC exposed to crocidolite asbestos, consistently with a high ROS production, thus confirming the response to oxidative stress induced by asbestos at the mesothelium level, which could drive MPM development.

Confirming our data, linearity was observed concerning Nrf2 in results proposed by other research groups on immortalized cell lines of mesothelioma, which showed an increased expression of this factor [32,36]. In some tumors, such as lung cancer, Nrf2 is found to be constitutively expressed primarily for mutations affecting the KEAP-1 suppressor [20]. So, in our MPM models, the expression of Nrf2, in mesothelioma, remains to be confirmed if it is associated with possible mutations of KEAP-1. As demonstrated, Nrf2 controls the transcription of many genes involved in the antioxidant response and in cellular ROS detoxification [18,19], by upregulating enzymes such as SOD2, GST, CAT, and HO-1, which, when overexpressed, protect cells to oxidative damage. We demonstrated clearly, in our experimental model, a significant overexpression of SOD2, GST, CAT, and HO-1 in MPM cells towards HMC, thus confirming the increase in antioxidant defense mediated by Nrf2 and a consequent alteration of redox balance, so increasing the survival of cancer cells. In the context of MPM therefore, in which there is a prolonged exposure to asbestos related oxidative stress induction, other studies have shown that an aberrant increase in the antioxidant systems, mediated by Nrf2 overexpression, may have a role in promoting tumorigenicity and chemoresistance [49], supporting the importance of this factor as a possible pharmacological target in many types of cancer [19].

Ref-1 still counteracts oxidative stress by activating a series of related factors [10], such as NF-kB. We demonstrated the p50 active subunit of NF-kB is overexpressed in MPM cells, thus enhancing antioxidant system against oxidative stress. This NF-kB upregulation in turn regulates p53 and PTEN oncosuppressors. In our cellular models, p53 and PTEN were overexpressed into the cytosol, but not in the nucleus, thus avoiding their role as tumor suppressors. Although p53 is considered a "guardian of the cell cycle" and is changed in many tumors, in the results obtained there is a confirmation of this event in MPM. However, from the literature, it emerges that the p53 mutation is present, although rare, in mesothelioma [50,51], and a similar point of view concerns PTEN, which has still not been well clarified in MPM [51], but it has been already demonstrated to be inactive in many tumors. However, previous studies have clarified that PTEN expression is not related to a better prognosis in patients with mesothelioma and its expression decreases with chemotherapeutic treatments [52].

FOXM1 mediates antioxidant defense via a dual mechanism. It can modulate the transcription of some genes involved in redox regulation, such as *SOD2* and *CAT* [27], via its induction by the active phosphorylated form of Erk, which in turn could be regulated by ROS increase [26,29]. As for Nrf2, our results demonstrated an overexpression of SOD2 and CAT proteins in MPM cells and not in the mesothelium, thus confirm also for this factor its strong involvement in MPM resistance against oxidative stress and its overexpression in cancer cells. It has been shown FOXM1 nuclear translocation is mediated by MAPK/Erk [29]. As for Nrf2, we demonstrated the mechanism of FOXM1 activation is mediated by Erk phosphorylation, which resulted upregulated in MPM cells and not in HMC. Therefore, from these data, it can be highlighted that there is the same mechanism underlying the activation of Nrf2 and FOXM1, mediated by Erk, and in this way it is possible to elicit a possible synergy or crosstalk between these two factors.

Mutagenesis, a phenomenon initiator of carcinogenesis, reflects DNA damage, which, in cells exposed to asbestos, is mediated by ROS. Therefore, the activation of Nrf2, Ref-1, and FOXM1 can be a key event in maintaining the right balance between apoptosis and carcinogenesis. Several studies have demonstrated the central role of Nrf2 signaling pathways in carcinogenesis and the potential benefit in inducing the inhibition of Nrf2 controlled enzymes [53]. Furthermore, MPM occurs following the accumulation of a series of acquired genetic events, which lead to the deactivation of tumor suppressor genes, by means of a complex cascade mechanism. Ref-1 is therefore necessary for cell survival, and its frequent overexpression in tumor cells strongly suggests a fundamental role of this protein in preventing apoptosis and in controlling cell proliferation. FOXM1, which is variously expressed in many tumors, controls not only the antioxidant defense, but it is widely involved in the control of cell cycle and proliferation [25,26], promoting neoplastic transformation, thus it is can also be rightly considered a possible mediator of MPM development after asbestos exposure.

Chronic oxidative stress and increased ROS production are present at the beginning of an inflammatory response of the mesothelium that involves still the High Mobility Group Box 1 (HMGB1). Until now, numerous studies have shown its relevance in the context of mesothelioma [5]. Our data confirmed an overexpression of this factor in our MPM models compared to the mesothelium (data not shown). This event can be associated to a crosstalk with Nrf2: ROS activates Nrf2 which consequently induces the transcription of antioxidant genes which in turn block the signaling pathway leading to HMGB1 activation. Therefore, the hyper-functioning antioxidant defenses are such that they cannot stem the emergence of the anti-inflammatory response triggered by HMGB1, exacerbating the molecular picture related to MPM. Moreover, redox-sensitive transcription factors, such as Nrf2, when overexpressed in cancer, contributed to contrast oxidative stress also when induced by chemotherapeutic agents [33,34], thus preserve tumor environment and contribute to make MPM resistant to therapeutic approach.

Redox-sensitive factors have long been studied in many tumors, since numerous studies report an important involvement of oxidative stress in neoplastic diseases. The cellular response to oxidative stress by these factors may therefore be representative of a key molecular mechanism related to the carcinogenic effects of asbestos, particularly crocidolite asbestos, which could explain the attempt by the mesothelial cells to counteract both oxidative stress and induced ROS production. The mesothelium probably cannot cope with this situation, and for this reason these factors, once deregulated, can probably be the potential "initiators" of the neoplastic process in the development of MPM. A peculiar aspect of asbestos-induced carcinogenesis, however, is the latency time between exposure and clinical manifestation [1]. This aspect can play a double role: on the one hand it could be important in the context of a therapeutic intervention, on the other hand it can become a major obstacle in the use of a mouse model for the study over time of the effects of a continuous exposure to asbestos.

Although there are still many aspects to be clarified, the present study proposes Nrf2, Ref-1, and FOXM1 as potential predictive markers of MPM associated with the primary toxic effect evoked by asbestos fibers at mesothelial level. Since MPM has a poor prognosis and a low survival, it is very crucial to detect new prognostic markers and to propose the use of new pharmacological treatments in the attempt to prevent and counteract this serious disease. Moreover, this aspect is important because there are no currently biomarkers predictive of mesothelioma development in asbestos-exposed people, so these potential predictive biomarkers and possible pharmacological targets are crucial in the fight against MPM, particularly important when foreseeing the growing increase in MPM in the next years.

4. Materials and Methods

4.1. Chemicals

Electrophoresis reagents were obtained from Bio-Rad Laboratories (Hercules, CA, USA). The protease inhibitor cocktail set III was obtained from Millipore (Billerica, MA, USA). Unless specified otherwise, all reagents were purchased from Sigma Chemicals Co. (St. Louis, MO, USA).

4.2. Cells

Primary human mesothelial cells (HMC) were isolated from three patients with pleural fluid secondary to congestive heart failure, with no history of a malignant disease, as detailed previously [54]. In total, nine primary human MPM samples (3 epithelioid MPM, 3 biphasic MPM, 3 sarcomatous MPM) were obtained from diagnostic thoracoscopies (see Table S1). MPM cells were obtained after written informed consent from the Biologic Bank of Malignant Mesothelioma, SS. Antonio e Biagio Hospital (Alessandria, Italy). MPM samples, identified with an Unknown Patient Number (UPN), were used within passage 6. The Ethical Committee of Biological Bank of Mesothelioma, S. Antonio e Biagio Hospital, Alessandria, Italy approved the study (#9/11/2011). HMC and MPM cells were grown in Ham's F10 nutrient mixture medium, supplemented with 10% v/v fetal bovine serum (FBS, Invitrogen Life Technologies, Carlsbad, CA, USA) and 1% v/v penicillin-streptomycin (Sigma Chemical Co). Cells were checked for Mycoplasma spp. contamination by PCR every three weeks and contaminated cells were discharged. The mesothelial origin of the isolated cells was confirmed by positive immunostaining, as detailed previously [55], and authenticated by the STR analysis method. Cells were used until passage 6.

The NSCLC cells (A549) were provided by the "Bruno Umbertini" experimental zooprophylactic institute (Brescia, Italy). Cells were grown in RPMI-1640, supplemented with 10% v/v FBS, and 1% of penicillin and streptomycin.

The plasticware for cell culture was provided by Falcon (Becton Dickinson, Franklin Lakes, NJ, USA).

4.3. Asbestos Fibers

Crocidolite fibers (from Union for International Cancer Control, UICC) were sonicated (Labsonic sonicator, Hielscher, Teltow, Germany, 100 W, 10 s) before incubation with cell cultures, to dissociate fibers bundles, and allow a better suspension and diffusion of fibers in the culture medium. Crocidolite fibers (at concentrations of 1–5-10–25 $\mu g/cm^2$) were incubated for 24 h in HMC.

4.4. Western Blot Analysis

Cytosolic and nuclear extracts were obtained using an Active Motif nuclear extraction kit (Active Motif, La Hulpe, Belgium) according to the manufacturer's instructions. The protein content in the cells was detected using a bicinchoninic acid assay (BCA) kit (Sigma Chemical Co., Saint Louis, MO, USA). Cytosolic and nuclear extracts were separated by sodium dodecyl sulfate-polyacrylamide gel electrophoresis (SDS-PAGE), transferred to polyvinylidene difluoride (PVDF) membrane sheets (Immobilon-P, Millipore, Billerica, MA) and probed with the required antibody diluted in 0.1% PBS-Tween with 5% nonfat dry milk. After 1 h of incubation, the membranes were washed with 0.1% PBS-Tween and then incubated for 1 h with peroxidase-conjugated sheep anti-mouse or sheep anti-rabbit IgG antibody (Amersham International, Little Chalfont, UK) diluted 1:3000 in 0.1% PBS-Tween with 5% nonfat dry milk. The membranes were washed again with 0.1% PBS-Tween, and proteins were detected by enhanced chemiluminescence (Perkin Elmer, Waltham, MA, USA). Ultrapure water (Millipore, Billerica, MA, USA) was used for all experiments.

Antibodies against Nrf2 and phospho-Nrf2 were purchased from Abcam (Cambridge, UK). Antibodies against Ref-1, FOXM1, p53, PTEN, SOD2, GST, HO-1 tubulin, and TATA-binding protein (TBP) were all provided by Santa Cruz Biotechnology, Inc. (Santa Cruz, CA, USA). The anti-Erk and anti-phospho Erk antibodies were provided by Millipore (Billerica, MA, USA). The anti-p50 antibody was provided by Sigma Chemical Co (St. Louis, MO, USA). Tubulin and TBP were used as loading controls for the cytosol and the nucleus, respectively. Band density was calculated using ImageJ software (http://www.rsb.info.nih.gov.bibliopass.unito.it/ij/, accessed date: 17 February 2021).

4.5. Statistical Analysis

The results were analyzed by a one-way analysis of variance (ANOVA) and Tukey's test, using GraphPad Prism software (v6.01, San Diego, CA, USA). $p < 0.05$ was considered significant. All data in the text and figures are provided as means $\pm$ SD.

5. Conclusions

Nrf2, Ref-1, and FOXM1 are upregulated in MPM and not in non-transformed mesothelium, presumably as consequence of the toxic effect evoked by asbestos fibers at the mesothelium level. These factors can therefore be considered potential candidates as predictive markers of the development of MPM, particularly important considering asbestos-related damages that predispose to mesothelioma development.

In conclusion, our results and proposed considerations lay and broaden the foundations for future studies in the context of MPM, a tumor that continues to be a public health problem.

Supplementary Materials: The following are available online at https://www.mdpi.com/2072-6694/13/5/1138/s1, Figure S1: Nuclear expression of PTEN and p53 proteins induced by Ref-1 in MPM cells, Figure S2: Expression of Nrf2, Ref-1 and FOXM1 in HMC, Figure S3: Intracellular ROS levels in all three histological types of MPM, epithelioid (EMM), sarcomatoid (SMM) and biphasic (BMM) forms, towards HMC and Table S1: analysis data on MPM cells obtained from total 9 MPM patients, 3 for each histotype (epithelioid, biphasic, sarcomatous), of the Biological Bank of Mesothelioma (AO Nazionale di Alessandria, Italy).

Author Contributions: Conceptualization, E.A.; methodology, M.S. and F.S.; software, L.B.; validation, M.S. and E.G.; formal analysis, M.S. and L.B.; investigation, E.A. and M.S.; resources, R.L.; data curation, M.S. and L.B.; Writing—Original draft preparation, E.A. and M.S.; Writing—Review and editing, E.A. and C.R.; visualization, M.S. and C.R.; supervision, E.A.; project administration, E.A.; funding acquisition, E.A. All authors have read and agreed to the published version of the manuscript.

Funding: This work was funded by Italian Ministry of University and Research (EX60% Funding 2019 to E.A.), grant "ALDE_RILO_19_01".

Institutional Review Board Statement: The study was conducted according to the guidelines of the Declaration of Helsinki and approved by the Ethical Committee of Biological Bank of Mesothelioma, SS. Antonio e Biagio Hospital, Alessandria, Italy (#9/11/2011).

Informed Consent Statement: Informed consent was obtained from all subjects involved in the study.

Data Availability Statement: All data generated or analyzed during this study are included in this published article.

Acknowledgments: We acknowledge Costanzo Costamagna, Department of Oncology, University of Torino, for the technical support.

Conflicts of Interest: The authors declare no conflict of interest.

References

1. Yap, T.A.; Aerts, J.G.; Popat, S.; Fennell, D.A. Novel insights into mesothelioma biology and implications for therapy. *Nat. Rev. Cancer* **2017**, *17*, 475–488. [CrossRef] [PubMed]
2. Alì, G.; Bruno, R.; Fontanini, G. The pathological and molecular diagnosis of malignant pleural mesothelioma: A literature review. *J. Thorac. Dis.* **2018**, *10*, S276–S284. [CrossRef] [PubMed]
3. Pira, E.; Donato, F.; Maida, L.; Discalzi, G. Exposure to asbestos: Past, present and future. *J. Thorac. Dis.* **2018**, *10*, S237–S245. [CrossRef] [PubMed]
4. Sun, H.H.; Vaynblat, A.; Pass, H.I. Diagnosis and prognosis—Review of biomarkers for mesothelioma. *Ann. Transl. Med.* **2017**, *5*, 244. [CrossRef] [PubMed]
5. Ledda, C.; Senia, P.; Rapisarda, V. Biomarkers for early diagnosis and prognosis of malignant pleural mesothelioma: The quest goes on. *Cancers* **2018**, *10*, 203. [CrossRef] [PubMed]
6. Chew, S.H.; Toyokuni, S. Malignant mesothelioma as an oxidative stress-induced cancer: An update. *Free Radic. Bio. Med.* **2015**, *86*, 166–178. [CrossRef]
7. Gào, X.; Schöttker, B. Reduction oxidation pathways involved in cancer development: A systematic review of literature reviews. *Oncotarget* **2017**, *8*, 51888–51906. [CrossRef]
8. Kumari, S.; Badana, A.K.; Murali Mohan, G.; Shailender, G.; Malla, R. Reactive Oxygen Species: A key constituent in cancer survival. *Biomark. Insights* **2018**, *13*, 1–9. [CrossRef]
9. Cloer, E.W.; Goldfarb, D.; Schrank, T.P.; Weissman, B.E.; Major, M.B. NRF2 activation in cancer: From DNA to protein. *Cancer Res.* **2019**, *79*, 889–898. [CrossRef] [PubMed]
10. Thakur, S.; Sarkar, B.; Cholia, R.P.; Gautam, N.; Dhiman, M.; Mantha, A.K. APE1/Ref-1 as an emerging therapeutic target for various human diseases: Phytochemical modulation of its functions. *Exp. Mol. Med.* **2014**, *46*, e106. [CrossRef] [PubMed]
11. Gartel, A.L. FOXM1 in cancer: Interactions and vulnerabilities. *Cancer Res.* **2017**, *77*, 3135–3139. [CrossRef]
12. Yangyang, G.; Luyan, S. Overexpression of NRF2 is correlated with prognoses of patients with malignancies: A meta-analysis. *Thorac. Cancer* **2017**, *8*, 558–564.
13. Yang, S.; Lai, Y.; Xiao, L.; Han, F.; Wu, W.; Long, S.; Li, W.; He, Y. Susceptibility and REF1 gene polymorphism towards colorectal cancer. *Cell Biochem. Biophys.* **2015**, *71*, 977–982. [CrossRef] [PubMed]
14. Park, H.J.; Carr, J.R.; Wang, Z.; Nogueira, V.; Hay, N.; Tyner, A.L.; Lau, L.F.; Costa, R.H.; Raychaudhuri, P. FoxM1, a critical regulator of oxidative stress during oncogenesis. *EMBO J.* **2009**, *28*, 2908–2918. [CrossRef]
15. Cui, Q.; Wang, J.Q.; Assaraf, Y.G.; Ren, L.; Gupta, P.; Wei, L.; Ashby, C.R.; Yang, D.H.; Chen, Z.S. Modulating ROS to overcome multidrug resistance in cancer. *Drug Resist. Updates* **2018**, *41*, 1–25. [CrossRef] [PubMed]
16. Bellezza, I.; Giambanco, I.; Minelli, A.; Donato, R. Nrf2-Keap1 signaling in oxidative and reductive stress. *Biochim. Biophys. Acta Mol. Cell Res.* **2018**, *1865*, 721–733. [CrossRef]
17. Dinkova-Kostova, A.T.; Kostov, R.V.; Canning, P. Keap1, the cysteine-based mammalian intracellular sensor for electrophiles and oxidants. *Arch. Biochem. Biophys.* **2017**, *617*, 84–93. [CrossRef]
18. Basak, P.; Sadhukhan, P.; Sarkar, P.; Sil, P.C. Perspectives of the Nrf-2 signaling pathway in cancer progression and therapy. *Toxicol. Rep.* **2017**, *4*, 306–318. [CrossRef] [PubMed]
19. Rojo de la Vega, M.; Chapman, E.; Zhang, D.D. NRF2 and the hallmarks of cancer. *Cancer Cell* **2018**, *34*, 21–43. [CrossRef] [PubMed]
20. Kitamura, H.; Motohashi, H. NRF2 addiction in cancer cells. *Cancer Sci.* **2018**, *109*, 900–911. [CrossRef] [PubMed]
21. Huang, H.C.; Nguyen, T.; Pickett, C.B. Phosphorylation of Nrf2 at Ser-40 by protein kinase C regulates antioxidant response element-mediated transcription. *J. Biol. Chem.* **2002**, *277*, 42769–42774. [CrossRef]
22. Park, J.S.; Kim, H.L.; Kim, Y.J.; Weon, J.I.; Sung, M.K.; Chung, H.W.; Seo, Y.R. Human AP Endonuclease 1: A potential marker for the prediction of environmental carcinogenesis risk. *Oxid. Med. Cell Longev.* **2014**, *2014*, 730301. [CrossRef] [PubMed]

23. Shah, F.; Logsdon, D.; Messmann, R.A.; Fehrenbacher, J.C.; Fishel, M.L.; Kelley, M.R. Exploiting the Ref-1-APE1 node in cancer signaling and other diseases: From bench to clinic. *NPJ Precis. Oncol.* **2017**, *1*, 19. [CrossRef] [PubMed]
24. Choi, S.; Joo, H.K.; Jeon, B.H. Dynamic regulation of APE1/Ref-1 as a therapeutic target protein. *Chonnam. Med. J.* **2016**, *52*, 75–80. [CrossRef] [PubMed]
25. Wierstra, I. The transcription factor FOXM1 (Forkhead box M1): Proliferation-specific expression, transcription factor function, target genes, mouse models, and normal biological roles. *Adv. Cancer Res.* **2013**, *118*, 97–398. [PubMed]
26. Liao, G.B.; Li, X.Z.; Zeng, S.; Liu, C.; Yang, S.M.; Yang, L.; Hu, C.J.; Bai, J.Y. Regulation of the master regulator FOXM1 in cancer. *Cell Commun. Signal.* **2018**, *16*, 57. [CrossRef]
27. Leone, A.; Roca, M.S.; Ciardiello, C.; Costantini, S.; Budillon, A. Oxidative stress gene expression profile correlates with cancer patient poor prognosis: Identification of crucial pathways might select novel therapeutic approaches. *Oxid. Med. Cell Longev.* **2017**, *2017*, 2597581. [CrossRef] [PubMed]
28. Halasi, M.; Gartel, A.L. FOX(M1) news—It is cancer. *Mol. Cancer Ther.* **2013**, *12*, 245–254. [CrossRef] [PubMed]
29. Ma, R.Y.M.; Tong, T.H.K.; Cheung, A.M.S.; Tsang, A.C.C.; Leung, W.Y.; Yao, K.M. Raf/MEK/MAPK signaling stimulates the nuclear translocation and transactivating activity of FOXM1c. *J. Cell Sci.* **2005**, *118*, 795–806. [CrossRef] [PubMed]
30. Shukla, A.; Gulumian, M.; Hei, T.K.; Kamp, D.; Rahman, Q.; Mossman, B.T. Multiple roles of oxidants in the pathogenesis of asbestos-induced diseases. *Free Radic. Biol. Med.* **2003**, *34*, 1117–1129. [CrossRef]
31. Hodgson, J.T.; Darnton, A. The quantitative risks of mesothelioma and lung cancer in relation to asbestos exposure. *Ann. Occup. Hyg.* **2000**, *44*, 565–601. [CrossRef]
32. Pietrofesa, R.; Chatterjee, S.; Park, K.; Arguiri, E.; Albelda, S.; Christofidou-Solomidou, M. Synthetic lignan secoisolariciresinol diglucoside (LGM2605) reduces asbestos-induced cytotoxicity in a Nrf2-dependent and -independent manner. *Antioxidants* **2018**, *7*, 38. [CrossRef]
33. Lee, Y.J.; Lee, D.M.; Lee, S.H. Nrf2 expression and apoptosis in quercetin-treated malignant mesothelioma cells. *Mol. Cells* **2015**, *38*, 416–425. [CrossRef] [PubMed]
34. Lee, Y.J.; Im, J.H.; Lee, D.M.; Park, J.S.; Won, S.Y.; Cho, M.K.; Nam, H.S.; Lee, Y.J.; Lee, S.H. Synergistic inhibition of mesothelioma cell growth by the combination of clofarabine and resveratrol involves Nrf2 downregulation. *BMB Rep.* **2012**, *45*, 647–652. [CrossRef]
35. Giusti, L.; Ciregia, F.; Bonotti, A.; Da Valle, Y.; Donadio, E.; Boldrini, C.; Foddis, R.; Giannaccini, G.; Mazzoni, M.R.; Canessa, P.A.; et al. Comparative proteomic analysis of malignant pleural mesothelioma: Focusing on the biphasic subtype. *EuPA Open Proteom.* **2016**, *10*, 42–49. [CrossRef]
36. Lee, Y.J.; Jeong, H.Y.; Kim, Y.B.; Lee, Y.J.; Won, S.Y.; Shim, J.H.; Cho, M.K.; Nam, H.S.; Lee, S.H. Reactive oxygen species and PI3K/Akt signaling play key roles in the induction of Nrf2-driven heme oxygenase-1 expression in sulforaphane-treated human mesothelioma MSTO-211H cells. *Food Chem. Toxicol.* **2012**, *50*, 116–123. [CrossRef]
37. Flaherty, D.M.; Monick, M.M.; Carter, A.B.; Peterson, M.W.; Hunninghake, G.W. Oxidant-mediated increases in redox factor-1 nuclear protein and activator protein-1 DNA binding in asbestos-treated macrophages. *J. Immunol.* **2002**, *168*, 5675–5681. [CrossRef]
38. Fung, H.; Kow, Y.W.; Houten, B.V.; Taatjes, D.J.; Hatahet, Z.; Janssen, Y.M.; Vacek, P.; Faux, S.P.; Mossman, B.T. Asbestos increases mammalian AP-endonuclease gene expression, protein levels, and enzyme activity in mesothelial cells. *Cancer Res.* **1998**, *58*, 189–194.
39. Cunniff, B.; Benson, K.; Stumpff, J.; Newick, K.; Held, P.; Taatjes, D.; Joseph, J.; Kalyanaraman, B.; Heintz, N.H. Mitochondrial-targeted nitroxides disrupt mitochondrial architecture and inhibit expression of peroxiredoxin 3 and FOXM1 in malignant mesothelioma cells. *J. Cell Physiol.* **2013**, *228*, 835–845. [CrossRef] [PubMed]
40. Cunniff, B.; Wozniak, A.N.; Sweeney, P.; DeCosta, K.; Heintz, N.H. Peroxiredoxin 3 levels regulate a mitochondrial redox setpoint in malignant mesothelioma cells. *Redox. Biol.* **2014**, *3*, 79–87. [CrossRef] [PubMed]
41. Mizuno, T.; Murakami, H.; Fujii, M.; Ishiguro, F.; Tanaka, I.; Kondo, Y.; Akatsuka, S.; Toyokuni, S.; Yokoi, K.; Osada, H.; et al. YAP induces malignant mesothelioma cell proliferation by upregulating transcription of cell cycle-promoting genes. *Oncogene* **2012**, *31*, 5117–5122. [CrossRef]
42. Romagnoli, S.; Fasoli, E.; Vaira, V.; Falleni, M.; Pellegrini, C.; Catania, A.; Roncalli, M.; Marchetti, A.; Santambrogio, L.; Coggi, G.; et al. Identification of potential therapeutic targets in malignant mesothelioma using cell-cycle gene expression analysis. *Am. J. Pathol.* **2009**, *174*, 762–770. [CrossRef] [PubMed]
43. Cigognetti, M.; Lonardi, S.; Fisogni, S.; Balzarini, P.; Pellegrini, V.; Tironi, A.; Bercich, L.; Bugatti, M.; Rossi, G.; Murer, B.; et al. BAP1 (BRCA1-associated protein 1) is a highly specific marker for differentiating mesothelioma from reactive mesothelial proliferations. *Mod. Pathol.* **2015**, *28*, 1043–1057. [CrossRef] [PubMed]
44. Janssen, Y.M.; Marsh, J.P.; Absher, M.P.; Hemenway, D.; Vacek, P.M.; Leslie, K.O.; Borm, P.J.; Mossman, B.T. Expression of antioxidant enzymes in rat lungs after inhalation of asbestos or silica. *J. Biol. Chem.* **1992**, *267*, 10625–10630. [CrossRef]
45. Shukla, A.; Hillegass, J.M.; MacPherson, M.B.; Beuschel, S.L.; Vacek, P.M.; Butnor, K.J.; Pass, H.I.; Carbone, M.; Testa, J.R.; Heintz, N.H.; et al. ERK2 is essential for the growth of human epithelioid malignant mesotheliomas. *Int. J. Cancer* **2011**, *129*, 1075–1086. [CrossRef] [PubMed]
46. Benedetti, S.; Nuvoli, B.; Catalani, S.; Galati, R. Reactive oxygen species a double-edged sword for mesothelioma. *Oncotarget* **2015**, *6*, 16848–16865. [CrossRef] [PubMed]

47. Aldieri, E.; Riganti, C.; Silvagno, F.; Orecchia, S.; Betta, P.G.; Doublier, S.; Gazzano, E.; Polimeni, M.; Bosia, A.; Ghigo, D. Antioxidants prevent the RhoA inhibition evoked by crocidolite asbestos in human mesothelial and mesothelioma cells. *Am. J. Respir. Cell Mol. Biol.* **2011**, *45*, 625–631. [CrossRef]
48. Kamp, D.W. Asbestos-induced lung diseases: An update. *Transl. Res.* **2009**, *153*, 143–152. [CrossRef] [PubMed]
49. DeNicola, G.M.; Karreth, F.A.; Humpton, T.J.; Gopinathan, A.; Wei, C.; Frese, K.; Mangal, D.; Yu, K.H.; Yeo, C.J.; Calhoun, E.S.; et al. Oncogene-induced Nrf2 transcription promotes ROS detoxification and tumorigenesis. *Nature* **2011**, *475*, 106–109. [CrossRef] [PubMed]
50. Hylebos, M.; Van Camp, G.; van Meerbeeck, J.P.; Op de Beeck, K. The genetic landscape of malignant pleural mesothelioma: Results from massively parallel sequencing. *J. Thorac. Oncol.* **2016**, *11*, 1615–1626. [CrossRef]
51. De Assis, L.V.; Isoldi, M.C. The function, mechanisms, and role of the genes PTEN and TP53 and the effects of asbestos in the development of malignant mesothelioma: A review focused on the genes' molecular mechanisms. *Tumor Biol.* **2014**, *35*, 889–901. [CrossRef]
52. Bitanihirwe, B.K.Y.; Meerang, M.; Friess, M.; Soltermann, A.; Frischknecht, L.; Thies, S.; Felley-Bosco, E.; Tsao, M.-S.; Allo, G.; de Perrot, M.; et al. PI3K/mTOR signaling in mesothelioma patients treated with induction chemotherapy followed by extrapleural pneumonectomy. *J. Thorac. Oncol.* **2014**, *9*, 239–247. [CrossRef] [PubMed]
53. Hammad, A.; Namani, A.; Elshaer, M.; Wang, X.J.; Tang, X. "NRF2 addiction" in lung cancer cells and its impact on cancer therapy. *Cancer Lett.* **2019**, *467*, 40–49. [CrossRef] [PubMed]
54. Riganti, C.; Lingua, M.F.; Salaroglio, I.C.; Falcomatà, C.; Righi, L.; Morena, D.; Picca, F.; Oddo, D.; Kopecka, J.; Pradotto, M.; et al. Bromodomain inhibition exerts its therapeutic potential in malignant pleural mesothelioma by promoting immunogenic cell death and changing the tumor immune-environment. *Oncoimmunology* **2017**, *7*, e1398874. [CrossRef] [PubMed]
55. Kopecka, J.; Salaroglio, I.C.; Righi, L.; Libener, R.; Orecchia, S.; Grosso, F.; Milosevic, V.; Ananthanarayanan, P.; Ricci, L.; Capelletto, E.; et al. Loss of C/EBP-β LIP drives cisplatin resistance in malignant pleural mesothelioma. *Lung Cancer* **2018**, *120*, 34–45. [CrossRef] [PubMed]

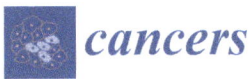

Article

Digital Gene Expression Analysis of Epithelioid and Sarcomatoid Mesothelioma Reveals Differences in Immunogenicity

Luka Brcic [1,†], Alexander Mathilakathu [2,†], Robert F. H. Walter [2], Michael Wessolly [2], Elena Mairinger [2], Hendrik Beckert [3], Daniel Kreidt [2], Julia Steinborn [2], Thomas Hager [2], Daniel C. Christoph [4], Jens Kollmeier [5], Thomas Mairinger [6], Jeremias Wohlschlaeger [7], Kurt Werner Schmid [2], Sabrina Borchert [2,‡] and Fabian D. Mairinger [2,*,‡]

1. Diagnostic and Research Institute of Pathology, Medical University of Graz, 8010 Graz, Austria; luka.brcic@medunigraz.at
2. Institute of Pathology, University Hospital Essen, University of Duisburg Essen, 45147 Essen, Germany; alexander.mathilakathu@stud.uni-due.de (A.M.); Robert.Walter@rlk.uk-essen.de (R.F.H.W.); Michael.Wessolly@uk-essen.de (M.W.); elena.mairinger@ruhrlandklinik.de (E.M.); daniel.kreidt@stud.uni-due.de (D.K.); Julia.Steinborn@uk-essen.de (J.S.); thomas.hager@uk-essen.de (T.H.); KW.Schmid@uk-essen.de (K.W.S.); Sabrina.Borchert@rlk.uk-essen.de (S.B.)
3. Department of Pulmonary Medicine, University Hospital Essen—Ruhrlandklinik, 45239 Essen, Germany; hendrik.beckert@rlk.uk-essen.de
4. Department of Medical Oncology, Evang. Kliniken Essen-Mitte, 45136 Essen, Germany; D.Christoph@kliniken-essen-mitte.de
5. Department of Pneumology, Helios Klinikum Emil von Behring, 14165 Berlin, Germany; jens.kollmeier@helios-kliniken.de
6. Department of Tissue Diagnostics, Helios Klinikum Emil von Behring, 14165 Berlin, Germany; thomas.mairinger@helios-gesundheit.de
7. Department of Pathology, Diakonissenkrankenhaus Flensburg, 24939 Flensburg, Germany; wohlschlaegerje@diako.de
* Correspondence: Fabian.Mairinger@uk-essen.de
† These authors contributed equally to this paper.
‡ These authors contributed equally to this paper.

Simple Summary: Malignant pleural mesothelioma (MPM) is a rare, biologically extremely aggressive tumor with an infaust prognosis. In this retrospective study, we aimed to assess the role of tumor-infiltrating immune cells and their activity in the respective histologic subtypes. We confirmed a substantial difference between epithelioid and sarcomatoid mesothelioma regarding the host's anti-cancer immune reaction. Whereas antigen processing and presentation to resident cytotoxic T cells as well as phagocytosis is highly affected in sarcomatoid mesothelioma, cell–cell interaction via cytokines seems to be of greater importance in epithelioid cases. Our work reveals the specific role of the immune system within the different histologic subtypes of MPM, providing a more detailed background of their immunogenic potential. This is of great interest regarding therapeutic strategies addressing immunotherapy in mesothelioma.

Abstract: Malignant pleural mesothelioma (MPM) is an aggressive malignancy associated with asbestos exposure. Median survival ranges from 14 to 20 months after initial diagnosis. As of November 2020, the FDA approved a combination of immune checkpoint inhibitors after promising intermediate results. Nonetheless, responses remain unsatisfying. Adequate patient stratification to improve response rates is still lacking. This retrospective study analyzed formalin fixed paraffin embedded specimens from a cohort of 22 MPM. Twelve of those samples showed sarcomatoid, ten epithelioid differentiation. Complete follow-up, including radiological assessment of response by modRECIST and time to death, was available with reported deaths of all patients. RNA of all samples was isolated and subjected to digital gene expression pattern analysis. Our study revealed a notable difference between epithelioid and sarcomatoid mesothelioma, showing differential gene expression for 304/698 expressed genes. Whereas antigen processing and presentation to resident cytotoxic T cells as well as phagocytosis is highly affected in sarcomatoid mesothelioma, cell–cell interaction via cytokines seems to be of greater importance in epithelioid cases. Our work reveals the specific role of the immune system within the different histologic subtypes of MPM, providing a more detailed background of their immunogenic potential. This is of great interest regarding therapeutic strategies including immunotherapy in mesothelioma.

Keywords: pleural mesothelioma; gene expression; immunogenicity; sarcomatoid; epithelioid

1. Introduction

Malignant pleural mesothelioma (MPM) is a rare type of cancer that is heavily associated with asbestos exposure [1,2]. This malignancy originates from the pleural mesothelium and is associated with a bad prognosis. Median survival times range from 14–20 months after initial diagnosis [3–5]. Generally, MPM can be differentiated into three major histologic subtypes, epithelioid (EMM), sarcomatoid (SMM), and biphasic (BMM). EMM accounts for up to 80% of all MPM cases [6]. It has also a more favorable outcome compared with the SMM or BMM, especially when surgery is applied [7]. Though it needs to be noted that epithelioid morphology can differ greatly [6,8], thereby also impacting clinical outcome [9–11]. The sarcomatoid subtype is the least prevalent subtype of mesothelioma (<10%) [8]. SMM is considered to be more aggressive in a clinical setting with a higher tendency of distant metastasis [6,12]. The BMM has a mixed composition of both epithelioid and sarcomatoid histology [8]. It is currently discussed whether a proportion of specific histology in biphasic MPM has a prognostic value [13,14].

As distinct biomarkers are lacking [15], early detection is often impeded, thereby worsening patients' outcome. Unfortunately, only a small fraction of patients is suitable for pleurectomy [16], while most patients are treated with a cisplatin/pemetrexed combination. The treatment may prolong overall survival by 3 months [5]. Meanwhile, patients undergoing palliative care including palliative chemotherapy may have an overall survival of 9 months. Immune checkpoint inhibitors are also used as a treatment option in MPM. These inhibitors target negative regulatory immune checkpoints on immune cells, thereby enhancing a prevalent immune response against the tumor. Single agents (pembrolizumab, a PD-1 inhibitor) have shown increased response rates; however, they have failed to show benefits for progression-free (PFS) or overall survival (OS) [17]. Despite this setback, the Checkmate 743 study revealed a four-month OS benefit (mOS, HR: 0.74, CI: 0.60–0.91, p-value: 0.0020) and increased two-year survival rate (41% vs. 27%), when comparing immune checkpoint doublet therapy (ipilimumab and nivolumab) with standard systematic chemotherapy [4]. Nonetheless, responses remain unsatisfying with only marginal improvements compared to the best supportive care [18]. With immune therapy now in the focus of current mesothelioma treatment, a deeper knowledge of the tumor's immunogenic potential may help to improve patient selection for this form of therapy.

Though the immune system is widely recognized for its anti-tumor activity, it plays a dual role in MPM and may also support tumor survival and progression. Inhaled microfibres, which are released during processing, corrosion, and weathering of asbestos, often reside in pleural tissue. Unfortunately, macrophages are unable to decompose them [3]. Over time, the persistent fibers damage adjacent cells, leading to necrosis and potentially triggering an immune response. The resulting chronic inflammatory reaction can induce tumor mutagenesis via release of reactive oxygen species (ROS) [19]. These macrophages, together with other various not-tumor-derived cell types essential for MPM development, constitute the so-called tumor microenvironment (TME) [20]. Three important immune cell types, known to infiltrate MPM, are tumor-associated macrophages (TAMs), T-lymphocytes, and myeloid-derived suppressor cells (MDSCs) [20]. TAMs are generally considered to be the largest subset of cells infiltrating MPM (up to 42%) [21,22]. Non-tissue resident macrophages are attracted to the tumor site via expression of the chemokine CCL2 [23].

Once within the tumor, growth factors expressed by the tumor (M-CSF, IL-34, TGF-b, and IL-10) induce an immunosuppressive macrophage phenotype (M2 macrophages) [23–25]. From a clinical perspective, the immune suppressive effects of macrophages are associated with poor prognosis and resistance to standard chemotherapy [23]. Some studies suggested macrophage-based biomarkers to estimate prognosis and outcome in EMM [26–28]. Despite next-generation sequencing studies identifying few mutations resulting in presented neoepitopes and increased immunogenicity [29], T-lymphocytes are the second biggest fraction of the immune cell infiltrate (20–42%), closely following TAMs [27,30,31]. It is speculated that the neoepitope load is higher than suggested, as chromosomal rearrangements can not be detected by targeted amplicon-based NGS, which are often present in MPM [32]. The infiltrating lymphocytes are mostly CD8-positive cytotoxic T lymphocytes (CTL), as well as CD4 and FoxP3 positive regulatory T cells (Tregs) [22,31]. Strikingly, based on pleural effusions of MPM, regulatory T-cells are less common when compared to other tumor entities [25]. Though high infiltration rates and activity of CTL are observed in MPM [25,33], they display signs of anergy or exhaustion [34]. MDSCs are the smallest fraction of the immune cell infiltrate (up to 9%) [30,35]. These cells are predominately associated with suppression of T-cells via releasing of ROS and PD-L1 expression [35–37]. Furthermore, a higher concentration of MDSCs can be linked to poor prognosis in EMM [27,38]. Based on these findings one can conclude that the majority of acting immune cells at the tumor site are either ineffective or are reprogrammed to support tumor growth and progression. Unfortunately, most studies did not distinguish between EMM and SMM when analyzing tumor immune infiltration or are only based on limited numbers of SMM samples. A recent study showed the infiltration of CD8+ T cells as being twice as high in SMM than in EMM but included only six SMM [39].

The above-mentioned points highlight the importance of the immune system for MPM development and progression and raise the question of how different immunogenicity contributes to the different outcomes between EMM and SMM. Deepening the understanding of the biological background of immune escape mechanisms in those histologic subtypes might carry the potential for new therapeutic approaches and improved clinical management of patients in the future.

2. Materials and Methods
2.1. Patient Cohort and Experimental Design

This retrospective study was performed on therapy-naïve, formalin-fixed paraffin-embedded samples of 22 patients with MPM treated at the West German Cancer Centre or the West German Lung Centre (Essen, Germany) between 2006 and 2009 and the Helios Klinikum Emil von Behring (Berlin, Germany) between 2002 and 2009. Twelve of those were diagnosed as SMM and 10 as EMM. The diagnosis was confirmed by two experienced pathologists (JWO, KWS), based on the current WHO classification [40]. Patients were staged according to the 2017 UICC/AJCC staging [41]. Inclusion criteria were the availability of sufficient tumor material and a complete set of clinical data concerning follow-up and treatment. All patients received platinum-based chemotherapy. The radiologic response rate was assessed by modified Response Evaluation Criteria in Solid Tumours (modRECIST) [42]. Surveillance for this study was stopped on August 31, 2014. Complete follow-up was available for all patients with reported deaths of all patients. Clinicopathological data of the study cohort are summarized in Table 1.

Table 1. Clinicopathological data of the study cohort.

Histology	Age	Sex	T Stage	N Status	M Status	UICC/AJCC	Overall Survival in Months	Outcome	Progression-Free Survival in Months	Initial Progression
EMM	52	M	2	2	0	3B	9.3	Death	5.5	Yes
EMM	56	M	3	0	1	4	43.2	Death	5.5	No
EMM	61	M	2	2	1	4	2.1	Death	1.2	Yes
EMM	65	M	2	2	0	3B	8.8	Death	4.9	Yes
EMM	68	F	2	0	1	4	3.7	Death	3.5	No
EMM	70	M	1	2	0	3B	14.5	Death	6.7	Yes
EMM	73	M	2	0	0	1B	18.0	Death	4.8	Yes
EMM	75	M	3	0	0	1B	21.7	Death	6.4	Yes
EMM	76	M	2	0	0	1B	44.2	Death	14.3	Yes
EMM	77	M	2	0	0	1B	4.6	Death	3.8	Yes
SMM	54	M	2	1	0	2	3.2	Death	2.6	No
SMM	59	M	2	0	0	1B	7.2	Death	7.1	No
SMM	61	m	3	0	0	1B	25.2	Death	11.6	Yes
SMM	62	F	3	1	0	3A	8.9	Death	2.8	Yes
SMM	64	M	3	0	1	4	12.2	Death	5.5	No
SMM	66	M	1	0	0	1A	11.3	Death	9.7	No
SMM	66	M	2	0	1	4	8.4	Death	3.5	Yes
SMM	69	M	4	2	0	3B	8.0	Death	1.4	Yes
SMM	70	M	3	0	0	1B	21.6	Death	11.6	Yes
SMM	71	M	2	2	0	3B	0.8	Death	0.2	No
SMM	79	F	3	2	1	4	13.6	Death	4.1	Yes
SMM	82	M	2	0	0	1B	13.3	Death	9.3	Yes

Legend: EMM—epithelioid malignant mesothelioma, SMM—sarcomatoid malignant mesothelioma.

2.2. RNA Isolation and Integrity Assessment

RNA was purified from 20 µm thick FFPE sections, using the Maxwell RSC RNA FFPE Kit supplied by Promega. Obtained RNA was eluted in 50 µL RNase-free water and stored at −80°C. Before the assessment, RNA concentration was determined via Qubit Fluorometric Quantification (Thermo Fisher Science, Waltham, MA, USA) undergoing manufacturer's instructions for the RNA broad range assay kit. Ultimately, 200 ng of each sample was processed.

2.3. Digital Gene Expression Analysis

For evaluation of the RNA expression pattern, the commercially available NanoString PanCancer Immune Profiling Panel including 770 immune-related as well as 30 reference genes was used. All code sets along with experiment reagents were designed and synthesized by NanoString Technologies (Seattle, WA, USA). The post-hybridization processing was performed using the nCounter MAX/FLEX System (NanoString) and cartridges were scanned on the Digital Analyzer (NanoString). Samples were analyzed on the NanoString nCounter PrepStation, using the high-sensitivity program, and cartridges were read at maximum sensitivity (555 FOV).

2.4. NanoString Data Processing

NanoString data processing was performed with the R statistical programming environment (v4.0.2) using NanoStringNorm [36] and NAPPA package, respectively. Considering the counts obtained for positive control probe sets, raw NanoString counts for each gene were subjected to a technical factorial normalization, carried out by subtracting the mean counts plus two-times standard deviation from the CodeSet inherent negative controls. Afterward, a biological normalization using the geometric mean of all reference genes was carried out. To overcome basal noise, all counts with $p > 0.05$ after one-sided t-test versus negative controls plus 2× standard deviations were interpreted as not expressed.

2.5. Statistical Analysis

Statistical analysis was carried out using the R statistical programming environment V 4.0.2. Prior to exploratory data analysis, the Shapiro–Wilks-test was applied to test for normal distribution of each dataset for ordinal and metric variables. The resulting dichotomous variables underwent either the Wilcoxon Mann–Whitney rank sum test (non-parametric) or the two-sided student's *t*-test (parametric). For comparison of ordinal variables and factors with more than two groups, either the Kruskal–Wallis test (non-parametric) or ANOVA (parametric) were used to detect group differences.

Double dichotomous contingency tables were analyzed using Fisher's exact test. To test the dependency of ranked parameters with more than two groups the Pearson's Chi-squared test was used. Correlations between metrics were tested applying Spearman's rank correlation test as well as Pearson's product-moment correlation testing for linearity.

Basic quality control of run data was performed by mean-vs-variances plotting to find outliers in target or sample level. True differences were calculated by correlation matrices analysis. Pathway analysis is based on the KEGG database and was performed using the "pathview" package of R. Differences were specified by −log2 fold changes between means (if parametric) or medians (if non-parametric) of compared groups. Significant pathway associations were identified by gene set enrichment analysis using the WEB-based GEne SeT AnaLysis Toolkit (WebGestalt) [43–45]. Each run was executed with 1000 permutations. Finally, all associations were ranked according to the false discovery rate ($p < 0.05$).

Due to the multiple statistical tests, the *p*-values were adjusted by using the false discovery rate (FDR). The level of statistical significance was defined as $p \leq 0.05$ after adjustment.

3. Results

3.1. Gene Expression Pattern of Immune-Related Genes

Overall, 304 out of 698 (43.6%) significantly expressed immune-related genes show differential expression between EMM and SMM, indicating an overall difference in interaction with the host's immune system. In particular, 90 of those 304 genes (29.6%) show expression only or in a much stronger manner in SMM compared to EMM cases, whereas 214 targets (70.4%) present with overexpression in EMM. In ranked order, ABCB1, SYCP1 und IFNA7 show most differences between both subtypes, with solid expression levels (between about 500 counts for SYCP1ˆ and up to nearly 3000 counts for IFNA7) in EMM but an absence of expression in SMM, whereas MAPK8, AXL und UBC show gene expression predominantly in sarcomatoid cases.

No differences in infiltration density of CD8+ CTL could be observed (FDR adj. $p = 0.901$). Of note, CD4+ T-cells, as well as CD68+ macrophages, were enriched in the SMM. CD20+ B cells tend to be denser in EMM than in SMM, but the overall expression of MS4A1 (CD20) is only slightly above background (20 vs. 100 counts in median) and the association did not reach statistical significance after adjustment (*p*-value: 0.050; FDR adj. *p*-value: 0.094).

An overview of all differences in gene expression pattern between the two histologic subtypes is illustrated in Figure 1, an overview of all *p*-values and statistical parameters can be found in Table S1.

3.2. Gene Set Enrichment Analysis (GSEA)

To identify biological background mechanisms (pathways and biological functions/categories) behind the different expression patterns regarding immune-related genes in EMM and SMM, a Gene Set Enrichment Analysis (GSEA) was performed (Figure 2).

In the SMM mainly the pathways for phagosome, antigen processing and presentation, lysosome, autoimmune thyroid disease, viral myocarditis, Fc gamma R-mediated phagocytosis, Epstein–Barr virus infection, endocytosis, focal adhesion, and proteoglycans in cancer show the strongest enrichment. On the other hand, cytokine–cytokine receptor interaction, salmonella infection, inflammatory mediator regulation of TRP channels, adrenergic signaling in cardiomyocytes, amoebiasis, African trypanosomiasis, parathyroid hormone synthesis, secretion and action, NF-kappa B signaling pathway, inflammatory bowel disease, and Kaposi sarcoma-associated herpesvirus infection are identified as enriched and thereby potentially activated in EMM.

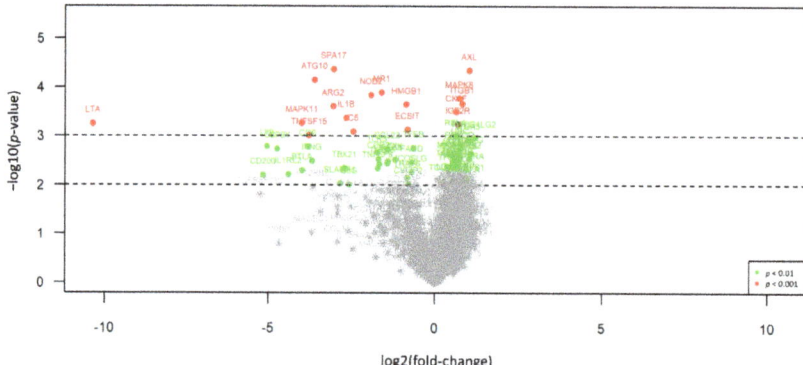

Figure 1. Volcano plot illustrating the differential expression between EMM and SMM. 90 of 304 differentially expressed genes (29.6%) show expression only or in a much stronger manner in SMM (right side) compared to EMM cases, whereas 214 targets (70.4%) present with overexpression in EMM (left side). Red dots indicate highly significant and green dots significant association identified by explorative data analysis using either Wilcoxon Mann–Whitney rank sum test (non-parametric) or the two-sided student's *t*-test (parametric).

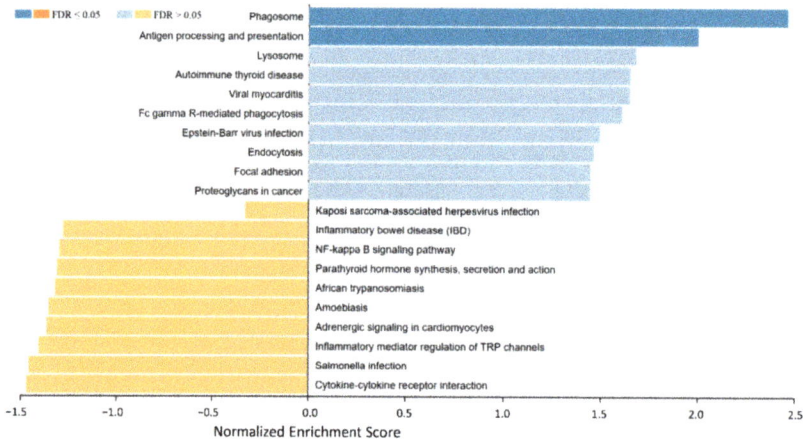

Figure 2. Gene set enrichment analysis of differential expressed genes between EMM and SMM presenting an overview of gene sets enriched in SMM (right side, blue bars) and EMM (left side, yellow bars). In the SMM the pathways for phagosome, Fc gamma R-mediated phagocytosis, antigen processing and presentation and proteoglycans in cancer show enrichment. Cytokine–cytokine receptor interaction is enriched and thereby potentially activated in EMM.

Details of the GSEA, including normalized enrichment score, the *p*-value of enrichment, exact targets included in the gene sets, and those differentially regulated, can be found in Table S2.

The main altered/influenced pathways are described in particular in the following paragraphs:

3.2.1. Phagocytosis and Antigen Presentation

All phagocytosis- and antigen-presentation associated signaling pathways, including phagosome (Figure S1), antigen processing and presentation (Figure S2), lysosome, Fc gamma R-mediated phagocytosis (Figure S3), and endocytosis are strongly enriched in SMM. For direct phagocytosis, this includes important factors involved in the phagolysosome, like LAMP or cathepsin β, antigen processing and cross-presentation, like TAP1/2 or MHC I/II molecules, or the cytochrome b558 mediated activation of NADPHoxidase, with strong overexpression of gp91 and p40phox. Furthermore, strong expression levels of most phagocytosis-promoting receptors, including Fc receptors, complement receptors, integrins, toll-like receptors, C-lectin receptors as well as Scavenger receptors, could be shown. Accumulation of CD45 positive cells, as activators of T cell response, expression of the Fcγ receptors FcγIIA and B, and downstream signaling via Src and Syk could be verified. Besides antigen processing via autophagy, the "classic" proteasome-associated mechanism for antigen processing and presentation via TAP1/2, TAPBP, and MHC1 binding showed strong activation on all levels of the MHC I pathway for antigen presentation to CD8+ CTL and KIR+ NK cells. Furthermore, the MHC II pathway, important for antigen presentation to CD4+ helper T-cells via MHC II, is overexpressed in total, including but not limited to Ii, MHC2, SLIP, CTSB/L/S, CLIP, and HLA-DM.

3.2.2. Cell–Cell Interaction and Communication within the Tumor Microenvironment

MPM subtypes show a clear difference in the communication networks used between the tumor cells and/or different immune cell types. This spans biological mechanisms and pathways from cytokine–cytokine receptor interactions over cell–cell interaction via proteoglycans up to differences in focal adhesion (Figures S4 and S5). This could be shown by highly increased expression levels of hyaluronan (HA, including CD44, CD44v3), heparan sulfate proteoglycans (HSPGs, including the integrins α2β1, αvβ3 or α5β1 and fibronectin) as well as chondroitin/dermatan sulfate proteoglycans (CSPG/DSPG, including TLR2 and TLR4) (Figure S4).

For cell communication via cytokines, especially γ-chain utilizing class I helical cytokine receptors (IL2RA, IL2RG, IL4R, IL15RA, IL21R, IL7R) and IL4-like receptors (IL3RA, CSF2RB, IL13RA1), significantly elevated gene expression in SMM compared to EMM was shown. In EMM samples, an enrichment of IL6/12-like (IL6R, IL11RA, IL12RB2) and IL1-like receptors (IL1R2, IL1RL2, Il18R1, ST2) could be observed.

On the side of chemokine secretion, markable differences in CXC subfamily member expression was observed, whereas those binding CXCR1 (CXCL1, CXCL5, CXCL6) and CXCR2 (CXCL2, CXCL3, CXCL7) are expressed in EMM and those binding CXCR3 (CXCL9, CXCL10, CXCL11) or CXCR5 (CXCL13) are expressed in SMM (Figure S5).

4. Discussion

For a long time, tumors have been widely underestimated in their complexity, viewed as a clustering of cancer cells on their own, and not considered in terms of the importance of extracellular signaling and complex interactions in the TME. Since then, extensive research has been conducted on the topic of tumor-associated immune events, revealing their enormous influence on tumor progression. In this study, we have approached MPM as a cancer entity with an especially heterogenous TME, whose composition might also be of prognostic value [46]. Our data analysis revealed numerous factors and pathways involved in the cell cycle progression, presumably acting in a synergistic effect and offering an explanation for the progression of MPM despite therapy.

4.1. Phagocytosis

Despite the understanding of the decisive role the phagosome pathway plays in cancer, it has not yet been described for MPM. GSEA in our study revealed the following phagocytotic pathways being affected with high significance: phagosome, Fc gamma R-mediated phagocytosis, lysosome, and endocytosis. As the phagosome pathway showed the highest enrichment (2.5), we focused on differences between gene expression of selected SMM and EMM genes in this pathway (Figures S1 and S3). The phagosome pathway is mainly involved in the response of the innate immune defense and includes endocytosis, phagocytosis, phagosome maturation, and the development of the lysosome [47]. Phagocytes (macrophages, granulocytes, or dendritic cells) use their plasma membrane to engulf a large particle (e.g., apoptotic cell or microbes) [47]. Tumor cells are also engulfed by phagocytes. The ensuing early endosome fuses with the lysosome into a late endosome, then diffused through the membrane of the phagolysosome. Cathepsins are key acid hydrolases within the lysosome. They are associated with the processes of the lysosome, including the process of antigen presentation [48]. Cathepsins represent the principal effectors of protein catabolism and autophagy and support the increased metabolic needs of proliferating cancer cells [48]. In this study, cathepsin was overexpressed in SMM. Overexpression of cathepsin is associated with poor prognosis [48,49]. LAMPs were also overexpressed in SMM. This family of glycosylated proteins is involved in supporting tumor growth and metastatic spread [50].

Toll-like receptors (TLRs) are involved in the response of the innate immunity, but can also organize several downstream signaling pathways leading to the formation or suppression of cancer cells [51]. Once synthesized, they are translocated to the Golgi complex and subsequently delivered to the plasma or endosomes [51]. Overexpression of TLRs has been reported for several cancers like prostate cancer, neuroblastoma, lung cancer, and ovarian cancer. While in some studies overexpression of TLRs has been associated with more aggressive forms of, e.g., squamous cell carcinoma [52], other studies revealed high expression being indicative of longer survival rates [53]. In our study, in contrast to SMM with increased expression of TLR2 and TLR4, EMM exhibited overexpression of TLR6. TLR6 is suggested to have an anticancer function, as described in the literature for colon cancer [54]. TLR2 and TLR4 have been associated with gastric cancer [55].

The TAP transporter and MHC class I and II molecules are involved in the process of antigen processing and cross-presentation. These are overexpressed in phagocytes of SMM. As these molecules are also involved in antigen processing and presentation, this finding is further discussed in Section 3.2.

4.2. Antigen Processing and Presentation

Modern immunotherapeutic approaches have already been investigated in clinical trials in MPM [56–58]. One possible explanation for different responses might be in the processing and presentation of tumor-specific epitopes [59,60] important for the activation of tumor-specific T-cells [61]. A complex intracellular pathway is involved in processing these antigenic peptides (Figure S2). It starts with the polyubiquitination of the protein, which is then degraded by the proteasome. We have previously demonstrated strong 20S proteasome expression in MPM [62]. Its function is to remove misfolded/dysfunctional proteins, but high expression might lead to an "overheated" proteasome with deficient antigen processing capabilities. This could explain why the high expression of proteasomal components is associated with worse outcomes in MPM [62]. Translocation of small fragments processed by the proteasome into the endoplasmatic reticulum is performed via the TAP-transporter, a homodimer composed of TAP1 and TAP2 [63]. These peptide fragments bind the HLA class I molecule, and the whole complex is transported to the cell surface where it is recognized by CTL [61]. Classically, three genes (HLA-A, HLA-B, HLA-C) with an ample number of alleles code for the HLA class I molecule, but inferior genes are also known [64]. In the present study, we demonstrated a markable upregulation of gene expression levels of the above-mentioned components in SMM. Elevated CD68 expression levels (higher amount of macrophages) increased the activation of antigen-presentation-associated pathways in macrophages and dendritic cells with simultaneously even levels of CD8+ CTL, and no signs of direct anti-cancer immune aggression (like an expression of perforin or granzymes), implies altered processing of tumor neoantigens. This results in a "last-ditch attempt" of antigen-presenting cells to stimulate cytotoxic lymphocytes and NK cells. Deficiencies of the antigen presentation resulting in immune evasion from CTL are well described in different tumors [65,66]. These include the deficiency of HLA/MHC class I molecules due to point mutations or large deletions, but also mutations in HLA/MHC class I subunits, like β-2 microglobulin [56]. Furthermore, tumors might be capable of regulating HLA/MHC class I expression on an epigenetic level via DNA hypermethylation [67]. Johnsen et al. observed the development of large and persistent tumors through TAP1-negative parental transformed murine fibroblast cell line. In the case of tumor progression, TAP1-negative cells have been reported to be selection-wise favored over TAP1-positive cells [68]. Already in 1993, Restifo et al. suggested a possible tumor escape mechanism through deficient antigen presentation and processing based on finding of low mRNA levels for LMP-2 and LMP-7 (proteasome subunits) and TAP1 and TAP2 in small lung cell carcinomas [69]. Additional escape mechanisms involving TAP-mutations and cofactors that interact with TAP have been described [63]. The missing potency of cytotoxic T lymphocytes activity against the tumor cells by altered antigen processing and presentation could explain the inhomogenous response rates in the Checkmate 743.

4.3. Proteoglycans in Cancer

In recent decades, extracellular matrix (ECM) and TME have been recognized as major factors of tumor development and progression. In ECM, many different proteins and molecules are regulating different processes important for carcinogenesis. One of the key players in ECM is fibronectin (FN), which was found to be overexpressed in SMM in this study. FN is a glycoprotein with a central role in tumor cell proliferation, angiogenesis, invasion, and metastasis development, but also in processes involved in tumor evasion of the immune system (for review see [70]). Furthermore, its overexpression in SMM is not surprising, since FN is an important mesenchymal marker, and when found in epithelial malignancies is used as a sign of epithelia-mesenchymal transition (EMT) [71]. Its activation of TGF-β induces a partial EMT phenotype, usually at the invasive front of the epithelial tumors [72]. We have also found increased expression of integrin receptors α5 β1, α2 β1 and αv β3 in SMM in our cohort. Integrins are cell adhesion receptors, and the main receptor for ECM proteins and FN, and therefore also involved in many pro-tumor activities like tumor cell proliferation, metastasis, tumor angiogenesis. Binding between FN and integrins is further enhanced by integrin clustering and interacting with urokinase plasminogen activator receptor (uPAR), also overexpressed in SMM [73,74].

Another overexpressed protein in SMM was CD44. CD44 is a transmembrane glycoprotein and primary receptor through which hyaluronan (HA) activates different intracellular pathways resulting in tumor cell growth, migration, invasion, and angiogenesis [75,76]. HA, the only proteoglycan which is not covalently attached to protein core is related to poor prognosis in breast, colon, and ovarian carcinoma [77], and its presence in tumor stroma is an indication of the more aggressive tumor [78–80]. It has been shown that HA in MPM is overexpressed in intracellular, but also in pleural, fluid [81]. Hanagiri et al. demonstrated that the interaction of HA with CD44 is important for the proliferation and migration of tumor cells in MPM [82]. Interestingly, overexpression of CD44 was not observed in the EMM group.

As previously mentioned, we have also found overexpression of TLR 2 and TLR4, which are receptors for decorin, proteoglycan important for growth control, usually with binding and inactivation of TGF-β [83–85], inhibition of angiogenesis, and inducing of apoptosis through EGFR down-regulation [86]. It has been shown that decorin, through TLR2 and TLR4, induces proinflammatory tumor suppressor programmed cell death 4 (PDCD4), whose degradation is further prevented through the TGF-β1 blockade [87].

Thrombospondin-1, overexpressed in SMM, is a very controversial ECM protein involved in cell survival, migration, invasion, angiogenesis, and inflammation. However, its role is not straightforward and depends on tumor and ECM type. It is regarded as an anti-angiogenic factor, but some studies have reported its angiogenic activity as well [88]. It was described as a pro-adhesive protein but can also decrease the adhesion of tumor cells and promote invasion and metastases [89,90].

Very similar is the role of lumican, keratan sulfate, in cancer. Its expression is correlated with poor outcome in lung carcinoma, and in colorectal carcinoma, but is a favorable prognostic factor for osteosarcoma and melanoma [91–93]. It is known that lumican induces FAS by binding FAS ligands and in this way plays a role in the initiation of apoptosis and suppresses cell proliferation [94–96]. FAS is highly expressed in our EMM cohort. At the same time, TGF-β2, which is involved in growth suppression and cell adhesion in osteosarcoma [97], and is negatively regulated by lumican, has been highly expressed in SMM.

4.4. Secretion of Cytokines and Communication with the Immune System

To establish themselves and progress properly, it is inevitable for cancer cells to shape their local microenvironment to their benefit. This goal is achieved through continuous inflammatory reactions and heavy modulations of the immune response [98]. With cytokines and out of those especially chemokines being essential mediators for such a process, changes in their expression patterns are of great interest if we are to develop a deeper understanding of MPMs acquired TME. Various ligands, as well as receptors within the CC chemokine subfamily, were overexpressed in both MPM subtypes. This upregulation might support the flourishment of MPM since these chemokines have already been considered to play a vital role in tumor genesis, while their overexpression also appears to modulate the hosts' immune response against cancer cells [99]. We found a more distinguishable expression pattern regarding the CXC chemokine family. The EMM cases overexpress ligands for CXCR1/2, whereas the sarcomatoid subtype appears to stimulate the CXCR3-pathway with CXCL 9–13. Especially, the activation patterns measured in the EMM stick out, as the CXCR1/2 pathways are thought to contribute massively to the development of, among others, prostate, lung, colorectal, and breast cancer, as well as inflammatory diseases such as COPD and asthma [100,101]. Furthermore, malignancies appear to increase their therapy resistance by overexpression of these receptors and their ligands. In fact, the CXCR1/2 axis has been unreveiled as a potential therapeutic target in malignant melanoma, with pathway-inhibition significantly improving sensitivity for chemotherapy in otherwise resistant melanoma cells in vitro [102], while also decreasing progression and metastasis even in advanced disease [103].

Interleukins are considered to play a key role in MPM development. It was shown that asbestos-exposed knockout mice bearing modified inflammasomes, resulting in a diminished IL-1β release, had a significantly reduced incidence of MPM and later disease onset compared to their wild-type counterparts [104]. Furthermore, IL-6 is thought to not only essentially contribute to MPMs asbestos-related development, but also to impede effective chemotherapy and inducing angiogenesis by increasing VEGF expression [105,106]. In our study, the SMM demonstrated a surprisingly broad spectrum of elevated receptor expressions throughout interleukin 2-, as well as interleukin 4-like receptors. Interestingly, both subtypes, epithelioid via receptor-, sarcomatoid via ligand-upregulation, heavily stimulate the IL-6R pathway.

Especially the recruitment of TAMs has already been considered as a promising therapeutic target in MPM [107]. This hypothesis is further substantiated by Blondy et al., who discovered that MPM cells are directly involved in the recruitment of immunosuppressive macrophages by stimulation of the M-CSF/IL-34/CSF-1R pathway [108]. This perfectly fits the above-mentioned narrative since we were also able to demonstrate an elevated expression of mentioned pathways in our GSEA. Moreover, particularly the SMM upregulates the production of TNF- related TWEAK and TRAIL, as well as TGF-β related ligands TGFB-1 and -2. While the role of TNF has already been established in various malignant processes [109], TGF-ß has even been unraveled as an essential factor in MPM genesis [110,111].

An interesting thought occurred while regarding our expression patterns in the light of modern therapeutic approaches. In a recent study, Horn et al. demonstrated improved immune response and prognostically favorable TME remodeling of breast and lung cancer in a murine model after simultaneous inhibition of the CXCR1/2 and TGF-ß pathway during PDL-1 therapy [112]. As PDL-1 treatment in combination with a cisplatin-pemetrexed based chemotherapy [4,113] has yielded relatively promising results in MPM therapy so far, and with us showing increased activation of the corresponding pathways, transferring this experimental approach to the MPM might be important for future multimodal treatment.

Our study has several technical and biological limitations. As the present study is only based on gene expression data, the final proof of differences in the composition and quantity of the infiltrating immune cells, and chemokine secretion described above is lacking. Furthermore, the relatively small sample sizes of SMM and EMM reduce study strength, as variability, especially between samples of different ethnical origins, may be underestimated. Furthermore, it would be of great interest to analyze the expression of genes involved in innate and acquired immunity in normal mesothelium and compare these findings with EMM and SMM. It is known that normal mesothelial cells form a protective barrier, and are involved in antigen presentation, inflammation, and cell adhesion [114,115]. However, normal pleural tissue from healthy patients can only rarely be provided, which makes it more difficult to characterize a "normal" state and define EMM and SMM-specific features.

5. Conclusions

Immune evasion as a hallmark of cancer and both in EMM and SMM can be problematic issue for therapeutic intervention. Our work reveals the specific gene expression pattern of genes involved in immunological and inflammatory processes within the different histologic subtypes of MPM, providing a more detailed background of their immunogenic potential and demonstrating their distinct pattern of immunogenicity. Those differences comprise genes associated with antigen processing and presentation to resident cytotoxic T cells as well as phagocytosis, but also cell–cell communication via the cytokine system. Knowledge about underlying biological processes has the potential to pave the ground for patient stratification for modern therapeutic approaches such as immune-checkpoint blockades and will be the key for improved clinical management of patients with MPM.

Supplementary Materials: The following are available online at https://www.mdpi.com/article/10.3390/cancers13081761/s1, Figure S1: Gene set enrichment analysis of differential expressed genes between EMM and SMM involved in phagosome pathway, Figure S2: Gene set enrichment analysis of differential expressed genes between EMM and SMM involved in antigen processing and presentation pathway, Figure S3: Gene set enrichment analysis of differential expressed genes between EMM and SMM involved in Fc gamma R-mediated phagocytosis, Figure S4: Gene set enrichment analysis of differential expressed genes for proteoglycans, Figure S5: Gene set enrichment analysis of differential expressed genes between EMM and SMM involved in cytokine-cytokine receptor interaction, Table S1: Overview of *p*-values and 95% CI of associations to histological subtype calculated for all genes, Table S2: Results of the gene set enrichment analysis between EMM and SMM.

Author Contributions: Conceptualization, L.B., S.B. and F.D.M.; Methodology, F.D.M. and R.F.H.W.; Software, M.W., F.D.M.; Validation, R.F.H.W., S.B. and F.D.M.; Formal analysis, R.F.H.W., M.W., and F.D.M.; Investigation, A.M., S.B., J.W. and F.D.M.; Resources, F.D.M., L.B. and K.W.S.; Data curation, A.M., L.B., M.W., E.M., H.B., D.K., J.S., T.H., D.C.C., J.K., T.M. and F.D.M.; Writing—original draft preparation, R.F.H.W., L.B., A.M., M.W. and F.D.M.; Writing—review and editing, R.F.H.W., L.B., A.M., M.W., E.M., A.M., H.B., D.K., L.B., J.S., T.H., D.C.C., J.K., T.M., J.W., S.B., K.W.S., F.D.M.; Visualization, M.W., and F.D.M.; Supervision, F.D.M.; Project administration, L.B. and F.D.M.; Funding acquisition, F.D.M. and K.W.S. (institutional). All authors have read and agreed to the published version of the manuscript.

Funding: This research received no external funding.

Institutional Review Board Statement: The study was conducted according to the guidelines of the Declaration of Helsinki and approved by the Ethics Committee of University Hospital Essen (protocol code 14-5775-BO).

Informed Consent Statement: As the majority of patients were deceased at the time of data collection and collection of follow-up data, a written informed consent has not been obtained from them. All patient data have been anonymized prior to analysis. The ethics committee of the University Hospital Essen waived the necessity for a written informed consent when they approved the present study.

Data Availability Statement: All data are available from the author directly.

Conflicts of Interest: The authors declare no conflict of interest.

References

1. Neumann, V.; Löseke, S.; Nowak, D.; Herth, F.J.; Tannapfel, A. Malignant pleural mesothelioma: Incidence, etiology, diagnosis, treatment, and occupational health. *Dtsch. Arztebl. Int.* **2013**, *110*, 319–326. [CrossRef]
2. Alpert, N.; van Gerwen, M.; Taioli, E. Epidemiology of mesothelioma in the 21(st) century in Europe and the United States, 40 years after restricted/banned asbestos use. *Transl. Lung Cancer Res.* **2020**, *9*, S28–S38. [CrossRef]
3. Gaudino, G.; Xue, J.; Yang, H. How asbestos and other fibers cause mesothelioma. *Transl. Lung Cancer Res.* **2020**, *9*, S39–S46. [CrossRef] [PubMed]
4. Baas, P.; Scherpereel, A.; Nowak, A.K.; Fujimoto, N.; Peters, S.; Tsao, A.S.; Mansfield, A.S.; Popat, S.; Jahan, T.; Antonia, S.; et al. First-line nivolumab plus ipilimumab in unresectable malignant pleural mesothelioma (CheckMate 743): A multicentre, randomised, open-label, phase 3 trial. *Lancet* **2021**, *397*, 375–386. [CrossRef]
5. Vogelzang, N.J.; Rusthoven, J.J.; Symanowski, J.; Denham, C.; Kaukel, E.; Ruffie, P.; Gatzemeier, U.; Boyer, M.; Emri, S.; Manegold, C.; et al. Phase III study of pemetrexed in combination with cisplatin versus cisplatin alone in patients with malignant pleural mesothelioma. *J. Clin. Oncol.* **2003**, *21*, 2636–2644. [CrossRef]
6. Brcic, L.; Kern, I. Clinical significance of histologic subtyping of malignant pleural mesothelioma. *Transl. Lung Cancer Res.* **2020**, *9*, 924–933. [CrossRef] [PubMed]
7. Meyerhoff, R.R.; Yang, C.F.; Speicher, P.J.; Gulack, B.C.; Hartwig, M.G.; D'Amico, T.A.; Harpole, D.H.; Berry, M.F. Impact of mesothelioma histologic subtype on outcomes in the Surveillance, Epidemiology, and End Results database. *J. Surg. Res.* **2015**, *196*, 23–32. [CrossRef]
8. Galateau-Salle, F.; Churg, A.; Roggli, V.; Travis, W.D. The 2015 World Health Organization Classification of Tumors of the Pleura: Advances since the 2004 Classification. *J. Thorac. Oncol.* **2016**, *11*, 142–154. [CrossRef] [PubMed]
9. Brčić, L.; Jakopović, M.; Brčić, I.; Klarić, V.; Milošević, M.; Sepac, A.; Samaržija, M.; Seiwerth, S. Reproducibility of histological subtyping of malignant pleural mesothelioma. *Virchows Arch.* **2014**, *465*, 679–685. [CrossRef]
10. Kadota, K.; Suzuki, K.; Sima, C.S.; Rusch, V.W.; Adusumilli, P.S.; Travis, W.D. Pleomorphic epithelioid diffuse malignant pleural mesothelioma: A clinicopathological review and conceptual proposal to reclassify as biphasic or sarcomatoid mesothelioma. *J. Thorac. Oncol.* **2011**, *6*, 896–904. [CrossRef] [PubMed]
11. Ordóñez, N.G. Pleomorphic mesothelioma: Report of 10 cases. *Mod. Pathol.* **2012**, *25*, 1011–1022. [CrossRef]
12. Cantin, R.; Al-Jabi, M.; McCaughey, W.T. Desmoplastic diffuse mesothelioma. *Am. J. Surg. Pathol.* **1982**, *6*, 215–222. [CrossRef] [PubMed]
13. Salle, F.G.; Le Stang, N.; Nicholson, A.G.; Pissaloux, D.; Churg, A.; Klebe, S.; Roggli, V.L.; Tazelaar, H.D.; Vignaud, J.M.; Attanoos, R.; et al. New Insights on Diagnostic Reproducibility of Biphasic Mesotheliomas: A Multi-Institutional Evaluation by the International Mesothelioma Panel From the MESOPATH Reference Center. *J. Thorac. Oncol.* **2018**, *13*, 1189–1203. [CrossRef] [PubMed]
14. Vigneswaran, W.T.; Kircheva, D.Y.; Ananthanarayanan, V.; Watson, S.; Arif, Q.; Celauro, A.D.; Kindler, H.L.; Husain, A.N. Amount of Epithelioid Differentiation Is a Predictor of Survival in Malignant Pleural Mesothelioma. *Ann. Thorac. Surg.* **2017**, *103*, 962–966. [CrossRef]
15. Chen, Z.; Gaudino, G.; Pass, H.I.; Carbone, M.; Yang, H. Diagnostic and prognostic biomarkers for malignant mesothelioma: An update. *Transl. Lung Cancer Res.* **2017**, *6*, 259–269. [CrossRef]
16. Bueno, R.; Opitz, I. Surgery in Malignant Pleural Mesothelioma. *J. Thorac. Oncol.* **2018**, *13*, 1638–1654. [CrossRef] [PubMed]
17. Popat, S.; Curioni-Fontecedro, A.; Polydoropoulou, V.; Shah, R.; O'Brien, M.; Pope, A.; Fisher, P.; Spicer, J.; Roy, A.; Gilligan, D.; et al. A multicentre randomized phase III trial comparing pembrolizumab (P) vs single agent chemotherapy (CT) for advanced pre-treated malignant pleural mesothelioma (MPM): Results from the European Thoracic Oncology Platform (ETOP 9-15) PROMISE-meso trial. *Ann. Oncol.* **2019**, *30*, v931. [CrossRef]
18. Scagliotti, G.V.; Gaafar, R.; Nowak, A.K.; Nakano, T.; van Meerbeeck, J.; Popat, S.; Vogelzang, N.J.; Grosso, F.; Aboelhassan, R.; Jakopovic, M.; et al. Nintedanib in combination with pemetrexed and cisplatin for chemotherapy-naive patients with advanced malignant pleural mesothelioma (LUME-Meso): A double-blind, randomised, placebo-controlled phase 3 trial. *Lancet Respir. Med.* **2019**, *7*, 569–580. [CrossRef]
19. Carbone, M.; Yang, H. Molecular pathways: Targeting mechanisms of asbestos and erionite carcinogenesis in mesothelioma. *Clin. Cancer Res.* **2012**, *18*, 598–604. [CrossRef]
20. Chu, G.J.; van Zandwijk, N.; Rasko, J.E.J. The Immune Microenvironment in Mesothelioma: Mechanisms of Resistance to Immunotherapy. *Front. Oncol.* **2019**, *9*, 1366. [CrossRef]
21. Lievense, L.A.; Cornelissen, R.; Bezemer, K.; Kaijen-Lambers, M.E.; Hegmans, J.P.; Aerts, J.G. Pleural Effusion of Patients with Malignant Mesothelioma Induces Macrophage-Mediated T Cell Suppression. *J. Thorac. Oncol.* **2016**, *11*, 1755–1764. [CrossRef] [PubMed]
22. Marcq, E.; Siozopoulou, V.; De Waele, J.; van Audenaerde, J.; Zwaenepoel, K.; Santermans, E.; Hens, N.; Pauwels, P.; van Meerbeeck, J.P.; Smits, E.L. Prognostic and predictive aspects of the tumor immune microenvironment and immune checkpoints in malignant pleural mesothelioma. *Oncoimmunology* **2017**, *6*, e1261241. [CrossRef]

23. Chéné, A.L.; d'Almeida, S.; Blondy, T.; Tabiasco, J.; Deshayes, S.; Fonteneau, J.F.; Cellerin, L.; Delneste, Y.; Grégoire, M.; Blanquart, C. Pleural Effusions from Patients with Mesothelioma Induce Recruitment of Monocytes and Their Differentiation into M2 Macrophages. *J. Thorac. Oncol.* **2016**, *11*, 1765–1773. [CrossRef] [PubMed]
24. Cioce, M.; Canino, C.; Goparaju, C.; Yang, H.; Carbone, M.; Pass, H.I. Autocrine CSF-1R signaling drives mesothelioma chemoresistance via AKT activation. *Cell Death Dis.* **2014**, *5*, e1167. [CrossRef] [PubMed]
25. DeLong, P.; Carroll, R.G.; Henry, A.C.; Tanaka, T.; Ahmad, S.; Leibowitz, M.S.; Sterman, D.H.; June, C.H.; Albelda, S.M.; Vonderheide, R.H. Regulatory T cells and cytokines in malignant pleural effusions secondary to mesothelioma and carcinoma. *Cancer Biol. Ther.* **2005**, *4*, 342–346. [CrossRef] [PubMed]
26. Burt, B.M.; Rodig, S.J.; Tilleman, T.R.; Elbardissi, A.W.; Bueno, R.; Sugarbaker, D.J. Circulating and tumor-infiltrating myeloid cells predict survival in human pleural mesothelioma. *Cancer* **2011**, *117*, 5234–5244. [CrossRef]
27. Chee, S.J.; Lopez, M.; Mellows, T.; Gankande, S.; Moutasim, K.A.; Harris, S.; Clarke, J.; Vijayanand, P.; Thomas, G.J.; Ottensmeier, C.H. Evaluating the effect of immune cells on the outcome of patients with mesothelioma. *Br. J. Cancer* **2017**, *117*, 1341–1348. [CrossRef]
28. Cornelissen, R.; Lievense, L.A.; Maat, A.P.; Hendriks, R.W.; Hoogsteden, H.C.; Bogers, A.J.; Hegmans, J.P.; Aerts, J.G. Ratio of Intratumoral Macrophage Phenotypes Is a Prognostic Factor in Epithelioid Malignant Pleural Mesothelioma. *PLoS ONE* **2014**, *9*, e106742. [CrossRef]
29. Bueno, R.; Stawiski, E.W.; Goldstein, L.D.; Durinck, S.; De Rienzo, A.; Modrusan, Z.; Gnad, F.; Nguyen, T.T.; Jaiswal, B.S.; Chirieac, L.R.; et al. Comprehensive genomic analysis of malignant pleural mesothelioma identifies recurrent mutations, gene fusions and splicing alterations. *Nat. Genet.* **2016**, *48*, 407–416. [CrossRef] [PubMed]
30. Awad, M.M.; Jones, R.E.; Liu, H.; Lizotte, P.H.; Ivanova, E.V.; Kulkarni, M.; Herter-Sprie, G.S.; Liao, X.; Santos, A.A.; Bittinger, M.A.; et al. Cytotoxic T Cells in PD-L1–Positive Malignant Pleural Mesotheliomas Are Counterbalanced by Distinct Immunosuppressive Factors. *Cancer Immunol. Res.* **2016**, *4*, 1038–1048. [CrossRef] [PubMed]
31. Anraku, M.; Cunningham, K.S.; Yun, Z.; Tsao, M.-S.; Zhang, L.; Keshavjee, S.; Johnston, M.R.; de Perrot, M. Impact of tumor-infiltrating T cells on survival in patients with malignant pleural mesothelioma. *J. Thorac. Cardiovasc. Surg.* **2008**, *135*, 823–829. [CrossRef] [PubMed]
32. Mansfield, A.S.; Peikert, T.; Smadbeck, J.B.; Udell, J.B.M.; Garcia-Rivera, E.; Elsbernd, L.; Erskine, C.L.; Van Keulen, V.P.; Kosari, F.; Murphy, S.J.; et al. Neoantigenic Potential of Complex Chromosomal Rearrangements in Mesothelioma. *J. Thorac. Oncol.* **2019**, *14*, 276–287. [CrossRef] [PubMed]
33. Kiyotani, K.; Park, J.-H.; Inoue, H.; Husain, A.; Olugbile, S.; Zewde, M.; Nakamura, Y.; Vigneswaran, W.T. Integrated analysis of somatic mutations and immune microenvironment in malignant pleural mesothelioma. *OncoImmunology* **2017**, *6*, e1278330. [CrossRef]
34. Marcq, E.; Waele, J.D.; Audenaerde, J.V.; Lion, E.; Santermans, E.; Hens, N.; Pauwels, P.; van Meerbeeck, J.P.; Smits, E.L.J. Abundant expression of TIM-3, LAG-3, PD-1 and PD-L1 as immunotherapy checkpoint targets in effusions of mesothelioma patients. *Oncotarget* **2017**, *8*, 89722–89735. [CrossRef]
35. Khanna, S.; Graef, S.; Mussai, F.; Thomas, A.; Wali, N.; Yenidunya, B.G.; Yuan, C.; Morrow, B.; Zhang, J.; Korangy, F.; et al. Tumor-Derived GM-CSF Promotes Granulocyte Immunosuppression in Mesothelioma Patients. *Clin. Cancer Res.* **2018**, *24*, 2859–2872. [CrossRef] [PubMed]
36. Nagaraj, S.; Gupta, K.; Pisarev, V.; Kinarsky, L.; Sherman, S.; Kang, L.; Herber, D.L.; Schneck, J.; Gabrilovich, D.I. Altered recognition of antigen is a mechanism of CD8+ T cell tolerance in cancer. *Nat. Med.* **2007**, *13*, 828–835. [CrossRef]
37. Schmielau, J.; Finn, O.J. Activated granulocytes and granulocyte-derived hydrogen peroxide are the underlying mechanism of suppression of t-cell function in advanced cancer patients. *Cancer Res.* **2001**, *61*, 4756–4760.
38. Kao, S.C.H.; Pavlakis, N.; Harvie, R.; Vardy, J.L.; Boyer, M.J.; van Zandwijk, N.; Clarke, S.J. High Blood Neutrophil-to-Lymphocyte Ratio Is an Indicator of Poor Prognosis in Malignant Mesothelioma Patients Undergoing Systemic Therapy. *Clin. Cancer Res.* **2010**, *16*, 5805–5813. [CrossRef]
39. Brockwell, N.K.; Alamgeer, M.; Kumar, B.; Rivalland, G.; John, T.; Parker, B.S. Preliminary study highlights the potential of immune checkpoint inhibitors in sarcomatoid mesothelioma. *Transl. Lung Cancer Res.* **2020**, *9*, 639–645. [CrossRef]
40. *WHO Classification of Tumours of the Lung, Pleura, Thymus and Heart*, 4th ed.; Travis, W.D.; Brambilla, E.; Burke, A.; Marx, A.; Nicholson, G. (Eds.) International Agency for Research on Cancer: Lyon, France, 2015.
41. *TNM Classification of Malignant Tumours*, 8th ed.; Brierley, J.D.; Gospodarowicz, M.K.; Wittekind, C. (Eds.) Wiley-Blackwell: Oxford, UK, 2017.
42. Byrne, M.J.; Nowak, A.K. Modified RECIST criteria for assessment of response in malignant pleural mesothelioma. *Ann. Oncol.* **2004**, *15*, 257–260. [CrossRef]
43. The R Project for Statistical Computing. Available online: https://www.r-project.org/ (accessed on 3 December 2020).
44. WEB-based GEne SeT AnaLysis Toolkit. Available online: http://www.webgestalt.org/ (accessed on 3 December 2020).
45. Waggott, D.; Chu, K.; Yin, S.; Wouters, B.G.; Liu, F.F.; Boutros, P.C. NanoStringNorm: an extensible R package for the pre-processing of NanoString mRNA and miRNA data. *Bioinformatics* **2012**, *28*, 1546–1548, doi:10.1093/bioinformatics/bts188
46. Minnema-Luiting, J.; Vroman, H.; Aerts, J.; Cornelissen, R. Heterogeneity in Immune Cell Content in Malignant Pleural Mesothelioma. *Int. J. Mol. Sci.* **2018**, *19*, 1041. [CrossRef] [PubMed]

47. Ambrose, C.T. The Osler slide, a demonstration of phagocytosis from 1876 Reports of phagocytosis before Metchnikoff's 1880 paper. *Cell Immunol.* **2006**, *240*, 1–4. [CrossRef]
48. Olson, O.C.; Joyce, J.A. Cysteine cathepsin proteases: Regulators of cancer progression and therapeutic response. *Nat. Rev. Cancer* **2015**, *15*, 712–729. [CrossRef] [PubMed]
49. Jedeszko, C.; Sloane, B.F. Cysteine cathepsins in human cancer. *Biol. Chem.* **2004**, *385*, 1017–1027. [CrossRef]
50. Alessandrini, F.; Pezze, L.; Ciribilli, Y. LAMPs: Shedding light on cancer biology. *Semin. Oncol.* **2017**, *44*, 239–253. [CrossRef] [PubMed]
51. Mokhtari, Y.; Pourbagheri-Sigaroodi, A.; Zafari, P.; Bagheri, N.; Ghaffari, S.H.; Bashash, D. Toll-like receptors (TLRs): An old family of immune receptors with a new face in cancer pathogenesis. *J. Cell Mol. Med.* **2020**. [CrossRef]
52. Kauppila, J.H.; Korvala, J.; Siirila, K.; Manni, M.; Makinen, L.K.; Hagstrom, J.; Atula, T.; Haglund, C.; Selander, K.S.; Saarnio, J.; et al. Toll-like receptor 9 mediates invasion and predicts prognosis in squamous cell carcinoma of the mobile tongue. *J. Oral. Pathol. Med.* **2015**, *44*, 571–577. [CrossRef] [PubMed]
53. Leppanen, J.; Helminen, O.; Huhta, H.; Kauppila, J.H.; Isohookana, J.; Haapasaari, K.M.; Lehenkari, P.; Saarnio, J.; Karttunen, T.J. High toll-like receptor (TLR) 9 expression is associated with better prognosis in surgically treated pancreatic cancer patients. *Virchows Arch.* **2017**, *470*, 401–410. [CrossRef] [PubMed]
54. Semlali, A.; Almutairi, M.; Pathan, A.A.K.; Azzi, A.; Parine, N.R.; AlAmri, A.; Arafah, M.; Aljebreen, A.M.; Alharbi, O.; Almadi, M.A.; et al. Toll-like receptor 6 expression, sequence variants, and their association with colorectal cancer risk. *J. Cancer* **2019**, *10*, 2969–2981. [CrossRef]
55. Tongtawee, T.; Simawaranon, T.; Wattanawongdon, W.; Dechsukhum, C.; Leeanansaksiri, W. Toll-like receptor 2 and 4 polymorphisms associated with Helicobacter pylori susceptibility and gastric cancer. *Turk. J. Gastroenterol.* **2019**, *30*, 15–20. [CrossRef] [PubMed]
56. Topfer, K.; Kempe, S.; Muller, N.; Schmitz, M.; Bachmann, M.; Cartellieri, M.; Schackert, G.; Temme, A. Tumor evasion from T cell surveillance. *J. Biomed. Biotechnol.* **2011**, *2011*, 918471. [CrossRef] [PubMed]
57. Brahmer, J.R.; Pardoll, D.M. Immune checkpoint inhibitors: Making immunotherapy a reality for the treatment of lung cancer. *Cancer Immunol. Res.* **2013**, *1*, 85–91. [CrossRef] [PubMed]
58. Pardoll, D.M. The blockade of immune checkpoints in cancer immunotherapy. *Nat. Rev. Cancer* **2012**, *12*, 252–264. [CrossRef] [PubMed]
59. Wessolly, M.; Stephan-Falkenau, S.; Streubel, A.; Werner, R.; Borchert, S.; Griff, S.; Mairinger, E.; Walter, R.F.H.; Bauer, T.; Eberhardt, W.E.E.; et al. A Novel Epitope Quality-Based Immune Escape Mechanism Reveals Patient's Suitability for Immune Checkpoint Inhibition. *Cancer Manag. Res.* **2020**, *12*, 7881–7890. [CrossRef] [PubMed]
60. Wessolly, M.; Walter, R.F.H.; Vollbrecht, C.; Werner, R.; Borchert, S.; Schmeller, J.; Mairinger, E.; Herold, T.; Streubel, A.; Christoph, D.C.; et al. Processing Escape Mechanisms Through Altered Proteasomal Cleavage of Epitopes Affect Immune Response in Pulmonary Neuroendocrine Tumors. *Technol. Cancer Res. Treat.* **2018**, *17*, 1533033818818418. [CrossRef]
61. Kloetzel, P.M. The proteasome and MHC class I antigen processing. *Biochim. Biophys. Acta* **2004**, *1695*, 225–233. [CrossRef] [PubMed]
62. Walter, R.F.H.; Sydow, S.R.; Berg, E.; Kollmeier, J.; Christoph, D.C.; Christoph, S.; Eberhardt, W.E.E.; Mairinger, T.; Wohlschlaeger, J.; Schmid, K.W.; et al. Bortezomib sensitivity is tissue dependent and high expression of the 20S proteasome precludes good response in malignant pleural mesothelioma. *Cancer Manag. Res.* **2019**, *11*, 8711–8720. [CrossRef] [PubMed]
63. Abele, R.; Tampe, R. The TAP translocation machinery in adaptive immunity and viral escape mechanisms. *Essays Biochem.* **2011**, *50*, 249–264. [CrossRef] [PubMed]
64. Choo, S.Y. The HLA system: Genetics, immunology, clinical testing, and clinical implications. *Yonsei Med. J.* **2007**, *48*, 11–23. [CrossRef]
65. Maleno, I.; Cabrera, C.M.; Cabrera, T.; Paco, L.; Lopez-Nevot, M.A.; Collado, A.; Ferron, A.; Garrido, F. Distribution of HLA class I altered phenotypes in colorectal carcinomas: High frequency of HLA haplotype loss associated with loss of heterozygosity in chromosome region 6p21. *Immunogenetics* **2004**, *56*, 244–253. [CrossRef]
66. Maleno, I.; Romero, J.M.; Cabrera, T.; Paco, L.; Aptsiauri, N.; Cozar, J.M.; Tallada, M.; Lopez-Nevot, M.A.; Garrido, F. LOH at 6p21.3 region and HLA class I altered phenotypes in bladder carcinomas. *Immunogenetics* **2006**, *58*, 503–510. [CrossRef]
67. Serrano, A.; Castro-Vega, I.; Redondo, M. Role of gene methylation in antitumor immune response: Implication for tumor progression. *Cancers* **2011**, *3*, 1672–1690. [CrossRef]
68. Johnsen, A.K.; Templeton, D.J.; Sy, M.; Harding, C.V. Deficiency of transporter for antigen presentation (TAP) in tumor cells allows evasion of immune surveillance and increases tumorigenesis. *J. Immunol.* **1999**, *163*, 4224–4231. [PubMed]
69. Restifo, N.P.; Esquivel, F.; Kawakami, Y.; Yewdell, J.W.; Mule, J.J.; Rosenberg, S.A.; Bennink, J.R. Identification of human cancers deficient in antigen processing. *J. Exp. Med.* **1993**, *177*, 265–272. [CrossRef]
70. Efthymiou, G.; Saint, A.; Ruff, M.; Rekad, Z.; Ciais, D.; Van Obberghen-Schilling, E. Shaping Up the Tumor Microenvironment With Cellular Fibronectin. *Front. Oncol.* **2020**, *10*, 641. [CrossRef] [PubMed]
71. Dongre, A.; Weinberg, R.A. New insights into the mechanisms of epithelial-mesenchymal transition and implications for cancer. *Nat. Rev. Mol. Cell Biol.* **2019**, *20*, 69–84. [CrossRef] [PubMed]

72. Puram, S.V.; Tirosh, I.; Parikh, A.S.; Patel, A.P.; Yizhak, K.; Gillespie, S.; Rodman, C.; Luo, C.L.; Mroz, E.A.; Emerick, K.S.; et al. Single-Cell Transcriptomic Analysis of Primary and Metastatic Tumor Ecosystems in Head and Neck Cancer. *Cell* **2017**, *171*, 1611–1624.e24. [CrossRef]
73. Naci, D.; Vuori, K.; Aoudjit, F. Alpha2beta1 integrin in cancer development and chemoresistance. *Semin. Cancer Biol.* **2015**, *35*, 145–153. [CrossRef] [PubMed]
74. Ivaska, J.; Heino, J. Cooperation between integrins and growth factor receptors in signaling and endocytosis. *Annu. Rev. Cell Dev. Biol.* **2011**, *27*, 291–320. [CrossRef]
75. Twarock, S.; Tammi, M.I.; Savani, R.C.; Fischer, J.W. Hyaluronan stabilizes focal adhesions, filopodia, and the proliferative phenotype in esophageal squamous carcinoma cells. *J. Biol. Chem.* **2010**, *285*, 23276–23284. [CrossRef] [PubMed]
76. Wang, S.J.; Bourguignon, L.Y. Role of hyaluronan-mediated CD44 signaling in head and neck squamous cell carcinoma progression and chemoresistance. *Am. J. Pathol.* **2011**, *178*, 956–963. [CrossRef]
77. Tammi, R.H.; Kultti, A.; Kosma, V.M.; Pirinen, R.; Auvinen, P.; Tammi, M.I. Hyaluronan in human tumors: Pathobiological and prognostic messages from cell-associated and stromal hyaluronan. *Semin. Cancer Biol.* **2008**, *18*, 288–295. [CrossRef]
78. Aaltomaa, S.; Lipponen, P.; Tammi, R.; Tammi, M.; Viitanen, J.; Kankkunen, J.P.; Kosma, V.M. Strong Stromal Hyaluronan Expression Is Associated with PSA Recurrence in Local Prostate Cancer. *Urol. Int.* **2002**, *69*, 266–272. [CrossRef]
79. Kosunen, A.; Ropponen, K.; Kellokoski, J.; Pukkila, M.; Virtaniemi, J.; Valtonen, H.; Kumpulainen, E.; Johansson, R.; Tammi, R.; Tammi, M.; et al. Reduced expression of hyaluronan is a strong indicator of poor survival in oral squamous cell carcinoma. *Oral. Oncol.* **2004**, *40*, 257–263. [CrossRef]
80. Pirinen, R.; Tammi, R.; Tammi, M.; Hirvikoski, P.; Parkkinen, J.J.; Johansson, R.; Böhm, J.; Hollmén, S.; Kosma, V.-M. Prognostic value of hyaluronan expression in non-small-cell lung cancer: Increased stromal expression indicates unfavorable outcome in patients with adenocarcinoma. *Int. J. Cancer* **2001**, *95*, 12–17. [CrossRef]
81. Thylén, A.; Hjerpe, A.; Martensson, G. Hyaluronan content in pleural fluid as a prognostic factor in patients with malignant pleural mesothelioma. *Cancer* **2001**, *92*, 1224–1230. [CrossRef]
82. Hanagiri, T.; Shinohara, S.; Takenaka, M.; Shigematsu, Y.; Yasuda, M.; Shimokawa, H.; Nagata, Y.; Nakagawa, M.; Uramoto, H.; So, T.; et al. Effects of hyaluronic acid and CD44 interaction on the proliferation and invasiveness of malignant pleural mesothelioma. *Tumour. Biol.* **2012**, *33*, 2135–2141. [CrossRef] [PubMed]
83. Yamaguchi, Y.; Ruoslahti, E. Expression of human proteoglycan in Chinese hamster ovary cells inhibits cell proliferation. *Nature* **1988**, *336*, 244–246. [CrossRef] [PubMed]
84. Yamaguchi, Y.; Mann, D.M.; Ruoslahti, E. Negative regulation of transforming growth factor-beta by the proteoglycan decorin. *Nature* **1990**, *346*, 281–284. [CrossRef]
85. Iozzo, R.V. Proteoglycans and neoplasia. *Cancer Metastasis Rev.* **1988**, *7*, 39–50. [CrossRef]
86. Seidler, D.G.; Goldoni, S.; Agnew, C.; Cardi, C.; Thakur, M.L.; Owens, R.T.; McQuillan, D.J.; Iozzo, R.V. Decorin protein core inhibits in vivo cancer growth and metabolism by hindering epidermal growth factor receptor function and triggering apoptosis via caspase-3 activation. *J. Biol. Chem.* **2006**, *281*, 26408–26418. [CrossRef]
87. Merline, R.; Moreth, K.; Beckmann, J.; Nastase, M.V.; Zeng-Brouwers, J.; Tralhao, J.G.; Lemarchand, P.; Pfeilschifter, J.; Schaefer, R.M.; Iozzo, R.V.; et al. Signaling by the matrix proteoglycan decorin controls inflammation and cancer through PDCD4 and MicroRNA-21. *Sci. Signal.* **2011**, *4*, ra75. [CrossRef] [PubMed]
88. Byrne, G.J.; Hayden, K.E.; McDowell, G.; Lang, H.; Kirwan, C.C.; Tetlow, L.; Kumar, S.; Bundred, N.J. Angiogenic characteristics of circulating and tumoural thrombospondin-1 in breast cancer. *Int. J. Oncol.* **2007**, *31*, 1127–1132. [CrossRef] [PubMed]
89. Tuszynski, G.P.; Rothman, V.; Murphy, A.; Siegler, K.; Smith, L.; Smith, S.; Karczewski, J.; Knudsen, K.A. Thrombospondin promotes cell-substratum adhesion. *Science* **1987**, *236*, 1570–1573. [CrossRef] [PubMed]
90. Albo, D.; Rothman, V.L.; Roberts, D.D.; Tuszynski, G.P. Tumour cell thrombospondin-1 regulates tumour cell adhesion and invasion through the urokinase plasminogen activator receptor. *Br. J. Cancer* **2000**, *83*, 298–306. [CrossRef] [PubMed]
91. Matsuda, Y.; Yamamoto, T.; Kudo, M.; Kawahara, K.; Kawamoto, M.; Nakajima, Y.; Koizumi, K.; Nakazawa, N.; Ishiwata, T.; Naito, Z. Expression and roles of lumican in lung adenocarcinoma and squamous cell carcinoma. *Int. J. Oncol.* **2008**, *33*, 1177–1185. [PubMed]
92. Nikitovic, D.; Berdiaki, A.; Zafiropoulos, A.; Katonis, P.; Tsatsakis, A.; Karamanos, N.K.; Tzanakakis, G.N. Lumican expression is positively correlated with the differentiation and negatively with the growth of human osteosarcoma cells. *FEBS J.* **2008**, *275*, 350–361. [CrossRef]
93. Brezillon, S.; Venteo, L.; Ramont, L.; D'Onofrio, M.F.; Perreau, C.; Pluot, M.; Maquart, F.X.; Wegrowski, Y. Expression of lumican, a small leucine-rich proteoglycan with antitumour activity, in human malignant melanoma. *Clin. Exp. Dermatol.* **2007**, *32*, 405–416. [CrossRef]
94. Vij, N.; Roberts, L.; Joyce, S.; Chakravarti, S. Lumican suppresses cell proliferation and aids Fas-Fas ligand mediated apoptosis: Implications in the cornea. *Exp. Eye Res.* **2004**, *78*, 957–971. [CrossRef]
95. Owen-Schaub, L.; Chan, H.; Cusack, J.C.; Roth, J.; Hill, L.L. Fas and Fas ligand interactions in malignant disease. *Int. J. Oncol.* **2000**, *17*, 5–12. [CrossRef]
96. Vij, N.; Roberts, L.; Joyce, S.; Chakravarti, S. Lumican regulates corneal inflammatory responses by modulating Fas-Fas ligand signaling. *Investig. Ophthalmol. Vis. Sci.* **2005**, *46*, 88–95. [CrossRef]

97. Nikitovic, D.; Aggelidakis, J.; Young, M.F.; Iozzo, R.V.; Karamanos, N.K.; Tzanakakis, G.N. The biology of small leucine-rich proteoglycans in bone pathophysiology. *J. Biol. Chem.* **2012**, *287*, 33926–33933. [CrossRef]
98. Heneberg, P. Paracrine tumor signaling induces transdifferentiation of surrounding fibroblasts. *Crit. Rev. Oncol. Hematol.* **2016**, *97*, 303–311. [CrossRef]
99. Vilgelm, A.E.; Richmond, A. Chemokines Modulate Immune Surveillance in Tumorigenesis, Metastasis, and Response to Immunotherapy. *Front. Immunol.* **2019**, *10*, 333. [CrossRef] [PubMed]
100. Liu, Q.; Li, A.; Tian, Y.; Wu, J.D.; Liu, Y.; Li, T.; Chen, Y.; Han, X.; Wu, K. The CXCL8-CXCR1/2 pathways in cancer. *Cytokine Growth Factor Rev.* **2016**, *31*, 61–71. [CrossRef]
101. Ha, H.; Debnath, B.; Neamati, N. Role of the CXCL8-CXCR1/2 Axis in Cancer and Inflammatory Diseases. *Theranostics* **2017**, *7*, 1543–1588. [CrossRef] [PubMed]
102. Wu, S.; Saxena, S.; Varney, M.L.; Singh, R.K. CXCR1/2 Chemokine Network Regulates Melanoma Resistance to Chemotherapies Mediated by NF-κB. *Curr. Mol. Med.* **2017**, *17*, 436–449. [CrossRef] [PubMed]
103. Sharma, B.; Singh, S.; Varney, M.L.; Singh, R.K. Targeting CXCR1/CXCR2 receptor antagonism in malignant melanoma. *Expert Opin. Ther. Targets* **2010**, *14*, 435–442. [CrossRef] [PubMed]
104. Kadariya, Y.; Menges, C.W.; Talarchek, J.; Cai, K.Q.; Klein-Szanto, A.J.; Pietrofesa, R.A.; Christofidou-Solomidou, M.; Cheung, M.; Mossman, B.T.; Shukla, A.; et al. Inflammation-Related IL1β/IL1R Signaling Promotes the Development of Asbestos-Induced Malignant Mesothelioma. *Cancer Prev. Res.* **2016**, *9*, 406–414. [CrossRef]
105. Rahim, S.N.A.; Ho, G.Y.; Coward, J.I. The role of interleukin-6 in malignant mesothelioma. *Transl. Lung Cancer Res.* **2015**, *4*, 55–66. [CrossRef]
106. Adachi, Y.; Aoki, C.; Yoshio-Hoshino, N.; Takayama, K.; Curiel, D.T.; Nishimoto, N. Interleukin-6 induces both cell growth and VEGF production in malignant mesotheliomas. *Int. J. Cancer* **2006**, *119*, 1303–1311. [CrossRef]
107. Horio, D.; Minami, T.; Kitai, H.; Ishigaki, H.; Higashiguchi, Y.; Kondo, N.; Hirota, S.; Kitajima, K.; Nakajima, Y.; Koda, Y.; et al. Tumor-associated macrophage-derived inflammatory cytokine enhances malignant potential of malignant pleural mesothelioma. *Cancer Sci.* **2020**, *111*, 2895–2906. [CrossRef]
108. Blondy, T.; d'Almeida, S.M.; Briolay, T.; Tabiasco, J.; Meiller, C.; Chéné, A.L.; Cellerin, L.; Deshayes, S.; Delneste, Y.; Fonteneau, J.F.; et al. Involvement of the M-CSF/IL-34/CSF-1R pathway in malignant pleural mesothelioma. *J. Immunother. Cancer* **2020**, *8*. [CrossRef] [PubMed]
109. Balkwill, F. TNF-alpha in promotion and progression of cancer. *Cancer Metastasis Rev.* **2006**, *25*, 409–416. [CrossRef] [PubMed]
110. Fujii, M.; Toyoda, T.; Nakanishi, H.; Yatabe, Y.; Sato, A.; Matsudaira, Y.; Ito, H.; Murakami, H.; Kondo, Y.; Kondo, E.; et al. TGF-β synergizes with defects in the Hippo pathway to stimulate human malignant mesothelioma growth. *J. Exp. Med.* **2012**, *209*, 479–494. [CrossRef] [PubMed]
111. Turini, S.; Bergandi, L.; Gazzano, E.; Prato, M.; Aldieri, E. Epithelial to Mesenchymal Transition in Human Mesothelial Cells Exposed to Asbestos Fibers: Role of TGF-β as Mediator of Malignant Mesothelioma Development or Metastasis via EMT Event. *Int. J. Mol. Sci.* **2019**, *20*, 150. [CrossRef]
112. Horn, L.A.; Riskin, J.; Hempel, H.A.; Fousek, K.; Lind, H.; Hamilton, D.H.; McCampbell, K.K.; Maeda, D.Y.; Zebala, J.A.; Su, Z.; et al. Simultaneous inhibition of CXCR1/2, TGF-β, and PD-L1 remodels the tumor and its microenvironment to drive antitumor immunity. *J. Immunother. Cancer* **2020**, *8*. [CrossRef] [PubMed]
113. de Gooijer, C.J.; Borm, F.J.; Scherpereel, A.; Baas, P. Immunotherapy in Malignant Pleural Mesothelioma. *Front. Oncol.* **2020**, *10*, 187. [CrossRef] [PubMed]
114. Mutsaers, S.E. The mesothelial cell. *Int. J. Biochem. Cell Biol.* **2004**, *36*, 9–16. [CrossRef]
115. Jantz, M.A.; Antony, V.B. Pathophysiology of the pleura. *Respiration* **2008**, *75*, 121–133. [CrossRef]

Article

Response to Immune Checkpoint Inhibitor Therapy in Patients with Unresectable Recurrent Malignant Pleural Mesothelioma Shown by FDG-PET and CT

Kazuhiro Kitajima [1,*], Mitsunari Maruyama [1], Hiroyuki Yokoyama [1], Toshiyuki Minami [2], Takashi Yokoi [2], Akifumi Nakamura [3], Masaki Hashimoto [3], Nobuyuki Kondo [3], Kozo Kuribayashi [2], Takashi Kijima [2], Seiki Hasegawa [3] and Koichiro Yamakado [1]

1. Department of Radiology, Hyogo College of Medicine, 1-1 Mukogawa-cho, Nishinomiya, Hyogo 663-8501, Japan; mit-maruyama@hyo-med.ac.jp (M.M.); yokoyama.h@meiwa-hospital.com (H.Y.); yamakado@hyo-med.ac.jp (K.Y.)
2. Department of Internal Medicine, Division of Respiratory Medicine, Hyogo College of Medicine, 1-1 Mukogawa-cho, Nishinomiya, Hyogo 663-8501, Japan; to-minami@hyo-med.ac.jp (T.M.); ta-yokoi@hyo-med.ac.jp (T.Y.); kuririn@hyo-med.ac.jp (K.K.); tkijima@hyo-med.ac.jp (T.K.)
3. Department of Thoratic Surgery, Hyogo College of Medicine, 1-1 Mukogawa-cho, Nishinomiya, Hyogo 663-8501, Japan; ak-nakamura@hyo-med.ac.jp (A.N.); masaki-h@hyo-med.ac.jp (M.H.); kondon@hyo-med.ac.jp (N.K.); hasegawa@hyo-med.ac.jp (S.H.)
* Correspondence: ka-kitajima@hyo-med.ac.jp; Tel.: +81-798-45-6883 (ext. 6104); Fax: +81-798-45-6262

Simple Summary: This is the first known study to compare three FDG-PET/CT criteria (EORTC, PERCIST, imPERCIST) with CT criteria (combined modified RECIST and RECIST 1.1) used to evaluate tumor response to ICI therapy in patients with recurrent MPM as well as prediction of prognosis. All of the FDG-PET/CT and CT criteria analyzed were found to be accurate for both evaluation of tumor response and prediction of progression free survival in the present cohort. In comparison with CT, all three FDG-PET/CT criteria judged a greater percentage of patients (16.7%) as CR, while two (EORTC, PERCIST) judged a greater percentage (10–13.3%) as PD.

Abstract: Background: To compare three FDG-PET criteria (EORTC, PERCIST, imPERCIST) with CT criteria (combined modified RECIST and RECIST 1.1) for response evaluation and prognosis prediction in patients with recurrent MPM treated with ICI monotherapy. Methods: Thirty MPM patients underwent FDG-PET/CT and contrast-enhanced CT at the baseline and during nivolumab therapy (median 10 cycles). Therapeutic response was evaluated according to EORTC, PERCIST, imPERCIST, and CT criteria. PFS and OS were examined using log-rank and Cox methods. Results: CMR/PMR/SMD/PMD numbered 5/3/4/18 for EORTC, 5/1/7/17 for PERCIST, and 5/3/9/13 for imPERCIST. With CT, CR/PR/SD/PD numbered 0/6/10/14. There was high concordance between EORTC and PERCIST (κ = 0.911), and PERCIST and imPERCIST (κ = 0.826), while that between EORTC and imPERCIST (κ = 0.746) was substantial, and between CT and the three PET criteria moderate (κ = 0.516–0.544). After median 14.9 months, 26 patients showed progression and nine died. According to both PET and CT findings, patients with no progression (CMR/PMR/SMD or CR/PR/SD) showed significantly longer PFS and somewhat longer OS than PMD and PD patients (EORTC $p = 0.0004$ and $p = 0.055$, respectively; PERCIST $p = 0.0003$ and $p = 0.052$; imPERCIST $p < 0.0001$ and $p = 0.089$; CT criteria $p = 0.0015$ and $p = 0.056$). Conclusions: Both FDG-PET and CT criteria are accurate for response evaluation of ICI therapy and prediction of MPM prognosis. In comparison with CT, all three FDG-PET/CT criteria judged a greater percentage of patients (16.7%) as CMR, while two (EORTC, PERCIST) judged a greater percentage (10–13.3%) as PMD. For predicting PFS, the three FDG-PET criteria were superior to the CT criteria, and imPERCIST demonstrated the highest rate of accurate prediction.

Keywords: mesothelioma; immunotherapy; therapy response; survival; FDG; PET-CT

1. Introduction

Individuals affected by malignant pleural mesothelioma (MPM), a rare type of aggressive malignancy, have a poor prognosis. Platinum-based chemotherapy has been commonly used as the standard first-line treatment in unresectable MPM cases, though few other treatment options are available for those not showing response. However, a paradigm shift has occurred in recent years because of development of immune checkpoint inhibitors (ICIs), and several groups have reported survival benefits for patients with recurrent MPM [1–5]. Those include a single-arm phase II study conducted in Japan (MERIT study) that examined nivolumab (anti-PD-1 monoclonal antibody) monotherapy for efficacy and safety in 34 MPM patients with a history of chemotherapy, with their findings leading to approval of nivolumab for unresectable recurrent MPM treatment in Japan [3].

A crucial factor for effective cancer treatment management is adequate assessment of systemic treatment response, with efficient monitoring of responsiveness to systemic therapy by the tumor vital for moderating the high risk of mortality and also cytotoxic effects associated with systemic therapeutic regimens. Classic methods have been developed for examining patients undergoing cytotoxic chemotherapy and given molecular targeted agents are used for evaluation of treatment response, such as the Response Evaluation Criteria in Solid Tumors version 1.1 (RECIST 1.1) [6] for computed tomography (CT), and the European Organization for Research and Treatment of Cancer (EORTC) criteria [7] and Positron Emission Tomography Response Criteria in Solid Tumors (PERCIST) [8] for [^{18}F]fluorodeoxyglucose positron emission tomography/computed tomography (FDG-PET/CT), as those treatments can directly result in reduced tumor cell viability. However, immunotherapy differs from classical cytotoxic drugs in regard to the action mechanism, as that mechanism of the former is based on stimulation of host immune response against cancer cells, possibly resulting in inflammation development at the tumor site, leading to a subsequent antitumor response [9].

ICI therapeutic efficacy is difficult to assess and the role of FDG-PET has not yet been established. An increase in FDG uptake or appearance of new lesions following therapy may represent infiltration of cancer foci by host immune cells (pseudo-progression) rather than true tumor progression, thus making evaluation of treatment response using FDG-PET/CT results challenging. As a result, another group recently proposed immunotherapy-modified PERCIST (imPERCIST) findings for this evaluation, in which new lesions are not considered to define progressive metabolic disease (PMD) during the early period of assessment (2–4 cycles) of ICI response in metastatic melanoma patients [10].

No other known studies have examined or compared use of FDG-PET/CT and CT for determining MPM patient response to ICI therapy. The present retrospective investigation compared three functional FDG-PET criteria (EORTC, PERCIST, imPERCIST) with morphological CT criteria (combined modified RECIST [11] and RECIST 1.1 [6]) to evaluate response to treatment and predict prognosis in patients with recurrent MPM undergoing nivolumab monotherapy treatment.

2. Materials and Methods

2.1. Patients

Approval from a local review board was received for this retrospective study, and the requirement for patient-informed consent was waived. A search of our database was used to obtain the records of patients with unresectable recurrent MPM and treated with nivolumab monotherapy between June 2018 and December 2019. For the present analysis, a total of 30 (mean 68.1 ± 7.2 years old, range 46–77 years) who underwent FDG-PET/CT and contrast-enhanced CT examinations at our institution at the baseline and during nivolumab monotherapy (after 4–6 cycles in 3, 7–9 in 9, 10–12 in 9, 13–15 in 4, 16–18 in 3, 19–21 in 2; median 10 cycles) for treatment response evaluation were included. Baseline FDG-PET/CT and baseline contrast-enhanced CT examinations were conducted at a median 1.0 months (1.0–2.2 months) and 1.4 months (0.7–2.3 months), respectively, before initiation of nivolumab therapy. The interval of FDG-PET/CT and contrast-enhanced CT was less than two weeks at the baseline and during nivolumab therapy in every patient. Table 1 shows patient and tumor characteristics. CT, FDG-PET/CT, and brain magnetic resonance imaging (MRI) results were used for diagnosis of disease recurrence, metastasis, and progression during the follow-up period. When disease progression or recurrence was suspected on the physical findings, CT or FDG-PET/CT was undertaken for the evaluating the whole-body state, and the brain MRI was carried out for the screening of the brain. In some patients without suspected progression or recurrence, those imaging examinations were undertaken every 6–12 months for surveillance.

Table 1. Study population characteristics.

Variable	Total Patients (n = 30)	%
Sex		
Male	24	80.0%
Female	6	20.0%
Age		
Mean	68.1 ± 7.2	
Range	46–77	
Histological subtypes		
Epithelial	24	80.0%
Sarcomatoid	4	13.3%
Biphasic	2	6.7%
Initial cStage		
I	9	30.0%
II	3	10.0%
III	14	46.7%
IV	4	13.3%
Previous treatment		
First line (Pemetrexed + cisplatin/carboplatin)	13	43.3%
First line + Second line (Pemetrexed)	3	10.0%
First line + Second line (Irinotecan + Gemcitabine)	2	6.7%
First line + Surgery	5	16.7%
First line + Surgery + second line (Pemetrexed + cisplatin/carboplatin)	5	16.7%
First line + Surgery + second line (Pemetrexed + cisplatin) + third line (Irinotecan + Gemcitabine)	1	3.3%
First line + Surgery + Second line (Pemetrexed)	1	3.3%

Data are presented as numbers.

Intravenous nivolumab was given at 3 mg/kg every two weeks until apparent disease progression or unacceptable toxicity was observed, or the patient or attending physician decided to discontinue treatment. Of the 30 enrolled patients, treatment-related adverse events were noted in nine (30.0%) (rash in two, hypothyroidism in two, interstitial lung disease in one, increased lipase level in one, diarrhea in one, hypoadrenocorticism in one, fatigue in one). After discontinuing nivolumab treatment, alternative treatment (cisplatin/carboplatin and pemetrexed, pemetrexed, or irinotecan and gemcitabine) was tried.

2.2. FDG-PET/CT

Four different PET/CT scanners installed at our institution (Gemini GXL16, Gemini TF64, Ingenuity TF: Philips Medical Systems, Eindhoven, The Netherlands; Discovery IQ: GE Healthcare, Waukesha, WI, USA) were used for performing the FDG-PET/CT examinations. Each patient was instructed to fast for five hours before the examination, and blood glucose was measured immediately prior to FDG injection (4.0 MBq/kg body weight for GXL16, 3.0 MBq/kg for TF64, 3.7 MBq/kg body weight for Ingenuity TF and Discovery IQ), with all in the present cohort showing a level lower than 160 mg/dL. Approximately 60 min after the injection, static emission images were obtained. For attenuation correction and anatomic localization, helical CT scan images from the top of the head to mid-thigh were obtained with the following parameters: tube voltage 120 kV (all four scanners), effective tube current auto-mA up to 120 mA (GXL16), 100 mA (TF64), 155 mA (Ingenuity TF), or 15–390 mA (Smart mA: noise index 25) (Discovery IQ), gantry rotation speed 0.5 s, detector configuration 16 × 1.5 mm (GXL16), 64 × 0.625 mm (TF64 and Ingenuity TF), or 16 × 1.25 mm (Discovery IQ), slice thickness 2 mm, and a transverse field of view 600 mm (GXL16, TF64, Ingenuity TF) or 700 mm (Discovery IQ). Immediately after completion of the CT examination, PET imaging was performed from the head to mid-thigh for 90 s (GXL16, TF64, Ingenuity TF) or 180 s (Discovery IQ) per bed position in three-dimensional mode. The patient was allowed to breathe normally during PET scanning. For the GXL16, attenuation-corrected PET images were reconstructed with a line-of-response row-action maximum likelihood algorithm, while for the TF64 and Ingenuity an ordered-subset expectation maximization (OSEM) iterative reconstruction algorithm (33 subsets, three iterations) was used, and Q.Clear (block sequential regularized expectation maximization (BSREM)) (β = 400) was utilized for the Discovery IQ.

2.3. Contrast-Enhanced CT

To obtain pre-contrast and contrast-enhanced CT images of the neck, chest, abdomen, and pelvis, a 128-detector row CT (SOMATOM Definition AS: Siemens Healthcare, Erlangen, Germany) was used at 120 kV, with an effective mA of 220 (CAREDose4D), beam pitch of 0.6, collimation of 1.2 × 32 mm, and B31 + medium smooth + image reconstruction. Details regarding the contrast-enhanced CT procedures have been previously presented. Briefly, blood creatinine level determined prior to the examination was ≤1.5 mg/dL in all of the patients. Iodinated contrast material (Iopamiron Inj, Syringe, Bayer Schering Pharma, Berlin, Germany) containing 300 mg of iodine per ml at a dose of 600 mg of iodine per kg of body weight was intravenously administered using a power injector, with scanning started at 120 s after the injection.

2.4. Image Analysis

A board-certified nuclear medicine expert with 12 years of oncologic FDG-PET/CT experience and without knowledge of the other imaging results, or clinical or histopathologic data for the present patients, retrospectively reviewed the FDG-PET/CT images. To assist the attending clinician with treatment response monitoring, the GI-PET software package (AZE Co., Ltd., Tokyo, Japan), which can harmonize standardized uptake values (SUVs) obtained with different PET/CT systems using phantom data [12], was employed. Maximum SUV (SUVmax) was defined as the maximum concentration in the target lesion (injected dose/body weight). For calculating SUVpeak, a 1.2-cm diameter volume region of interest (ROI) placed on the hottest site of the tumor was used, then normalized to SUV corrected for lean body mass (SULpeak) (SUVpeak × [lean body mass]/[total body mass]).

A board-certified radiologist with 12 years of experience with CT retrospectively evaluated the contrast-enhanced CT images and made determinations, in the absence of knowledge of the other imaging results or clinical data for the present patients. Coronal, axial, and sagittal section images were viewed and analyzed, with appropriate winding applied.

2.5. EORTC

Using the EORTC guidelines [7], complete resolution of FDG uptake within the tumor volume indistinguishable from surrounding normal tissue was determined as complete metabolic response (CMR), while PMD was the classification for appearance of new FDG uptake in another region in the second FDG-PET/CT scan. The EORTC recommends defining regions of high FDG uptake that represent a viable tumor by use of pre-treatment scan findings and also utilization of the same ROI volumes in subsequent scanning examinations positioned as close to the original tumor as possible, as well as determination of maximal tumor ROI count per pixel per second calibrated as MBq/L [7]. The number of lesions to be measured is not recommended by the EORTC, thus up to five with the highest level of FDG uptake and up to two per organ, with same lesions measured in subsequent follow-up scan imaging results, were the parameters used in the present study [13]. The values for all five targets used for SUVmax measurement were summed for each scan, resulting in ΣSUVmax. Percentage changes from baseline to second summed SUVmax were calculated, with a reduction of ≥25% in summed SUVmax value defined as partial metabolic response (PMR). PMD was classified as an increase in tumor summed SUVmax value ≥25% within the ROI defined based on the baseline scan, while stable metabolic disease (SMD) was defined as an increase in the summed SUVmax value of <25% or a decrease <25%.

2.6. PERCIST

For therapeutic response determination according to PERCIST [8], SUL values were calculated using a 1.2-cm diameter volume ROI placed on the target lesion, and SUL values were calculated. Additionally, the SULpeak value of the tumor was determined and noted if it was 1.5 times or more greater than that of the liver SUL (mean ± 2 standard deviations) in a 3-cm diameter spherical ROI on the normal right lobe. When complete resolution of FDG uptake within the target lesion was lower than mean liver activity and indistinguishable from the background blood-pool level, CMR was the classification. For cases with metabolically active lesions noted in follow-up scan findings, the SULpeak of up to five lesions at the baseline and follow-up examinations was summed (maximum two per organ) [8]. The hottest lesions in each scan were selected; thus, the target lesions detected in follow-up imaging were not necessarily the same as those in the baseline images. When the SULpeak sum was decreased by ≥30%, tumor response for that case was classified as PMR. Conversely, an increase in SULpeak sum ≥30% or appearance of new hypermetabolic lesions or ≥75% increase in total lesion glycolysis (TLG) in follow-up FDG PET/CT scan imaging was defined as PMD. Any cases not defined as CMR, PMR, or PMD were classified as SMD.

2.7. imPERCIST

imPERCIST was performed in the same manner as used for PERCIST, though appearance of new lesions alone did not result in a classification of PMD [10], as that was defined only by increase in sum of SULpeaks of ≥30%. New lesions were included in the SULpeak sum when a higher uptake level than the existing target lesions was shown or when fewer than five target lesions were detected in baseline scan results.

2.8. Combined Modified RECIST and RECIST 1.1

Pleural tumor thickness perpendicular to the chest wall or mediastinum was measured at two different points at three different levels for evaluations with modified RECIST [11]. For assessing the morphological response of nonpleural lesions, RECIST 1.1 was used [6]. The target lesion was defined as a well-defined soft tissue lesion with the longest axis for the lymph node ≥ 1 cm and the shortest axis ≥1.5 cm, and the greatest sum of the diameter of five target lesions, maximum two lesions per organ, and used for evaluation. Sclerotic or lytic/sclerotic (mixed type) bone metastasis was considered to be a non-measurable lesion. With both modified RECIST and RECIST 1.1, a decrease ≥30% in largest diameter sum was considered to be partial response (PR), while progressive disease (PD) was determined in cases with an increase ≥20%. Stable disease (SD) was considered to be any change between PR and PD of <−30% to <+20%; complete response (CR) was determined in cases with disappearance of nonpleural target lesions and lymph nodes in the shortest axis <1 cm, and PD when there was appearance of a new lesion. In a comparison of mRECIST and RECIST 1.1 results, the worst objective response was chosen as the final classification shown by CT.

2.9. Statistical Analysis

Cohen's κ coefficient was used to examine concordance between criteria methods was assessed using [14], with a slight (κ < 0.21), fair (κ = 0.21–0.40), moderate (κ = 0.41–0.60), substantial (κ = 0.61–0.80), or nearly perfect (κ > 0.80) level of agreement noted. Progression-free survival (PFS) was defined based on time elapsed from start of nivolumab therapy to date of disease progression shown in radiological and/or clinical examination results, or death from any cause. Any patient with no evidence of progressive disease was censored at the date of the last follow-up examination. Time from start of nivolumab therapy until death from any cause was used to determine overall survival (OS). Patients living at the final follow-up examination were censored, and classified as alive with disease or no evidence of progression. The Kaplan–Meier method was used to generate actuarial survival curves, with a log-rank test employed to examine differences between groups. Statistical analyses were performed with the SAS software package, version 9.3 (SAS Institute Inc., Cary, NC, USA), with p values < 0.05 considered to be significant.

3. Results

3.1. Treatment Response Assessment

Using EORTC criteria with FDG-PET/CT findings resulted in CMR being noted in five patients (16.7%), PMR in three (10.0%), SMD in four (13.3%), and PMD in 18 (60.0%), while use of PERCIST with FDG-PET/CT findings showed CMR in five (16.7%), PMR in one (3.3%), SMD in seven (23.3%), and PMD in 17 (56.7%) patients, respectively, and use of imPERCIST with FDG-PET/CT findings showed CMR in five (16.7%), PMR in three (10.0%), SMD in nine (30.0%), and PMD in 13 (43.3%) patients, respectively. When the combination of modified RECIST and RECIST 1.1 with CT was used, no patients (0%) had CR, six (20.0%) had PR, 10 (33.3%) had SD, and 14 (46.7%) had PD. Figures 1 and 2 present data of two representative cases.

Prior to nivolumab treatment, FDG-PET/CT examinations showed only pleural lesions in 25 patients, while two had pleural and nodal lesions, one had only nodal lesions, one had pleural and lung lesions, and one had pleural, nodal, and peritoneal lesions. Tiny nodal or peritoneal lesions were not detected with contrast-enhanced CT in two patients before starting nivolumab treatment, though those are not included as target lesions in the RECIST criteria due to their small size. The second FDG-PET/CT examination detected new lesions in eight patients (lung metastasis in two; pleural lesions in one; lymph node metastasis in one; bone metastasis in one; small intestine metastasis in one; lymph node and peritoneal dissemination in one; lymph node, peritoneal, bone, and muscle metastasis in one). Of those eight cases with new lesions revealed in the second FDG-PET/CT examination, the CT reader was unable to detect new lesions in three (bone metastasis in one; small intestine metastasis in one; lymph node, peritoneal, bone, and muscle metastasis in one).

3.2. Treatment Response Assessment Comparisons among Criteria Methods

Twenty-seven (90%) of the cases demonstrated concordance between the EORTC criteria and PERCIST response classifications, while discordance was noted in three (10.0%), with nearly perfect agreement (κ = 0.911) for response classification between them (Table 2). As for EORTC and imPERCIST, concordance between them was seen in 23 (76.7%) cases and discordance was noted in seven (23.3%), with substantial agreement (κ = 0.746) for response classification found between them (Table 3). Furthermore, in 26 (86.7%) cases, concordance between PERCIST and imPERCIST was seen, and discordance was noted in four (13.3%), with nearly perfect agreement (κ = 0.826) for response classification found between them (Table 3). Four PMD patients defined by PERCIST were classified as SMD (two patients) and PMR (two patients) based on imPERCIST due to the definition of the latter.

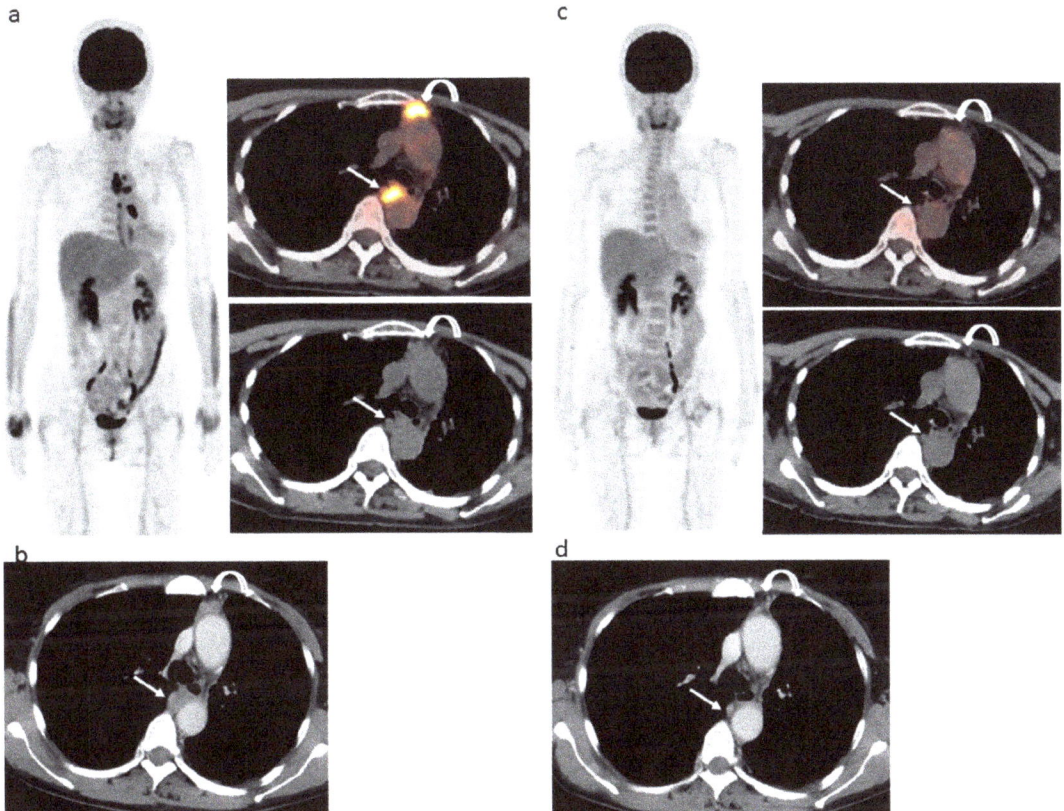

Figure 1. 61 year-old woman with left epithelioid malignant pleural mesothelioma who previously received neoadjuvant chemotherapy (pemetrexed + cisplatin), pleurectomy, and decortication surgery (pT3N1M0), then six cycles of chemotherapy (pemetrexed + cisplatin) after the operation, followed by 10 cycles of second-line therapy (irinotecan + gemcitabine) and then nivolumab as third-line chemotherapy. (**a**) Pre-nivolumab treatment FDG-PET/CT shows several areas of strong FDG uptake related to a pleural lesion (curved arrow) and mediastinal lymph nodal lesion (arrow). (**b**) Pre-nivolumab treatment contrast-enhanced CT shows mass-forming thickness of pleura lesion (curved arrow) and mediastinal lymph nodal lesion (arrow). (**c**) During-treatment FDG-PET/CT after 13 cycles of nivolumab shows FDG uptake disappearance in both pleural (curved arrow) and nodal (arrow) lesions. (**d**) During-treatment contrast-enhanced CT after 13 cycles of nivolumab shows remarkable improvements of both pleural (curved arrow) and nodal (arrow) lesions. EORTC, PERCIST, and imPERCIST indicated CMR. Interpretation of combined modified RECIST and RECIST 1.1 indicated a classification of PR, with the sum pleural lesion size decreasing by 45.5% and the sum mediastinal node size decreasing by 78.3%. The patient continued with 29 more cycles of nivolumab and was alive without progression at 15.1 months after nivolumab initiation.

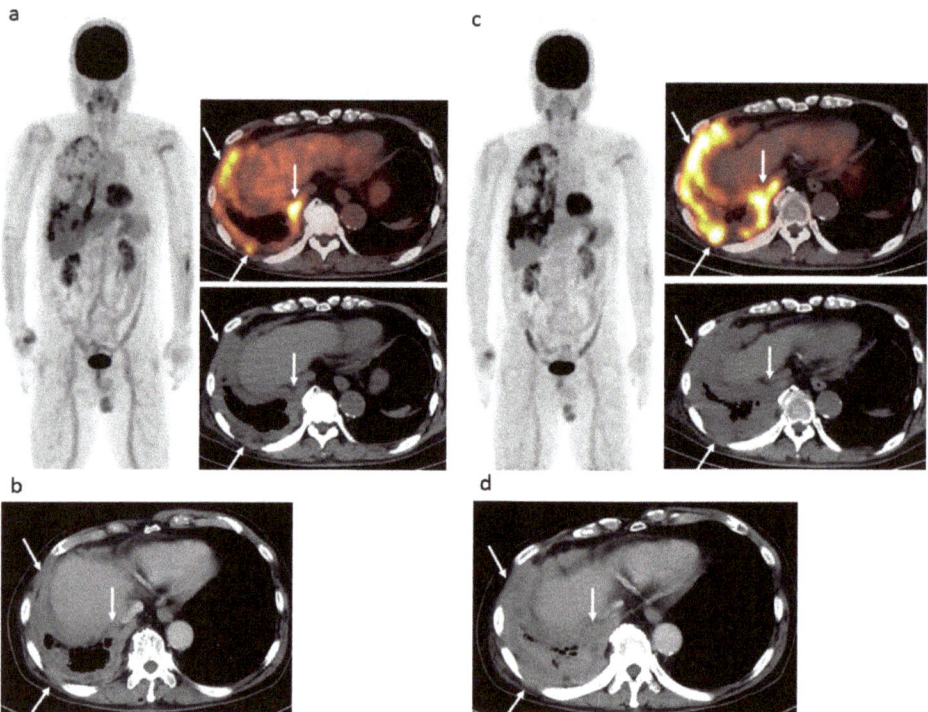

Figure 2. 74 year-old man with right epithelioid malignant pleural mesothelioma (cT2N0M0), who previously received six cycles of first-line chemotherapy (pemetrexed + cisplatin) and then 12 cycles of nivolumab as second-line chemotherapy. (**a**) Pre-nivolumab treatment FDG-PET/CT shows multiple areas of strong FDG uptake in areas of right pleural lesions (arrows). (**b**) Pre-nivolumab treatment contrast-enhanced CT shows mass-forming thickness of right pleura (arrows). (**c**) Post-treatment FDG-PET/CT after 12 cycles of nivolumab shows remarkable progression of multiple pleural lesions (arrows) and appearance of new pleural lesions. (**d**) Post-treatment contrast-enhanced CT after 12 cycles of nivolumab shows remarkable progression of pleural lesions (arrows). EORTC, PERCIST, imPERCIST, and CT criteria (modified RECIST and RECIST 1.1) indicated PMD or PD due to remarkable progression and appearance of new lesions. In FDG-PET/CT results, the SULpeak sum of the five highest level pleural lesions was increased by 98.6%. In CT findings, the sum size of six pleural lesions perpendicular to the chest wall was increased by 40.3%. According to the second (**c**) FDG-PET/CT and (**d**) contrast-enhanced CT result, the patient started another chemotherapy series (irinotecan + gemcitabine), though was alive at 13.9 months after initiation of nivolumab.

Table 2. Comparison of treatment response assessments in EORTC criteria and PERCIST.

	EORTC Criteria				
	PMD	SMD	PMR	CMR	Total
PERCIST					
PMD	17	0	0	0	17
SMD	1	4	2	0	7
PMR	0	0	1	0	1
CMR	0	0	0	5	5
Total	18	4	3	5	30

Data are presented as numbers. Abbreviations: EORTC: European Organization for Research and Treatment of Cancer, PERCIST: Positron Emission Tomography Response Criteria in Solid Tumors, PMD: progressive metabolic disease, SMD: stable metabolic disease, PMR: partial metabolic response, CMR: complete metabolic response.

Table 3. Comparison of treatment response assessments in imPERCIST and two other PET citeria (EORTC criteria and PERCIST).

	EORTC Criteria					PERCIST				
	PMD	SMD	PMR	CMR	Total	PMD	SMD	PMR	CMR	Total
imPERCIST										
PMD	13	0	0	0	13	13	0	0	0	13
SMD	3	4	2	0	9	2	7	0	0	9
PMR	2	0	1	0	3	2	0	1	0	3
CMR	0	0	0	5	5	0	0	0	5	5
Total	18	4	3	5	30	17	7	1	5	30

Data are presented as numbers. Abbreviations: EORTC: European Organization for Research and Treatment of Cancer, PERCIST: Positron Emission Tomography Response Criteria in Solid Tumors, imPERCIST: immunotherapy-modified Positron Emission Tomography Response Criteria in Solid Tumors, PMD: progressive metabolic disease, SMD: stable metabolic disease, PMR: partial metabolic response, CMR: complete metabolic response.

Finally, in 18 (60.0%) cases concordance was noted between the CT criteria (combined modified RECIST and RECIST 1.1) and three PET response classifications (EORTC, PERCIST, imPERCIST), while discordance was noted in 12 (40.0%), with moderate agreement ($\kappa = 0.516$ between CT criteria and EORTC, $\kappa = 0.529$ between CT criteria and PERCIST, $\kappa = 0.544$ between CT criteria and imPERCIST) noted between them for response classification (Table 4). Five (16.7%) of the present 30 patients were classified as CMR based on the EORTC, PERCIST, and imPERCIST criteria, which was not demonstrated by CT criteria (combined modified RECIST and RECIST 1.1).

Table 4. Comparison of treatment response assessments in CT criteria (combined modified RECIST and RECIST1.1) and three PET criteria (EORTC criteria, PERCIST, imPERCIST).

	EORTC Criteria					PERCIST					imPERCIST				
	PMD	SMD	PMR	CMR	Total	PMD	SMD	PMR	CMR	Total	PMD	SMD	PMR	CMR	Total
CT criteria															
PD	13	0	1	0	14	13	1	0	0	14	11	2	1	0	14
SD	4	4	1	1	10	3	5	1	1	10	2	6	1	1	10
PR	1	0	1	4	6	1	1	0	4	6	0	1	1	4	6
CR	0	0	0	0	0	0	0	0	0	0	0	0	0	0	0
Total	18	4	3	5	30	17	7	1	5	30	13	9	3	5	30

Data are presented as numbers. Abbreviations: EORTC: European Organization for Research and Treatment of Cancer, PERCIST: Positron Emission Tomography Response Criteria in Solid Tumors, imPERCIST: immunotherapy-modified Positron Emission Tomography Response Criteria in Solid Tumors, PMD: progressive metabolic disease, SMD: stable metabolic disease, PMR: partial metabolic response, CMR: complete metabolic response, PD: progressive disease, SD: stable disease, PR: partial response, CR: complete response.

3.3. Progression Free Survivals (PFS)

Twenty-six (86.7%) of the 30 patients had progressive disease noted after a median period of 8.0 months (3.3–22.4 months). Both PET (EORTC, PERCIST, imPERCIST) and CT (combined modified RECIST and RECIST 1.1) criteria indicated a significantly longer PFS in patients with no progression (CMR/PMR/SMD, CR/PR/SD) as compared to those with PMD or PD (EORTC: $p = 0.0004$, PERCIST: $p = 0.0003$, imPERCIST: $p < 0.0001$, combined modified RECIST and RECIST 1.1: $p = 0.0015$) (Figure 3). Similarly, responders (CMR/PMR) based on PET criteria (EORTC, PERCIST, imPERCIST) showed significantly longer PFS than non-responders (SMD/PMD) (EORTC: $p = 0.0064$, PERCIST: $p = 0.0007$, imPERCIST: $p = 0.0005$), whereas use of CT criteria (combined modified RECIST and RECIST 1.1) showed that responders (CR/PR) had a tendency for longer PFS as compared to non-responders (SD/PD), though the difference was not significant ($p = 0.074$) (Figure 4).

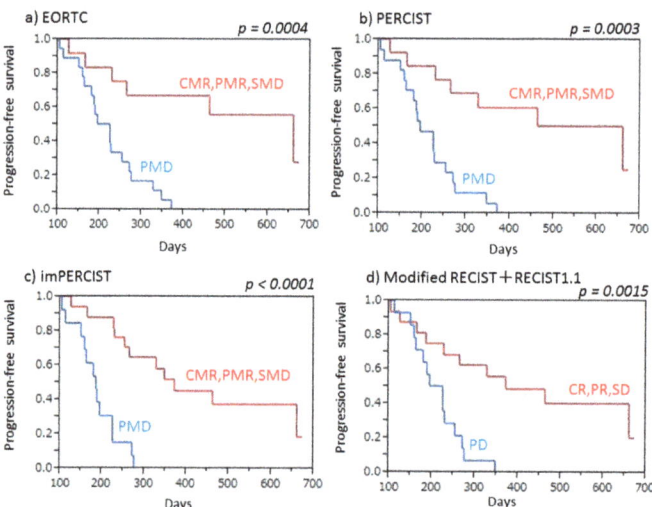

Figure 3. Progression-free survival (PFS) of malignant pleural mesothelioma patients treated by nivolumab therapy, with and without progression. (**a**) EORTC demonstrated that patients with no progression (CMR/PMR/SMD) showed significantly longer PFS than those with PMD ($p = 0.0004$). (**b**) PERCIST demonstrated that patients with no progression (CMR/PMR/SMD) showed significantly longer PFS than those with PMD ($p = 0.0003$). (**c**) imPERCIST demonstrated that patients with no progression (CMR/PMR/SMD) showed significantly longer PFS than those with PMD ($p < 0.0001$). (**d**) Combined modified RECIST and RECIST 1.1 demonstrated that patients with no progression (CR/PR/SD) showed significantly longer PFS than those with PD ($p = 0.0015$).

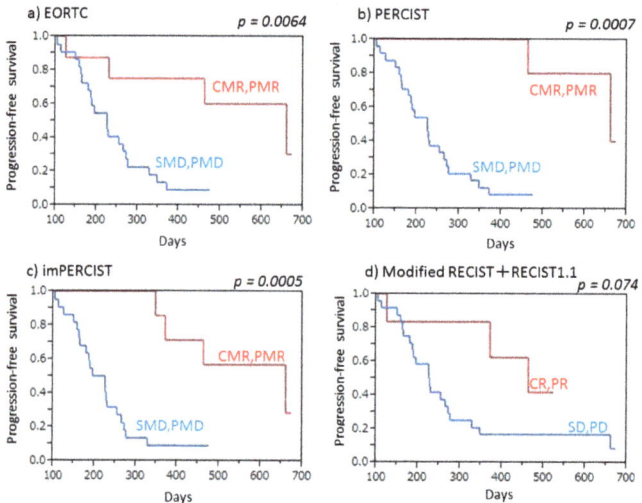

Figure 4. Progression-free survival (PFS) of malignant pleural mesothelioma patients treated by nivolumab therapy, with and without response. (**a**) EORTC demonstrated that responders (CMR/PMR) showed significantly longer PFS than non-responders (SMD/PMD) ($p = 0.0064$). (**b**) PERCIST demonstrated that responders (CMR/PMR) showed significantly longer PFS than non-responders (SMD/PMD) ($p = 0.0007$). (**c**) imPERCIST demonstrated that responders (CMR/PMR) showed significantly longer PFS than non-responders (SMD/PMD) ($p = 0.0005$). (**d**) Combined modified RECIST and RECIST 1.1 demonstrated that responders (CR/PR) tended to show longer PFS than non-responders (SD/PD), without a significant difference ($p = 0.074$).

3.4. Overall Survival (OS)

Nine (30.0%) of the 30 patients died from MPM after a median 14.9 months (5.8–25.6 months). Both PET (EORTC, PERCIST, imPERCIST) and CT (combined modified RECIST and RECIST 1.1) criteria indicated that patients without progression (CMR/PMR/SMD, CR/PR/SD) had a tendency for longer OS as compared to patients with PMD or PD (EORTC: $p = 0.055$, PERCIST: $p = 0.052$, imPERCIST: $p = 0.089$, combined modified RECIST and RECIST 1.1: $p = 0.056$), though the difference was not significant (Figure 5). Similarly, according to both PET (EORTC, PERCIST, imPERCIST) and CT (combined modified RECIST and RECIST 1.1) criteria, responders (CMR/PMR, CR/PR) showed longer OS than non-responders (SMD/PMD, SD/PD) (EORTC: $p = 0.055$, PERCIST: $p = 0.052$, imPERCIST: $p = 0.053$) without a significant difference, whereas CT criteria (combined mRECIST and RECIST 1.1) indicated that OS values for responders (CR/PR) and non-responders (SD/PD) were not different ($p = 0.87$) (Figure 6).

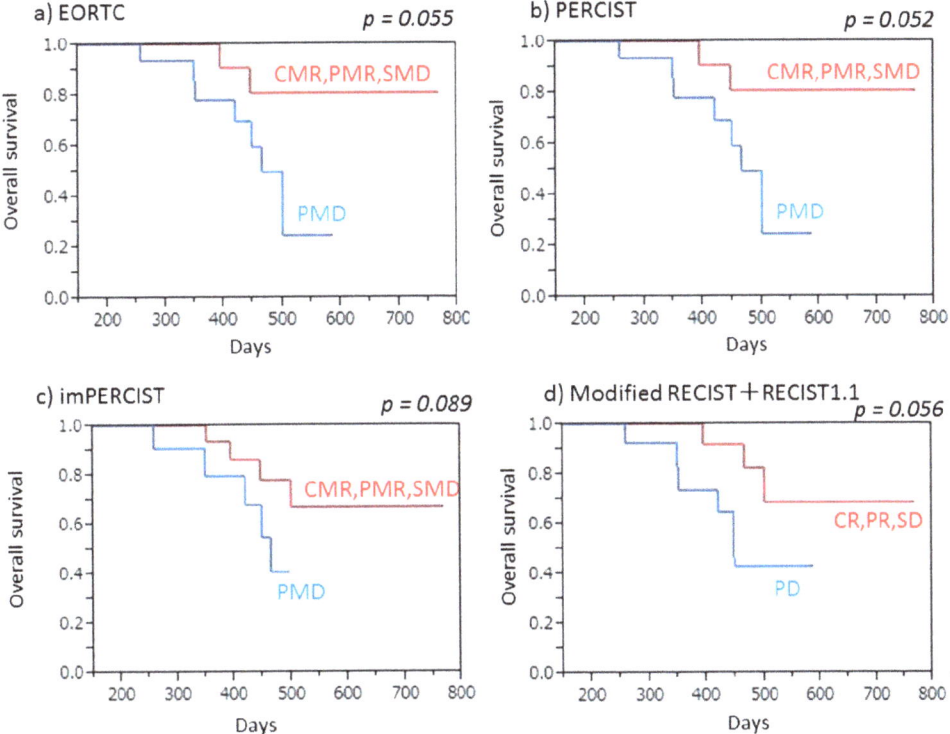

Figure 5. Overall survival (OS) of malignant pleural mesothelioma patients treated by nivolumab therapy, with and without progression. (**a**) EORTC demonstrated that patients with no progression (CMR/PMR/SMD) tended to show longer OS than those with PMD, without a significant difference ($p = 0.055$). (**b**) PERCIST demonstrated that patients with no progression (CMR/PMR/SMD) tended to show longer OS than those with PMD, without a significant difference ($p = 0.052$). (**c**) imPERCIST demonstrated that patients with no progression (CMR/PMR/SMD) tended to show longer OS than those with PMD, without a significant difference ($p = 0.089$). (**d**) Combined modified RECIST and RECIST 1.1 demonstrated that patients with no progression (CR/PR/SD) tended to show longer OS than those without PD, without a significant difference ($p = 0.056$).

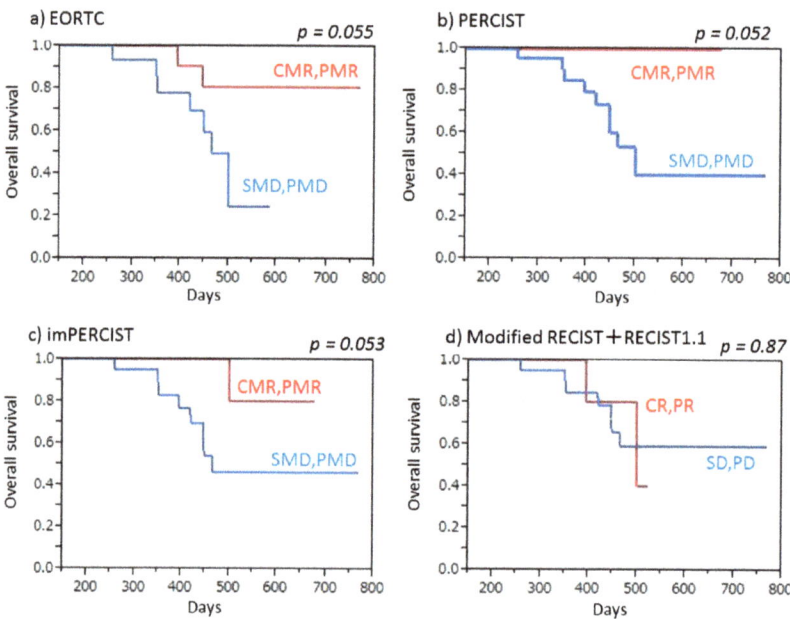

Figure 6. Overall survival (OS) of malignant pleural mesothelioma patients treated by nivolumab therapy, with and without response. (**a**) EORTC demonstrated that responders (CMR/PMR) tended to show longer OS than non-responders (SMD/PMD), without a significant difference ($p = 0.055$). (**b**) PERCIST demonstrated that responders (CMR/PMR) tended to show longer OS than non-responders (SMD/PMD), without a significant difference ($p = 0.052$). (**c**) imPERCIST demonstrated that responders (CMR/PMR) tended to show longer OS than non-responders (SMD/PMD), without a significant difference ($p = 0.053$). (**d**) Combined modified RECIST and RECIST 1.1 demonstrated no significant difference for OS between responders (CR/PR) and non-responders (SD/PD) ($p = 0.87$).

4. Discussion

This is the first known study to compare three FDG-PET/CT criteria (EORTC, PERCIST, imPERCIST) with CT criteria (combined modified RECIST and RECIST 1.1) used to evaluate tumor response to ICI therapy in patients with recurrent MPM as well as prediction of prognosis. All of the FDG-PET/CT and CT criteria analyzed were found to be accurate for both evaluation of tumor response and prediction of PFS in the present cohort, though the FDG-PET/CT criteria showed a slight superiority. FDG-PET/CT is known as an accurate tool for evaluating tumor viability, and the results are useful for clear diagnosis of CMR when a residual tumor does not have abnormal FDG uptake during or after treatment. We noted that the EORTC, PERCIST, and imPERCIST criteria classified five (16.7%) of the present 30 patients as CMR, which was not obtained with use of the contrast-enhanced CT criteria (combined modified RECIST and RECIST 1.1). Additionally, FDG-PET/CT findings are known to be accurate for detecting bone/muscle and tiny lymph node metastasis, as well as very small dissemination in a second FDG-PET/CT examination. This study found that the EORTC and PERCIST criteria were able to classify four and three more patients (10–13.3%) as PMD in comparison to contrast-enhanced CT results with use of the combined modified RECIST and RECIST 1.1 criteria. The number of PMD cases determined by imPERCIST was lower than that by the EORTC and PERCIST criteria, due to the imPERCIST definition (new lesions do not result in PMD and are included in the sum of SULpeak if they showed a higher uptake level than existing target lesions).

In summary, all three FDG-PET/CT criteria clearly judged more patients (16.7%) as CMR and two of those, EORTC and PERCIST, were able to judge more patients (10–13.3%) as PMD in comparison with CT criteria. For predicting PFS, the three FDG-PET criteria were superior to the CT criteria and imPERCIST demonstrated the highest rate of accurate prediction. It is considered that FDG-PET/CT might be a powerful tool for late (≥4 cycles) response assessment when evaluating ICI therapy and able to identify MPM patients who can most benefit from that. If MPM patients undergoing nivolumab were judged as non-PMD, nivolumab is continued. Unfortunately, MPM patients undergoing nivolumab were judged as PMD, alternative treatment (cisplatin/carboplatin and pemetrexed, pemetrexed, or irinotecan and gemcitabine) is tried in order to improve patient outcome.

Tumor infiltration by immune cells can delay tumor shrinkage or even cause a temporary increase in size (pseudoprogression), making assessment of tumor response to ICI treatment challenging. Although several criteria have been proposed for use with CT findings to determine response to that treatment, such as immune-related response criteria (irRC) [15], immune-related RECIST (irRECIST) [9], and immune RECIST (iRECIST) [16], as well as for use with FDG-PET results, including PET/CT criteria for early prediction of Response to Immune checkpoint inhibitor Therapy (PECRIT) [17], PET Response Evaluation Criteria for Immunotherapy (PERCIMT) [18], imPERCIST [10], and immune PERCIST (iPERCIST) [19], an optimal evaluation method has yet to be determined. Although pseudoprogression must be considered in the early phase following initiation of ICI treatment, that was not observed in any of the present 30 patients, probably due to late (≥4 cycles) response assessment.

There have been several articles demonstrating the usefulness of FDG-PET/CT for assessing the ICI therapeutic response, especially early response (2~4 cycles of ICI) in metastatic melanoma patients [10,17,18,20]. Cho et al. [17] analyzed PECRIT, which includes change in lesion size combined with change in FDG avidity shown by FDG-PET/CT after one cycle of ICI monotherapy (ipilimumab, nivolumab, or BMS-936559), in a study of 20 advanced melanoma patients. They found that criteria including SD shown by RECIST 1.1 and an SULpeak increase >15.5% in the hottest lesion shown by FDG-PET/CT were accurate for predicting treatment response after four months, with values for sensitivity, specificity, and accuracy of 100%, 93%, and 95%, respectively. In another study, PERCIMT, which uses absolute number of new lesions rather than changes in metabolic parameters (i.e., SUV) shown by FDG-PET/CT, was introduced by Anwar et al. [18] to evaluate 41 patients with metastatic melanoma after four cycles of ipilimumab. Those criteria, which include four or more new lesions <1 cm in functional diameter, were found to be accurate for clinical benefit prediction, with a sensitivity of 84% and specificity of 100%. Ito et al. [10] originally presented imPERCIST, in which the appearance of new lesions is not used to define PMD. Those authors noted that an increase in SULpeak sum of ≥30% in up to five measured lesions in FDG-PET/CT results accurately reflected PMD after 2–4 cycles of ipilimumab treatment in 60 metastatic melanoma patients. Although the significant and apparent superiority of FDG-PET/CT was not observed in our series, the potential reason may be biological difference between malignant melanoma and MPM, late (≥4 cycles) response assessment, or small sample size. With iPERCIST, Goldfarb et al. [19] introduced two new categories used for response to PMD, unconfirmed (UPMD) and confirmed (CPMD). Results of 28 non-small cell lung cancer patients who were receiving nivolumab were analyzed and indicated that any metabolic progression observed at eight weeks (after four cycles) should be confirmed by another FDG-PET/CT examination performed four weeks later, while they also noted that iPERCIST was useful for differentiation of responders from non-responders and OS prediction ($p = 0.0003$).

The present study has some limitations, including its retrospective nature, performance at a single center, and small sample size. Thus, generalization of the findings is limited and statistical errors are possible. To clarify the roles of FDG-PET/CT and CT for decision making, as well as predicting long-term outcomes in clinical settings a prospective multicenter trial with a larger cohort will be necessary. Additionally, the enrolled cohort was heterogeneous, as patients who underwent nivolumab monotherapy and received the second FDG-PET/CT examination after from four to 21 cycles were included; thus, confounding factors were likely introduced. The impact of PET/CT is primarily early within the course of treatment, because metabolic changes proceed volumetric changes [20]. This cannot be demonstrated in this study due to the very large and relatively late variation of the time points for the follow-up study. We are planning a prospective study to clarify both early and late response evaluation with less variation of the time to second and third FDG-PET/CT examinations from ICI treatment start, using three times of FDG-PET/CT examinations in MPM patients receiving ICI treatment Although we used four different PET/CT scanners, we harmonized PET quantitative values by a software, which can harmonize SUVs obtained with different PET/CT systems using phantom data [12]. Finally, irRC, irRECIST, iRECIST, and iPERCIST were not evaluated, because regular and follow-up CT and FDG-PET/CT examinations were not performed in every case.

5. Conclusions

In conclusion, results obtained with the use of three FDG-PET/CT (EORTC, PERCIST, and imPERCIST) and one CT (combined modified RECIST and RECIST 1.1) criteria were found useful to evaluate tumor response to ICI therapy as well as prediction of progression in recurrent MPM patients. In comparison with CT, all three FDG-PET/CT criteria judged a greater percentage of patients (16.7%) as CMR, while two (EORTC, PERCIST) judged a greater percentage (10–13.3%) as PMD. For predicting PFS, the three FDG-PET criteria were superior to the CT criteria, and imPERCIST demonstrated the highest rate of accurate prediction. Further validation in a prospective study with a larger cohort is warranted.

Author Contributions: Conceptualization: K.K. (Kazuhiro Kitajima), H.Y., and K.Y.; methodology: K.K. (Kazuhiro Kitajima) and M.M.; recruiting of patients: T.M., T.Y., K.K. (Kazuhiro Kitajima), T.K., A.N., M.H., N.K., and S.H.; statistical analysis: H.Y.; resources: K.K. (Kazuhiro Kitajima); data curation: K.K. (Kazuhiro Kitajima) and K.K. (Kozo Kuribayashi); writing—original draft preparation: K.K. (Kazuhiro Kitajima); writing—review and editing: T.M., K.K. (Kozo Kuribayashi), and K.Y.; supervision: K.Y. and T.M.; project administration: K.K. (Kazuhiro Kitajima); All authors have read and agreed to the published version of the manuscript.

Funding: This work was supported by a JSPS KAKENHI grant (No. 19K08187).

Institutional Review Board Statement: The study was conducted according to the guidelines of the Declaration of Helsinki, and approved by the Institutional Review Board of Hyogo College of Hospital (protocol code 3315 and date of approval 2019/12/26).

Informed Consent Statement: Patient consent was waived due to the retrospective study by IRB.

Conflicts of Interest: The authors declare no conflict of interest.

References

1. Alley, E.W.; Lopez, J.; Santoro, A.; Morosky, A.; Saraf, S.; Piperdi, B.; van Brummelen, E. Clinical safety and activity of pembrolizumab in patients with malignant pleural mesothelioma (KEYNOTE-028): Preliminary results from a non-randomised, open-label, phase 1B trial. *Lancet Oncol.* **2017**, *18*, 623–630. [CrossRef]
2. Quispel-Janssen, J.; van der Noort, V.; de Vries, J.F.; Zimmerman, M.; Lalezari, F.; Thunnissen, E.; Monkhorst, K.; Schouten, R.; Schunselaar, L.; Disselhorst, M.; et al. Programmed death 1 blockade with nivolumab in patients with recurrent malignant pleural mesothelioma. *J. Thorac. Oncol.* **2018**, *13*, 1569–1576. [CrossRef] [PubMed]
3. Okada, M.; Kijima, T.; Aoe, K.; Kato, T.; Fujimoto, N.; Nakagawa, K.; Takeda, Y.; Hida, T.; Kanai, K.; Imamura, F.; et al. Clinical Efficacy and Safety of Nivolumab: Results of a Multicenter, Open-label, Single-arm, Japanese Phase II study in Malignant Pleural Mesothelioma (MERIT). *Clin. Cancer Res.* **2019**, *25*, 5485–5492. [CrossRef] [PubMed]
4. Scherpereel, A.; Mazieres, J.; Greillier, L.; Lantuejoul, S.; Dô, P.; Bylicki, O.; Monnet, I.; Corre, R.; Audigier-Valette, C.; Locatelli-Sanchez, M.; et al. French Cooperative Thoracic Intergroup. Nivolumab or Nivolumab plus ipilimumab in patients with relapsed malignant pleural mesothelioma (IFCT-1501 MAPS2): A multicentre, open-Label, randomised, non-comparative, Phase 2 Trial. *Lancet Oncol.* **2019**, *20*, 239–253. [CrossRef]
5. Nakamura, A.; Kondo, N.; Nakamichi, T.; Kuroda, A.; Hashimoto, M.; Matsumoto, S.; Yokoi, T.; Kuribayashi, K.; Kijima, T.; Hasegawa, S. Initial evaluation of nivolumab in patients with post-operative recurrence of malignant pleural mesothelioma. *Jpn. J. Clin. Oncol.* **2020**, *50*, 920–925. [CrossRef] [PubMed]
6. Eisenhauer, E.A.; Therasse, P.; Bogaerts, J.; Schwartz, L.H.; Sargent, D.; Ford, R.; Dancey, J.; Arbuck, S.; Gwyther, S.; Mooney, M.; et al. New response evaluation criteria in solid tumours: Revised RECIST guideline (version 1.1). *Eur. J. Cancer* **2009**, *45*, 228–247. [CrossRef] [PubMed]

7. Young, H.; Baum, R.; Cremerius, U.; Herholz, K.; Hoekstra, O.; Lammertsma, A.A.; Pruim, J.; Price, P. Measurement of clinical and subclinical tumour response using [^{18}F]-fluorodeoxyglucose and positron emission tomography: Review and 1999 EORTC recommendations. *Eur. J. Cancer* **1999**, *35*, 1773–1782. [CrossRef]
8. Wahl, R.L.; Jacene, H.; Kasamon, Y.; Lodge, M.A. From RECIST to PERCIST: Evolving considerations for PET response criteria in solid tumors. *J. Nucl. Med.* **2009**, *50* (Suppl. 1), 122S–150S. [CrossRef] [PubMed]
9. Chiou, V.L.; Burotto, M. Pseudoprogression and immune-related response in solid tumors. *J. Clin. Oncol.* **2015**, *33*, 3541–3543. [CrossRef] [PubMed]
10. Ito, K.; Teng, R.; Schöder, H.; Humm, J.L.; Ni, A.; Michaud, L.; Nakajima, R.; Yamashita, R.; Wolchok, J.D.; Weber, W.A. ^{18}F-FDG PET/CT for Monitoring of Ipilimumab Therapy in Patients with Metastatic Melanoma. *J. Nucl. Med.* **2019**, *60*, 335–341. [CrossRef] [PubMed]
11. Byrne, M.J.; Nowak, A.K. Modified RECIST criteria for assessment of response in malignant pleural mesothelioma. *Ann. Oncol.* **2004**, *15*, 257–260. [CrossRef] [PubMed]
12. Kitajima, K.; Nakatani, K.; Yamaguchi, K.; Nakajo, M.; Tani, A.; Ishibashi, M.; Hosoya, K.; Morita, T.; Kinoshita, T.; Kaida, H.; et al. Response to neoadjuvant chemotherapy for breast cancer judged by PERCIST—multicenter study in Japan. *Eur. J. Nucl. Med. Mol. Imaging* **2018**, *45*, 1661–1671. [CrossRef] [PubMed]
13. Depardon, E.; Kanoun, S.; Humbert, O.; Bertaut, A.; Riedinger, J.M.; Tal, I.; Vrigneaud, J.M.; Lasserre, M.; Toubeau, M.; Berriolo-Riedinger, A.; et al. FDG PET/CT for prognostic stratification of patients with metastatic breast cancer treated with first line systemic therapy: Comparison of EORTC criteria and PERCIST. *PLoS ONE* **2018**, *13*, e0199529. [CrossRef]
14. Kundel, H.L.; Polansky, M. Measurement of observer agreement. *Radiology* **2003**, *228*, 303–308. [CrossRef] [PubMed]
15. Wolchok, J.D.; Hoos, A.; O'Day, S.; Weber, J.S.; Hamid, O.; Lebbé, C.; Maio, M.; Binder, M.; Bohnsack, O.; Nichol, G.; et al. Guidelines for the evaluation of immune therapy activity in solid tumors: Immune-related response criteria. *Clin. Cancer Res.* **2009**, *15*, 7412–7420. [CrossRef] [PubMed]
16. Seymour, L.; Bogaerts, J.; Perrone, A.; Ford, R.; Schwartz, L.H.; Mandrekar, S.; Lin, N.U.; Litière, S.; Dancey, J.; Chen, A.; et al. RECIST working group. RECIST working group. iRECIST: Guidelines for response criteria for use in trials testing immunotherapeutics. *Lancet Oncol.* **2017**, *18*, e143–e152. [CrossRef]
17. Cho, S.Y.; Lipson, E.J.; Im, H.J.; Rowe, S.P.; Gonzalez, E.M.; Blackford, A.; Chirindel, A.; Pardoll, D.M.; Topalian, S.L.; Wahl, R.L. Prediction of response to immune checkpoint inhibitor therapy using early-time-point ^{18}F-FDG PET/CT imaging in patients with advanced melanoma. *J. Nucl. Med.* **2017**, *58*, 1421–1428. [CrossRef] [PubMed]
18. Anwar, H.; Sachpekidis, C.; Winkler, J.; Kopp-Schneider, A.; Haberkorn, U.; Hassel, J.C.; Dimitrakopoulou-Strauss, A. Absolute number of new lesions on ^{18}F-FDG PET/CT is more predictive of clinical response than SUV changes in metastatic melanoma patients receiving ipilimumab. *Eur. J. Nucl. Med. Mol. Imaging* **2018**, *45*, 376–383. [CrossRef] [PubMed]
19. Goldfarb, L.; Duchemann, B.; Chouahnia, K.; Zelek, L.; Soussan, M. Monitoring anti-PD-1-based immunotherapy in non-small cell lung cancer with FDG PET: Introduction of iPERCIST. *Ejnmmi Res.* **2019**, *9*, 8. [CrossRef] [PubMed]
20. Dimitrakopoulou-Strauss, A. Monitoring of patients with metastatic melanoma treated with immune checkpoint inhibitors using PET-CT. *Cancer Immunol. Immunother.* **2019**, *68*, 813–822. [CrossRef] [PubMed]

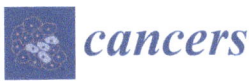

Article

VATS Pleurectomy Decortication Is a Reasonable Alternative for Higher Risk Patients in the Management of Malignant Pleural Mesothelioma: An Analysis of Short-Term Outcomes

Dong-Seok Lee *, Andrea Carollo, Naomi Alpert, Emanuela Taioli and Raja Flores

Thoracic Surgery Department, Icahn School of Medicine at Mount Sinai, Mount Sinai Health System, New York, NY 10029, USA; Andrea.Carollo@mountsinai.org (A.C.); Naomi.Alpert@mountsinai.org (N.A.); Emanuela.Taioli@mountsinai.org (E.T.); Raja.Flores@mountsinai.org (R.F.)
* Correspondence: Dong-Seok.Lee@mountsinai.org

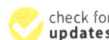

Citation: Lee, D.-S.; Carollo, A.; Alpert, N.; Taioli, E.; Flores, R. VATS Pleurectomy Decortication Is a Reasonable Alternative for Higher Risk Patients in the Management of Malignant Pleural Mesothelioma: An Analysis of Short-Term Outcomes. *Cancers* 2021, *13*, 1068. https://doi.org/10.3390/cancers13051068

Academic Editors: Daniel L. Pouliquen and Joanna Kopecka

Received: 20 January 2021
Accepted: 23 February 2021
Published: 3 March 2021

Publisher's Note: MDPI stays neutral with regard to jurisdictional claims in published maps and institutional affiliations.

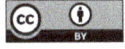

Copyright: © 2021 by the authors. Licensee MDPI, Basel, Switzerland. This article is an open access article distributed under the terms and conditions of the Creative Commons Attribution (CC BY) license (https://creativecommons.org/licenses/by/4.0/).

Simple Summary: Malignant pleural mesothelioma (MPM) is an aggressive malignancy that drastically affects a patient's quality of life. Surgery typically entails radical resection with or without the removal of the underlying lung. In an era where minimally invasive surgery is sought after, MPM remains an anomaly. The purpose of this study is to assess the feasibility of minimally invasive surgery as an alternative to more radical surgery in MPM. We examined short-term outcomes between the radical approaches and minimally invasive surgery and minimally invasive surgery had improved outcomes. Minimally invasive surgery can be considered in patients with MPM.

Abstract: Surgery is a mainstay of treatment allowing for debulking of tumor and expansion of the lung for improvement in median survival and quality of life for patients with malignant pleural mesothelioma (MPM). Although optimal surgical technique remains open for debate—extrapleural pneumonectomy (EPP) vs. pleurectomy/decortication (P/D)—minimally invasive surgery (VATS-P/D) remains underutilized in the management of MPM. We examined whether VATS-P/D is a feasible alternative to EPP and P/D. We evaluated the New York Statewide Planning and Research Cooperative System (SPARCS) from 2007–2017 to assess the short-term complications of EPP vs. P/D, including a subanalysis of open P/D vs. VATS-P/D. There were 331 patients with open surgery; 269 with P/D and 62 with EPP. There were 384 patients with P/D; 269 were open and 115 VATS. Rates of any complication were similar between EPP and P/D patients, but EPP had significantly higher rates of cardiovascular complications. After adjusting for confounders, those with a VATS approach were less likely to have any complication, compared to an open approach and significantly less likely to have a pulmonary complication. VATS-P/D remains a viable alternative to radical surgery in MPM patients allowing for improved short-term outcomes.

Keywords: malignant mesothelioma; VATS; extrapleural pneumonectomy; pleurectomy decortication

1. Introduction

Malignant pleural mesothelioma (MPM) is a rare but aggressive cancer with an overall poor prognosis. Treatment frequently involves multimodal therapy, of which surgical resection remains an essential component, significantly improving median survival compared to patients who do not undergo surgery [1]. However, there remains debate about the optimal surgical technique. Extrapleural pneumonectomy (EPP) theoretically offers the better chance at complete resection and was considered the standard. However, lung-sparing pleurectomy/decortication (P/D) has become more common, as research has indicated decreased perioperative morbidity and mortality and similar survival compared to EPP [2–6]. In addition, quality of life appears better as physical and social function and global health measures are better at 12 months with P/D over EPP [7,8].

Despite the increasing utilization of minimally invasive techniques in many oncologic surgical procedures, MPM-directed surgeries have historically been performed as open procedures. Although minimally invasive lung surgery has improved short-term outcomes with equivalent long-term survival compared to open surgery [9,10], its use in MPM is more challenging. Video-assisted thoracoscopic surgery (VATS) has been primarily focused on diagnosis or palliation of symptoms. Although there is extensive literature comparing outcomes of EPP to P/D, there is a paucity of data examining outcomes of minimally invasive surgery for MPM. Our group had previously reported improved short-term outcomes for patients with P/D compared to EPP using New York State hospital discharge data [3]. The aims of this study were to utilize the same large database to provide updated results of our prior study, with an added focus on comparing a minimally invasive approach to open surgery.

2. Materials and Methods

2.1. Data Source and Sample Selection

This analysis used the New York Statewide Planning and Research Cooperative System (SPARCS) from 2007–2017. SPARCS includes all hospital discharges in the state, and has information on patient demographics, diagnoses, procedures, admission and discharge type. This research was approved by the Mount Sinai Institutional Review Board (IRB# 18-00947, FWA #00005656).

There were 4,959,270 patients at least 50 years old, with a patient identifier who had an inpatient discharge between 1 January 2007 and 31 December 2017. Those with an admission accompanied by a diagnosis of pleural mesothelioma (n = 2169) and who had either EPP or P/D (See Supplementary Materials Table S1 for ICD-9 and ICD-10 diagnosis and procedures codes) were included (n = 589) for analysis. For patients with multiple mesothelioma-related surgeries, the first surgery was chosen. Patients where the surgical approach (open or minimally invasive) was unknown were excluded, as were the few who were coded as having minimally invasive EPP (n_{excl} = 143). The initial analysis was limited to patients with an open EPP or P/D surgery (n = 331), while a secondary analysis compared surgical approach among those with P/D (n = 384) (Figure 1).

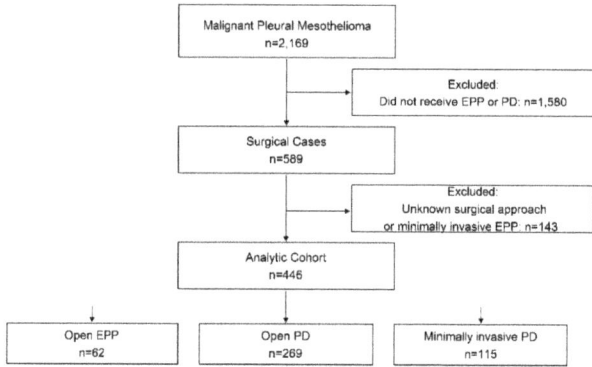

Abbreviations: EPP, Extrapleural Pneumonectomy; PD, Pleurectomy/Decortication

Figure 1. Patient Selection.

2.2. Predictors and Outcomes

The primary predictors of interest were the type of surgery and surgical approach. Outcomes of interest were short-term complications after surgery. In-hospital complications were defined based on diagnosis codes that were not present at the time of admission

(Supplementary Materials Table S2), and were categorized as cardiovascular, pulmonary, infectious or intraoperative complications. Patient comorbidities were defined using the algorithm described by Elixhauser, et al. [11], and a count of non-cancer-related comorbidities was created. Other covariates of interest included age, gender, race (Non-Hispanic White (NHW) vs. Hispanic or Non-White), primary insurance payer (government vs. non-government), type of admission to the hospital (urgent/emergency vs. elective), and the year of surgery.

2.3. Statistical Analysis

Patients were compared across surgical type on all variables, using t-tests for continuous variables, and χ^2-tests for categorical variables. Univariate and multivariable logistic regressions were used to model the independent associations between covariates and type of surgery, using Odds Ratios (ORs) and 95% Confidence Intervals (CI). Multivariable logistic regression models were also used to assess the association of surgical type with having complications (any, cardiovascular, or pulmonary), adjusting for possible confounders. Supraventricular arrhythmia was examined individually as a subset of cardiovascular complications. As there were a very small number of infectious and intraoperative complications, these were individually assessed only at the univariate level. Multivariable models were adjusted for age, gender, race/ethnicity, admission type, insurance, number of comorbidities, and year of surgery, to account for changes over time. Outcomes were also assessed using an optimal propensity matching analysis, with a maximum difference of 0.01, matching on all variables.

Analyses were repeated on the subset of patients with P/D, in order to compare outcomes in patients with minimally invasive and open approaches. All analyses were conducted using SAS software, v 9.4 (SAS Institute, Cary, NC, USA).

3. Results

3.1. Extrapleural Pneumonectomy vs. Pleurectomy Decortication

There were 331 patients with open surgery; 269 (81.3%) with P/D and 62 (18.7%) with EPP. EPP patients were significantly younger (mean age: 64.6 vs. 69.1 years, $p < 0.0001$), more likely to have non-government insurance coverage (61.3% vs. 44.6%, $p = 0.0217$), and had fewer comorbidities (29.0% vs. 55.4% with ≥ 2 comorbidities; $p = 0.0002$). EPP patients also more frequently had elective admissions ($p = 0.0552$) (Table 1).

Table 1. Demographics of the sample, according to surgery type.

Variable	P/D (*n* = 269)	EPP (*n* = 62)	*p*-Value
Patient and Admission Characteristics	N (%)	N (%)	
Mean Age, years (SE)	69.1 (0.5)	64.6 (0.8)	<0.0001
Gender			0.9314
Male	201 (74.7)	46 (74.2)	
Female	68 (25.3)	16 (25.8)	
Race			0.1726
NHW	214 (79.6)	$\geq$11 *	
Hispanic or Non-White	55 (20.4)	<11 *	
Primary Insurance Payer			0.0217
Non-Government	120 (45.1)	38 (61.3)	

Table 1. *Cont.*

Variable	P/D (n = 269)	EPP (n = 62)	p-Value
Government	146 (54.9)	24 (38.7)	
Type of Admission			0.0552
Elective	237 (88.8)	≥11 *	
Urgent/Emergency	30 (11.2)	<11 *	
Number of Comorbidities			0.0002
0–1	120 (44.6)	44 (71.0)	
≥2	149 (55.4)	18 (29.0)	
Complications			
Cardiovascular	36 (13.4)	20 (32.3)	0.0004
Pulmonary	92 (34.2)	13 (21.0)	0.0439
Infection	13 (4.8)	<11 *	0.1395
Bleeding	<11 *	<11 *	0.4381
Supraventricular arrhythmia			0.0003
No	242 (90.0)	45 (72.6)	
Yes	27 (10.0)	17 (27.4)	
Any Complication			0.8248
No	156 (58.0)	35 (56.5)	
Yes	113 (42.0)	27 (43.5)	

Abbreviations: P/D, Pleurectomy Decortication; EPP, Extrapleural pneumonectomy. * Exact cell sizes masked to protect against identification of patients.

After adjustment, those with EPP were significantly younger (ORadj: 0.91, 95% CI: 0.86–0.96) and significantly less likely to have an urgent or emergency surgery (ORadj: 0.21, 95% CI: 0.05–0.97). There was no significant difference in gender, race/ethnicity, type of insurance, or number of comorbidities (Table 2).

Table 2. Independent Factors Associated with Receipt of EPP vs. P/D (n = 326).

	EPP vs. P/D	
Variable	OR_{adj} * (95% CI)	p-Value
Age (years)	0.91 (0.86–0.96)	0.0011
Gender		
Female vs. Male	0.88 (0.42–1.84)	0.7347
Race/Ethnicity		
Hispanic or Non-White vs. Non-Hispanic White	0.57 (0.22–1.45)	0.2354
Admission Type		
Urgent/Emergency vs. Elective	0.21 (0.05–0.97)	0.0450
Insurance		
Non-Government vs. Government	0.82 (0.37–1.79)	0.6103
Number of Comorbidities		
≥2 vs. 0–1	0.62 (0.32–1.22)	0.1637

* Adjusted for all variables listed and year of surgery.

At the univariate level, rates of any complication were similar between EPP and P/D patients (43.5% for EPP vs. 42.0% for P/D; $p = 0.8248$), but EPP had significantly higher rates of cardiovascular complications (32.3% vs. 13.4%; $p = 0.0004$) supraventricular arrhythmia (27.4% vs. 10.0%; $p = 0.0003$), and lower rates of pulmonary complications (21.0% vs. 34.2%; $p = 0.0439$) (Table 1).

In the multivariable analysis, those with EPP were significantly more likely to have any complication (ORadj: 2.12, 95% CI: 1.08–4.18), as well as have cardiovascular complications (ORadj: 5.00, 95% CI: 2.23–11.24), and supraventricular arrhythmia specifically (ORadj: 6.63, 95% CI: 2.64–16.64). There was no significant difference in the odds of a pulmonary complication (Table 3).

Table 3. Odds of Complications in EPP vs. P/D patients, multivariable and propensity-matched analyses.

	Any Complication (Y vs. N)	Cardiovascular Complication (Y vs. N)	Supraventricular Arrhythmia (Y vs. N)	Pulmonary Complication (Y vs. N)
	OR_{adj} * (95% CI); p-Value	OR_{adj} * (95% CI); p-Value	OR_{adj} * (95% CI); p-Value	OR_{adj} * (95% CI); p-Value
Multivariable Analysis (n = 326)				
EPP vs. P/D	2.12 (1.08–4.18); 0.0302	5.00 (2.23–11.24); <0.0001	6.63 (2.64–16.64); <0.0001	0.89 (0.41–1.91); 0.7619
Propensity-Matched Analysis (n = 100)				
EPP vs. P/D	1.11 (0.45–2.73); 0.8186	2.60 (0.93–7.29); 0.0694	2.75 (0.88–8.64); 0.0832	0.58 (0.23–1.48); 0.2571

Abbreviations: EPP, extrapleural pneumonectomy; P/D, Pleurectomy Decortication. * Adjusted for/propensity matched on age, gender, race/ethnicity, admission type, insurance, number of comorbidities, and year of surgery. Adjusted models were not conducted for infection or intraoperative complication due to an insufficient number of outcomes.

After propensity matching, there were 50 EPP and 50 P/D patients, who were well matched on all covariates (range of p-values: 0.5637 to 1). Although not statistically significant, patients with EPP continued to have more cardiovascular complications in general (OR: 2.60, 95% CI: 0.93–7.29), and specifically supraventricular arrhythmia (OR: 2.75, 95% CI: 0.88–8.64) (Table 3).

3.2. Minimally Invasive vs. Open P/D

There were 384 patients with P/D; 269 (70.1%) with an open surgical approach, and 115 (29.9%) with a minimally invasive approach. Patients with a minimally invasive surgical approach were significantly older (mean age: 71.8 vs. 69.1 years; $p = 0.0132$) and more likely to have an urgent/emergency admission (47.0% vs. 11.2%; $p < 0.0001$). They were also less often NHW ($p = 0.0524$) (Table 4).

Table 4. Demographics of the sample according to surgical approach among P/D patients.

Variable	Open (n = 269)	Minimally Invasive (n = 115)	p-Value
Patient and Admission Characteristics	N (%)	N (%)	
Mean Age, years (SE)	69.1 (0.5)	71.8 (1.0)	0.0132
Gender			0.5773
Male	201 (74.7)	89 (77.4)	
Female	68 (25.3)	26 (22.6)	
Race			0.0524
NHW	214 (79.6)	81 (70.4)	

Table 4. Cont.

Variable	Open (n = 269)	Minimally Invasive (n = 115)	p-Value
Hispanic or Non-White	55 (20.4)	34 (29.6)	
Primary Insurance Payer			0.1194
Non-Government	120 (45.1)	42 (36.5)	
Government	146 (54.9)	73 (63.5)	
Type of Admission			<0.0001
Elective	237 (88.8)	60 (52.6)	
Urgent/Emergency	30 (11.2)	54 (47.4)	
Number of Comorbidities			0.7899
0–1	120 (44.6)	53 (46.1)	
≥2	149 (55.4)	62 (53.9)	
Complications			
Cardiovascular	36 (13.4)	11 (9.6)	0.2958
Pulmonary	92 (34.2)	31 (27.0)	0.1635
Infection	13 (4.8)	<11 *	0.8369
Bleeding	<11 *	<11 *	0.7296
Any Complication			0.0995
No	156 (58.0)	77 (67.0)	
Yes	113 (42.0)	38 (33.0)	

Abbreviations: P/D, Pleurectomy Decortication * Exact cell sizes masked to protect against identification of patients. Percentages and p-values are presented for non-missing values.

After adjustment, those with a minimally invasive approach remained significantly older (ORadj: 1.05, 95% CI: 1.01–1.08) and more likely to have an urgent/emergency admission (ORadj: 7.18, 95% CI: 4.07–12.64), compared to those with an open approach (Table 5).

Table 5. Independent Factors Associated with Receipt of Minimally Invasive vs. Open Surgery (n = 378).

	Minimally Invasive vs. Open	
Variable	OR$_{adj}$ * (95% CI)	p-Value
Age (years)	1.05 (1.01–1.08)	0.0106
Gender		
Female vs. Male	0.90 (0.49–1.64)	0.7343
Race/Ethnicity		
Hispanic or Non-White vs. Non-Hispanic White	1.37 (0.76–2.49)	0.3008
Admission Type		
Urgent/Emergency vs. Elective	7.18 (4.07–12.64)	<0.0001
Insurance		
Non-Government vs. Government	1.11 (0.61–2.00)	0.7353
Number of Comorbidities		
≥2 vs. 0–1	0.66 (0.40–1.10)	0.1126

* Adjusted for all variables listed and year of surgery.

After adjusting for confounders, those with a minimally invasive approach were less likely to have any complication, compared to those with an open approach (ORadj: 0.58, 95% CI: 0.34–1.01) and significantly less likely to have a pulmonary complication (ORadj: 0.55, 95% CI: 0.31–0.99) (Table 6).

Table 6. Odds of complications in minimally invasive vs. open P/D patients, multivariable and propensity-matched analyses.

	Any Complication (Y vs. N)	Cardiovascular Complication (Y vs. N)	Pulmonary Complication (Y vs. N)
	OR_{adj} * (95% CI); p-Value	OR_{adj} * (95% CI); p-Value	OR_{adj} * (95% CI); p-Value
Multivariable Analysis (n = 378)			
Minimally Invasive vs. Open	0.58 (0.34–1.01); 0.0524	0.88 (0.40–1.95); 0.7518	0.55 (0.31–0.99); 0.0448
Propensity-Matched analysis (n = 150)			
Minimally Invasive vs. Open	0.70 (0.37–1.32); 0.2649	1.13 (0.43–2.92); 0.8085	0.65 (0.30–1.38); 0.2606

Abbreviations: P/D, Pleurectomy Decortication. * adjusted for/propensity matched on age, gender, race/ethnicity, admission type, insurance, number of comorbidities, and year of surgery. Adjusted models were not conducted for infection or intraoperative complication, due to an insufficient number of outcomes.

The propensity-matched analysis was well balanced on all covariates (range of p-values: 0.3980–1) with 75 patients per group. Although not significant, results were similar, with minimally invasive surgery having lower risk of overall complications (OR: 0.70, 95% CI: 0.37–1.32) and pulmonary complications (OR: 0.65, 95% CI: 0.30–1.38) (Table 6).

4. Discussion

Our study utilized the New York SPARCS database in order to compare perioperative morbidity with EPP, P/D, and VATS-P/D for MPM. Complications examined were cardiovascular, pulmonary, infectious, and intraoperative complications. The majority of complications were either cardiovascular or pulmonary. Perioperative mortality was not included in the present analysis due to limited observations. Generally, the more radical resection was associated with younger age, elective procedure, and increased incidence of complications. EPP patients were more likely to have cardiovascular complications, primarily supraventricular arrhythmias, than P/D patients on multivariable analysis and propensity matching. On the other hand, cardiovascular complications were similar in open and minimally invasive P/D patients but open patients were more prone to pulmonary complications on multivariable analysis and propensity matching.

The goal of oncologic surgery with curative intent is removal of all macroscopic and, if possible, microscopic disease. This is challenging in MPM as it is an insidious diffuse disease throughout the pleura and often requires radical resection. Therefore, the mainstay of surgical treatment for MPM includes extrapleural pneumonectomy and pleurectomy/decortication. A number of studies have been performed showing that EPP and P/D confer similar overall survival but that the short-term mortality and morbidity associated with EPP is greater than P/D [2–6]. Less radical and more minimally invasive surgery has primarily been limited to diagnostic biopsy or symptom management with talc pleurodesis or indwelling pleural catheters. VATS-P/D has not achieved widespread use in the management of MPM, as it is primarily considered to be a palliative surgical option [12] as opposed to a potentially curative one. The goal of VATS-P/D is the debulking of enough pleural disease and decortication of the underlying trapped lung in order to obliterate the pleural space to allow pleural apposition.

The only randomized control trial to date, MesoVATS, compared VATS partial pleurectomy (VATS-PP) to talc pleurodesis [13]. The primary endpoint was overall survival at

12 months and no significant difference was noted between the two groups. Although VATS-PP had a non-significant trend towards increased morbidity, the authors noted a 70% resolution of pleural effusion with VATS-PP compared to 77% resolution with talc pleurodesis but significantly improved quality of life scores at 6 and 12 months for the VATS-PP group. A follow-up study, currently in progress, aims to address VATS-PP against the use of indwelling pleural catheters for patients with MPM and trapped lung [14].

In addition to providing a palliative benefit, VATS-P/D appears to confer a survival benefit as cytoreduction and post-resection tumor volume may play a role in long-term outcomes [15,16]. It is unclear how it compares with more radical surgery. A previously published single institutional study looking at VATS P/D showed a modest non-significant improvement in survival with VATS versus EPP (14 months vs. 11.5 months). They also noted symptomatic improvement in the majority of patients and statistically significant advantage in 30-day mortality versus EPP [17].

Our study is the first to utilize a large population-based database in order to assess short-term outcomes in EPP, P/D, and minimally invasive P/D. However, it is not without its limitations. Despite the extensive size of the dataset, MPM remains an uncommon disease such that it accounts for a very small percentage of admissions, and thus, numbers remain relatively small. There may be selection bias in regards to surgical technique due to both surgeon preference and elective versus emergent presentation. Confounders that are unable to be addressed include information that could not be ascertained from the database, such as tumor grade, oncologic stage, long-term outcomes, surgeon experience, and potential use of induction therapy. However, this analysis includes a greater number of patients than would be available from a single-center study.

In confirmation of our previous analysis, P/D was associated with improved short-term outcomes compared to EPP and likely explains the shift from equivalent amounts of EPP and P/D performed (46.6% EPP, 53.4% P/D) from 1995–2012 [3] to predominantly P/D (81.3% P/D, 18.7% EPP) performed for the treatment of MPM from 2007–2017. Despite the increasing age of patients with less radical surgery, VATS P/D patients exhibited improved short-term outcomes, when controlling for this difference. Further investigation in regards to long-term survival with VATS P/D in comparison to EPP and P/D is needed.

5. Conclusions

Malignant pleural mesothelioma remains a challenging cancer to treat. Surgical options range from the more radical curative techniques such as EPP and P/D to the less invasive palliative VATS P/D. Patients who undergo VATS P/D have better short-term outcomes compared to those who undergo curative attempts at surgery. Therefore, VATS P/D should be considered in the armamentarium of treatment for MPM, especially in older and frailer patients who may not tolerate more radical surgery.

Supplementary Materials: The following are available online at https://www.mdpi.com/2072-6694/13/5/1068/s1, Table S1: Diagnosis and Procedure Codes to Identify Surgical Pleural Mesothelioma Patients, Table S2: Diagnosis Codes to Identify Complications.

Author Contributions: Conceptualization, D.-S.L., A.C., N.A.; Methodology, N.A.; Formal Analysis, N.A.; Resources, R.F., E.T.; Data Curation, N.A.; Writing—Original Draft Preparation, D.-S.L.; A.C.; Writing—Review & Editing, D.-S.L., N.A.; Supervision, E.T., R.F. All authors have read and agreed to the published version of the manuscript.

Funding: This research received no external funding.

Institutional Review Board Statement: This research was approved by the Mount Sinai Institutional Review Board (IRB# 18-00947, FWA #00005656).

Informed Consent Statement: Patient consent was waived due to utilization of a retrospective population-based database where researchers had no method of contact for included subjects.

Data Availability Statement: No new data was generated by the authors of this study. The data used and analyzed during the current study are available from the New York State Department of Health.

Conflicts of Interest: The authors declare no conflict of interest.

References

1. Taioli, E.; Wolf, A.S.; Camacho-Rivera, M.; Kaufman, A.; Lee, D.S.; Nicastri, D.; Rosenzweig, K.; Flores, R.M. Determinants of survival in malignant pleural mesothelioma: A Surveillance, Epidemiology, and End Results (SEER) study of 14,228 patients. *PLoS ONE* **2015**, *10*, e0145039. [CrossRef] [PubMed]
2. Flores, R.M.; Pass, H.I.; Seshan, V.E.; Dycoco, J.; Zakowski, M.; Carbone, M.; Bains, M.S.; Rusch, V.W. Extrapleural pneumonectomy versus pleurectomy/decortication in the surgical management of malignant pleural mesothelioma: Results in 663 patients. *J. Thorac. Cardiovasc.* **2008**, *135*, 620–626. [CrossRef] [PubMed]
3. Van Gerwen, M.; Wolf, A.; Liu, B.; Flores, R.; Taioli, E. Short-term outcomes of pleurectomy decortication and extrapleural pneumonectomy in mesothelioma. *J. Surg. Oncol.* **2018**, *118*, 1178–1187. [CrossRef] [PubMed]
4. Taioli, E.; Wolf, A.S.; Flores, R.M. Meta-analysis of survival after pleurectomy decortication versus extrapleural pneumonectomy in mesothelioma. *Ann. Thorac. Surg.* **2015**, *99*, 472–480. [CrossRef] [PubMed]
5. Magouliotis, D.E.; Tasiopoulou, V.S.; Athanassiadi, K. Updated meta-analysis of survival after extrapleural pneumonectomy versus pleurectomy/decortication in mesothelioma. *Gen. Thorac. Cardiovasc. Surg.* **2019**, *67*, 312–320. [CrossRef] [PubMed]
6. Burt, B.M.; Cameron, R.B.; Mollberg, N.M.; Kosinski, A.S.; Schipper, P.H.; Shrager, J.B.; Vigneswaran, W.T. Malignant pleural mesothelioma and the Society of Thoracic Surgeons Database: An analysis of surgical morbidity and mortality. *J. Thorac. Cardiovasc. Surg.* **2014**, *148*, 30–35. [CrossRef] [PubMed]
7. Rena, O.; Casadio, C. Extrapleural pneumonectomy for early stage malignant pleural mesothelioma: A harmful procedure. *Lung Cancer* **2012**, *77*, 151–155. [CrossRef] [PubMed]
8. Schwartz, R.M.; Lieberman-Cribbin, W.; Wolf, A.; Flores, R.M.; Taioli, E. Systematic review of quality of life following pleurectomy decortication and extrapleural pneumonectomy for malignant pleural mesothelioma. *BMC Cancer* **2018**, *18*, 1188. [CrossRef] [PubMed]
9. Whitson, B.A.; Groth, S.S.; Duval, S.J.; Swanson, S.J.; Maddaus, M.A. Surgery for early-stage non-small cell lung cancer: A systematic review of the video-assisted thoracoscopic surgery versus thoracotomy approaches to lobectomy. *Ann. Thorac. Surg.* **2008**, *86*, 2008–2016. [CrossRef] [PubMed]
10. Taioli, E.; Lee, D.S.; Lesser, M.; Flores, R.M. Long-term survival in video-assisted thoracoscopic lobectomy versus open lobectomy in lung-cancer patients: A meta-analysis. *Eur. J. Cardiothorac. Surg.* **2013**, *44*, 591–597. [CrossRef] [PubMed]
11. Elixhauser, A.; Steiner, C.; Harris, D.R.; Coffey, R.M. Comorbidity measures for use with administrative data. *Med. Care* **1998**, *36*, 8–27. [CrossRef] [PubMed]
12. Martin-Ucar, A.E.; Edwards, J.G.; Rengajaran, A.; Muller, S.; Waller, D.A. Palliative surgical debulking in malignant mesothelioma. Predictors of survival and symptom control. *Eur. J. Cardio Thorac. Surg.* **2001**, *20*, 1117–1121. [CrossRef]
13. Rintoul, R.C.; Ritchie, A.J.; Edwards, J.G.; Waller, D.A.; Coonar, A.S.; Bennett, M.; Lovato, E.; Hughes, V.; Fox-Rushby, J.A.; Sharples, L.D.; et al. Efficacy and cost of video-assisted thoracoscopic partial pleurectomy versus talc pleurodesis in patients with malignant pleural mesothelioma (MesoVATS): An open-label, randomised, controlled trial. *Lancet* **2014**, *384*, 1118–1127. [CrossRef]
14. Matthews, C.; Freeman, C.; Sharples, L.D.; Fox-Rushby, J.; Tod, A.; Maskell, N.A.; Edwards, J.G.; Coonar, A.S.; Sivasothy, P.; Hughes, V.; et al. MesoTRAP: A feasibility study that includes a pilot clinical trial comparing video-assisted thoracoscopic partial pleurectomy decortication with indwelling pleural catheter in patients with trapped lung due to malignant pleural mesothelioma designed to address recruitment and randomisation uncertainties and sample size requirements for a phase III trial. *BMJ Open Respir. Res.* **2019**, *6*, e000368. [CrossRef] [PubMed]
15. Halstead, J.C.; Lim, E.; Venkateswaran, R.M.; Charman, S.C.; Goddard, M.; Ritchie, A.J. Improved survival with VATS pleurectomy-decortication in advanced malignant mesothelioma. *Eur. J. Surg. Oncol.* **2005**, *31*, 314–320. [CrossRef] [PubMed]
16. Pass, H.I.; Temeck, B.K.; Kranda, K.; Steinberg, S.M.; Feuerstein, I.R. Preoperative tumour volume is associated with outcome in malignant pleural mesothelioma. *J. Thorac. Cardiovasc. Surg.* **1998**, *115*, 310–317. [CrossRef]
17. Nakas, A.; Martin Ucar, A.E.; Edwards, J.G.; Waller, D.A. The role of video-assisted thoracoscopic pleurectomy/decortication in the therapeutic management of malignant pleural mesothelioma. *Eur. J. Cardio Thorac. Surg.* **2008**, *33*, 83–88. [CrossRef] [PubMed]

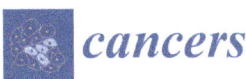

Article

Radical Hemithoracic Radiotherapy Induces Systemic Metabolomics Changes That Are Associated with the Clinical Outcome of Malignant Pleural Mesothelioma Patients

Emanuela Di Gregorio [1], Gianmaria Miolo [2], Asia Saorin [1], Elena Muraro [1], Michela Cangemi [1], Alberto Revelant [3], Emilio Minatel [3], Marco Trovò [4], Agostino Steffan [1] and Giuseppe Corona [1,*]

[1] Immunopathology and Cancer Biomarkers Unit, Centro di Riferimento Oncologico di Aviano (CRO), IRCCS, 33081 Aviano, Italy; emanuela.digregorio@cro.it (E.D.G.); asia.saorin@cro.it (A.S.); emuraro@cro.it (E.M.); michela.cangemi@cro.it (M.C.); asteffan@cro.it (A.S.)
[2] Medical Oncology and Cancer Prevention Unit, Centro di Riferimento Oncologico di Aviano (CRO), IRCCS, 33081 Aviano, Italy; gmiolo@cro.it
[3] Radiation Oncology Department, Centro di Riferimento Oncologico di Aviano (CRO), IRCCS, 33081 Aviano, Italy; alberto.revelant@cro.it (A.R.); eminatel@cro.it (E.M.)
[4] Radiation Oncology Department, Azienda Sanitaria Integrata, 33100 Udine, Italy; marco.trovo@asufc.sanita.fvg.it
* Correspondence: giuseppe.corona@cro.it; Tel.: +39-0434-659-666

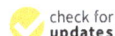

Citation: Di Gregorio, E.; Miolo, G.; Saorin, A.; Muraro, E.; Cangemi, M.; Revelant, A.; Minatel, E.; Trovò, M.; Steffan, A.; Corona, G. Radical Hemithoracic Radiotherapy Induces Systemic Metabolic Changes That Are Associated with the Clinical Outcome of Malignant Pleural Mesothelioma Patients. *Cancers* **2021**, *13*, 508. https://doi.org/10.3390/cancers13030508

Academic Editors: Daniel L. Pouliquen and Joanna Kopecka
Received: 23 December 2020
Accepted: 25 January 2021
Published: 29 January 2021

Publisher's Note: MDPI stays neutral with regard to jurisdictional claims in published maps and institutional affiliations.

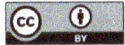

Copyright: © 2021 by the authors. Licensee MDPI, Basel, Switzerland. This article is an open access article distributed under the terms and conditions of the Creative Commons Attribution (CC BY) license (https://creativecommons.org/licenses/by/4.0/).

Simple Summary: Radical hemithoracic radiotherapy represents a promising new advance in the field of radiation oncology and encouraging results have been achieved in the treatment of malignant pleural mesothelioma patients. This study showed that this radiotherapy modality produces significant changes in serum metabolomics profile mainly affecting arginine and polyamine biosynthesis pathways. Interestingly, individual metabolomics alterations were found associated with the clinical overall survival outcome of the radiotherapy treatment. These results highlight metabolomics profile analysis as a powerful prognostic tool useful to better understand the mechanisms underlying the interpatients variability and to identify patients who may receive the best benefit from this specific radiotherapy treatment.

Abstract: Radical hemithoracic radiotherapy (RHRT) represents an advanced therapeutic option able to improve overall survival of malignant pleural mesothelioma patients. This study aims to investigate the systemic effects of this radiotherapy modality on the serum metabolome and their potential implications in determining the individual clinical outcome. Nineteen patients undergoing RHRT at the dose of 50 Gy in 25 fractions were enrolled. Serum targeted metabolomics profiles were investigated at baseline and the end of radiotherapy by liquid chromatography and tandem mass spectrometry. Univariate and multivariate OPLS-DA analyses were applied to study the serum metabolomics changes induced by RHRT while PLS regression analysis to evaluate the association between such changes and overall survival. RHRT was found to affect almost all investigated metabolites classes, in particular, the amino acids citrulline and taurine, the C14, C18:1 and C18:2 acyl-carnitines as well as the unsaturated long chain phosphatidylcholines PC ae 42:5, PC ae 44:5 and PC ae 44:6 were significantly decreased. The enrichment analysis showed arginine metabolism and the polyamine biosynthesis as the most perturbed pathways. Moreover, specific metabolic changes encompassing the amino acids and acyl-carnitines resulted in association with the clinical outcome accounting for about 60% of the interpatients overall survival variability. This study highlighted that RHRT can induce profound systemic metabolic effects some of which may have a significant prognostic value. The integration of metabolomics in the clinical assessment of the malignant pleural mesothelioma could be useful to better identify the patients who can achieve the best benefit from the RHRT treatment.

Keywords: metabolomics; mesothelioma; radiotherapy; biomarkers; cancers

1. Introduction

Malignant pleural mesothelioma (MPM) is a rare primary carcinoma originating from the pleural cavity, strongly linked to asbestos exposure [1]. The long latency after exposure and its characteristics of invasiveness and high aggressiveness contribute to make MPM a silent and invariable fatal disease with a median survival of less than 1 year when untreated [2]. The trimodal therapeutic approach that combines surgery, chemotherapy, and sequential radiotherapy (RT) represents the mainstream of current therapeutic protocols for MPM [3,4]. Over the last decades, RT technology has evolved [5], and the intensity-modulated radiation therapy (IMRT) has become one of the most interesting advance allowing the delivery of highly conformal radiation doses to the whole hemithorax limiting the normal tissue exposure. In MPM patients, this new RT modality referred as radical hemithoracic radiotherapy (RHRT) is delivered with a curative intent. However, despite its potential, its wide application is still debated especially for its possible severe toxicity [6], even if recent clinical investigations have shown encouraging results in enhancing patients' survival with acceptable toxicity [7–9]. Despite the relevant overall survival gain, the clinical outcome of the RHRT was very heterogeneous among patients and there is an urgent need for prognostic biomarkers to guide clinical decision-making and to tailor the RHRT treatment. The knowledge of the molecular mechanisms involved in tumour and normal tissue response to RT has retained an important footstep to improve the efficacy of the treatment through the identification of specific molecular signatures useful to recognize patients who may achieve the best benefit from RT. In order to get more insight into the role of RHRT in the treatment of MPM patients, we investigated the host response to this specific treatment evaluating the systemic metabolic changes by the application of metabolomics and searched for potential new prognostic biomarkers.

Metabolomics is a rapidly advancing field that aims to characterize the concentration changes of all metabolites (<1 KDa) present in biological fluids or tissues [10]. The metabolomics profile describes the biochemical events occurring in an organism and reflects the complex interactions among age, sex, gene transcription, protein expression, physio-pathological conditions, and environmental effects as well as chemical or physical interventions such as the RT [11,12]. The radiation treatments may induce whole-body responses that can be mirrored and observed at the blood metabolome level. Hence, the blood metabolites composition represents a hypothetical source of biomarkers and the understanding of how metabolites and their concentrations change under RT interventions may allow the discovery of potential biomarkers for RT efficacy and toxicity. The effect of anticancer drug treatments on local and systemic metabolism have been widely investigated in different cancer types by the metabolomics tool [13–16]. Nevertheless, only a few broad-based metabolomics studies have been so far reported about the effects of RT on the host system [17–23] and none in the specific MPM field.

In attempt to fill this gap, this study aims to investigate the RHRT effects on the systemic metabolism by the analysis of changes in serum metabolomics profiles consequent to the treatment. The investigation provides new insights on the host biochemical alterations induced by the RHRT treatment and on their potential role in determining the individual clinical outcome. The results of this explorative translational investigation indicate that RHRT can produce profound effects on the serum metabolomics profile engaging amino acids and lipids metabolic pathways that could be relevant to establish the effective clinical benefit of the treatment.

2. Results

2.1. Demographic and Clinical Baseline Patients' Characteristics

This translational study investigated 19 nonmetastatic MPM patients who underwent RHRT treatment consisting of 50 Gy in 25 fractions with a simultaneous integrated boost of 60 Gy in residual active disease. The clinical and demographic characteristics of the 19 MPM patients are reported in Table 1. The median age of the patients was 70 years (range: 33–79) with a great prevalence of male patients (89%). At baseline, 31% of patients presented adequate clinical conditions reporting an ECOG performance status (PS) score of 0, the majority of patients (53%) presented a PS score of 1 and only 16% had a PS score of 2. At the diagnosis, 95% of the MPM tumours had an epithelioid origin, while only 5% showed a biphasic histotype. Stage I–II characterized 47% of tumours, while the remaining 53% were classified as stage III–IV. The majority of the patients underwent previously nonradical surgical intervention for diagnostic purposes as biopsy (63%), and lung-sparing surgery pleurectomy/decortication (26%) or decortication (11%) leaving gross residual disease. All patients received systemic pharmacological treatment based on the pemetrexed and cisplatin chemotherapy. The RHRT was administered 4–6 weeks from the chemotherapy treatment.

Table 1. Clinical characteristics of 19 malignant pleural mesothelioma (MPM) patients.

Characteristics	n (%)
Age (years), median, range	70 (33–79)
Sex	
Female	2 (11%)
Male	17 (89%)
Performance Status *	
0	6 (31%)
1	10 (53%)
2	3 (16%)
Histology	
Epithelioid	18 (95%)
Nonepithelioid	1 (5%)
Stage	
I–II	9 (47%)
III–IV	10 (53%)
Chemotherapy	
Pemetrexed, cisplatin	19 (100%)
Surgery	
Pleurectomy/decortication (P/D)	5 (26%)
Decortication	2 (11%)
Biopsy	12 (63%)

* Evaluated by ECOG, Eastern Cooperative Oncology Group.

The baseline characteristics of a reference group consisted of 15 MPM patients treated with standard palliative local RT (LRT). They are reported in Table S2. This reference group was characterized by superimposable demographic and clinical characteristics and underwent sparing surgery and chemotherapy treatment analogously to the RHRT group.

2.2. RHRT Effect on Serum Metabolome

The study of baseline and post-RHRT serum metabolomics profiles aimed to investigate the complex biochemical effects that RT may induce in the host. A targeted serum profile of 188 metabolites covering wide biochemical metabolic pathways was considered for this investigation (Table S1). Twenty-seven metabolites showed concentrations lower than the limit of detection and were excluded from further statistical analyses. Exploratory data analysis performed using principal component analysis (PCA) (Figure S1) did not detect any outliers. The metabolomics profile at baseline and after RHRT resulted homogeneous without any clusters of patients associated with the different diagnostic intervention as well as patients' outliers. However, when the metabolomics profile at baseline and post-RHRT where compared, the PCA model explained only 22% of total variance and did not allow to characterize differences, supporting the application of supervised orthogonal partial least squares discriminant analysis (OPLS-DA) approach. Multivariate OPLS-DA model clearly differentiated the baseline serum metabolomic profiles from those post-RHRT with a significant discrimination power (Figure 1a) ($p = 0.007$, CV-ANOVA). OPLS-DA model showed good performance when internal leave-one-out cross-validation (LOOCV) was assessed ($R^2 = 0.77$, $Q^2 = 0.54$) without any potential risk of over-fitting verified by permutation test (Figure 1b). The extent of the RHRT effects on the serum metabolomics profile was estimated by determining the relative percentage of variation (Δ%) of serum concentrations of the metabolites with VIP > 1 that most contribute to the OPLS-DA model (Figure 1c). After RHRT, the 52% of investigated metabolites showed a serum variation of ≥10%; among them, 14 were upregulated, while 69 were downregulated. All these changes were not found associated with the gross residual disease indicating that they could not be attributed to the tumour extent but likely to host metabolic response.

The wide decrease in serum metabolites concentrations after RHRT is clearly indicated by the heat map for the selected statistically significant metabolites (Figure 1d). Only a small set of metabolites, mainly belonging to the amino acids class, significantly increased after irradiation. It included the aromatic AA phenylalanine and tryptophan, the branched amino acids (BCAA) valine and leucine and alpha aminoadipic acid, methionine and carnitine. Conversely, almost all the phospholipids, encompassing PC, lysoPC and SM, significantly decreased after RHRT. Among amino acids, citrulline resulted the most altered metabolite ($p = 9 \times 10^{-6}$, $q = 0.001$), followed by taurine ($p = 3 \times 10^{-5}$, $q = 0.002$) and the acyl-carnitines C14 ($p = 0.002$, $q = 0.04$), C18:1 ($p = 0.002$, $q = 0.05$) and C18:2 ($p = 2.8 \times 10^{-4}$, $q = 0.02$), while for phospholipids, the significant changes regarded the PC ae C42:5 ($p = 0.001$, $q = 0.03$), PC ae C44:5 ($p = 0.001$, $q = 0.03$) and PC ae C44:6 ($p = 3.7 \times 10^{-4}$, $q = 0.02$) derivatives (Table 2). The individual concentration variations of such metabolites are shown in Figure S3 where it is possible to appreciate the homogeneous decreasing trend for each patient as a consequence of the RHRT treatment.

2.3. Metabolic Patterns Influenced by RHRT

All the metabolites significantly altered after RHRT were considered for the metabolic set enrichment analysis addressed to elucidate the biochemical pathways most influenced by RHRT. The Over Representation Analysis (ORA) indicates that polyamines biosynthesis, urea cycle as well as arginine and proline metabolism were the pathways more significantly perturbed by RHRT (Figure 2a). The polyamines biosynthesis pathway resulted downregulated, indeed the serum concentrations of putrescine, spermidine and spermine were significantly lower in post-RHRT serum samples (Figure 2b). Polyamines biosynthesis is linked to the urea cycle through ornithine whose serum level was found 12.3% lower post-RHRT ($p = 0.02$, $q = 0.113$). This latter amino acid is also the precursor of both citrulline and arginine. However, while arginine concentration remained constant and independent from the RHRT, citrulline underwent a dramatic drop (33%) ($p = 9.0 \times 10^{-6}$, $q = 0.001$). Such citrulline depletion was found highly correlated with that of ornithine ($r = 0.72$, $p = 0.0005$) but it was not associated with the common precursor glutamine, which did not undergo significant variations after RHRT. Analogously, proline, a further ornithine precursor, resulted in 19.2% lower post-RHRT compared with its baseline level ($p = 5.3 \times 10^{-3}$, $q = 0.078$).

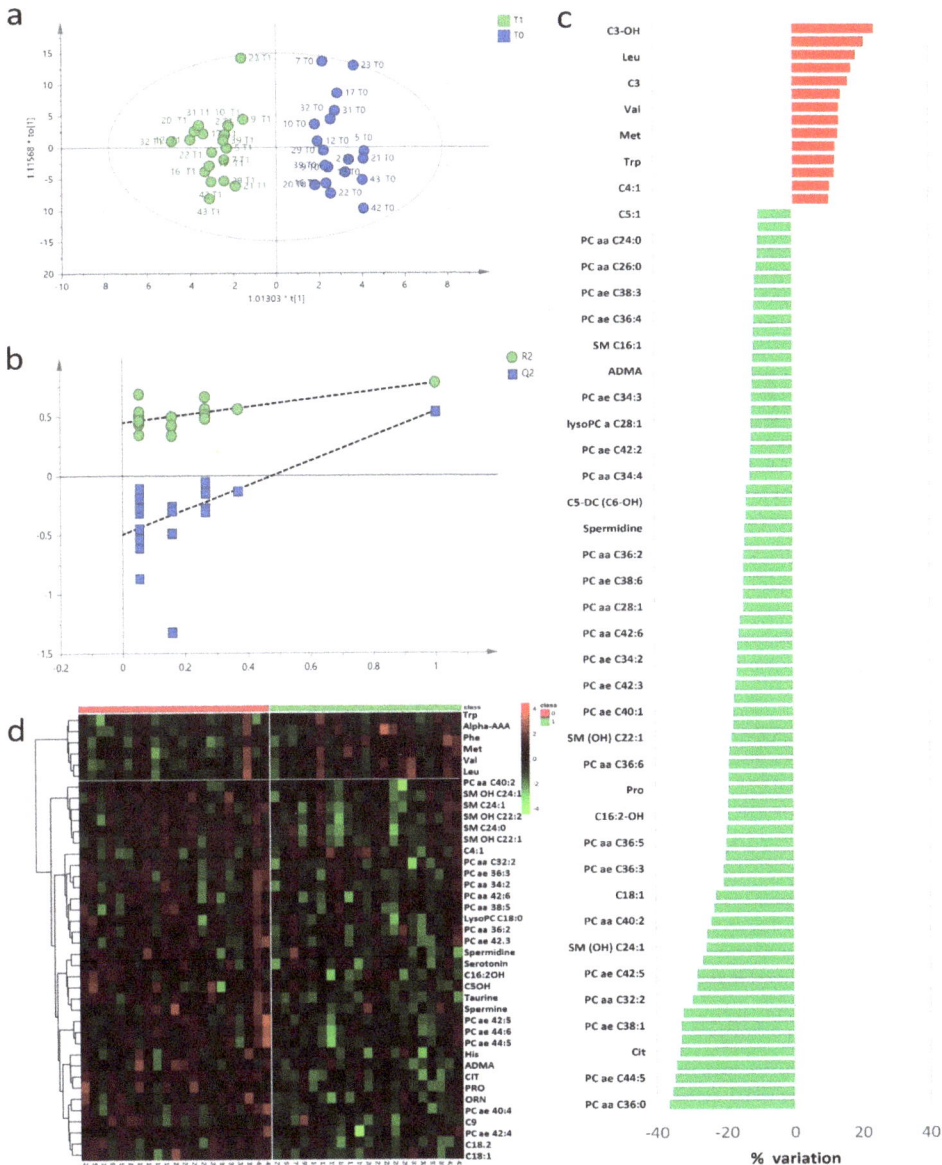

Figure 1. Orthogonal partial least squares discriminant analysis (OPLS-DA) score plot discriminated serum metabolomics profiles ($n = 19$) at baseline (T_0, blue) and post-radical hemithoracic radiotherapy (RHRT) (T_1, green) (**a**). Internal validation by permutation test showed R^2 (green) and Q^2 (blue) values from the permuted models (bottom left) significantly lower than the corresponding original model (top right) (**b**). Percentage variations of metabolites altered by RHRT (**c**). Heat map plot of the significantly changed serum metabolites between T_0 samples (left) and T_1 samples (right) ranked by t-test. Metabolites significantly decreased were in green, while metabolites significantly increased were in red. The brightness of the colour corresponded to the magnitude of the difference with the mean value (**d**).

Table 2. Metabolites significantly altered as effect of radical hemithoracic radiotherapy (RHRT) in 19 MPM patients.

Class	Name	Mean (µM) ± SD		Fold Change	Trend	p-Value	q-Value
		Baseline	Post-HRT				
Amino acids and derivatives	Cit	33.22 ± 7.02	22.19 ± 7.15	0.67	↓	9.0×10^{-6}	0.001
	ADMA	0.57 ± 0.06	0.5 ± 0.09	0.88	↓	0.007	0.085
	Orn	71.74 ± 9.56	62.89 ± 13.15	0.88	↓	0.017	0.113
	Pro	220.95 ± 36.99	178.47 ± 63.76	0.81	↓	0.005	0.078
	Putrescine	0.14 ± 0.03	0.13 ± 0.04	0.89	↓	0.027	0.149
	Serotonin	0.48 ± 0.22	0.36 ± 0.22	0.75	↓	0.005	0.078
	Spermidine	0.13 ± 0.03	0.11 ± 0.03	0.86	↓	0.010	0.099
	Spermine	0.19 ± 0.01	0.18 ± 0.01	0.96	↓	0.016	0.113
	Taurine	104.05 ± 18.69	74.49 ± 22.79	0.72	↓	3.0×10^{-5}	0.002
	total DMA	1.06 ± 0.31	0.94 ± 0.34	0.88	↓	0.024	0.139
	Phe	70.96 ± 11.05	79.71 ± 8.17	1.14	↑	0.009	0.095
	Val	178.21 ± 38.35	202.63 ± 36.56	1.12	↑	0.035	0.176
	alpha-AAA	1.17 ± 0.58	1.42 ± 0.34	1.21	↑	0.035	0.176
	Trp	46.96 ± 9.37	52.78 ± 10.89	1.12	↑	0.039	0.176
Acyl-carnitines	C10:2	0.08 ± 0.01	0.06 ± 0.04	0.73	↓	0.012	0.104
	C14	0.06 ± 0.02	0.04 ± 0.02	0.79	↓	0.002	0.038
	C14:1-OH	0.02 ± 0.01	0.02 ± 0.01	0.83	↓	0.032	0.174
	C:16	0.15 ± 0.03	0.12 ± 0.05	0.81	↓	0.012	0.104
	C16:2-OH	0.01 ± 0.005	0.01 ± 0.005	0.81	↓	0.037	0.176
	C18:1	0.19 ± 0.04	0.14 ± 0.06	0.77	↓	0.002	0.048
	C18:2	0.06 ± 0.02	0.04 ± 0.02	0.66	↓	2.8×10^{-4}	0.015
	C0	37.26 ± 6.11	41.23 ± 6.00	1.11	↑	0.022	0.138
Phospholipids	lysoPC a C18:0	24.71 ± 6.45	20.01 ± 6.61	0.81	↓	0.005	0.078
	PC aa C28:1	2.85 ± 0.84	2.43 ± 0.95	0.85	↓	0.007	0.085
	PC aa C36:2	203.53 ± 51.70	173.58 ± 42.35	0.85	↓	0.012	0.104
	PC aa C38:0	3.04 ± 1.00	2.44 ± 1.58	0.8	↓	0.024	0.139
	PC aa C40:2	0.29 ± 0.11	0.22 ± 0.12	0.76	↓	0.043	0.185
	PC ae C36:3	6.23 ± 1.31	4.94 ± 2.11	0.79	↓	0.036	0.176
	PC ae C38:6	6.95 ± 2.27	5.92 ± 3.08	0.85	↓	0.046	0.195
	PC ae C40:1	1.38 ± 0.42	1.14 ± 0.60	0.82	↓	0.015	0.113
	PC ae C40:4	2.22 ± 0.32	1.77 ± 0.68	0.8	↓	0.015	0.113
	PC ae C42:3	0.74 ± 0.23	0.61 ± 0.29	0.83	↓	0.039	0.176
	PC ae C42:4	0.71 ± 0.25	0.47 ± 0.41	0.67	↓	0.007	0.085
	PC ae C42:5	2.33 ± 0.30	1.67 ± 0.92	0.72	↓	0.001	0.026
	PC ae C44:5	2.1 ± 0.42	1.37 ± 1.22	0.65	↓	0.001	0.026
	PC ae C44:6	1.25 ± 0.31	0.85 ± 0.65	0.68	↓	3.7×10^{-4}	0.015
Sphyngomielyns	SM C24:0	18.29 ± 5.87	14.75 ± 4.30	0.81	↓	0.018	0.113
	SM C24:1	48.12 ± 13.66	41.99 ± 11.09	0.87	↓	0.047	0.195
	SM-OH C24:1	1.25 ± 0.3	0.93 ± 0.49	0.74	↓	0.014	0.113

Fold change, metabolite concentration after RHRT divided by baseline concentration; Cit, citrulline; Orn, ornithine; Pro, proline; Phe, phenylalanine; Val, valine; alpha-AAA, alpha-amino adipic acid; Trp, tryptophan; Cn:z, acylcarnitine, n = number of carbons, z = number of unsaturations; lysoPC Cn:z, lysophosphatidylcholine; PC Cn:z, phosphatidylcholine; SM Cn:z, sphingomyelins; SM OH Cn:z, hydroxylated sphingomyelins. In bold are metabolites with q-values < 0.05. ↓, down-regulated; ↑, up-regulated.

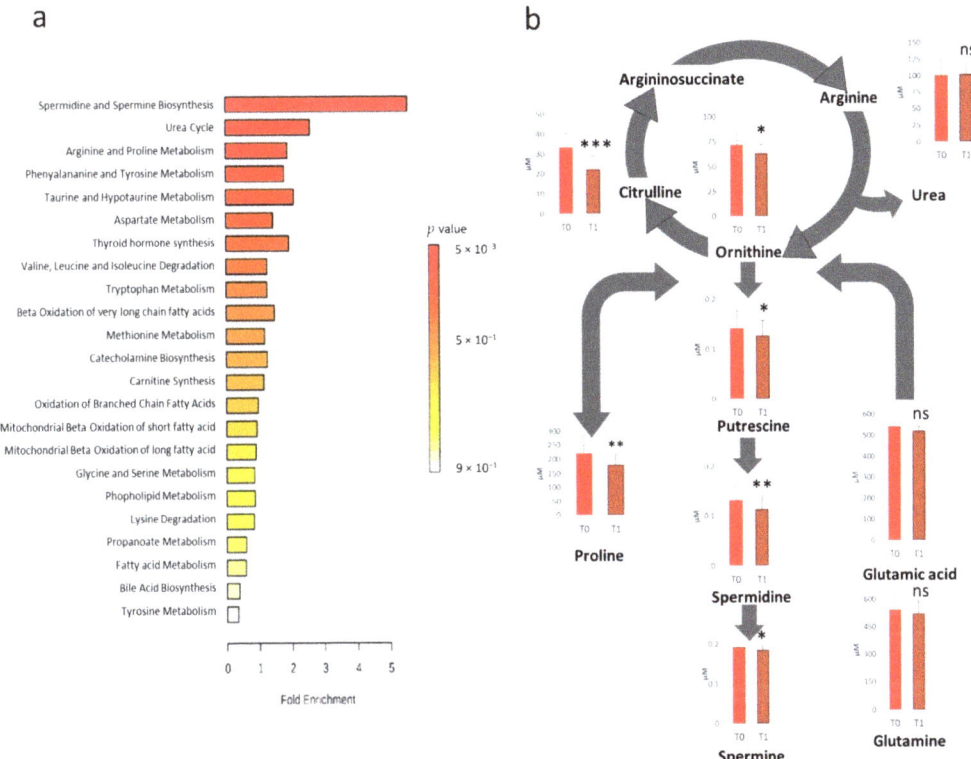

Figure 2. Over Representation Analysis plot from enrichment analysis. Bars represent matched pathways coloured according to their significance values, with gradations from yellow (low significance) to red (high significance) (**a**). Metabolic pathways altered as effect of RHRT and relative metabolites concentrations prior- (T_0) and post-RHRT (T_1) in 19 malignant pleural mesothelioma (MPM) patients. p-values derive from the Student's t-test, *** $p < 0.001$, ** $p < 0.01$, * $p < 0.05$ (**b**).

2.4. Serum Metabolome Variations as Function of Radiation Dose

The amino acids class resulted mostly influenced by the RHRT since 14 out of 36 quantified amino acids and derivatives were significantly altered. Conversely, such widespread effect did not occur in the reference group subjected to palliative LRT at the dose of 21 Gy in 3 fractions. In this latter group, none of the metabolites included in the metabolomics profile analysis underwent significant variations, except citrulline that showed a slight (<10%) decrease ($p = 0.04$, $q = 0.72$) (Figure S4a). The mean fold changes of the metabolites belonging to the amino acids class in the two investigated groups are displayed in Figure S4b where it is evident that the RHRT produced higher variations on serum amino acid metabolites as compared with the LRT. The mean absolute variation of amino acids derivatives was 11.8% (range: 0.44–31.76%) and 4.0% (range: 0.26–11.8%) for RHRT and LRT treatments, respectively.

2.5. RHRT Metabolomics Alterations and Clinical Outcome

The clinical outcome, expressed as median overall survival (OS), was 24 months (95% CI, 17–43 months) for the patients who underwent RHRT. At last follow-up, before the metabolomics data analysis, all investigated patients succumbed to the MPM disease. Their overall OS outcome was not found associated with age, tumour stage or performance status. Conversely, OS was significantly correlated with the serum metabolomics variations induced by RHRT. When partial least square (PLS) analysis was applied, the regression model showed a relevant association between the metabolites' fold changes and the OS, which explained about 60% of interpatients OS variability (Figure 3a). The metabolites that most contributed to the model, as emerged by the loading plot (Figure 3b) and by Pearson correlation analysis were: asymmetric dimethyl-arginine (ADMA), threonine, symmetric dimethyl-arginine (SDMA), putrescine, serine, asparagine and the acyl-carnitines C2, C10:1, C16:2 and C18:1 whose serum variations were positively correlated with OS (Figure 3c).

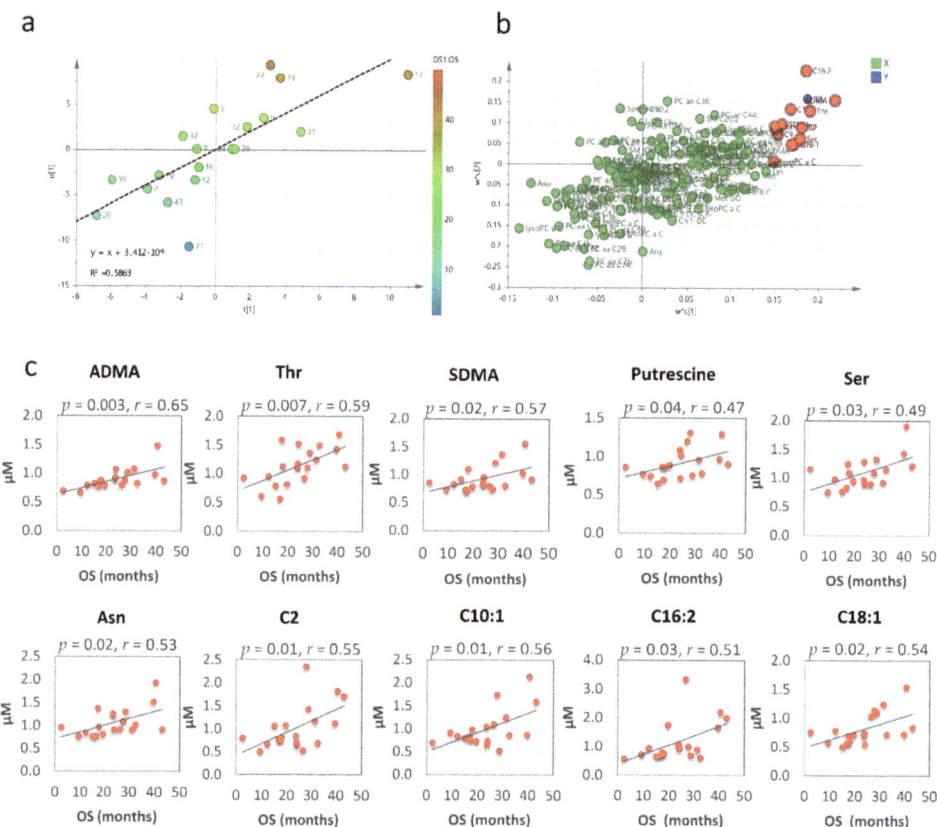

Figure 3. Partial least square (PLS) score plot for the first two latent variables t(1) and u(1), in which each point represents one patient, plotted as scores (or coefficients) from the metabolomics fold changes data (X block) vs. the score from the overall survival (OS) (Y block). Colour gradations from blue to red represents increasing values of OS (**a**). PLS loading plot. Each point is a metabolite plotted as the coefficient from PLS LV1 (first latent variable) vs. the coefficient from LV2 (second latent variable). Metabolites in the top right (highest positive coefficient) or in the bottom left (lowest negative coefficient) have a strong correlation with the OS (**b**). Metabolites fold changes most correlated with OS by Pearson correlation analysis (**c**).

When the patients' population was stratified according to OS quartiles, the mean fold-changes of these specific metabolites were 0.77 ± 0.07 (range: 0.64–0.90) for the patients' group with OS < 16.9 months (Q1), 1.01 ± 0.14 (range: 0.81–1.26) and 1.23 ± 0.17 (range: 0.98–1.47) for those with OS between 16.9 and 28.8 months (IQ) and > 28.8 months (Q4), respectively (Figure S5). Interestingly, when the analysis was focused on the entire class of amino acids, the overall variations for the long survival patients (16.9–43.17 months) resulted 22% higher than that observed for short survival patients (OS < 16.9) (Figure 4).

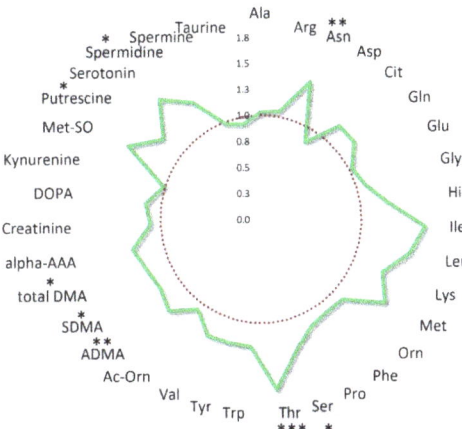

Figure 4. Amino acids mean overall variations of long survival patients normalized to those of short survival patients. Long survival patients belong to IQ (interquartile) and Q4 OS groups; short survival patients belong to the Q1 OS group. Amino acids statistically significant ($p < 0.05$) are highlighted in grey *** $p < 0.001$; ** $p < 0.01$, * $p < 0.05$.

3. Discussion

The application of the ionizing radiation to tumour and surrounding normal tissues elicits complex responses that, behind the DNA cytotoxic activity, disrupt tumour metabolic processes and influence the overall host biochemistry [24].

The present study highlighted that in MPM patients the RHRT treatment is able to produce remarkable systemic metabolomics alterations involving a large set of biochemical pathways as a result of its activity on both normal and tumour tissues. This RT modality was found to produce an overall serum decrease in almost all investigated metabolites. Such depleting effect was commonly observed also for other RT treatment and cancer types suggesting that these serum metabolome drop phenomena could represent a distinctive tract of the host systemic metabolic response to irradiation [18,20–23,25]. Among the metabolites found altered after RHRT, only a small set that included valine and leucine was upregulated. These BCAAs are involved in protein metabolism, energy production and in various biosynthetic pathways which are all overactivated in tumour cells [26,27]. The high BCAA catabolism reported in tumour tissues has been found associated with a systemic deprivation of these amino acids [27–29]. In this context, the post-RHRT increase in valine and leucine may suggest a reduced tumour demand of BCAA as analogously observed in breast cancer patients where a specific raise of serum isoleucine, leucine and valine to normal range was reported after RT treatment [17]. Beyond BCAA, phenylalanine was another essential amino acid significantly increased post-RHRT. This amino acid increases during inflammation conditions [30,31] and its serum levels were found correlated with those of immune activation markers such as neopterin and isoprostane-8 [32,33]. The radiation exposure is known to promote oxidative stress leading to an acute inflammatory status [34,35] and mounting evidence indicates as the RT itself could also stimulate the immune system [36–39] that may be indirectly mirrored by the increase in serum phenylalanine observed after RHRT.

Notably, RHRT was found to influence extensively the lipid metabolism, and in particular, choline-containing phospholipids such as PC, lysoPC and SM derivatives, which underwent a significant serum concentration drop likely associated with the elevated lipids membrane turnover consequent to radiation tissue damage. Thus, this effect may not be specific for RHRT treatment but rather a common trait of the radiation exposure, since a wide lipids drop was also reported in other metabolomics studies regarding different RT treatments [18,19,22,40]. Phospholipids have not only a structural role in the cellular membrane but they also act as signal-transducer metabolites in different cellular pathways including apoptosis [41–43]. In this context, their downregulation, consequent to the RHRT treatment, may contribute to disrupt tumour signalling pathways and synergize with the radiation cellular killing effect [44]. Beyond phospholipids, the acyl-carnitines metabolite class was also found perturbed by RHRT. These lipids derivatives play a critical role in energy production working as a shuttle of fatty acids into the mitochondria, where they undergo β-oxidation for ATP production. In the investigated series of patients, the concomitant increase in carnitine precursor and the overall decrease in acyl-carnitines derivatives may suggest an alteration in their synthesis likely due to low availability of free fatty acids or acetyl-CoA intermediates that may be diverted to restore the phospholipids pool. Despite the broad perturbation of lipid metabolism, only amino acids-related pathways emerged from the set enrichment analysis. These involved the polyamine biosynthesis, urea cycle, and the arginine and proline metabolism that are strictly interconnected to each other sharing arginine as central metabolite. This latter is synthesized in the kidney and, besides its involvement in the urea cycle for ammonia detoxification, it is the substrate for other essential cellular metabolic pathways such as nitric oxide (NO) production [45]. The main endogenous source of arginine is citrulline that was the metabolite subjected to the highest decrease after RHRT. This nonproteogenic amino acid is synthesized in the small intestine from glutamine and ornithine precursors, but it can be also produced in other tissues as a recycled product of the NO synthesis [46]. The citrulline depletion after RHRT might be attributed to the reduction in its enterocytes biosynthesis as a side effect of the high-dose radiations that partially reach the hemithorax surrounding organs. Indeed, citrulline is a well-known biomarker of intestinal failure and a decrease in its blood concentration was registered in inflammatory bowel diseases [47] as well as in patients who received chemotherapy [14,48–50] or RT [51,52]. The systemic loss of citrulline does not seem to affect the arginine synthesis, since its level was unvaried by RHRT, suggesting that the host metabolism maintains a systemic reservoir of such semiessential amino acid at the expense of citrulline.

The RHRT effect is not limited only to arginine pathways but encompasses the whole class of amino acids likely consequent to the high dose of RHRT. Indeed, the patients treated with a low palliative dose of LRT did not show such significant alterations in the observed time-frame compared with those who received the high dose of RHRT. However, a modest but significant citrulline serum shortage was detected also in the LRT group where the involvement of the intestine was negligible suggesting other citrulline fates. Interestingly, citrulline has been revealed to exhibit antioxidant properties working as a suicidal radical-scavenger [53,54], thus in both RHRT and LRT groups, it may be oxidized by the reactive oxygen species (ROS) produced over the RT treatments. In addition, the radiolysis of the protein lysine-residuals leads to the release of alpha-aminoadipic acid [55,56] that was significantly high in the serum post-RHRT. Radiation oxidative injuries could be also suppressed by the sulphur amino acid taurine that works as antioxidant by reinforcing the endogenous radical-scavenger cellular systems [57–60] as recently demonstrated in lung tissues animal model [61]. Therefore, the taurine serum exhaustion after RHRT may indicate an increased tissue up-take of this amino acid as a consequence of the oxidative stress induced by the treatment.

Ornithine, another amino acid belonging to the arginine metabolism, was found significantly affected by RHRT treatment. Its serum decrease was found significantly correlated with that of citrulline being ornithine, together with glutamine, the principal precursor of citrulline [46]. Ornithine can be synthetized also from proline [62], which significantly decreased post-RHRT, suggesting that the radiation treatment can influence the whole ornithine biosynthetic pathways. The ornithine shortage may have relevant consequences because it represents an important precursor of putrescine, spermidine and spermine, collectively called polyamines. These cationic amino acid derivatives play a key role in cell proliferation [63] and the pharmacological inhibition of their synthesis has been demonstrated to induce tumour growth suppression in xenograft models of MPM [64].

In the context of this study, the significant downregulation of the polyamines, due to the low availability of their common precursor ornithine, may be translated into a potential inhibition of tumour growth with beneficial effect on MPM disease control.

Taken all together, these serum metabolomics changes seem to reflect the overall host metabolic mobilization not only to deal with the radiotoxic effects but also to indirectly control the MPM tumour growth. In agreement with this hypothesis, the individual metabolic response to RHRT could have implications in determining the patients' clinical outcome. Indeed, a significant association between the metabolic profile variations and the OS was found for the amino acids and acyl-carnitines derivatives such as ADMA, threonine, SDMA, putrescine, asparagine and serine as well as the acylcarnitines C2, C10:1, C16:2 and C18:1. The patients' groups with medium and high OS showed a higher increase in these metabolites after RHRT indicating that a greater metabolic response to RHRT may yield a better outcome. This observation can be extended to the whole amino acids metabolism further supporting that in long survival patients, the RHRT stimulates a highly dynamic metabolic response likely associated with a superior individual biochemical resilience. Such metabolic activity can be attributed to their high biological reserves availability that allows not only to better contrast the stress but also to integrate the potential stimulating effects of RHRT.

The low sample size of the present investigation does not allow to properly validate the results, and longitudinal studies with a larger cohort of patients are needed before the discovered systemic metabolomics signatures may find definitive clinical applications. Further investigations have to include time-series analyses along the RT treatment and the patients' follow-up to distinguish the acute and long-term effects of RHRT on patients' metabolomics profiles as well as to better identify the most powerful prognostic biomarkers. Moreover, the extension of the coverage of the metabolome considering other biological matrix such urine would allow having a full view of the metabolic response to RHRT.

4. Materials and Methods

4.1. Patients' Population

This metabolomics study enrolled 34 patients from 2014 to 2018 with histologically confirmed MPM referred to Centro di Riferimento Oncologico of Aviano, Italy, for RT after nonradical surgery and systemic chemotherapy. All patients were enrolled within an ongoing randomized phase III study addressed to assess the OS advantages of RHRT over palliative LRT treatment. A test group of 19 patients received RHRT while a reference group of 15 patients underwent standard palliative LTR. The RHRT treatment was delivered with curative intent by IMRT technique to the hemithorax at the pleural surface level from the lung apex to the upper abdomen at the dose of 50 Gy in 25 fractions. The dose was delivered so that 95% of the planned target volume (PTV) was covered by 95% of the prescription dose. Tumour sites with high-fluorodeoxyglucose avidity received simultaneous integrated boosts of 60 Gy. The LRT for the reference group of patients was delivered at 21 Gy in 3 fractions at the thoracotomy scar level. All patients belonging to the test and the reference groups had good respiratory function and normal baseline renal, hepatic and bone marrow functions. The investigation was carried out in accordance with the principles of the Declaration of Helsinki and with approval from Ethics Committee of Centro di Riferimento Oncologico di Aviano (Clinical Trial code ID: CRO-2013-38). All subjects gave written informed consent.

4.2. Sample Collection

Overnight fasting sample (5 mL) was collected from peripheral venous blood at the baseline and at the end of RHRT and LRT treatments. The blood was allowed to clot for 30 min at room temperature and then centrifuged at room temperature for 15 min at 2100 rpm. Serum samples were immediately stored at $-80\ °C$ until metabolomics analysis.

4.3. Study Design

The study aims to explore the systemic metabolomics effects induced by RHRT in a group of 19 MPM patients. For each enrolled patient, serum targeted metabolomics profile was investigated both at the baseline, before the delivery of the RHRT and at the end of the daily 50 Gy/25 fractions administration. The significant metabolomics changes induced by such RT modality were analysed by univariate and multivariate analysis. The serum metabolomics alterations consequent to RHRT were compared with those of a reference group who received LRT to better distinguish the metabolic pathways specifically induced by RHRT.

4.4. Targeted Serum Metabolomics Profile Analysis

Metabolomics analysis of serum samples was performed using the Biocrates Absolute-IDQ P180 kit (Life Science AG, Innsbruck, Austria) targeted to 188 metabolites belonging to the following classes: amino acids ($n = 21$), biogenic amines and polyamines ($n = 19$), acylcarnitines ($n = 40$), lysophosphatidylcholines ($n = 15$), phosphatidylcholines ($n = 77$), sphingolipids ($n = 15$) and hexoses ($n = 1$). The list of all measured metabolites is reported in Table S1. Sample preparation was carried out following the manufacturer's instructions. Briefly, after thawing, 10 μL of serum was transferred into a filter on the upper well of a 96-well sandwich plate. A mixture of internal standards labelled isotopically with deuterium, ^{13}C or ^{15}N was already present in each well. Nitrogen steam drying of filters was followed by derivatization of amino acids with 5% phenyl isothiocyanate (PTC) and a second drying step. Metabolites were then extracted with 500 μL of 5 mM ammonium acetate in methanol and the extraction solution was filtered and diluted with MS running solvent for the analysis.

The instrumentation consisted of a LC ultimate 3000 (Thermo Fisher Scientific, Milan, Italy) coupled with a 4000 QTAP (AB Sciex Framingham, MA, USA) mass spectrometer. Flow injection analysis coupled with tandem mass spectrometry (FIA-MS/MS) was used for the analysis of carnitine, acylcarnitines, lipids and hexoses, while liquid chromatography with tandem mass spectrometry (LC-MS/MS) was used for amino acids and biogenic amines PTC-derivatives separated in a ZORBAX SB 100×2.1 mm column (Agilent, Santa Clara, CA, USA). The triple quadruple operated in multiple reaction monitoring, neutral loss and precursor ion scan modes in positive and negative polarity. The MS/MS signals were integrated by Analyst 1.6.1 software (AB Sciex, Framingham, MA, USA) and quantified using a calibration curve according to the manufacturer's instructions. Quality controls (QCs) at three concentration levels, low (QC1), medium (QC2) and high (QC3), were used to evaluate the performance of the analytical assay using the MetIQ software. Metabolites with serum concentration under the limit of detection were excluded for the statistical analysis.

4.5. Statistical Data Analysis

Quantitative metabolomics data were preprocessed by log transformation and autoscaling normalization. Unsupervised multivariate PCA of serum metabolomics data was applied to identify outliers. Supervised OPLS-DA was used to classify the metabolomics dataset and build a model able to differentiate serum metabolomics profiles at baseline (T_0) and post-RHRT (T_1). The OPLS-DA was validated to exclude data over-fitting using LOOCV by evaluation of the goodness of fit (R^2) and predictive ability (Q^2) values and by random permutation test to verify the true predictive ability of the model. Analysis of variance of cross-validated predictive residuals (CV-ANOVA) was computed for assessing model reliability. Variable Importance in Projection (VIP) that ranks the metabolites contribution in the OPLS-DA model and paired univariate Student's *t*-test were used to identify metabolites whose concentrations differed significantly between T_0 and T_1. Multiple testing false discovery rate (FDR) correction was performed according to Benjamini–Hochberg method and a $q < 0.05$ was considered statistically significant unless otherwise specified.

Metabolite Set Enrichment Analysis was applied to detect the relevant metabolic pathways significantly altered by RHRT. All the metabolites selected by VIP > 1 and $p < 0.05$ were imported and matched in HMDB, PUBCHEM, SMPDB and KEGG databases, thus categorized according to SMPDB library. The most meaningful biochemical patterns altered by RHRT were inferred by the ORA plot where the metabolic pathways were ranked according to their significance values.

Association between the serum metabolomics fold-change (ratio T_1/T_0) and the OS of the patients, calculated from the date of first radiation fraction administration to the death date, was investigated by multivariate PLS analysis between two groups of variables. The Y variable (OS) was predicted using a few linear combinations of X variables (metabolites fold-changes) called latent variables (LVs). The extent of the correlation was evaluated by the regression coefficient of the PLS model (R^2), while the validation of PLS regression model was performed by LOOCV and permutation test. The metabolites that best contributed to the PLS model were identified and selected by the loading plot for the component w*c [1] >0.15 and <−0.15. Data analysis and the statistical evaluations were carried out using SIMCA (Umetrics, v. 14.1) software, GraphPad Prism 7 and MetaboAnalyst v. 4.0 [65].

5. Conclusions

The results of this first exploratory study support the integration of metabolomics for the clinical evaluation of MPM patients. The metabolomics investigation may contribute to better understand the mechanisms underlying the interpatients OS variability to RHRT treatment and to recognize frail patients as a function of their specific metabolic phenotypes. Further validation of such powerful diagnostic tool could effectively improve the selection of the patients who could not receive clinical benefit from the RHRT treatment moving toward alternative personalized treatments.

Supplementary Materials: The following are available online at https://www.mdpi.com/2072-6694/13/3/508/s1, Figure S1: Principal component analysis (PCA) of metabolomics profiles of 19 malignant pleural mesothelioma (MPM) patients before (T_0) and after (T_1) radical hemithoracic radiotherapy (RHRT), Figure S2: Metabolites ranked according to their Variable Importance in Projection (VIP) scores in the orthogonal partial least squares discriminant analysis (OPLS-DA) model, Figure S3: Serum concentrations at baseline (T_0) and post-RHRT (T_1) for metabolites resulted significantly altered in 19 MPM patients, Figure S4: Citrulline serum concentrations at baseline (T_0) and post-RHRT (T_1) in MPM patients underwent local radiotherapy (LRT) and RHRT, Figure S5: Fold changes of serum amino acids and derivatives expressed in MPM patients under RHRT and LRT treatments, Table S1: Metabolites included in the targeted metabolomics analysis, Table S2: Clinical characteristics of LRT group's patients.

Author Contributions: Conceptualization, G.C.; methodology, E.D.G.; G.C.; E.M. (Elena Muraro), A.S. (Asia Saorin), A.R., E.M. (Emilio Minatel) and M.C.; formal analysis, E.D.G., G.C., G.M., and A.R.; investigation, E.D.G., A.S., E.M. (Asia Saorin), E.M. (Elena Muraro), A.R., E.M. (Emilio Minatel), M.C., and M.T.; data curation, A.R., G.C., and E.D.G.; writing original draft preparation, E.D.G., G.M., and G.C.; supervision, G.C. and A.S. (Agostino Steffan); visualization, E.D.G., G.C.; G.M., E.M. (Elena Muraro), A.S. (Asia Saorin), A.R., E.M. (Emilio Minatel), M.C., M.T., and A.S. (Agostino Steffan); project administration, G.C.; funding acquisition, G.C. and A.S. (Agostino Steffan). All authors have read and agreed to the published version of the manuscript.

Funding: This work was supported by the Italian Ministry of Health (Ricerca Corrente).

Institutional Review Board Statement: The study was conducted according to the guidelines of the Declaration of Helsinki and approved by the Ethics Committee of Centro di Riferimento Oncologico di Aviano (Clinical Trial code ID: CRO-2013-38, December 2013).

Informed Consent Statement: Informed consent was obtained from all subjects involved in the study.

Data Availability Statement: The data presented in this study are available on request from the corresponding author.

Conflicts of Interest: The authors declare no conflict of interest.

References

1. Noonan, C.W. Environmental Asbestos Exposure and Risk of Mesothelioma. *Ann. Transl. Med.* **2017**, *5*. [CrossRef] [PubMed]
2. Musk, A.W.; Olsen, N.; Alfonso, H.; Reid, A.; Mina, R.; Franklin, P.; Sleith, J.; Hammond, N.; Threlfall, T.; Shilkin, K.B.; et al. Predicting Survival in Malignant Mesothelioma. *Eur. Respir. J.* **2011**, *38*, 1420–1424. [CrossRef] [PubMed]
3. Fahrner, R.; Ochsenbein, A.; Schmid, R.A.; Carboni, G.L. Long Term Survival after Trimodal Therapy in Malignant Pleural Mesothelioma. *Swiss Med. Wkly.* **2012**, *142*. [CrossRef] [PubMed]
4. Hasegawa, S.; Okada, M.; Tanaka, F.; Yamanaka, T.; Soejima, T.; Kamikonya, N.; Tsujimura, T.; Fukuoka, K.; Yokoi, K.; Nakano, T. Trimodality Strategy for Treating Malignant Pleural Mesothelioma: Results of a Feasibility Study of Induction Pemetrexed plus Cisplatin Followed by Extrapleural Pneumonectomy and Postoperative Hemithoracic Radiation (Japan Mesothelioma Interest Group 0601 Trial). *Int. J. Clin. Oncol.* **2016**, *21*, 523–530. [CrossRef]
5. Rosenzweig, K.E. Malignant Pleural Mesothelioma: Adjuvant Therapy with Radiation Therapy. *Ann. Transl. Med.* **2017**, *5*. [CrossRef]
6. Foroudi, F.; Smith, J.G.; Putt, F.; Wada, M. High-Dose Palliative Radiotherapy for Malignant Pleural Mesothelioma. *J. Med. Imaging Radiat. Oncol.* **2017**, *61*, 797–803. [CrossRef]
7. Parisi, E.; Romeo, A.; Sarnelli, A.; Ghigi, G.; Bellia, S.R.; Neri, E.; Micheletti, S.; Dipalma, B.; Arpa, D.; Furini, G.; et al. High Dose Irradiation after Pleurectomy/Decortication or Biopsy for Pleural Mesothelioma Treatment. *Cancer Radiother.* **2017**, *21*, 766–773. [CrossRef]
8. Minatel, E.; Trovo, M.; Bearz, A.; Maso, M.D.; Baresic, T.; Drigo, A.; Barresi, L.; Furlan, C.; Conte, A.D.; Bruschi, G.; et al. Radical Radiation Therapy after Lung-Sparing Surgery for Malignant Pleural Mesothelioma: Survival, Pattern of Failure, and Prognostic Factors. *Int. J. Radiat. Oncol. Biol. Phys.* **2015**, *93*, 606–613. [CrossRef] [PubMed]
9. Rosenzweig, K.E.; Zauderer, M.G.; Laser, B.; Krug, L.M.; Yorke, E.; Sima, C.S.; Rimner, A.; Flores, R.; Rusch, V. Pleural Intensity-Modulated Radiation Therapy (IMRT) for Malignant Pleural Mesothelioma (MPM). *Int. J. Radiat. Oncol. Biol. Phys.* **2012**, *83*, 1278–1283. [CrossRef]
10. Clish, C.B. Metabolomics: An Emerging but Powerful Tool for Precision Medicine. *Cold Spring Harb. Mol. Case Stud.* **2015**, *1*. [CrossRef]
11. Corona, G.; Rizzolio, F.; Giordano, A.; Toffoli, G. Pharmaco-Metabolomics: An Emerging "Omics" Tool for the Personalization of Anticancer Treatments and Identification of New Valuable Therapeutic Targets. *J. Cell. Physiol.* **2012**, *227*, 2827–2831. [CrossRef] [PubMed]
12. Wishart, D.S. Metabolomics for Investigating Physiological and Pathophysiological Processes. *Physiol. Rev.* **2019**, *99*, 1819–1875. [CrossRef] [PubMed]
13. Debik, J.; Euceda, L.R.; Lundgren, S.; von der Lippe Gythfeldt, H.; Garred, Ø.; Borgen, E.; Engebraaten, O.; Bathen, T.F.; Giskeødegård, G.F. Assessing Treatment Response and Prognosis by Serum and Tissue Metabolomics in Breast Cancer Patients. *J. Proteome Res.* **2019**, *18*, 3649–3660. [CrossRef] [PubMed]
14. Miolo, G.; Di Gregorio, E.; Saorin, A.; Lombardi, D.; Scalone, S.; Buonadonna, A.; Steffan, A.; Corona, G. Integration of Serum Metabolomics into Clinical Assessment to Improve Outcome Prediction of Metastatic Soft Tissue Sarcoma Patients Treated with Trabectedin. *Cancers* **2020**, *12*, 1983. [CrossRef]
15. Vignoli, A.; Muraro, E.; Miolo, G.; Tenori, L.; Turano, P.; Di Gregorio, E.; Steffan, A.; Luchinat, C.; Corona, G. Effect of Estrogen Receptor Status on Circulatory Immune and Metabolomics Profiles of HER2-Positive Breast Cancer Patients Enrolled for Neoadjuvant Targeted Chemotherapy. *Cancers* **2020**, *12*, 314. [CrossRef]
16. Xu, P.-P.; Xiong, J.; Cheng, S.; Zhao, X.; Wang, C.-F.; Cai, G.; Zhong, H.-J.; Huang, H.-Y.; Chen, J.-Y.; Zhao, W.-L. A Phase II Study of Methotrexate, Etoposide, Dexamethasone and Pegaspargase Sandwiched with Radiotherapy in the Treatment of Newly Diagnosed, Stage IE to IIE Extranodal Natural-Killer/T-Cell Lymphoma, Nasal-Type. *EBioMedicine* **2017**, *25*, 41–49. [CrossRef]
17. Arenas, M.; Rodríguez, E.; García-Heredia, A.; Fernández-Arroyo, S.; Sabater, S.; Robaina, R.; Gascón, M.; Rodríguez-Pla, M.; Cabré, N.; Luciano-Mateo, F.; et al. Metabolite Normalization with Local Radiotherapy Following Breast Tumor Resection. *PLoS ONE* **2018**, *13*, e0207474. [CrossRef]
18. Jelonek, K.; Krzywon, A.; Jablonska, P.; Slominska, E.M.; Smolenski, R.T.; Polanska, J.; Rutkowski, T.; Mrochem-Kwarciak, J.; Skladowski, K.; Widlak, P. Systemic Effects of Radiotherapy and Concurrent Chemo-Radiotherapy in Head and Neck Cancer Patients—Comparison of Serum Metabolome Profiles. *Metabolites* **2020**, *10*, 60. [CrossRef]
19. Jelonek, K.; Pietrowska, M.; Ros, M.; Zagdanski, A.; Suchwalko, A.; Polanska, J.; Marczyk, M.; Rutkowski, T.; Skladowski, K.; Clench, M.R.; et al. Radiation-Induced Changes in Serum Lipidome of Head and Neck Cancer Patients. *Int. J. Mol. Sci.* **2014**, *15*, 6609–6624. [CrossRef]
20. Laiakis, E.C.; Mak, T.D.; Anizan, S.; Amundson, S.A.; Barker, C.A.; Wolden, S.L.; Brenner, D.J.; Fornace, A.J. Development of a Metabolomic Radiation Signature in Urine from Patients Undergoing Total Body Irradiation. *Radiat. Res.* **2014**, *181*, 350–361. [CrossRef]
21. Mörén, L.; Wibom, C.; Bergström, P.; Johansson, M.; Antti, H.; Bergenheim, A.T. Characterization of the Serum Metabolome Following Radiation Treatment in Patients with High-Grade Gliomas. *Radiat. Oncol.* **2016**, *11*, 51. [CrossRef] [PubMed]
22. Nalbantoglu, S.; Abu-Asab, M.; Suy, S.; Collins, S.; Amri, H. Metabolomics-Based Biosignatures of Prostate Cancer in Patients Following Radiotherapy. *OMICS J. Integr. Biol.* **2019**, *23*, 214–223. [CrossRef] [PubMed]

23. Ng, S.S.W.; Jang, G.H.; Kurland, I.J.; Qiu, Y.; Guha, C.; Dawson, L.A. Plasma Metabolomic Profiles in Liver Cancer Patients Following Stereotactic Body Radiotherapy. *EBioMedicine* **2020**, *59*, 102973. [CrossRef] [PubMed]
24. Bentzen, S.M. Preventing or Reducing Late Side Effects of Radiation Therapy: Radiobiology Meets Molecular Pathology. *Nat. Rev. Cancer* **2006**, *6*, 702–713. [CrossRef]
25. Wojakowska, A.; Zebrowska, A.; Skowronek, A.; Rutkowski, T.; Polanski, K.; Widlak, P.; Marczak, L.; Pietrowska, M. Metabolic Profiles of Whole Serum and Serum-Derived Exosomes Are Different in Head and Neck Cancer Patients Treated by Radiotherapy. *J. Pers. Med.* **2020**, *10*, 229. [CrossRef]
26. Ananieva, E.A.; Wilkinson, A.C. Branched-Chain Amino Acid Metabolism in Cancer. *Curr. Opin. Clin. Nutr. Metab. Care* **2018**, *21*, 64–70. [CrossRef]
27. Thewes, V.; Simon, R.; Hlevnjak, M.; Schlotter, M.; Schroeter, P.; Schmidt, K.; Wu, Y.; Anzeneder, T.; Wang, W.; Windisch, P.; et al. The Branched-Chain Amino Acid Transaminase 1 Sustains Growth of Antiestrogen-Resistant and ERα-Negative Breast Cancer. *Oncogene* **2017**, *36*, 4124–4134. [CrossRef]
28. Mayers, J.R.; Torrence, M.E.; Danai, L.V.; Papagiannakopoulos, T.; Davidson, S.M.; Bauer, M.R.; Lau, A.N.; Ji, B.W.; Dixit, P.D.; Hosios, A.M.; et al. Tissue of Origin Dictates Branched-Chain Amino Acid Metabolism in Mutant Kras-Driven Cancers. *Science* **2016**, *353*, 1161–1165. [CrossRef]
29. Tönjes, M.; Barbus, S.; Park, Y.J.; Wang, W.; Schlotter, M.; Lindroth, A.M.; Pleier, S.V.; Bai, A.H.C.; Karra, D.; Piro, R.M.; et al. BCAT1 Promotes Cell Proliferation through Amino Acid Catabolism in Gliomas Carrying Wild-Type IDH1. *Nat. Med.* **2013**, *19*, 901–908. [CrossRef]
30. Geisler, S.; Gostner, J.M.; Becker, K.; Ueberall, F.; Fuchs, D. Immune Activation and Inflammation Increase the Plasma Phenylalanine-to-Tyrosine Ratio. *Pteridines* **2013**, *24*, 27–31. [CrossRef]
31. Murr, C.; Grammer, T.B.; Meinitzer, A.; Kleber, M.E.; März, W.; Fuchs, D. Immune Activation and Inflammation in Patients with Cardiovascular Disease Are Associated with Higher Phenylalanine to Tyrosine Ratios: The Ludwigshafen Risk and Cardiovascular Health Study. *J. Amino Acids* **2014**, *2014*. [CrossRef] [PubMed]
32. Neurauter, G.; Grahmann, A.V.; Klieber, M.; Zeimet, A.; Ledochowski, M.; Sperner-Unterweger, B.; Fuchs, D. Serum Phenylalanine Concentrations in Patients with Ovarian Carcinoma Correlate with Concentrations of Immune Activation Markers and of Isoprostane-8. *Cancer Lett.* **2008**, *272*, 141–147. [CrossRef] [PubMed]
33. Ploder, M.; Neurauter, G.; Spittler, A.; Schroecksnadel, K.; Roth, E.; Fuchs, D. Serum Phenylalanine in Patients Post Trauma and with Sepsis Correlate to Neopterin Concentrations. *Amino Acids* **2008**, *35*, 303–307. [CrossRef] [PubMed]
34. Jelonek, K.; Pietrowska, M.; Widlak, P. Systemic Effects of Ionizing Radiation at the Proteome and Metabolome Levels in the Blood of Cancer Patients Treated with Radiotherapy: The Influence of Inflammation and Radiation Toxicity. *Int. J. Radiat. Biol.* **2017**, *93*, 683–696. [CrossRef]
35. McKelvey, K.J.; Hudson, A.L.; Back, M.; Eade, T.; Diakos, C.I. Radiation, Inflammation and the Immune Response in Cancer. *Mamm. Genome* **2018**, *29*, 843–865. [CrossRef]
36. Deloch, L.; Derer, A.; Hartmann, J.; Frey, B.; Fietkau, R.; Gaipl, U.S. Modern Radiotherapy Concepts and the Impact of Radiation on Immune Activation. *Front. Oncol.* **2016**, *6*, 141. [CrossRef]
37. Di Maggio, F.M.; Minafra, L.; Forte, G.I.; Cammarata, F.P.; Lio, D.; Messa, C.; Gilardi, M.C.; Bravatà, V. Portrait of Inflammatory Response to Ionizing Radiation Treatment. *J. Inflamm.* **2015**, *12*, 14. [CrossRef]
38. Huang, J.; Li, J.J. Cell Repopulation, Rewiring Metabolism, and Immune Regulation in Cancer Radiotherapy. *Radiat. Med. Prot.* **2020**, *1*, 24–30. [CrossRef]
39. Muraro, E.; Furlan, C.; Avanzo, M.; Martorelli, D.; Comaro, E.; Rizzo, A.; Fae, D.A.; Berretta, M.; Militello, L.; Del Conte, A.; et al. Local High-Dose Radiotherapy Induces Systemic Immunomodulating Effects of Potential Therapeutic Relevance in Oligometastatic Breast Cancer. *Front. Immunol.* **2017**, *8*, 1476. [CrossRef]
40. Boguszewicz, Ł.; Bieleń, A.; Mrochem-Kwarciak, J.; Skorupa, A.; Ciszek, M.; Heyda, A.; Wygoda, A.; Kotylak, A.; Składowski, K.; Sokół, M. NMR-Based Metabolomics in Real-Time Monitoring of Treatment Induced Toxicity and Cachexia in Head and Neck Cancer: A Method for Early Detection of High Risk Patients. *Metabolomics* **2019**, *15*, 110. [CrossRef]
41. Bartke, N.; Hannun, Y.A. Bioactive Sphingolipids: Metabolism and Function. *J. Lipid Res.* **2009**, *50*, S91–S96. [CrossRef] [PubMed]
42. Eyster, K.M. The Membrane and Lipids as Integral Participants in Signal Transduction: Lipid Signal Transduction for the Non-Lipid Biochemist. *Adv. Physiol. Educ.* **2007**, *31*, 5–16. [CrossRef] [PubMed]
43. Wright, M.M.; Howe, A.G.; Zaremberg, V. Cell Membranes and Apoptosis: Role of Cardiolipin, Phosphatidylcholine, and Anticancer Lipid Analogues. *Biochem. Cell Biol.* **2004**, *82*, 18–26. [CrossRef] [PubMed]
44. Verheij, M.; van Blitterswijk, W.J.; Bartelink, H. Radiation-Induced Apoptosis: The Ceramide-SAPK Signaling Pathway and Clinical Aspects. *Acta Oncol.* **1998**, *37*, 575–581. [CrossRef] [PubMed]
45. Wu, G.; Morris, S.M. Arginine Metabolism: Nitric Oxide and Beyond. *Biochem. J.* **1998**, *336*, 1–17. [CrossRef] [PubMed]
46. Curis, E.; Nicolis, I.; Moinard, C.; Osowska, S.; Zerrouk, N.; Bénazeth, S.; Cynober, L. Almost All about Citrulline in Mammals. *Amino Acids* **2005**, *29*, 177. [CrossRef]
47. Crenn, P.; Messing, B.; Cynober, L. Citrulline as a Biomarker of Intestinal Failure Due to Enterocyte Mass Reduction. *Clin. Nutr.* **2008**, *27*, 328–339. [CrossRef]
48. Blijlevens, N.M.A.; Lutgens, L.C.H.W.; Schattenberg, A.V.M.B.; Donnelly, J.P. Citrulline: A Potentially Simple Quantitative Marker of Intestinal Epithelial Damage Following Myeloablative Therapy. *Bone Marrow Transplant.* **2004**, *34*, 193–196. [CrossRef]

49. Ouaknine Krief, J.; Helly de Tauriers, P.; Dumenil, C.; Neveux, N.; Dumoulin, J.; Giraud, V.; Labrune, S.; Tisserand, J.; Julie, C.; Emile, J.-F.; et al. Role of Antibiotic Use, Plasma Citrulline and Blood Microbiome in Advanced Non-Small Cell Lung Cancer Patients Treated with Nivolumab. *J. Immunother. Cancer* **2019**, *7*, 176. [CrossRef]
50. Bachmayr-Heyda, A.; Aust, S.; Auer, K.; Meier, S.M.; Schmetterer, K.G.; Dekan, S.; Gerner, C.; Pils, D. Integrative Systemic and Local Metabolomics with Impact on Survival in High-Grade Serous Ovarian Cancer. *Clin. Cancer Res.* **2017**, *23*, 2081–2092. [CrossRef]
51. Lutgens, L.C.H.W.; Deutz, N.E.P.; Gueulette, J.; Cleutjens, J.P.M.; Berger, M.P.F.; Wouters, B.G.; von Meyenfeldt, M.F.; Lambin, P. Citrulline: A Physiologic Marker Enabling Quantitation and Monitoring of Epithelial Radiation-Induced Small Bowel Damage. *Int. J. Radiat. Oncol.* **2003**, *57*, 1067–1074. [CrossRef]
52. Onal, C.; Kotek, A.; Unal, B.; Arslan, G.; Yavuz, A.; Topkan, E.; Yavuz, M. Plasma Citrulline Levels Predict Intestinal Toxicity in Patients Treated with Pelvic Radiotherapy. *Acta Oncol.* **2011**, *50*, 1167–1174. [CrossRef] [PubMed]
53. Akashi, K.; Miyake, C.; Yokota, A. Citrulline, a Novel Compatible Solute in Drought-Tolerant Wild Watermelon Leaves, Is an Efficient Hydroxyl Radical Scavenger. *FEBS Lett.* **2001**, *508*, 438–442. [CrossRef]
54. Ginguay, A.; Regazzetti, A.; Laprevote, O.; Moinard, C.; De Bandt, J.-P.; Cynober, L.; Billard, J.-M.; Allinquant, B.; Dutar, P. Citrulline Prevents Age-Related LTP Decline in Old Rats. *Sci. Rep.* **2019**, *9*, 20138. [CrossRef]
55. Requena, J.R.; Chao, C.-C.; Levine, R.L.; Stadtman, E.R. Glutamic and Aminoadipic Semialdehydes Are the Main Carbonyl Products of Metal-Catalyzed Oxidation of Proteins. *PNAS* **2001**, *98*, 69–74. [CrossRef]
56. Sell, D.R.; Strauch, C.M.; Shen, W.; Monnier, V.M. 2-Aminoadipic Acid Is a Marker of Protein Carbonyl Oxidation in the Aging Human Skin: Effects of Diabetes, Renal Failure and Sepsis. *Biochem. J.* **2007**, *404*, 269–277. [CrossRef]
57. Das, J.; Sil, P.C. Taurine Ameliorates Alloxan-Induced Diabetic Renal Injury, Oxidative Stress-Related Signaling Pathways and Apoptosis in Rats. *Amino Acids* **2012**, *43*, 1509–1523. [CrossRef]
58. Jong, C.J.; Azuma, J.; Schaffer, S. Mechanism Underlying the Antioxidant Activity of Taurine: Prevention of Mitochondrial Oxidant Production. *Amino Acids* **2012**, *42*, 2223–2232. [CrossRef]
59. Sevin, G.; Ozsarlak-Sozer, G.; Keles, D.; Gokce, G.; Reel, B.; Ozgur, H.H.; Oktay, G.; Kerry, Z. Taurine Inhibits Increased MMP-2 Expression in a Model of Oxidative Stress Induced by Glutathione Depletion in Rabbit Heart. *Eur. J. Pharmacol.* **2013**, *706*, 98–106. [CrossRef]
60. Tabassum, H.; Rehman, H.; Banerjee, B.D.; Raisuddin, S.; Parvez, S. Attenuation of Tamoxifen-Induced Hepatotoxicity by Taurine in Mice. *Clin. Chim. Acta* **2006**, *370*, 129–136. [CrossRef]
61. Gao, Y.; Li, X.; Gao, J.; Zhang, Z.; Feng, Y.; Nie, J.; Zhu, W.; Zhang, S.; Cao, J. Metabolomic Analysis of Radiation-Induced Lung Injury in Rats: The Potential Radioprotective Role of Taurine. *Dose Response* **2019**, *17*. [CrossRef] [PubMed]
62. Marini, J.C. Interrelationships between Glutamine and Citrulline Metabolism. *Curr. Opin. Clin. Nutr. Metab. Care* **2016**, *19*, 62–66. [CrossRef] [PubMed]
63. Casero, R.A.; Murray Stewart, T.; Pegg, A.E. Polyamine Metabolism and Cancer: Treatments, Challenges and Opportunities. *Nat. Rev. Cancer* **2018**, *18*, 681–695. [CrossRef] [PubMed]
64. Lam, S.-K.; Yan, S.; Xu, S.; Ho, J.C.-M. Targeting Polyamine as a Novel Therapy in Xenograft Models of Malignant Pleural Mesothelioma. *Lung Cancer* **2020**, *148*, 138–148. [CrossRef]
65. Chong, J.; Wishart, D.S.; Xia, J. Using MetaboAnalyst 4.0 for Comprehensive and Integrative Metabolomics Data Analysis. *Curr. Protoc. Bioinform.* **2019**, *68*, e86. [CrossRef] [PubMed]

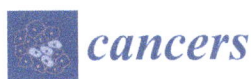

Article

Systematic Analysis of Aberrant Biochemical Networks and Potential Drug Vulnerabilities Induced by Tumor Suppressor Loss in Malignant Pleural Mesothelioma

Haitang Yang [1,2], Duo Xu [1], Zhang Yang [1], Feng Yao [2], Heng Zhao [2], Ralph A. Schmid [1,*] and Ren-Wang Peng [1,*]

1. Division of General Thoracic Surgery, Department of BioMedical Research (DBMR), Inselspital, Bern University Hospital, University of Bern, Murtenstrasse 50, CH3008 Bern, Switzerland; haitang.yang@dbmr.unibe.ch (H.Y.); duo.xu@dbmr.unibe.ch (D.X.); zhang.yang@dbmr.unibe.ch (Z.Y.)
2. Department of Thoracic Surgery, Shanghai Chest Hospital, Shanghai Jiao Tong University, Shanghai 200030, China; feng.yao@shchest.org (F.Y.); zh148@shchest.org (H.Z.)
* Correspondence: Ralph.Schmid@insel.ch (R.A.S.); Renwang.Peng@insel.ch (R.-W.P.)

Received: 13 June 2020; Accepted: 4 August 2020; Published: 17 August 2020

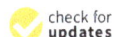

Abstract: *Background*: Malignant pleural mesothelioma (MPM) is driven by the inactivation of tumor suppressor genes (TSGs). An unmet need in the field is the translation of the genomic landscape into effective TSG-specific therapies. *Methods*: We correlated genomes against transcriptomes of patients' MPM tumors, by weighted gene co-expression network analysis (WGCNA). The identified aberrant biochemical networks and potential drug targets induced by tumor suppressor loss were validated by integrative data analysis and functional interrogation. *Results*: CDKN2A/2B loss activates G2/M checkpoint and PI3K/AKT, prioritizing a co-targeting strategy for CDKN2A/2B-null MPM. CDKN2A deficiency significantly co-occurs with deletions of anti-viral type I interferon (IFN-I) genes and BAP1 mutations, that enriches the IFN-I signature, stratifying a unique subset, with deficient IFN-I, but proficient BAP1 for oncolytic viral immunotherapies. Aberrant p53 attenuates differentiation and SETD2 loss acquires the dependency on EGFRs, highlighting the potential of differentiation therapy and pan-EGFR inhibitors for these subpopulations, respectively. LATS2 deficiency is linked with dysregulated immunoregulation, suggesting a rationale for immune checkpoint blockade. Finally, multiple lines of evidence support Dasatinib as a promising therapeutic for LATS2-mutant MPM. *Conclusions*: Systematic identification of abnormal cellular processes and potential drug vulnerabilities specified by TSG alterations provide a framework for precision oncology in MPM.

Keywords: mesothelioma; tumor suppressor; targeted therapy; immunotherapy

1. Introduction

Malignant pleural mesothelioma (MPM) is a deadly cancer with incidence and mortality still increasing globally [1]. The leading cause for the poor prognosis of MPM is the extreme dearth of effective treatment options. The great majority of MPM patients present with advanced diseases, for whom a chemotherapy regimen (cisplatin plus pemetrexed) established in 2003 remains the only clinically approved first-line therapy [2].

Comprehensive genomic studies in MPM have revealed a rarity of pharmacologically tractable mutations in oncogenes [3–5], but the prevalence of inactivating alterations in tumor suppressor genes (TSGs), e.g., cyclin-dependent kinase inhibitor 2A/2B (*CDKN2A/2B*), BRCA1-associated protein-1 (*BAP1*), neurofibromin 2 (*NF2*), tumor protein p53 (*TP53*), SET domain containing 2 histone lysine methyltransferase (*SETD2*) and large tumor suppressor kinase 2 (*LATS2*). While the pharmacological inhibition of oncoproteins is successful, targeted therapies that exploit abnormal TSGs have proven far more difficult. Precision oncology, a burgeoning effort aimed at targeting unique molecular alterations of individual patients, has achieved great success in many cancers, but significantly lags behind in MPM. Consequently, clinical trials in MPM without biomarker-directed stratifications have generally failed [6–9].

Although the direct intervention of tumor suppressors is challenging, aberrant TSGs induce the reprogramming of biochemical networks, which creates cancer-specific vulnerabilities and provides an alternative venue for precision oncology in TSG-driven cancer [10]. Systematic correlation analysis is a powerful tool to identify rewired cellular processes, potential therapeutic targets, and associated biomarkers [11]. Here, by implementing weighted gene co-expression network analysis (WGCNA) [12], paralleled by comprehensive data mining and functional interrogation, we systematically delineated the biochemical networks induced by the inactivation of major TSGs (*CDKN2A/2B*, *BAP1*, *NF2*, *TP53*, *SETD2*, and *LATS2*) in MPM, and the underlying implications for precision oncology. Identification of molecular traits and the associated drug vulnerabilities co-selected by the functional loss of specific TSGs provides unprecedented insights into MPM pathobiology and may promote personalized treatment of MPM patients with molecularly guided, targeted- and immuno-therapy.

2. Results

2.1. Systematic Analysis of Rewired Biochemical Networks and Therapeutic Vulnerabilities Enabled by Tumor Suppressor Loss in MPM

All the major genetic alterations (>10%) occurring in TCGA MPM cohort are TSGs, including *CDKN2A/2B* (homozygous deletions (HDs)), *BAP1* (HDs and point mutations), *NF2* (HDs and point mutations), *TP53* (point mutations), *SETD2* (HDs and point mutations), and *LATS2* (HDs and point mutations) (Figure 1A). Notably, there are substantial overlaps of alterations in different TSGs (Figure 1B). For instance, the majority (67.6%) of the MPM tumors that harbor HDs of *CDKN2A/2B* have co-occurring alterations in other TSGs, e.g., *BAP1* (40.5%) or *NF2* (37.8%). Importantly, analyses of RPPA data of TCGA MPM cohort ($n = 61$) showed that genetic alterations remarkably decreased the levels of the encoded proteins or downstream effectors (Figure 1C).

To uncover fundamental molecular features associated with the functional loss of TSGs in MPM, we performed WGCNA, based on the transcriptomic data of TCGA MPM cohort (Figure 1D and Figure S1A–D), and delineated a network of multiple modules or clusters, that are significantly positively or negatively correlated with genetic inactivation of the top six TSGs in MPM (Figure S1E). Genes in the positively correlated modules indicate the abundance of the module-specified traits conferred by individual TSG loss, while those in the negatively correlated ones indicate the attenuation. Genes in the gray module are those that cannot be clustered.

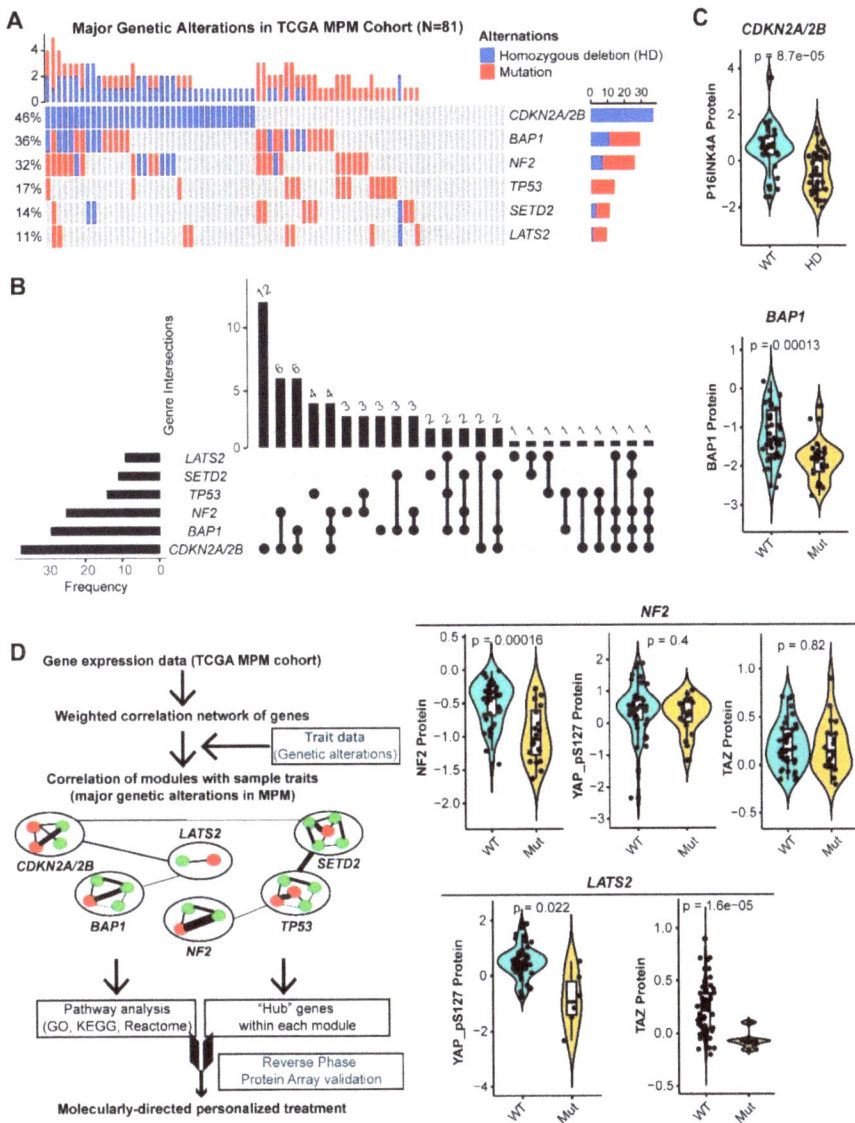

Figure 1. Major genetic alterations in The Cancer Genome Atlas (TCGA) MPM cohort. (**A**,**B**), Percentage (**A**) and overlap (**B**) of major (>10%) genetic alterations in The Cancer Genome Atlas (TCGA) malignant pleural mesothelioma (MPM) cohort ($N = 81$). (**C**), the association between the major genetic alterations (**A**) and the corresponding protein level in TCGA MPM cohort ($N = 61$). Protein array data were downloaded and reanalyzed from The Cancer Proteome Atlas (TCPA) database (https://tcpaportal.org/tcpa/). Of note, protein quantification data of LATS2 and SETD2 were not available in the TCPA database. Phospho-YAP (S127) and TAZ are two critical factors, indicating the activity of Hippo pathway. (**D**), Workflow of weighted gene correlation networks analysis (WGCNA).

2.2. CDKN2A/2B

CDKN2A/2B encodes three tumor suppressors, p16^{INK4a} and p14^{ARF} (by *CDKN2A*) and p15^{INK4b} (by *CDKN2B*), that play critical roles in cell cycle regulation. Moreover, p16^{INK4a} and p15^{INK4b} are functionally redundant by inhibiting cyclin-dependent kinase (CDK) 4/6 and cyclin D, and consequently blocking cell cycle progression from G1 to S [13].

The correlation network showed that *CDKN2A/2B* loss in MPM was significantly positively correlated with the green module (508 genes; correlation coefficient Pearson's r = 0.55; *p*-value = 2 × 10^{-7}, followed by the yellow (543 genes; r = 0.34; *p*-value = 0.002), but negatively with the red (356 genes; r = −0.36; *p*-value = 0.001) (Figure S1E). Pathway analyses (GO, KEGG, Reactome) revealed that the green module enriched the genes involved in cell cycle regulation, particularly checkpoints and mitosis (Figure 2A,B and Figure S2A), consistent with the function of *CDKN2A/2B* in cell-cycle regulation. The yellow module significantly enriched the genes of extracellular matrix (ECM)-receptor interaction, PI3K/AKT, and focal adhesion pathways (Figure 2C,D and Figure S2B,C). Interrogation of the RPPA data revealed that MPM deficient in *CDKN2A/2B* had significantly higher levels of proteins involved in the cell cycle (e.g., Cyclin B1, Cyclin E2, CDK1 (p-Y15), FOXM1) and PI3K (e.g., 4EBP1 and PKC-delta (p-S664)) pathways, but decreased p16^{INK4a} and PTEN (a negative regulator of PI3K) (Figure 2E), further supporting our results.

The red module negatively correlated with *CDKN2A/2B* loss enriched genes of anti-viral type I interferon (IFN-I, mainly IFN-α and IFN-β) signaling pathway, suggesting a link between *CDKN2A/2B* inactivation and impaired IFN-I pathway (Figure 2E–G and Figure S2D). To explore the underlying mechanisms, we analyzed co-occurring alterations in MPM samples, which revealed that *CDKN2A* and genes of the IFN family were significantly co-deleted (Figure 2H), consistent with a recent study, showing that defects in the IFN-I pathway mainly co-occur with *CDKN2A* loss [14].

We then analyzed intramodular connectivity, given that highly connected genes may serve as the hub with core regulatory roles. The top 20 best-connected genes in the green module are *KIF23, KIF4A, KIF2C, HJURP, KIF18B, MYBL2, BUB1, NUF2, UBE2C, CDCA8, CKAP2L, PLK1, DLGAP5, CDC20, TOP2A, DEPDC1, ANLN, CENPA, CDCA2, CEP55*. Most of these genes regulate the mitotic process and predict dismal prognosis in MPM (Figure S2E). Notably, the transcription factor MYBL2 is a central regulator of cell survival, proliferation and differentiation in cancer [15], and PLK1 and TOP2A are druggable by clinically advanced inhibitors. The top 20 best-connected genes in the yellow module are *COL5A1, VCAN, COL1A2, DACT1, FN1, CTHRC1, ITGA11, COL5A2, FAP, PODNL1, TGFB1I1, COL1A1, MMP2, COL3A1, LTBP1, MATN3, CHST6, POSTN, COL16A1, SRPX2*. Most of the genes are involved in ECM and associated with the suppression of anticancer immunity [16,17]. Supporting this notion, examining RPPA data revealed significantly decreased LCK, a key molecule in the selection and maturation of developing T-cells [18] (Figure 2E). Moreover, MPM has a high ECM signature compared to other solid tumors (Figure S3A), which predicts poor prognosis in patients (Figure S3B). However, the genetic underpinning for the high ECM of MPM has been unclear. Our data showed that the high ECM might be due to the high percentage (~46%) of MPM tumors with *CDKN2A/2B* alterations. The top 20 most connective genes in the red module are *OAS2, MX1, RSAD2, HERC6, IFIT3, CMPK2, IFI6, ISG15, USP18, IFIT2, OASL, IFI44, MX2, DDX60, IFI44L, OAS1, LAMP3, CYP39A1, IFIT1, RUFY4*, with the vast majority involved in the IFN-I pathway.

Collectively, these results reveal cellular processes that may represent therapeutic vulnerabilities in *CDKN2A/2B* deficient MPM. The enriched green and yellow modules indicate that *CDKN2A/2B*-mutant MPM may benefit from the co-targeting of the G2/M checkpoint or mitosis (e.g., PLK1) with PI3K/AKT, but might be associated with suppressive anticancer immunity due to high ECM. Oncolytic viral immunotherapy, a novel anticancer strategy preferentially killing proliferating cancer cells but sparing normal ones, might be particularly effective for the red module-marked subset, in which the IFN-I pathway genes are often co-deleted.

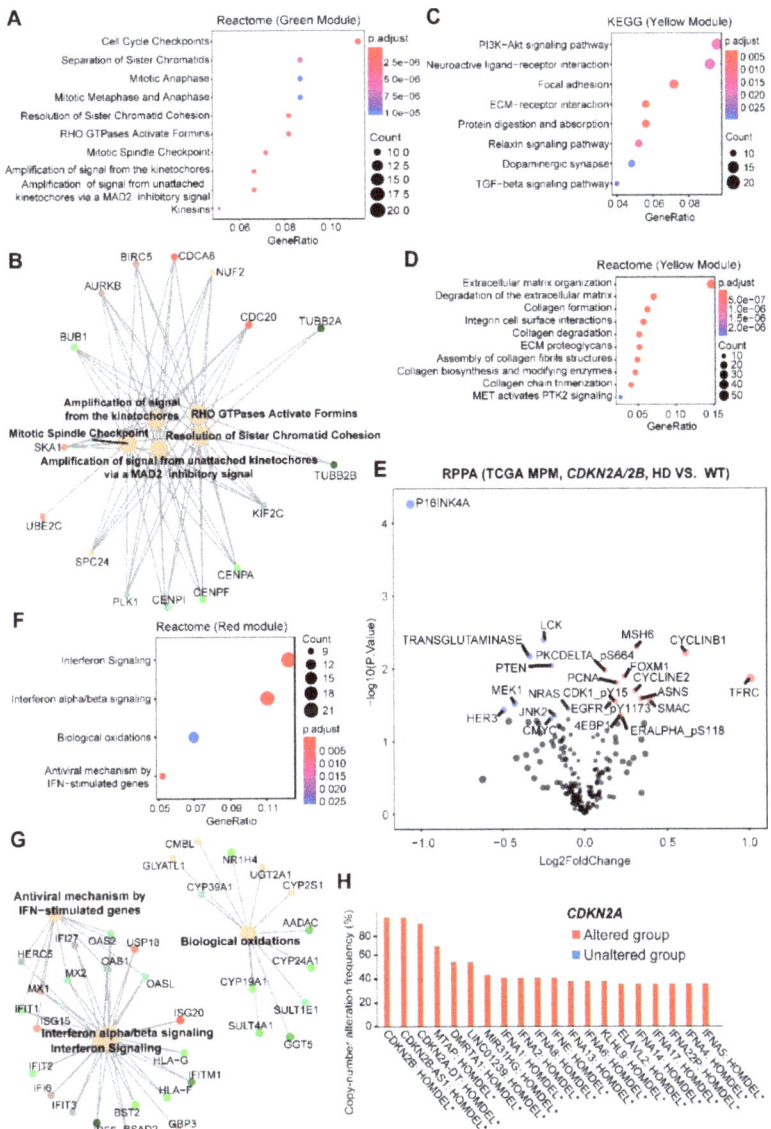

Figure 2. Enrichment analyses of genes significantly correlated with MPM tumors harboring HDs in *CDKN2A/2B*. (**A**,**B**), Top 10 significantly enriched Reactome pathways based on genes in the green module. In B, genes in the enriched Reactome pathways were listed. (**C**,**D**), Top 10 significantly enriched Kyoto Encyclopedia of Genes and Genomes (KEGG) (**C**) and Reactome (**D**) pathways based on genes in the yellow module. (**E**), Volcano plot showing the significantly (adjusted *p*-value < 0.05) upregulated (red) and downregulated (blue) proteins in malignant pleural mesothelioma (MPM) tumors harboring homozygous deletions (HDs) in CDKN2A/2B (versus wild-type), based on The Cancer Genome Atlas (TCGA) MPM cohort (*N* = 61). Data were downloaded and reanalyzed from The Cancer Proteome Atlas (TCPA) database (https://tcpaportal.org/tcpa/). (**F**,**G**), significantly enriched Reactome pathways based on genes in the red module. In (**G**), genes in the enriched Reactome pathways (**F**) were listed. (**H**), Genes significantly co-deleted with CDKN2A/2B in TCGA MPM samples. Data were downloaded from cBioPortal (https://www.cbioportal.org/). * $p < 0.05$. 2.3. BAP1.

BAP1 has pleiotropic roles, ranging from the maintenance of genomic stability to the repair of DNA double-strand breaks (DSBs) [19,20]. Our analysis showed that *BAP1* alterations in MPM are positively correlated with the red module only ($r = 0.41$; p-value $= 2 \times 10^{-4}$) that enriches the IFN-I pathway (Figure 2F,G), and negatively correlated with *CDKN2A/2B* loss (Figure S1E). This finding is supported by our recent study, showing that *BAP1* is negatively correlated with the IFN-I gene signature [21]. Thus, *CDKN2A/2B* deficiency plus *BAP1* proficiency defines a unique MPM subset that might particularly be sensitive to oncolytic viral immunotherapy.

2.3. NF2

NF2 is a plasma membrane protein binding to α-catenin and tight junctions to suppress cell growth. NF2 loss deregulates multiple signal pathways, although a prevalent notion holds that the Hippo pathway is central to the phenotype of *NF2*-mutant MPM.

Akin to *CDKN2A* loss, *NF2* alterations are positively correlated with the green ($r = 0.34$; p-value $= 0.002$) and the yellow ($r = 0.26$; p-value $= 0.02$) modules (Figure S1E), suggesting that NF2 might regulate cell cycle [22,23] and PI3K/AKT/mTORC1 (yellow module) [24], in addition to the canonical Hippo pathway. Supporting the notion, mining the public dataset that elaborates on protein-protein interactions revealed that the proteins involved in the ribosome, tight junction, Hippo and DNA repair are enriched in NF2-binding partners (Figure S4). The similarity between *CDKN2A*- and *NF2*-associated gene expression can alternatively be because *CDKN2A* and *NF2* alterations overlap in MPM (Figure 1B). However, *CDKN2A* and *BAP1* deficiency co-occurs at an even greater extent (Figure 1B) but rewires different gene networks (Figure 2) argues against this possibility.

Thus, like *CDKN2A/2B*, the genetic inactivation of *NF2* deregulates cell cycle, ECM and PI3K/AKT pathways, which prioritizes the co-targeting of the G2/M checkpoint/mitosis and PI3K/AKT pathway for *NF2*-altered MPM.

2.4. TP53

TP53 mutations are negatively correlated with the purple module (125 genes; $r = -0.37$; p-value $= 9 \times 10^{-4}$), to a less extent with the turquoise (1143 genes; $r = -0.29$; p-value $= 0.01$) and the green-yellow (108 genes; $r = -0.27$; p-value $= 0.02$), but positively with the salmon (57 genes; $r = 0.23$; p-value $= 0.04$), implying that *TP53* mutations deregulate multiple biological processes in MPM (Figure S1E). Notably, the turquoise is also significantly correlated with *LATS2* alterations (Figure S1E); we therefore focused on the purple and green-yellow module in the context of *TP53* mutations.

The purple module enriches genes of adipocyte differentiation/lipid metabolism, suggesting that *TP53*-mutant MPM might have attenuated activity of the processes (Figure 3A,B and Figure S5A) and benefit from differentiation therapy, e.g., peroxisome proliferator-activated receptor (PPAR) activator (Figure S5A). Supporting this notion, PPAR activator has been shown to promote the differentiation of mesenchymal therapy-resistant cancer cells to adipocytes [25]. Furthermore, the green-yellow module negatively correlated with *TP53* mutations enrich genes involved in lung epithelial cell differentiation (Figure 3C,D and Figure S5B), and the positively correlated salmon module enriches for genes of the neuronal system (Figure 3E,F). However, the marginal significance (p-value $= 0.04$) limits the value of this module.

The top 20 best-connected genes within the purple module are AQP7, PLIN1, ADIPOQ, TUSC5, CIDEA, THRSP, PLIN4, CIDEC, C14orf180, AQP7P1, CD300LG, C6, LIPE, LEP, NTRK2, SLC7A10, KCNIP2, GPD1, PDK4, and LPL, among which chemical agonists for PDK4, PRKAR2B and LPL are available. The top 20 best-connected genes of the green-yellow module include PDK4, TUSC5, LIPE, CIDEC, KCNIP2, CTSG, THRSP, CIDEA, AQP7P1, CD300LG, C7, C6, FREM1, THSD7B, MS4A2, TPSB2, C14orf180, FAM107A, TPSAB1, and TNMD.

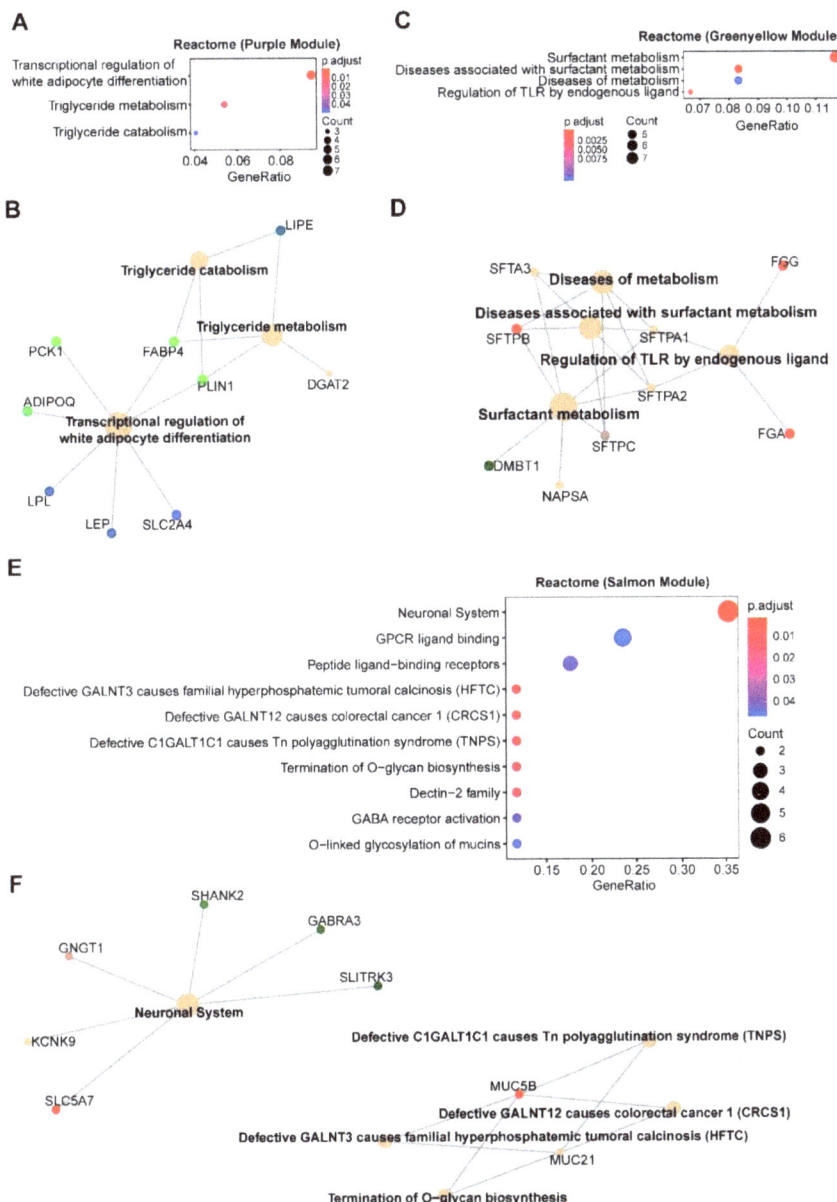

Figure 3. Enrichment analyses of genes significantly correlated with MPM tumors with TP53 alterations. (**A**,**E**), Significantly enriched Reactome pathways based on genes in the purple (**A**,**B**), green-yellow (**C**,**D**) and salmon (**E**,**F**) modules. Cnetplots in (**B**), (**D**) and (**F**) listed genes in the enriched Reactome pathways (**A**, **C** and **E**, respectively).

2.5. SETD2

SETD2 is a histone-modifying enzyme responsible for trimethylation of the lysine 36 residue on Histone 3 (H3K36me3) in humans. Impaired H3K36me3 causes aberrant gene regulation and chromosomal instability [26].

MPM with *SETD2* alterations is exclusively abundant ($r = 0.25$; *p*-value = 0.03) in the turquoise module, consisting of 1143 genes, with functions spanning from neuronal biology and receptor tyrosine kinases (particularly EGFR family) to the potassium channel, the Hippo and Wnt (Figure 4A–C). The Hippo and Wnt pathways are tumor-suppressive, precluding the potential as therapeutic targets. However, our results suggest that targeting EGFR might be a novel strategy for *SETD2*-altered MPM (Figure 4A,B).

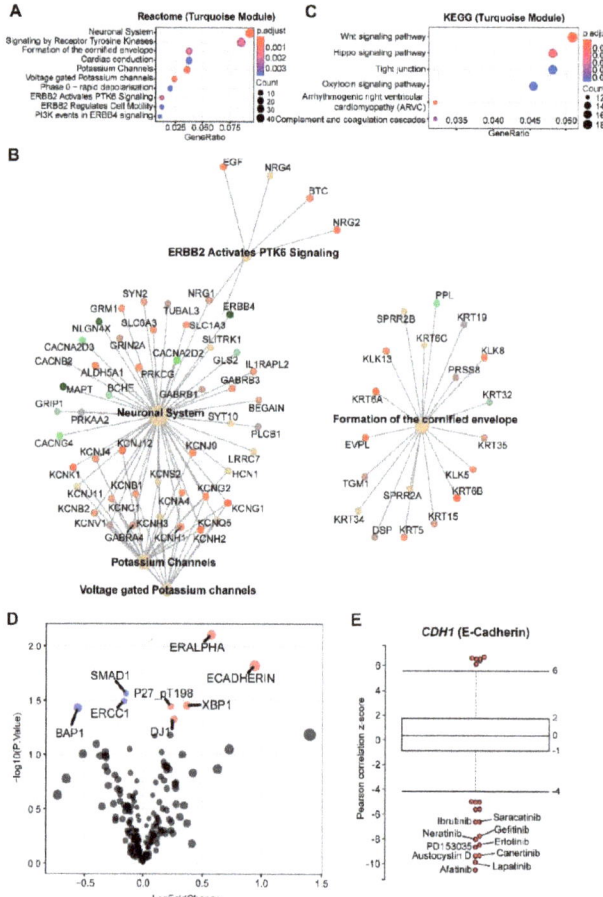

Figure 4. Enrichment analyses of genes significantly correlated with MPM tumors with *SETD2* alterations. (**A**,**C**) Top 10 significantly enriched Reactome (**A**,**B**) and Kyoto Encyclopedia of Genes and Genomes (KEGG) (**C**) pathways based on genes in the turquoise module. Cnetplot in (**B**) listed genes in the enriched Reactome pathways (**A**). (**D**) Volcano plot showing the significantly (adjusted *p*-value < 0.05) upregulated (red) and downregulated (blue) proteins in malignant pleural mesothelioma (MPM) tumors with SETD2 alterations (versus wild-type), based on The Cancer Genome Atlas (TCGA) MPM cohort ($N = 61$). Data were downloaded and reanalyzed from The Cancer Proteome Atlas (TCPA) database (https://tcpaportal.org/tcpa/). (**E**) Box-and-whisker plots show the extent of correlation between cytotoxic effects of each compound and with CDH1 (encoding E-cadherin) mRNA level, across 670 solid cancer cell lines. The y-axis indicates z scored Pearson's correlation coefficients; line, median; box, 25–75th percentile; whiskers, 2.5th and 97.5th percentile expansion; Here, only significantly ($p < 0.05$) correlated inhibitors were shown (in red dots). Labeled dots indicated the most negatively correlated drugs.

Genetic/molecular co-occurrence in tumor samples implies that progression to malignancy is a consequence of cooperative genetic/molecular dysregulations. Indeed, genetic alterations in *EGFR* and *SETD2* frequently co-occur in glioma [27] and TCGA pan-cancer cohort (Figure S6), supporting the notion that co-occurring *EGFR* and *SETD2* alterations cooperate to promote tumor progression, and that *SETD2*-mutant cancer may evolve a dependency on EGFR signaling. To further confirm the link between *SETD2* alterations and sensitivity to EGFR inhibition, we performed integrated analyses of proteomic (RPPA) and drug sensitivity data, which revealed that E-cadherin is significantly upregulated in *SETD2*-altered MPM (Figure 4D) and the expression of *CDH1* (encoding E-cadherin) is most negatively correlated with sensitivity to various EGFR inhibitors (Figure 4E). Of note, the red module, abundant in the IFN-I signature and positively correlated with *BAP1* alterations, is also positively correlated with *SETD2* mutations in MPM. This can be explained by considerably co-occurring *BAP1* and *SETD2* mutations, as 8 of 11 *SETD2*-altered MPM also have aberrant *BAP1* (Figure 1B). RPPA analysis confirmed significantly downregulated BAP1 in *SETD2*-altered MPM (Figure 4D).

The top 20 best-connected genes in the turquoise module are KLK11, CCDC64, CARNS1, CGN, BNC1, CLDN15, COBL, PARD6B, PLLP, PRR15, IGSF9, PRR15L, ANXA9, SELENBP1, PDZK1IP1, TGM1, SOX6, HOOK1, MSLN, NRG4. One of the hub genes in this module is MSLN, encoding mesothelin, a well-characterized biomarker for mesothelial tissue, and commonly overexpressed in epithelial mesotheliomas.

2.6. LATS2

At the heart of the Hippo pathway stands a core kinase cassette: MST1/2, LATS1/2, and adaptor proteins SAV1, MOB1A/B, which converges at LATS1/2-dependent phosphorylation of Yes-associated protein (YAP) and transcriptional co-activator with TAZ.

LATS2 alterations show a negative correlation with the turquoise module (Figure 2, $r = -0.45$; p-value $= 4 \times 10^{-5}$), which is opposite to *SETD2* alterations (positively correlated with the turquoise), but expected, in that genes involved in the Hippo and tight junction pathways are enriched in the turquoise module. Importantly, *LATS2* alterations in MPM are exclusively positively correlated ($r = 0.33$; p-value $= 0.004$) with the brown module (Figure S1E and Figure 5A), which significantly enriches for genes involved in immunoregulation (Figure 5B,C). These results suggest an immunoregulatory role beyond the canonical Hippo pathway by LATS2 and a rationale of immunotherapy for *LATS2*-altered MPM. Supporting the notion, PD-L1 (encoded by *CD274*) is the most significantly upregulated protein in *LATS2*-mutant MPM (Figure S7A), and LATS1/2 deletion has recently been shown to enhance anti-tumor immune responses [28]. Strikingly, a retrospective analysis of patients after being treated with immune checkpoint blockade showed that mutations of *LATS1/2*, rather than of *NF2*, predict significantly better survival (Figure 6A and Figure S7B).

The top 20 best-connected genes in the brown module are LCK, CD3E, IL2RG, SLAMF6, CD2, CD3D, SIT1, SH2D1A, CXCR3, TIGIT, TRAT1, CD6, GZMK, CD247, SIRPG, CD27, ZAP70, TBC1D10C, CD96, CD5. Of these, CD3E, IL2RG, CD2, CD3D, CD6, CD247, CD5, ITK, and CD3G are pharmacologically tractable.

Protein domains are important functional units and crucial for deconvolution of drug targets; we thus explored functional domains of the proteins encoded by the top 20 hub genes. Using SMART and PFAM protein fomains, we found that immunoreceptor tyrosine-based activation motif and Src homology 2 (SH2) domains are significantly enriched (false discovery rate < 0.05) in the hub proteins (Figure S7C). By correlating drug sensitivity with the gene expression of cancer cell lines ($n = 670$), we identified Dasatinib, a potent Abl/Src inhibitor, with the efficacy negatively correlated with several immune biomarkers (*CD274*, *CD47*, *PDCD1LG2*), that are preferentially expressed by cancer cells (Figure 6B). These results suggest that a role by LATS2 in cancer immunity and the potential of Dasatinib to target *LATS2*-altered MPM.

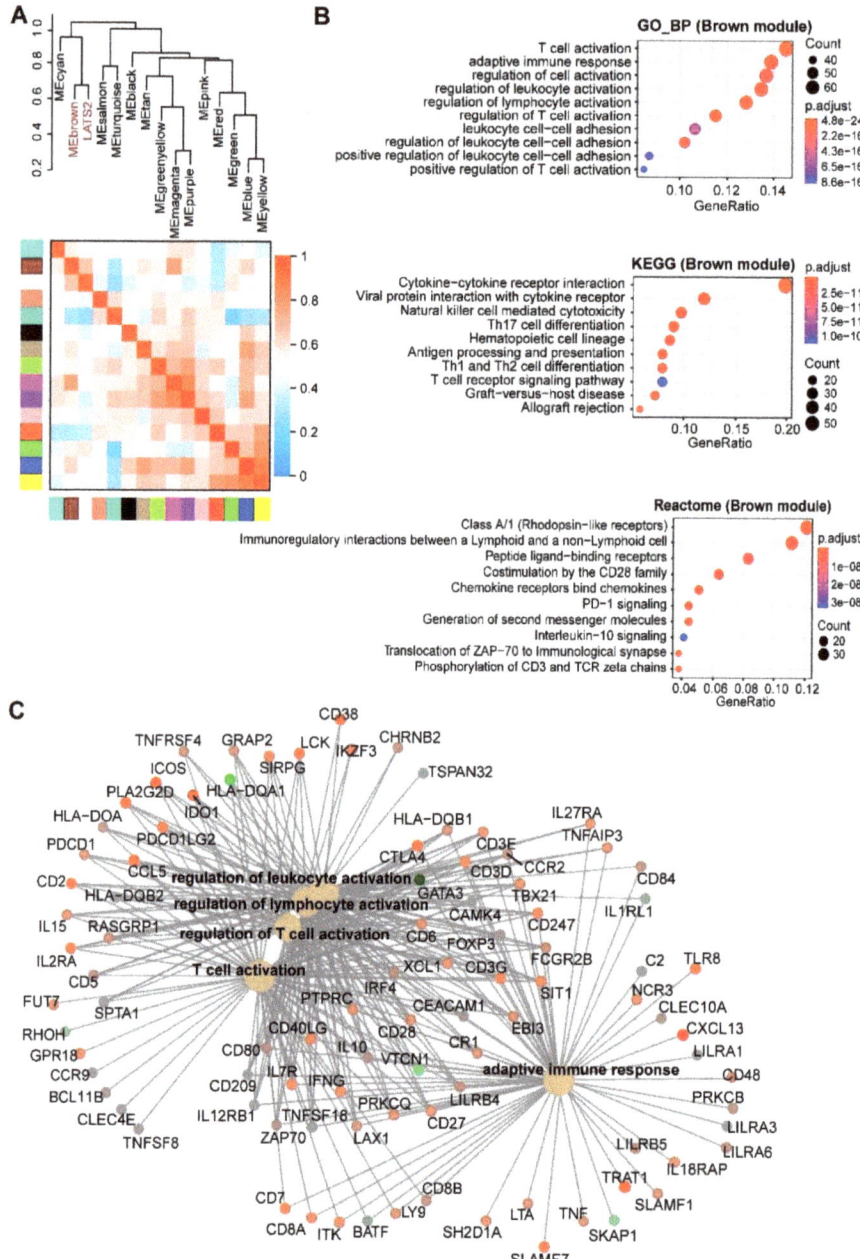

Figure 5. Enrichment analyses of genes significantly correlated with MPM tumors with LATS2 alterations. (**A**), Hierarchical clustering dendrogram of module eigengenes (labeled by their colors) and the sample trait (genetic alterations). Heatmap plot of the adjacencies in the eigengene network. In the heatmap, each row and column corresponds to one module eigengene (labeled by colors) or the trait. In the heatmap, green color indicates a negative correlation, while red represents a positive correlation. (**B**,**C**), Top 10 significantly enriched GO (biological process, BP), Kyoto Encyclopedia of Genes and Genomes (KEGG) and Reactome (**C**) pathways based on genes in the brown module. Cnetplot in C listed genes in the enriched Reactome pathways (**B**).

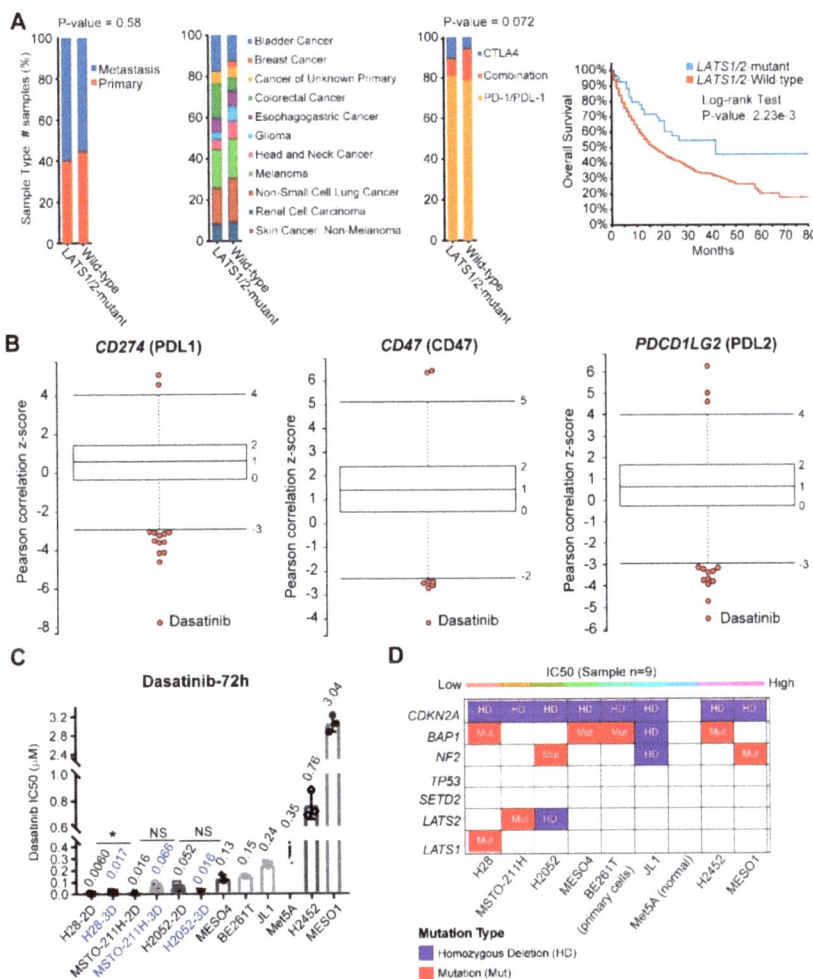

Figure 6. Identify Dasatinib as a promising therapeutic drug for MPM with *LATS2* alterations. (**A**) *LATS1/2* mutational status is associated with significantly improved overall survival in cancer patients after immune checkpoint blockage. The distribution of sample type (primary vs. metastatic; left panel), cancer type (middle panel) and drug type (anti-CTLA4; anti-PD1/PDL1; right panel) between *LATS1/2*-mutant and wild-type cancer. (**B**) Box-and-whisker plots show the extent of correlation between cytotoxic effects of Dasatinib and with several well-characterized immune markers (PDL1, PDL2, CD47), preferentially expressed by cancer cells. The y-axis indicates z scored Pearson's correlation coefficients; line, median; box, 25–75th percentile; whiskers, 2.5th and 97.5th percentile expansion; Here, only significantly ($p < 0.05$) correlated inhibitors were shown (in red dots). Notably, Dasatinib is the most negatively correlated drug. (**C**,**D**) the median inhibitory concentration (IC50) values of a panel of MPM cell lines treated with Dasatinib (72 h). MPM cells seeded in triplicate at 96-well plates were drugged 24 h later, over a 12-point concentration range (two-fold dilution). DMSO-treated cells were used as control. IC50 was determined using GraphPad Prism 7. IC50 values of Dasatinib in three MPM cell lines (H28, MSTO-211H, H2052) cultured in 2D and 3D were compared. * $p < 0.05$ by Welch's *t*-test. $N = 3$ biological replicates. In D, the genetic annotations of MPM cell lines (**C**) were shown.

As preclinical proof of the concept, we found that *LATS1/2*-altered MPM cells exhibited the highest sensitivity to Dasatinib (Figure 6C,D). Importantly, the *LATS1/2*-altered MPM cells cultured in 3D retain a high sensitivity to Dasatinib (Figure 6C). Surprisingly, the mutational status of NF2, an upstream factor of LATS1/2 in the Hippo pathway, appeared not to predict the sensitivity to Dasatinib, which may suggest that NF2 and LATS1/2 have distinct and uncoupled functions in MPM. Further supporting our finding, Dasatinib was reported to show durable anticancer effects by promoting anti-tumor T cell responses, besides direct targeting of Abl/Src [29,30].

Finally, by analyzing RPPA data, we identified several antioxidant and anti-ferroptotic proteins, e.g., TFRC, GP6D, and PRDX1, that are significantly enriched in *LATS2*-altered MPM (Figure S7) [31]. In line with this observation, MPM with the aberrant Hippo pathway was reported to be susceptible to ferroptosis induction [32].

These results uncover an unexpected role for LATS2 in modulating immune contexture, suggesting a rationale for Dasatinib to treat *LATS2*-mutant MPM. Our data also argue that LATS2 and NF2 may exert distinct roles in MPM, at odds with the long-held assumption that they act as tumor suppressors through the Hippo pathway.

3. Discussion

Cancer patients vary in prognosis and response to therapy due to tumor heterogeneity [33,34], highlighting the need for personalized treatment. Unlike many other solid tumors, MPM is characterized by a pharmacologically intractable abnormal tumor genome, mainly TSGs, for which targeted therapy has been poorly established. In this study, we presented, for the first time, a systematic analysis of biochemical networks and associated vulnerabilities induced by the functional loss of TSGs in MPM, which not only sheds light on the mechanisms of MPM biology but also provides a framework of biomarker-guided targeted therapy in MPM (Figure S8).

3.1. CDKN2A/2B and NF2

An important finding of this study is that *CDKN2A* and *NF2* loss leads to similar changes in cellular pathways in MPM. Despite the evidence for targeting PI3K/AKT/mTOR pathway in MPM subsets [3,35–38], whether the deregulation of the pathway is associated with specific genetic events is unclear. Our results reveal the molecular underpinning of *CDKN2A* and *NF2* deficiencies, and further suggest therapeutic options for these MPM subsets. As p16INK4a (product of *CDKN2A*) inhibits CDK4/6 [13], CDK4/6 activation upon *CDKN2A* loss renders *CDKN2A*-deficient MPM particularly vulnerable to CDK4/6 inhibitors [36,39], and co-targeting CDK4/6 and PI3K/AKT/mTOR induce synergistic anti-MPM effects [36]. PI3K/mTOR inhibitors as monotherapy failed in unselected MPM patients [7], highlighting the importance of biomarker-guided stratification in future clinical trials.

Oncolytic viral immunotherapy shows promises in MPM [40], partly due to the special location of the malignancy that facilitates viral administration. We showed that IFN-I pathway genes are often co-deleted with *CDKN2A*, suggesting a rational by oncolytic viral immunotherapy for *CDKN2A*-altered MPM, which is supported by a recent report [14]. As *CDKN2A/2B* loss is widely used in pathological diagnosis to distinguish MPM from benign pleural lesions, analyzing the mutations of IFN-I–related genes will improve MPM diagnosis and patient stratification.

MPM has a high ECM signature, which may drive immunotherapy resistance [16,17]. Here, we provided evidence that high ECM in MPM is mainly attributable to *CDKN2A/2B* and *NF2* deficiency, that accounts for ~55.6% (45 of 81) of MPM cases (Figure 1B).

3.2. BAP1

BAP1 loss is frequent in MPM, renal cell carcinoma, peritoneal mesothelioma, and uveal melanoma [41]. Given the role of BAP1 in the maintenance of genomic stability, the association between *BAP1* mutations and sensitivity to PARP1-targeted therapy has been demonstrated in the chicken model of DT40 cells [19]. However, we and others have recently shown that *BAP1* mutations cannot precisely predict the response to PARP1-targeted therapy in MPM [20,42]. In addition, BAP1 status has been shown to determine the sensitivity to Gemcitabine treatment in MPM [43,44]. Here, *BAP1* alterations show significant abundance in IFN-I pathway only, consistent with our finding that *BAP1* is negatively correlated with the IFN-I signature in MPM [21]. Our data suggest that *CDKN2A* deficiency and *BAP1* proficiency should be considered to stratify MPM for oncolytic viral immunotherapy.

3.3. TP53

Mutant p53 has been proposed to drive metabolic reprogramming, thereby promoting cancer progression [45–48]. Our data reveal a potential role for *TP53* mutation in lipid metabolism, by deregulating the PPAR signaling pathway. Supporting our finding, p53 interacts with PPAR-γ co-activator 1α (PGC-1α) [45–47], and PPAR activator promotes the differentiation of mesenchymal therapy-resistant breast cancer cells [25]. These results warrant further studies to test differentiation therapy for *TP53*-mutant MPM.

Notably, synthetic lethal targets with p53 inactivation have been investigated [49–51]. In particular, MDM2, a nuclear E3 ubiquitin ligase that binds and targets p53 for proteasomal degradation, is detected in 21.3% of clinical MPM samples, and its expression is significantly associated with poor survival [52]. To restore p53 function, several small molecules, such as the Nutlin-like drugs that disrupt MDM2/p53 interaction, have been tested in MPM [53–55]. Moreover, we and others have shown that the inactivation of *CDKN2A/2B* and *TP53* is associated with an increased dependence on the G2/M checkpoint, which represents a targetable vulnerability in MPM [56,57].

3.4. SETD2

We showed that SETD2 might have roles beyond histone modifications. Of note, RTKs, particularly EGFR members (HER1 (EGFR, ERBB1), HER2 (NEU, ERBB2), HER3 (ERBB3), and HER4 (ERBB4)) were exclusively enriched in *SETD2*-altered MPM, suggesting the potential of pan-EGFR inhibitors for this MPM subset. Indeed, co-mutant *EGFR* and *SETD2* are common in glioma and pan-cancer [27], suggesting that *SETD2*-mutant cancer might have evolved a unique dependence on EGFR signaling.

EGFR is not mutated, but overexpressed in MPM [58–60]. A previous study showed that MPM expressed EGFR (79.2%), ErbB4 (49.0%) and HER2 (6.3%), but lacked ErbB3 [61]. In line with this, anti-HER-2 antibody synergizes with cisplatin in a subset of MPM cell lines [62]. However, the first-generation EGFR/ERBB1 inhibitor erlotinib [9] and gefitinib [8] show no clinical benefit, suggesting that pan-EGFR inhibitors might be necessary. To be noted, EGFR and other RTKs (MET, AXL) have been demonstrated to contribute to the activation of the downstream PI3K/AKT/mTOR in MPM [35], and the targeting PI3K/AKT/mTOR pathway, alone or in combination with other agents, have been investigated in MPM [7,36–38]. We showed that E-Cadherin is overexpressed in *SETD2*-altered MPM and predicts the sensitivity to EGFR-targeted therapies. Our finding that E-cadherin is significantly negatively correlated with EGFR inhibitor efficacy prioritizes the need for biomarker-driven selection and pan-EGFR inhibitors that target ERBB2/3/4 as well.

3.5. LATS2

LATS1/2 are key players of the Hippo pathway, but only LATS2 is frequently mutated in MPM. We identified the significant enrichment of immunoregulatory pathways in *LATS2*-mutant MPM, suggesting an unanticipated role for LATS2 in immunoregulation. Supporting our finding, LATS1/2 can suppress cancer immunity, and their deletion improves tumor immunogenicity by enhancing anti-tumor immune responses [28]. These results support a rationale of immunotherapy to target *LATS2*-altered MPM, although how LATS1/2 modulates the immune response awaits further studies.

Immunotherapy shows promises in MPM, but with low and heterogeneous response rates [63,64], arguing for biomarker-guided stratifications of MPM subsets responsive to immunotherapies. Our data suggest that *LATS2* mutational status might be a critical factor in selecting MPM patients who can benefit from immunotherapies.

Strikingly, our study identified Dasatinib, a clinically approved RTK inhibitor, as a promising therapeutic for *LATS2*-altered MPM. Dasatinib shows the potential to modulate anticancer immunity (Figure 6B), and selectively impairs *LATS2*-altered MPM cells (Figure 6C), in line with the evidence that Dasatinib enhances anti-PDL1 efficacy in cancer [30]. These data suggest a rationale, by combining Dasatinib with immune checkpoint blockades to treat *LATS2*-altered MPM. Indeed, *LATS2* mutations are associated with beneficial survival in immunotherapy-treated patients (Figure 6A), but Dasatinib as monotherapy failed in unselected MPM patients [6,65], supporting the use of *LATS2* mutational status for patient stratification in clinical trials with Dasatinib.

Finally, we reveal a significant enrichment of proteins regulating ferroptosis in *LATS2*-mutant MPM, but not in those with *NF2* alterations, which is at odds with a recent report, showing that aberrant NF2-Hippo pathway is selectively susceptible to ferroptosis induction [32]. The observation that NF2 and LATS2 likely play different roles in MPM is supported by several lines of evidence. First, *LATS2* rather than *NF2* alterations are associated dysregulated YAP and TAZ (Figure 1C); secondly, *LATS2*- and *NF2*-mutant tumors show strikingly different enrichment of gene and protein signatures (Figures S1E and S7 and Figure 5); thirdly, Dasatinib selectively impairs *LATS2*- but not *NF2*-altered MPM (Figure 6); fourthly, *LATS1/2* mutations but not *NF2* alterations predict better survival in patients after immune checkpoint blockade therapy (Figure 6A and Figure S7B). Together, our data suggest that LATS2 and NF2 might have distinct roles in MPM, despite the long-held notion that both function through the Hippo pathway.

4. Materials and Methods

4.1. WGCNA and Function Enrichment Analyses

To identify the gene expression profiling associated with the major genetic alterations in MPM, The R package "WGCNA" was applied to the RNA-sequencing data retrieved from TCGA MPM cohort. In WGCNA, genes are clustered based on co-expression patterns to construct a gene co-expression network, which was transformed into the adjacency matrix and then topological overlap matrix (TOM) [12]. According to the TOM-based dissimilarity measure, genes were grouped into different modules (clusters) using the dynamic tree cut algorithm. For each module, the module eigengene (ME) was calculated; the first principal component representative of the module. The ME values were correlated with sample traits defined by specific genetic alterations in MPM samples. Here, we set the soft-thresholding power at 5 (scale-free $R2 = 0.86$), cut height at 0.25, and minimal module size to 30, to identify key modules. The module significantly correlated with sample traits was selected to explore its biological functions, such as gene ontology (GO), Kyoto Encyclopedia of Genes and Genomes (KEGG) and reactome pathway enrichment analyses, using the R package "clusterprofiler" [66]. Hub genes were defined as top 20 intramodular connected genes.

4.2. Cell Viability Assay

All normal human mesothelial cells Met-5A (MeT-5A, RRID: CVCL_3749), MPM cell lines H28 (NCI-H28, RRID: CVCL_1555), H2452 (NCI-H2452, RRID: CVCL_1553), and H2052 (NCI-H2052, RRID: CVCL_1518) were obtained from ATCC (American Type Culture Collection, Manassas, VA, USA) [67]. MPM cell lines MESO-1 (ACC-MESO-1, RRID: CVCL_5113) and MESO-4 (ACC-MESO-4, RRID: CVCL_5114) were obtained from RIKEN Cell Bank (Ibaraki, Japan). MPM cell lines MSTO-211H (RRID: CVCL_1430) and JL-1 (RRID: CVCL_2080) were purchased from DSMZ (German Collection of Microorganisms and Cell Cultures, Brunswick, Germany). A primary MPM cell culture (BE261T) was established from surgically resected tumors of a 67-year-old male patient, using the same protocol as described in [67] and used for short-term studies (up to eight passages in vitro). The human study was performed under the auspices of protocols approved by institutional review board (KEK number:

042/15), and informed consent was obtained from patients. Cells were cultured in RPMI-1640 medium (Cat. #8758; Sigma-Aldrich, St. Louis, MO, USA), supplemented with 10% fetal bovine serum/FBS (Cat. #10270-106; Life Technologies, Grand Island, NY, USA) and 1% penicillin/streptomycin (P/S) solution (Cat. #P0781, Sigma-Aldrich, St. Louis, MO, USA). For 3D culture, cells were cultured in ultra-low attachment plate (Sigma-Aldrich, #CLS3474-24EA) with FBS-free RPMI-1640 medium supplemented with EGF (20 ng/mL; Cat. #PHG0311; Thermo Fisher Scientific (Waltham, MA, USA), bFGF (20 ng/mL; Cat. #PHG6015; Thermo Fisher Scientific), 4µg/mL insulin (Cat. #I9278; Sigma-Aldrich), 1× B-27 (Cat. #17504044; Thermo Fisher Scientific), 1% P/S. All human cell lines have been authenticated using STR profiling within the last three years, and are confirmed free from mycoplasma contamination (Microsynth, Bern, Switzerland).

MPM cells seeded in triplicate at 96-well plates (for 2D: 1000–1500 cells/well in tissue-culture treated plate (Corning, #353072); for 3D: 4000–5000 cells/well in ultra-low attachment plate) were drugged 24 h later, over a 12-point concentration range (two-fold dilution), with DMSO as vehicle. Cell viability was determined 72 h post-treatment by the Acid Phosphatase Assay Kit (ab83367; Abcam) [68]. The median inhibitory concentration (IC50) was calculated using GraphPad Prism 7.

4.3. Public Databases

RNA-sequencing data of MPM samples ($n = 87$) were downloaded from TCGA (https://portal.gdc.cancer.gov/), in which 81 samples were provided with genetic alterations data. Normalized level 4 data of reverse phase protein array (RPPA) were downloaded from The Cancer Proteome Atlas (TCPA) database (https://tcpaportal.org/tcpa/) [69], which quantified 218 proteins in 61 out of the 87 MPM samples in TCGA. R packages "limma" and "edgeR" were used to normalize the data and identify the differential gene or protein expression, respectively [70]. Protein-interacting data were downloaded from Agile Protein Interactomes DataServer (http://cicblade.dep.usal.es:8080/APID/init.action) [71], and co-occurring analysis data were downloaded from cBioPortal (https://www.cbioportal.org/). Processed drug ($n = 481$) screening and gene expression data across solid cancer cell lines ($n = 659$) were downloaded and reanalyzed from a published study [11]. Fisher's z-transformation was applied to the correlation coefficients to adjust for (normalize) variations in cancer cell line numbers across small molecules and cell lineages. Genetic and survival data of patients after immunotherapies (anti-PD1/PDL1, anti-CTLA4) were from TMB and immunotherapy (MSKCC) cohort in cBioPortal [72].

4.4. Survival Analysis

Survival analysis was performed using "survminer" and "survival" R packages. Tumor samples within the TCGA MPM cohort were divided into two groups, based on each hub gene's best-separation cut-off value to plot the Kaplan–Meier survival curves.

4.5. ECM Gene Signature

The extracellular matrix (ECM)/stromal gene signature was scored as the sum of an ECM/stromal gene set (*VCAN, FAP, POSTN, FBLN1, COL1A1, PDPN, THY1, CSPG4, IL6, TGFB1, HGF, SERPINE1*). The gene list was curated based on previous studies across different cancer lineages [16,17].

4.6. Statistical Analysis

Data were presented as mean ± SD, with the indicated sample size (n) representing biological replicates. Gene expression and survival data derived from the public database, as well as the correlation coefficient, were analyzed using *R* (version 3.6.0). $p < 0.05$ was considered statistically significant.

5. Conclusions

Overall, we report the systematic identification of biochemical networks and therapeutic potential linked with aberrant TSGs, which provides a framework for biomarker-guided precision oncology for MPM subsets. Our work warrants further studies that verify the drug vulnerabilities and the stratification approaches for future clinical trials.

Supplementary Materials: The following are available online at http://www.mdpi.com/2072-6694/12/8/2310/s1, Figure S1: Weighted gene correlation network analysis (WGCNA) reveal gene modules linked with major genetic alterations in MPM; Figure S2: Pathway enrichment analyses of the genes significantly correlated with CDKN2A/2B loss; Figure S3: MPM has a high extracellular matrix (ECM) gene signature; Figure S4: Pathway enrichment analyses of the genes significantly correlated with NF2 alterations; Figure S5: Pathway enrichment analyses of the genes significantly correlated with TP53 mutations; Figure S6: Mutually exclusive and co-occurring analyses of STED2 and EGFR family genes across TCGA pan-cancer solid tumors; Figure S7: LATS2-altered MPM tumors enrich for the immune-regulatory signature; Figure S8: Tumor suppressor genes (TSGs)-guided precision oncology in MPM.

Author Contributions: Conceptualization, H.Y. and R.-W.P. Methodology, H.Y., D.X., Z.Y. Formal Analysis, H.Y. Investigation, H.Y., D.X., Z.Y. Data Curation, F.Y., H.Z., R.A.S., R.-W.P. Writing—Original Draft Preparation, H.Y. Writing—Review and Editing, all authors. Supervision, R.A.S., R.-W.P. Project Administration, R.A.S., R.-W.P. Funding Acquisition, H.Y., Z.Y., R.-W.P. All authors have read and agreed to the published version of the manuscript.

Funding: This work was supported by grants from Swiss Cancer League/Swiss Cancer Research Foundation (#KFS-4851-08-2019; to R.-W.P.), Swiss National Science Foundation (SNSF; #310030_192648; to R.-W.P.) and PhD fellowships from China Scholarship Council (to H.Y. and Z.Y.).

Acknowledgments: This study used TCGA Program database. The interpretation and reporting of these data are the sole responsibility of the authors. The authors acknowledge the efforts of the National Cancer Institute.

Conflicts of Interest: The authors have declared no conflicts of interest.

References

1. Mutti, L.; Peikert, T.; Robinson, B.W.S.; Scherpereel, A.; Tsao, A.S.; De Perrot, M.; Woodard, G.A.; Jablons, D.M.; Wiens, J.; Hirsch, F.R.; et al. Scientific Advances and New Frontiers in Mesothelioma Therapeutics. *J. Thorac. Oncol.* **2018**, *13*, 1269–1283. [CrossRef] [PubMed]
2. Vogelzang, N.J.; Rusthoven, J.J.; Symanowski, J.; Denham, C.; Kaukel, E.; Ruffié, P.; Gatzemeier, U.; Boyer, M.; Emri, S.; Manegold, C.; et al. Phase III Study of Pemetrexed in Combination with Cisplatin Versus Cisplatin Alone in Patients with Malignant Pleural Mesothelioma. *J. Clin. Oncol.* **2003**, *21*, 2636–2644. [CrossRef] [PubMed]
3. Bueno, R.; Stawiski, E.W.; Goldstein, L.D.; Durinck, S.; De Rienzo, A.; Modrusan, Z.; Gnad, F.; Nguyen, T.T.; Jaiswal, B.S.; Chirieac, L.R.; et al. Comprehensive genomic analysis of malignant pleural mesothelioma identifies recurrent mutations, gene fusions and splicing alterations. *Nat. Genet.* **2016**, *48*, 407–416. [CrossRef] [PubMed]
4. Hmeljak, J.; Sanchez-Vega, F.; Hoadley, K.A.; Shih, J.; Stewart, C.; Heiman, D.; Tarpey, P.; Danilova, L.; Drill, E.; Gibb, E.A.; et al. Integrative Molecular Characterization of Malignant Pleural Mesothelioma. *Cancer Discov.* **2018**, *8*, 1548–1565. [CrossRef] [PubMed]
5. Guo, G.; Chmielecki, J.; Goparaju, C.; Heguy, A.; Dolgalev, I.; Carbone, M.; Seepo, S.; Meyerson, M.; Pass, H.I. Whole-Exome Sequencing Reveals Frequent Genetic Alterations in BAP1, NF2, CDKN2A, and CUL1 in Malignant Pleural Mesothelioma. *Cancer Res.* **2014**, *75*, 264–269. [CrossRef]
6. Dudek, A.Z.; Pang, H.; Kratzke, R.A.; Otterson, G.A.; Hodgson, L.; Vokes, E.E.; Kindler, H.L.; Cancer and Leukemia Group B. Phase II Study of Dasatinib in Patients with Previously Treated Malignant Mesothelioma (Cancer and Leukemia Group B 30601): A Brief Report. *J. Thorac. Oncol.* **2012**, *7*, 755–759. [CrossRef]
7. Ou, S.-H.I.; Moon, J.; Garland, L.L.; Mack, P.C.; Testa, J.R.; Tsao, A.S.; Wozniak, A.J.; Gandara, D.R. SWOG S0722: Phase II study of mTOR inhibitor everolimus (RAD001) in advanced malignant pleural mesothelioma (MPM). *J. Thorac. Oncol.* **2015**, *10*, 387–391. [CrossRef]
8. Govindan, R. Gefitinib in Patients with Malignant Mesothelioma: A Phase II Study by the Cancer and Leukemia Group B. *Clin. Cancer Res.* **2005**, *11*, 2300–2304. [CrossRef]
9. Garland, L.L.; Rankin, C.; Gandara, D.R.; Rivkin, S.E.; Scott, K.M.; Nagle, R.B.; Klein-Szanto, A.J.; Testa, J.R.; Altomare, D.A.; Borden, E.C. Phase II Study of Erlotinib in Patients with Malignant Pleural Mesothelioma: A Southwest Oncology Group Study. *J. Clin. Oncol.* **2007**, *25*, 2406–2413. [CrossRef]

10. Ding, H.; Zhao, J.; Zhang, Y.; Yu, J.; Liu, M.; Li, X.; Xu, L.; Lin, M.; Liu, C.; He, Z.; et al. Systematic Analysis of Drug Vulnerabilities Conferred by Tumor Suppressor Loss. *Cell Rep.* **2019**, *27*, 3331–3344.e6. [CrossRef]
11. Rees, M.G.; Seashore-Ludlow, B.; Cheah, J.H.; Adams, D.J.; Price, E.V.; Gill, S.; Javaid, S.; Coletti, M.E.; Jones, V.L.; Bodycombe, N.E.; et al. Correlating chemical sensitivity and basal gene expression reveals mechanism of action. *Nat. Methods* **2015**, *12*, 109–116. [CrossRef] [PubMed]
12. Langfelder, P.; Horvath, S. WGCNA: An R package for weighted correlation network analysis. *BMC Bioinform.* **2008**, *9*, 559. [CrossRef] [PubMed]
13. Zhao, R.; Choi, B.Y.; Lee, M.-H.; Bode, A.M.; Surh, Y.-J. Implications of Genetic and Epigenetic Alterations of CDKN2A (p16(INK4a)) in Cancer. *EBioMedicine* **2016**, *8*, 30–39. [CrossRef]
14. Delaunay, T.; Achard, C.; Boisgerault, N.; Grard, M.; Petithomme, T.; Chatelain, C.; Dutoit, S.; Blanquart, C.; Royer, P.-J.; Minvielle, S.; et al. Frequent Homozygous Deletions of Type I Interferon Genes in Pleural Mesothelioma Confer Sensitivity to Oncolytic Measles Virus. *J. Thorac. Oncol.* **2020**, *15*, 827–842. [CrossRef] [PubMed]
15. Musa, J.; Aynaud, M.-M.; Mirabeau, O.; Delattre, O.; Grünewald, T.G.P. MYBL2 (B-Myb): A central regulator of cell proliferation, cell survival and differentiation involved in tumorigenesis. *Cell Death Dis.* **2017**, *8*, e2895. [CrossRef]
16. Mushtaq, M.U.; Papadas, A.; Pagenkopf, A.; Flietner, E.; Morrow, Z.; Chaudhary, S.G.; Asimakopoulos, F. Tumor matrix remodeling and novel immunotherapies: The promise of matrix-derived immune biomarkers. *J. Immunother. Cancer* **2018**, *6*, 65. [CrossRef]
17. Chakravarthy, A.; Khan, L.; Bensler, N.P.; Bose, P.; De Carvalho, D.D. TGF-β-associated extracellular matrix genes link cancer-associated fibroblasts to immune evasion and immunotherapy failure. *Nat. Commun.* **2018**, *9*, 4692. [CrossRef]
18. Bommhardt, U.; Schraven, B.; Simeoni, L. Beyond TCR Signaling: Emerging Functions of Lck in Cancer and Immunotherapy. *Int. J. Mol. Sci.* **2019**, *20*, 3500. [CrossRef]
19. Yu, H.; Pak, H.; Hammond-Martel, I.; Ghram, M.; Rodrigue, A.; Daou, S.; Barbour, H.; Corbeil, L.; Hébert, J.; Drobetsky, E.; et al. Tumor suppressor and deubiquitinase BAP1 promotes DNA double-strand break repair. *Proc. Natl. Acad. Sci. USA* **2013**, *111*, 285–290. [CrossRef]
20. Yang, H.; Xu, D.; Gao, Y.; Schmid, R.A.; Peng, R.-W. The Association of BAP1 Loss-of-Function with the Defect in Homologous Recombination Repair and Sensitivity to PARP-Targeted Therapy. *J. Thorac. Oncol.* **2020**, *15*, e88–e90. [CrossRef]
21. Yang, H. Co-Occurring LKB1 Deficiency Determinates the Susceptibility to ERK-Targeted Therapy in RAS-Mutant Lung Cancer. *J. Thorac. Oncol.* **2020**, *15*, e58–e59. [CrossRef] [PubMed]
22. Xiao, G.-H.; Gallagher, R.; Shetler, J.; Skele, K.; Altomare, D.A.; Pestell, R.G.; Jhanwar, S.; Testa, J.R. The NF2 Tumor Suppressor Gene Product, Merlin, Inhibits Cell Proliferation and Cell Cycle Progression by Repressing Cyclin D1 Expression. *Mol. Cell. Biol.* **2005**, *25*, 2384–2394. [CrossRef] [PubMed]
23. Shi, Y.; Bollam, S.R.; White, S.M.; Laughlin, S.Z.; Graham, G.T.; Wadhwa, M.; Chen, H.; Nguyen, C.; Vitte, J.; Giovannini, M.; et al. Rac1-Mediated DNA Damage and Inflammation Promote Nf2 Tumorigenesis but Also Limit Cell-Cycle Progression. *Dev. Cell* **2016**, *39*, 452–465. [CrossRef] [PubMed]
24. López-Lago, M.A.; Okada, T.; Murillo, M.M.; Socci, N.; Giancotti, F.G. Loss of the Tumor Suppressor Gene NF2, Encoding Merlin, Constitutively Activates Integrin-Dependent mTORC1 Signaling. *Mol. Cell. Biol.* **2009**, *29*, 4235–4249. [CrossRef] [PubMed]
25. Ishay-Ronen, D.; Diepenbruck, M.; Kalathur, R.K.R.; Sugiyama, N.; Tiede, S.; Ivanek, R.; Bantug, G.; Morini, M.F.; Wang, J.; Hess, C.; et al. Gain Fat—Lose Metastasis: Converting Invasive Breast Cancer Cells into Adipocytes Inhibits Cancer Metastasis. *Cancer Cell* **2019**, *35*, 17–32. [CrossRef] [PubMed]
26. Li, J.; Duns, G.; Westers, H.; Sijmons, R.; Berg, A.V.D.; Kok, K. SETD2: An epigenetic modifier with tumor suppressor functionality. *Oncotarget* **2016**, *7*, 50719–50734. [CrossRef] [PubMed]
27. Viaene, A.N.; Santi, M.; Rosenbaum, J.; Li, M.M.; Surrey, L.F.; Nasrallah, M.L.P. SETD2 mutations in primary central nervous system tumors. *Acta Neuropathol. Commun.* **2018**, *6*, 123. [CrossRef]
28. Moroishi, T.; Hayashi, T.; Pan, W.-W.; Fujita, Y.; Holt, M.V.; Qin, J.; Carson, D.A.; Guan, K.-L. The Hippo Pathway Kinases LATS1/2 Suppress Cancer Immunity. *Cell* **2016**, *167*, 1525–1539.e7. [CrossRef]
29. Yang, Y.; Liu, C.; Peng, W.; Lizée, G.; Overwijk, W.W.; Liu, Y.; Woodman, S.E.; Hwu, P. Antitumor T-cell responses contribute to the effects of dasatinib on c-KIT mutant murine mastocytoma and are potentiated by anti-OX40. *Blood* **2012**, *120*, 4533–4543. [CrossRef]

30. Tu, M.M.; Lee, F.Y.F.; Jones, R.T.; Kimball, A.K.; Saravia, E.; Graziano, R.F.; Coleman, B.; Menard, K.; Yan, J.; Michaud, E.; et al. Targeting DDR2 enhances tumor response to anti–PD-1 immunotherapy. *Sci. Adv.* **2019**, *5*, eaav2437. [CrossRef]
31. Dixon, S.J.; Lemberg, K.M.; Lamprecht, M.R.; Skouta, R.; Zaitsev, E.M.; Gleason, C.E.; Patel, D.N.; Bauer, A.J.; Cantley, A.M.; Yang, W.S.; et al. Ferroptosis: An Iron-Dependent Form of Nonapoptotic Cell Death. *Cell* **2012**, *149*, 1060–1072. [CrossRef] [PubMed]
32. Wu, J.; Minikes, A.; Gao, M.; Bian, H.; Li, Y.; Stockwell, B.R.; Chen, Z.-N.; Jiang, X. Intercellular interaction dictates cancer cell ferroptosis via Merlin-YAP signalling. *Nature* **2019**, *572*, 402–406. [CrossRef] [PubMed]
33. Yang, H.; Liang, S.-Q.; Schmid, R.A.; Peng, R.-W. New Horizons in KRAS-Mutant Lung Cancer: Dawn after Darkness. *Front. Oncol.* **2019**, *9*. [CrossRef] [PubMed]
34. Hausser, J.; Alon, U. Tumour heterogeneity and the evolutionary trade-offs of cancer. *Nat. Rev. Cancer* **2020**, *20*, 247–257. [CrossRef]
35. Zhou, S.; Liu, L.; Li, H.; Eilers, G.; Kuang, Y.; Shi, S.; Yan, Z.; Li, X.; Corson, J.M.; Meng, F.; et al. Multipoint targeting of the PI3K/mTOR pathway in mesothelioma. *Br. J. Cancer* **2014**, *110*, 2479–2488. [CrossRef]
36. Bonelli, M.; Digiacomo, G.; Fumarola, C.; Alfieri, R.; Quaini, F.; Falco, A.; Madeddu, D.; La Monica, S.; Cretella, D.; Ravelli, A.; et al. Combined Inhibition of CDK4/6 and PI3K/AKT/mTOR Pathways Induces a Synergistic Anti-Tumor Effect in Malignant Pleural Mesothelioma Cells. *Neoplasia* **2017**, *19*, 637–648. [CrossRef]
37. Altomare, D.A.; You, H.; Xiao, G.-H.; Ramos-Nino, M.E.; Skele, K.L.; De Rienzo, A.; Jhanwar, S.C.; Mossman, B.T.; Kane, A.B.; Testa, J.R. Human and mouse mesotheliomas exhibit elevated AKT/PKB activity, which can be targeted pharmacologically to inhibit tumor cell growth. *Oncogene* **2005**, *24*, 6080–6089. [CrossRef]
38. Yamaji, M.; Ota, A.; Wahiduzzaman, M.; Karnan, S.; Hyodo, T.; Konishi, H.; Tsuzuki, S.; Hosokawa, Y.; Haniuda, M. Novel ATP-competitive Akt inhibitor afuresertib suppresses the proliferation of malignant pleural mesothelioma cells. *Cancer Med.* **2017**, *6*, 2646–2659. [CrossRef]
39. Sobhani, N.; Corona, S.P.; Zanconati, F.; Generali, D. Cyclin dependent kinase 4 and 6 inhibitors as novel therapeutic agents for targeted treatment of malignant mesothelioma. *Genes Cancer* **2017**, *8*, 495–496. [CrossRef]
40. Pease, D.F.; Kratzke, R.A. Oncolytic Viral Therapy for Mesothelioma. *Front. Oncol.* **2017**, *7*. [CrossRef]
41. Carbone, M.; Yang, H.; Pass, H.I.; Krausz, T.; Testa, J.R.; Gaudino, G. BAP1 and Cancer. *Nat. Rev. Cancer* **2013**, *13*, 153–159. [CrossRef] [PubMed]
42. Rathkey, D.; Khanal, M.; Murai, J.; Zhang, J.; Sengupta, M.; Jiang, Q.; Morrow, B.; Evans, C.N.; Chari, R.; Fetsch, P.; et al. Sensitivity of Mesothelioma Cells to PARP Inhibitors Is Not Dependent on BAP1 but Is Enhanced by Temozolomide in Cells With High-Schlafen 11 and Low-O6-methylguanine-DNA Methyltransferase Expression. *J. Thorac. Oncol.* **2020**, *15*, 843–859. [CrossRef] [PubMed]
43. Guazzelli, A.; Meysami, P.; Bakker, E.; Demonacos, C.; Giordano, A.; Demonacos, C.; Mutti, L. BAP1 Status Determines the Sensitivity of Malignant Mesothelioma Cells to Gemcitabine Treatment. *Int. J. Mol. Sci.* **2019**, *20*, 429. [CrossRef]
44. Okonska, A.; Bühler, S.; Rao, V.; Ronner, M.; Blijlevens, M.; Van Der Meulen-Muileman, I.H.; De Menezes, R.X.; Wipplinger, M.; Oehl, K.; Smit, E.F.; et al. Functional Genomic Screen in Mesothelioma Reveals that Loss of Function of BRCA1-Associated Protein 1 Induces Chemoresistance to Ribonucleotide Reductase Inhibition. *Mol. Cancer Ther.* **2019**, *19*, 552–563. [CrossRef]
45. Sen, N.; Satija, Y.K.; Das, S. PGC-1α, a Key Modulator of p53, Promotes Cell Survival upon Metabolic Stress. *Mol. Cell* **2011**, *44*, 621–634. [CrossRef]
46. Assaily, W.; Rubinger, D.A.; Wheaton, K.; Lin, Y.; Ma, W.; Xuan, W.; Brown-Endres, L.; Tsuchihara, K.; Mak, T.W.; Benchimol, S. ROS-Mediated p53 Induction of Lpin1 Regulates Fatty Acid Oxidation in Response to Nutritional Stress. *Mol. Cell* **2011**, *44*, 491–501. [CrossRef]
47. Goldstein, I.; Rotter, V. Regulation of lipid metabolism by p53—Fighting two villains with one sword. *Trends Endocrinol. Metab.* **2012**, *23*, 567–575. [CrossRef]
48. Lacroix, M.; Riscal, R.; Arena, G.; Linares, L.K.; Le Cam, L. Metabolic functions of the tumor suppressor p53: Implications in normal physiology, metabolic disorders, and cancer. *Mol. Metab.* **2020**, *33*, 2–22. [CrossRef]

49. Tian, K.; Bakker, E.; Hussain, M.; Guazzelli, A.; Alhebshi, H.; Meysami, P.; Demonacos, C.; Schwartz, J.-M.; Mutti, L.; Krstic-Demonacos, M. p53 modeling as a route to mesothelioma patients stratification and novel therapeutic identification. *J. Transl. Med.* **2018**, *16*, 282. [CrossRef]
50. Wang, X.; Simon, R. Identification of potential synthetic lethal genes to p53 using a computational biology approach. *BMC Med. Genom.* **2013**, *6*, 30. [CrossRef]
51. Aning, O.A.; Cheok, C.F. Drugging in the absence of p53. *J. Mol. Cell Biol.* **2019**, *11*, 255–264. [CrossRef]
52. Mairinger, F.D.; Walter, R.F.; Ting, S.; Vollbrecht, C.; Kollmeier, J.; Griff, S.; Hager, T.; Mairinger, T.; Christoph, D.C.; Theegarten, D.; et al. Mdm2 protein expression is strongly associated with survival in malignant pleural mesothelioma. *Future Oncol.* **2014**, *10*, 995–1005. [CrossRef]
53. Di Marzo, D.; Forte, I.M.; Indovina, P.; Di Gennaro, E.; Rizzo, V.; Giorgi, F.; Mattioli, E.; Ianuzzi, C.A.; Budillon, A.; Giordano, A.; et al. Pharmacological targeting of p53 through RITA is an effective antitumoral strategy for malignant pleural mesothelioma. *Cell Cycle* **2013**, *13*, 652–665. [CrossRef] [PubMed]
54. Walter, R.F.; Werner, R.; Wessolly, M.; Mairinger, E.; Borchert, S.; Schmeller, J.; Kollmeier, J.; Mairinger, T.; Hager, T.; Bankfalvi, A.; et al. Inhibition of MDM2 via Nutlin-3A: A Potential Therapeutic Approach for Pleural Mesotheliomas with MDM2-Induced Inactivation of Wild-Type P53. *J. Oncol.* **2018**, *2018*, 1–10. [CrossRef] [PubMed]
55. Urso, L.; Cavallari, I.; Silic-Benussi, M.; Biasini, L.; Zago, G.; Calabrese, F.; Conte, P.; Ciminale, V.; Pasello, G. Synergistic targeting of malignant pleural mesothelioma cells by MDM2 inhibitors and TRAIL agonists. *Oncotarget* **2017**, *8*, 44232–44241. [CrossRef] [PubMed]
56. Xu, D.; Liang, S.-Q.; Yang, H.; Bruggmann, R.; Berezowska, S.; Yang, Z.; Marti, T.M.; Hall, S.R.R.; Gao, Y.; Kocher, G.J.; et al. CRISPR Screening Identifies WEE1 as a Combination Target for Standard Chemotherapy in Malignant Pleural Mesothelioma. *Mol. Cancer Ther.* **2019**, *19*, 661–672. [CrossRef] [PubMed]
57. Indovina, P.; Marcelli, E.; Di Marzo, D.; Casini, N.; Forte, I.M.; Giorgi, F.; Alfano, L.; Pentimalli, F.; Giordano, A. Abrogating G2/M checkpoint through WEE1 inhibition in combination with chemotherapy as a promising therapeutic approach for mesothelioma. *Cancer Biol. Ther.* **2014**, *15*, 380–388. [CrossRef]
58. Destro, A.; Ceresoli, G.; Falleni, M.; Zucali, P.; Morenghi, E.; Bianchi, P.; Pellegrini, C.; Cordani, N.; Vaira, V.; Alloisio, M.; et al. EGFR overexpression in malignant pleural mesothelioma. *Lung Cancer* **2006**, *51*, 207–215. [CrossRef]
59. Mezzapelle, R.; Miglio, U.; Rena, O.; Paganotti, A.; Allegrini, S.; Antona, J.; Molinari, F.; Frattini, M.; Monga, G.; Alabiso, O.; et al. Mutation analysis of the EGFR gene and downstream signalling pathway in histologic samples of malignant pleural mesothelioma. *Br. J. Cancer* **2013**, *108*, 1743–1749. [CrossRef]
60. Horvai, A.E.; Li, L.; Xu, Z.; Kramer, M.J.; Jablons, D.; Treseler, P.A. Malignant mesothelioma does not demonstrate overexpression or gene amplification despite cytoplasmic immunohistochemical staining for c-Erb-B2. *Arch. Pathol. Lab. Med.* **2003**, *127*, 465–469.
61. Klampatsa, A.; Achkova, D.Y.; Davies, D.M.; Parente-Pereira, A.C.; Woodman, N.; Rosekilly, J.; Osborne, G.; Thayaparan, T.; Bille, A.; Sheaf, M.; et al. Intracavitary 'T4 immunotherapy' of malignant mesothelioma using pan-ErbB re-targeted CAR T-cells. *Cancer Lett.* **2017**, *393*, 52–59. [CrossRef] [PubMed]
62. Toma, S.; Colucci, L.; Scarabelli, L.; Scaramuccia, A.; Emionite, L.; Betta, P.G.; Mutti, L. Synergistic effect of the anti-HER-2/neu antibody and cisplatin in immortalized and primary mesothelioma cell lines. *J. Cell. Physiol.* **2002**, *193*, 37–41. [CrossRef]
63. Popat, S.; Curioni-Fontecedro, A.; Polydoropoulou, V.; Shah, R.; O'Brien, M.; Pope, A.; Fisher, P.; Spicer, J.; Roy, A.; Gilligan, D.; et al. A multicentre randomized phase III trial comparing pembrolizumab (P) vs single agent chemotherapy (CT) for advanced pre-treated malignant pleural mesothelioma (MPM): Results from the European Thoracic Oncology Platform (ETOP 9-15) PROMISE-meso trial. *Ann. Oncol.* **2019**, *30*, v931. [CrossRef]
64. Maio, M.; Scherpereel, A.; Calabrò, L.; Aerts, J.; Perez, S.C.; Bearz, A.; Nackaerts, K.; A Fennell, D.; Kowalski, D.; Tsao, A.S.; et al. Tremelimumab as second-line or third-line treatment in relapsed malignant mesothelioma (DETERMINE): A multicentre, international, randomised, double-blind, placebo-controlled phase 2b trial. *Lancet Oncol.* **2017**, *18*, 1261–1273. [CrossRef]
65. Tsao, A.S.; Lin, H.; Carter, B.W.; Lee, J.J.; Rice, D.; Vaporcyan, A.; Swisher, S.; Mehran, R.; Heymach, J.; Nilsson, M.; et al. Biomarker-Integrated Neoadjuvant Dasatinib Trial in Resectable Malignant Pleural Mesothelioma. *J. Thorac. Oncol.* **2018**, *13*, 246–257. [CrossRef]

66. Yu, G.; Wang, L.-G.; Han, Y.; He, Q.-Y. clusterProfiler: An R Package for Comparing Biological Themes Among Gene Clusters. *OMICS A J. Integr. Biol.* **2012**, *16*, 284–287. [CrossRef]
67. Xu, D.; Yang, H.; Berezowska, S.; Gao, Y.; Liang, S.-Q.; Marti, T.M.; Hall, S.R.R.; Dorn, P.; Kocher, G.J.; Schmid, R.A.; et al. Endoplasmic Reticulum Stress Signaling as a Therapeutic Target in Malignant Pleural Mesothelioma. *Cancers* **2019**, *11*, 1502. [CrossRef]
68. Yang, H.; Liang, S.-Q.; Xu, D.; Yang, Z.; Marti, T.M.; Gao, Y.; Kocher, G.J.; Zhao, H.; Schmid, R.A.; Peng, R.-W. HSP90/AXL/eIF4E-regulated unfolded protein response as an acquired vulnerability in drug-resistant KRAS-mutant lung cancer. *Oncogenesis* **2019**, *8*, 45. [CrossRef]
69. Li, J.; Lu, Y.; Akbani, R.; Ju, Z.; Roebuck, P.L.; Liu, W.; Yang, J.-Y.; Broom, B.M.; Verhaak, R.G.W.; Kane, D.W.; et al. TCPA: A resource for cancer functional proteomics data. *Nat. Methods* **2013**, *10*, 1046–1047. [CrossRef]
70. Yang, H.; Zhao, L.; Yao, F.; Gao, Y.; Marti, T.M.; Schmid, R.A.; Peng, R.-W. Integrative Pharmacogenomic Profiling Identifies Novel Cancer Drugs and Gene Networks Modulating Ferroptosis Sensitivity in Pan-Cancer. 2020. Available online: https://doi.org/10.21203/rs.3.rs-34574/v1 (accessed on 3 July 2020).
71. Alonso-López, D.; Campos-Laborie, F.J.; A Gutiérrez, M.; Lambourne, L.; Calderwood, M.A.; Vidal, M.; Rivas, J.D. APID database: Redefining protein–protein interaction experimental evidences and binary interactomes. *Database* **2019**, *2019*. [CrossRef] [PubMed]
72. Samstein, R.M.; Lee, C.-H.; Shoushtari, A.N.; Hellmann, M.D.; Shen, R.; Janjigian, Y.Y.; Barron, D.A.; Zehir, A.; Jordan, E.J.; Omuro, A.; et al. Tumor mutational load predicts survival after immunotherapy across multiple cancer types. *Nat. Genet.* **2019**, *51*, 202–206. [CrossRef] [PubMed]

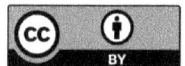

© 2020 by the authors. Licensee MDPI, Basel, Switzerland. This article is an open access article distributed under the terms and conditions of the Creative Commons Attribution (CC BY) license (http://creativecommons.org/licenses/by/4.0/).

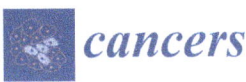

Article

Evaluation of the Preclinical Efficacy of Lurbinectedin in Malignant Pleural Mesothelioma

Dario P. Anobile [1,†], Paolo Bironzo [1,2,†], Francesca Picca [1,3], Marcello F. Lingua [4], Deborah Morena [1,3], Luisella Righi [1,5], Francesca Napoli [1,5], Mauro G. Papotti [1,6,7], Alessandra Pittaro [1,6], Federica Di Nicolantonio [1,8], Chiara Gigliotti [1,8], Federico Bussolino [1,7,8], Valentina Comunanza [1,8], Francesco Guerrera [9,10], Alberto Sandri [11], Francesco Leo [1,11], Roberta Libener [12], Pablo Aviles [13], Silvia Novello [1,2], Riccardo Taulli [1,3], Giorgio V. Scagliotti [1,2,7,*] and Chiara Riganti [1,7,14,*]

1. Department of Oncology, University of Torino, 10043 Orbassano, Italy; dario.anobile@edu.unito.it (D.P.A.); paolo.bironzo@unito.it (P.B.); francesca.picca@unito.it (F.P.); deborah.morena@unito.it (D.M.); luisella.righi@unito.it (L.R.); francesca.napoli@unito.it (F.N.); mauro.papotti@unito.it (M.G.P.); apittaro@cittadellasalute.to.it (A.P.); federica.dinicolantonio@unito.it (F.D.N.); chiara.gigliotti@unito.it (C.G.); federico.bussolino@unito.it (F.B.); valentina.comunanza@unito.it (V.C.); francesco.leo@unito.it (F.L.); silvia.novello@unito.it (S.N.); riccardo.taulli@unito.it (R.T.)
2. Thoracic Unit and Medical Oncology Division, Department of Oncology at San Luigi Hospital, University of Torino, 10043 Orbassano, Italy
3. Center for Experimental Research and Medical Studies (CeRMS), City of Health and Science University Hospital di Torino, University of Torino, 10126 Torino, Italy
4. Department of Medical Sciences, University of Torino, 10126 Torino, Italy; marcello.lingua@edu.unito.it
5. Pathology Unit, San Luigi Hospital, University of Torino, 10043 Orbassano, Italy
6. Pathology Unit, City of Health and Science University Hospital, 10126 Torino, Italy
7. Interdepartmental Centre for Studies on Asbestos and Other Toxic Particulates, University of Torino, 10125 Torino, Italy
8. Candiolo Cancer Institute—FPO, IRCCS, 10060 Candiolo, Italy
9. Department of Surgical Science, University of Torino, 10126 Torino, Italy; francesco.guerrera@unito.it
10. Department of Thoracic Surgery, City of Health and Science University Hospital, 10126 Torino, Italy
11. Thoracic Surgery Division, San Luigi Hospital, University of Torino, 10043 Orbassano, Italy; al.sandri@sanluigi.piemonte.it
12. Department of Integrated Activities Research and Innovation, Azienda Ospedaliera SS. Antonio e Biagio e Cesare Arrigo, 15121 Alessandria, Italy; rlibener@ospedale.al.it
13. Research and Development Department, PharmaMar, 28770 Colmenar Viejo, Madrid, Spain; paviles@pharmamar.com
14. Interdepartmental Research Center of Molecular Biotechnology, University of Torino, 10126 Torino, Italy
* Correspondence: giorgio.scagliotti@unito.it (G.V.S.); chiara.riganti@unito.it (C.R.)
† These authors contributed equally to this work.

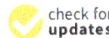

Citation: Anobile, D.P.; Bironzo, P.; Picca, F.; Lingua, M.F.; Morena, D.; Righi, L.; Napoli, F.; Papotti, M.G.; Pittaro, A.; Di Nicolantonio, F.; et al. Evaluation of the Preclinical Efficacy of Lurbinectedin in Malignant Pleural Mesothelioma. *Cancers* **2021**, *13*, 2332. https://doi.org/10.3390/cancers13102332

Academic Editor: Daniel L. Pouliquen

Received: 20 April 2021
Accepted: 10 May 2021
Published: 12 May 2021

Publisher's Note: MDPI stays neutral with regard to jurisdictional claims in published maps and institutional affiliations.

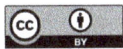

Copyright: © 2021 by the authors. Licensee MDPI, Basel, Switzerland. This article is an open access article distributed under the terms and conditions of the Creative Commons Attribution (CC BY) license (https://creativecommons.org/licenses/by/4.0/).

Simple Summary: The marine drug lurbinectedin revealed an unprecedented efficacy against patient-derived malignant pleural mesothelioma cells, regardless of the histological type and the BAP1 mutation status. By inducing strong DNA damages, it dramatically arrested cell cycle progression and induced apoptosis. These results may be translated into the use of lurbinectedin as an effective agent for malignant pleural mesothelioma patients.

Abstract: Background: Malignant pleural mesothelioma (MPM) is a highly aggressive cancer generally diagnosed at an advanced stage and characterized by a poor prognosis. The absence of alterations in druggable kinases, together with an immune-suppressive tumor microenvironment, limits the use of molecular targeted therapies, making the treatment of MPM particularly challenging. Here we investigated the in vitro susceptibility of MPM to lurbinectedin (PM01183), a marine-derived drug that recently received accelerated approval by the FDA for the treatment of patients with metastatic small cell lung cancer with disease progression on or after platinum-based chemotherapy. Methods: A panel of primary MPM cultures, resembling the three major MPM histological subtypes (epithelioid, sarcomatoid, and biphasic), was characterized in terms of BAP1 status and histological markers. Subsequently, we explored the effects of lurbinectedin at nanomolar concentration on cell cycle, cell viability, DNA damage, genotoxic stress response, and proliferation. Results: Stabilized

MPM cultures exhibited high sensitivity to lurbinectedin independently from the BAP1 mutational status and histological classification. Specifically, we observed that lurbinectedin rapidly promoted a cell cycle arrest in the S-phase and the activation of the DNA damage response, two conditions that invariably resulted in an irreversible DNA fragmentation, together with strong apoptotic cell death. Moreover, the analysis of long-term treatment indicated that lurbinectedin severely impacts MPM transforming abilities in vitro. Conclusion: Overall, our data provide evidence that lurbinectedin exerts a potent antitumoral activity on primary MPM cells, independently from both the histological subtype and BAP1 alteration, suggesting its potential activity in the treatment of MPM patients.

Keywords: MPM; lurbinectedin; DNA damage response

1. Introduction

Malignant pleural mesothelioma (MPM) is a rare but extremely aggressive type of cancer arising from pleural mesothelium and is highly associated with asbestos exposure. The disease is characterized by a long latency between initial exposure to asbestos and the clinical onset of the disease (30–50 years) and, although in Western regions the peak was expected in the 2020s [1], the ongoing use of asbestos in developing countries could lead to a persistence of new cases in the next decades [2]. MPM is classified into three major histological subtypes: epithelioid, sarcomatoid, and biphasic. While the epithelioid subtype occurs more frequently, accounting for approximately 60% of cases, and correlates with a better outcome, the sarcomatoid subgroup represents 10–20% of the cases and is characterized by a worse prognosis [3,4]. Independently from the morphology, the MPM tumor microenvironment is particularly enriched of immunosuppressive cells, which makes this tumor particularly refractory to different therapies [5–10]. Moreover, MPM is generally diagnosed in advanced stage, minimizing the role of curative treatments. For advanced-stage disease, the first-line systemic treatment consists of cisplatin and pemetrexed [11], a combination that prolongs the median survival time of only 3 months. Recently, the combination of immune checkpoint inhibitors directed against programmed death-1 (PD-1) and cytotoxic-T-lymphocyte-associated protein 4 (CTLA-4) showed its superiority over chemotherapy in previously untreated and unresectable MPM, especially in non-epithelioid tumors [12]. Conversely, no second-line standard therapy has been approved, despite the pre-clinical and the clinical evaluation of different therapeutic agents [13,14].

The genomic landscape of MPM reveals a low mutational burden with inactivating alterations mainly on oncosuppressors (BAP1, CDKN2A, NF2, TP53, LATS2, and SETD2) [15–18] thus precluding the use of molecular therapies against activated oncogenes. Among the oncosuppressors, BAP1 (BRCA1-associated protein) alterations account from 30% to 60% of cases [15,17,19,20]. Indeed, BAP1 germline mutations are known to predispose to mesothelioma and other cancer-associated syndromes [21,22] thus indicating a critical role for this deubiquitinase in suppressing tumor development. BAP1 regulates different biological processes among which chromatin modification, cell cycle, apoptosis, ferroptosis, cell metabolism, and differentiation [23]. Notably, BAP1 is involved in DNA synthesis, DNA duplication under stress conditions [24,25], and DNA damage response, by modulating the function of the BRCA1/BARD1 (BRCA1 Associated RING Domain 1) complex and coordinating the recruitment of RAD51 to the damaged DNA loci [26,27].

Lurbinectedin (PM01183) is a marine-derived anticancer drug that exerts a potent antitumor activity in different cancer cell lines and xenografts models and is currently under clinical evaluation in several tumor types [28–35]. Recently, the FDA has released a conditional approval for lurbinectedin for the treatment of second-line metastatic small cell lung cancer patients [36] while promising antitumor activity has been reported in MPM patients in second- and third-line [37]. However, there are no data available on the role of lurbinectedin as monotherapy or in combination in the first-line treatment of MPM. At the molecular level, lurbinectedin covalently binds CG-rich sequences in the DNA minor groove. The presence of the drug on the DNA helix inhibits the transcriptional process and is associated with the generation of DNA breaks [28]. Moreover, the interaction of lurbinectedin with both DNA strand breaks also interferes with the enzymes involved in the DNA damage response [38].

Here, we report about the potential efficacy of lurbinectedin in a panel of primary MPM cultures. Specifically, we demonstrated that lurbinectedin is strongly effective at nanomolar concentration and interferes with the transforming properties of MPM in a way that is independent of the BAP1 status and histological classification. With the caveat that our cell cultures were derived from diagnostic biopsies or surgical resections, our data indicate that lurbinectedin could potentially be explored in the management of patients with advanced MPM as second-line treatment or part of combination treatment in first-line.

2. Results

2.1. Primary Mesothelioma Cell Cultures Characterization

Twelve primary MPM cell lines, derived from patients with different histology, were stabilized as 2D cultures (Figure 1A). Flow cytometry for pan-cytokeratin (Figure 1B), immunohistochemical analysis (Figure 1C and Table 1), and immunoblotting for the BAP1 status (Figure 1D) were used to characterize the MPM cell lines. Notably, our panel (6 BAP1+ and 6 BAP1− cultures) was representative of the three major MPM histological subtypes (epithelioid, sarcomatoid, and biphasic) (Table S1).

Table 1. Histological characterization of MPM cultures.

UPN	BAP1	Pan-CK	WT1	CALR
1	POS	POS	POS	POS
2	POS	POS	NEG	NEG
3	POS	POS	POS	NEG
4	POS	POS	POS	POS
5	POS	NEG	POS	POS
6	POS	POS	NEG	NEG
7	NEG	POS	POS	POS
8	NEG	POS	POS	NEG
9	NEG	POS	POS	POS
10	NEG	POS	POS	POS
11	NEG	POS	NEG	POS
12	NEG	POS	NEG	NEG

Results of the immunohistochemical stainings of MPM samples for BRCA1 associated protein-1 (BAP1), pancytokeratin (pan-CK), Wilms tumor-1 antigen (WT1), calretinin (CALR). POS: positive; NEG: negative.

2.2. Lurbinectedin Exerts Anti-Proliferative Effects in Patient-Derived Mesothelioma Cells

As shown in Figure 2, lurbinectedin decreased the viability of MPM cells in a dose-dependent manner, with an IC_{50} in the low nanomolar range for all cell lines (Table 2), independently from the BAP1 status and the histological subtype (Figure 2A–D). Indeed, although the IC_{50} was slightly higher in BAP1− vs. BAP1+ cells (Figure 2C) as well as in the sarcomatoid/biphasic vs epithelioid histotype (Figure 2D), the difference was not statistically significant. Notably, UPN6, UPN10, and UPN12 received trabectedin as second-line treatment and their overall survival was <12 months (Table S1). The cell lines derived from these patients had indeed the highest IC_{50} in the panel analyzed, but it was below 5 nM for all of them (Table 2).

2.3. Long-Term Lurbinectedin Treatment Impacts on MPM Transforming Abilities

Since mesothelioma is particularly resistant to conventional chemotherapy, we evaluated the long-term effect of lurbinectedin in terms of inhibiting cell proliferation by performing a crystal violet viability assay. Also in this setting, nanomolar concentrations of lurbinectedin dramatically reduced cell growth (Figure 3A,B). Furthermore, we extended our analysis by testing lurbinectedin ability to interfere with the anchorage-independent growth of MPM cells. The number of visible colonies was markedly decreased upon treatment, showing long-term anticancer efficacy (Figure 3C,D). Importantly, the consistent reduction in anchorage-independent growth showed no differences between BAP1+ and BAP1− cells, suggesting that lurbinectedin strongly impairs the tumorigenic potential of MPM cells, independently from the BAP1 status.

Table 2. IC_{50} values of MPM cell lines treated with lurbinectedin.

UPN	IC_{50} L (nM)
1	0.073
2	0.33
3	0.28
4	0.35
5	1.09
6	1.13
7	0.085
8	0.65
9	0.23
10	3.29
11	0.76
12	4.54

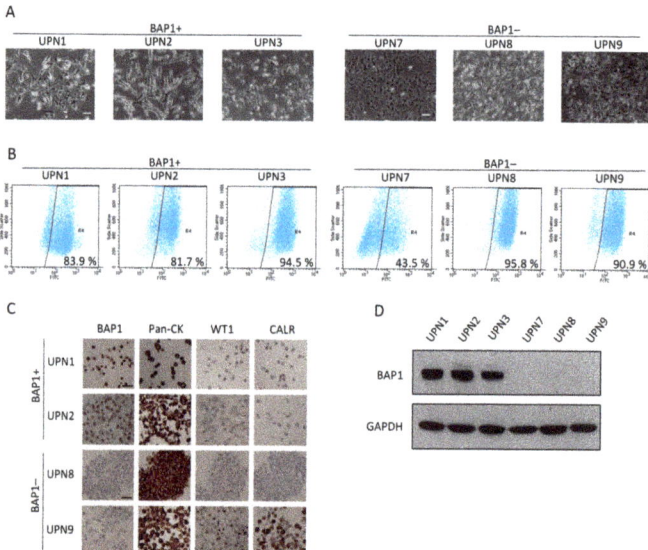

Figure 1. Characterization of patient-derived MPM cell lines. (**A**) Representative images showing different morphology of three BAP1 positive (BAP1+) and three BAP1 negative (BAP1−) MPM cell lines (scale bar = 100 µm). (**B**) Flow cytometry plot representing the percentage of pancytokeratine positive cells in the indicated MPM cell lines. (**C**) Immunohistochemical analysis of BAP1, pan-cytokeratin (pan-CK), Wilms tumor-1 antigen (WT1), and calretinin (CALR) in the indicated MPM cell lines (scale bar = 100 µm). (**D**) Western blot analysis showing BAP1 status of the reported MPM cell lines.

2.4. Lurbinectedin Treatment Interferes with Cell Cycle Progression

To study the molecular basis of this anti-proliferative activity, we analyzed the effect of lurbinectedin on cell cycle regulation. While we observed variable changes in the percentage of cells in the G2/M-phase, indicating an unlikely strong mitotic arrest, we observed a constant accumulation of cells in the S-phase (Figure 4 and Supplementary Figure S1). This event occurred in both BAP1+ and BAP1− cells, suggesting that lurbinectedin-mediated perturbation of the cell cycle is BAP1-independent.

2.5. Lurbinectedin Induces a Profound DNA Damage Coupled with Strong Apoptosis

Among the pleiotropic mechanisms of action of lurbinectedin [28,38] the increase of S-phase arrested cells is suggestive of irreversible DNA damage. Indeed, lurbinectedin induced a significant increase in round-shaped and dense cells (Supplementary Figure S2). The presence of irreversible DNA fragmentation was evaluated by the Single Cell Gel Electrophoresis (SCGE). Specifically, in both BAP1+ and BAP1− cells lurbinectedin induced a dose-dependent genomic fragmentation (Figure 5A,B). The presence of genotoxic stress was confirmed by the increase in the phospho (Ser345) Chk1 and phospho (Thr68) Chk2 (Figure 5C,D), two cell cycle checkpoints that block DNA replication after being phosphorylated by the DNA-damaging sensors ATM/ATR kinases [39]. Moreover, in lurbinectedin-treated cells, we observed the accumulation of phospho (Ser15) p53 and phospho (Ser139) H2AX (Figure 5C,D), two additional targets of ATM/ATR kinases that are generally phosphorylated in response to DNA strand breaks and stalled replication [40,41]. This provided additional evidence of the strong DNA damage induced by lurbinectedin, which is also responsible for cell growth arrest (Figure 4 and Supplementary Figure S1). Such mitotic catastrophe is often coupled with apoptosis [40]. Accordingly, lurbinectedin treatment resulted in a strong induction of apoptosis (Figure 6A,B) as also shown by the dose-dependent activation of caspase 3 (Figure 6C,D).

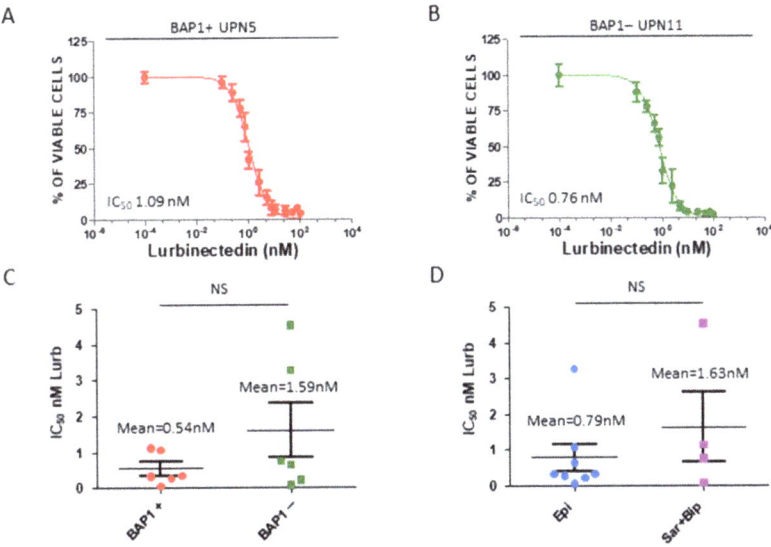

Figure 2. Patient-derived MPM cell lines sensitivity to lurbinectedin. (**A,B**) Representative dose-response curves and corresponding IC$_{50}$ values of the two indicated MPM cell lines treated with lurbinectedin (0.1 nM–100 nM) for 72 h. (**C**) Dot plot of IC$_{50}$ values measured in lurbinectedin-treated MPM cell lines positive or negative for BAP1 expression. ^{NS} $p > 0.05$. (**D**) Dot plot of IC$_{50}$ values measured in lurbinectedin-treated MPM cell lines grouped according to the histological subtype. ^{NS} $p > 0.05$.

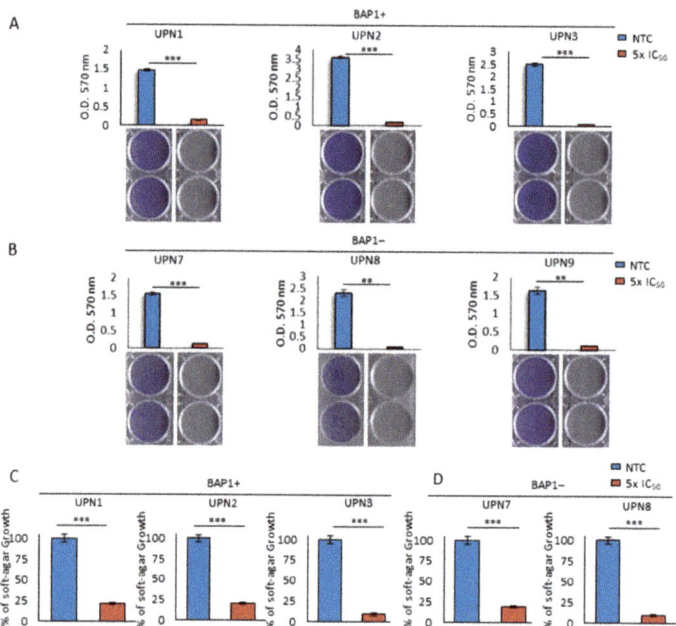

Figure 3. Lurbinectedin impairs long-term proliferation and anchorage-independent growth of MPM cell lines. (**A**,**B**) Representative pictures (lower panels) and quantification (upper panels) of crystal violet staining performed on the indicated MPM cell lines treated or not with lurbinectedin (5-fold the IC_{50}) for 10 days. Data are expressed as means ± SEM; ** $p < 0.01$; *** $p < 0.001$. (**C**,**D**) Soft agar growth assay quantification of the indicated MPM cell lines treated or not with lurbinectedin (5-fold the IC_{50}) for 20 days. The number of colonies obtained from untreated cells was set at 100%. Data are expressed as means ± SEM; *** $p < 0.001$.

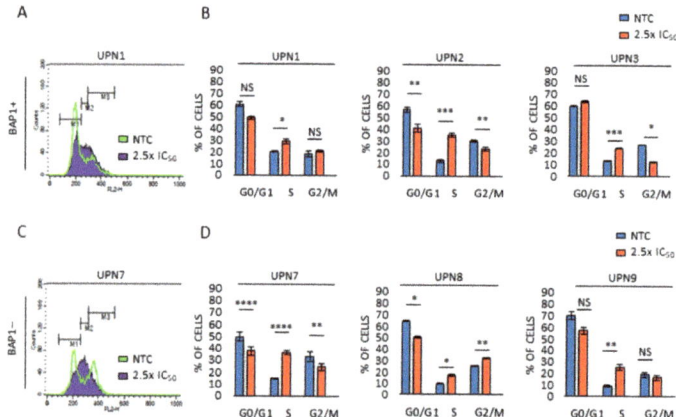

Figure 4. Lurbinectedin effects on cell cycle distribution. (**A**,**C**) Representative flow cytometry histogram showing the cell cycle distribution of the indicated MPM cell lines, treated (purple) or not (green) with lurbinectedin (2.5-fold the IC_{50}) for 24 h. (**B**,**D**) Histograms displaying cell number percentage in each cell cycle phase (G0/G1, S and G2/M) of the indicated MPM cell lines, treated or not with lurbinectedin (2.5-fold the IC_{50}) for 24 h. Data are expressed as means ± SEM; ^{NS} $p > 0.05$; * $p < 0.05$; ** $p < 0.01$; *** $p < 0.001$; **** $p < 0.0001$.

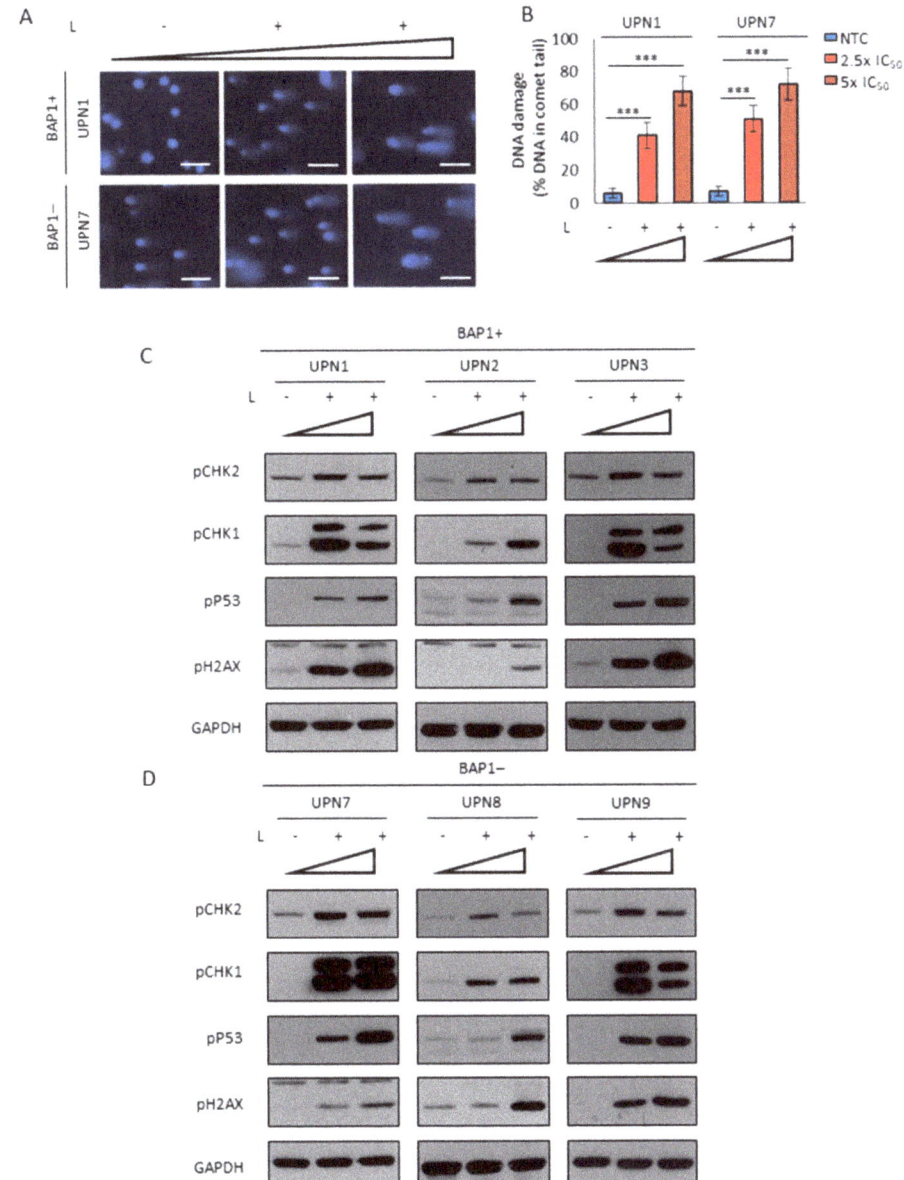

Figure 5. Lurbinectedin actively induces DNA damage response in MPM cell lines. (**A**) Representative Comet assay images of the indicated BAP1+ and BAP1− MPM cell lines treated or not with increasing lurbinectedin (L) concentrations (2.5-fold and 5-fold the IC$_{50}$) for 24h (scale bar = 5 μm). (**B**) Histograms showing Comet assay data quantitation by CometScore software. Bars represent a percentage of total DNA in the tail. Data are expressed as means ± SEM; *** $p < 0.001$. (**C,D**) Western blot analysis for the indicated proteins in BAP1+ and BAP1- MPM cell lines treated or not with increasing lurbinectedin (L) concentrations (2.5-fold and 5-fold the IC$_{50}$) for 24 h. GAPDH was used as a loading control.

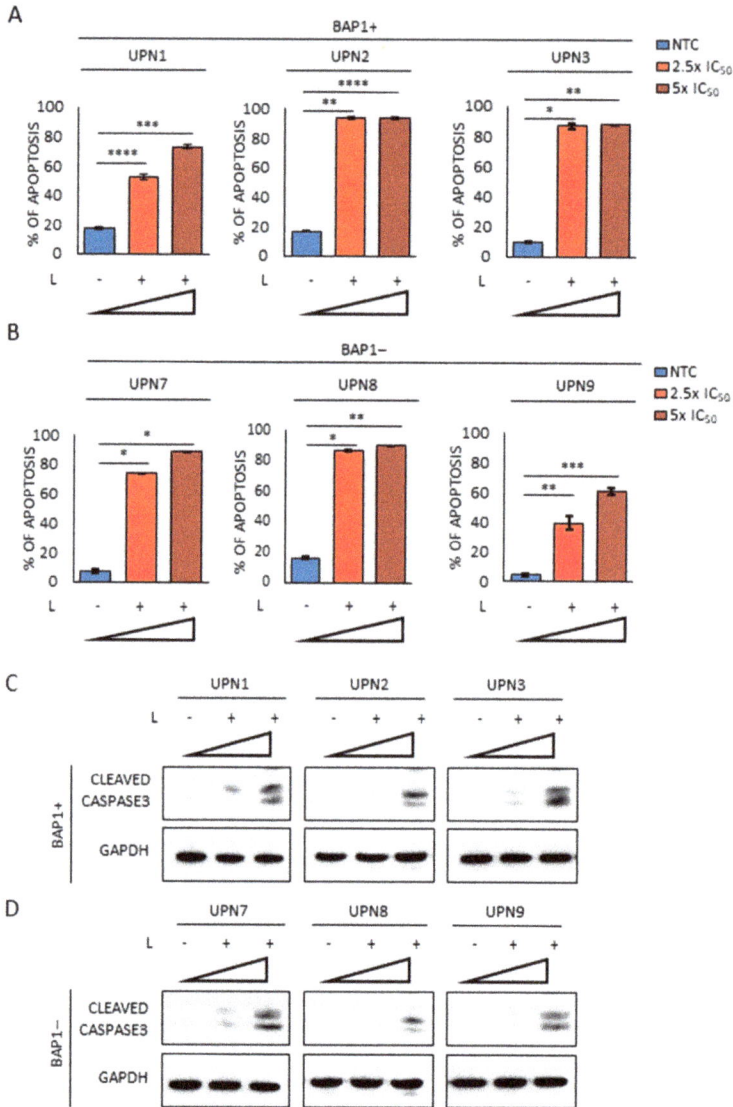

Figure 6. Lurbinectedin treatment strongly induces apoptosis in MPM cell lines. (**A,B**) Histograms representing the percentage of apoptotic MPM cells treated or not with increasing lurbinectedin (L) concentrations (2.5-fold and 5-fold the IC_{50}) for 72 h. The apoptotic rate was measured by TMRM assay. Data are expressed as means ± SEM; * $p < 0.05$; ** $p < 0.01$; *** $p < 0.001$, **** $p < 0.0001$. (**C,D**) Western blot analysis of cleaved caspase 3 in MPM cell lines treated or not with increasing lurbinectedin (L) concentrations (2.5-fold and 5-fold the IC_{50}) for 24 h. GAPDH was used as a loading control.

3. Discussion

Malignant Pleural Mesothelioma (MPM) is an aggressive tumor marginally impacted by standard chemotherapy regimens. Moreover, the lack of effective molecular therapies as well as the immune-evasive tumor microenvironment makes the treatment of MPM particularly challenging [5–10,42]. Because MPM currently lacks peculiar oncogenic drivers, we have explored the potential therapeutic efficacy of lurbinectedin, an alkylating agent which recently received FDA-conditional approval for the treatment of metastatic small cell lung cancer patients relapsing after chemotherapy [36].

We investigated the antitumor activity of lurbinectedin in a panel of 12 recently established primary MPM cell cultures. Our panel included all three MPM histotypes as well as cultures BAP1 positive and negative. Thus, although limited in terms of absolute number of cell lines, this panel is potentially representative of the different MPM phenotypes. Interestingly, we initially observed that lurbinectedin was effective at nanomolar concentrations and, as reported for other agents, its efficacy was independent of the BAP1 status. These data are particularly encouraging, although we are aware that freshly stabilized cultures could be potentially more sensitive to cytotoxic agents than what is usually observed at the clinical level. It is worthy of note, however, that three patients (UPN6, UPN10, UPN12) subsequently received trabectedin, a previous generation drug binding the minor groove of DNA, as second-line treatment. They did not show a superior clinical benefit compared to patients undergoing other treatments, indicating a limited efficacy of trabectedin. Interestingly, the MPM cells derived from these three patients had the highest IC_{50} to lurbinectedin. These data may suggest that the response obtained in our stabilized cultures is a good surrogate of the potential effect of drugs binding the DNA minor groove and targeting the DNA repair observed in vivo.

Our experiments revealed that, as a consequence of the intrinsic ability of lurbinectedin to bind the minor groove of DNA, the drug interferes with the cell cycle, delaying progression through the S-phase. Interestingly, MPM cells immediately responded to genotoxic stress as demonstrated by the phosphorylation of H2AX, an early marker of the cellular response triggered by DNA double-strand breaks. Moreover, we observed the activation of Chk1 and Chk2 as a direct consequence of the stalled replication induced by DNA damage, responsible for the accumulation of MPM cells in the S-phase of the cell cycle. Finally, in our setting, p53 stabilization was not associated with DNA repair but invariably resulted in a massive apoptotic response, as revealed by cleaved caspase 3 activity and irreversible DNA fragmentation detected by Comet assay.

Notably, the efficacy of lurbinectedin against MPM was maintained also upon long-term treatment, as assessed by both crystal violet viability and anchorage-independent growth assays, providing further evidence of its anticancer potential.

As a consequence of DNA damage, replication arrest, and induction of apoptosis, we propose that lurbinectedin impairs the tumorigenic potential of MPM cells, and our results provide support to the clinical data recently reported in a multicentric phase II trial in second- or third-line palliative therapy [37]. Speculatively, considering the high anti-proliferative effect, if the results of the present study will be confirmed in MPM PDXs, lurbinectedin could be potentially investigated in the front line setting, for instance for a short pre-operative treatment in the early stages of MPM. Indeed, the reduction of anchorage-independent growth ability suggests lurbinectedin as a potential cytoreductive agent that, if proven in animal models and at the clinical level, will allow more conservative/less invasive surgery. Finally, the efficacy in all histotypes, independently from the BAP1 status, confers to lurbinectedin a strong advantage compared to other drugs currently used in MPM treatment, since its use could be potentially considered for all patients.

4. Materials and Methods

4.1. Reagents and Chemicals

Cell culture plasticware was obtained from Falcon (Glendale, AZ, USA), Biofil (Indore, India), and Costar (Washingtone, DC, USA). Lurbinectedin (PM01183) was kindly provided by PharmaMar (Madrid, Spain).

4.2. Cells

Primary MPM cells were obtained from biopsies during explorative thoracoscopy or pleurectomy, performed at the Thoracic Surgery Division of AOU Città della Salute e della Scienza, Torino, Italy; AOU San Luigi Gonzaga, Orbassano, Italy, and AO of Alessandria, Biological Bank of Mesothelioma, Alessandria, Italy. Samples were anonymized by assigning an unknown patient number (UPN). Histological features of the original tumors and clinical features, including the first- and second-line treatment and the overall survival, of the corresponding patients are reported in Table S1. Samples were minced in 1 mm^3-pieces, enzymatically digested for 1 h at 37 °C with 0.2 mg/mL hyaluronidase and 1 mg/mL collagenase [5], centrifuged at 1200× g for 5 min and seeded at 1×10^6 cells/mL density in DMEM advanced/F12 (Gibco, Dublin, Ireland) until passage #5, when cultures were shifted to DMEM/F12 nutrient mixture medium (Sigma, Saint Louis, MO, USA). All media were supplemented with 10% heat-inactivated fetal bovine serum (FBS) (Sigma), 1% L-glutamine, 1% penicillin/streptomycin. Cells reached a stabilization (i.e., rate of cell subculture ≤1/week) in 2 to 7 months. UPN#3, UPN#4, UPN#5, UPN#6, UPN#10, UPN#11, UPN #12 were directly put in culture. UPN#1, UPN#2, UPN#7, UPN#8, UPN#9 were established from patient-derived xenografts. All cell lines were cultured in a humidified incubator at 37 °C in 5% CO_2 and routinely checked for Mycoplasma spp. contamination.

4.3. Patient-Derived Xenograft Generation

MPM patient-derived xenografts (PDXs) models were established from diagnostic tissue samples obtained at videothoracoscopy or during surgical pleurectomy. Each sample was implanted in the left or right side of the dorsal region of female NOD scid gamma (NSG) mice. A small piece of tumor was implanted subcutaneously and the wound was then stitched by surgical glue (Vetbond, Alcyon Italia, Cherasco, Italy). The tumor growth was monitored until the mass reached 2000 mm^3. Then the animal was sacrificed by cervical dislocation, after anesthesia. The tumor area was shaved and disinfected with alcohol and the skin around the tumor was cut off. The tumor was divided into smaller pieces for re-implanting and collecting materials for further investigations. In the present work, the PDX platform was used as a tool to generate primary MPM cell cultures, stabilized in a shorter period (i.e., 2–3 months) than cells obtained directly from surgical procedures and used for pharmacological screening. To this aim, 0.2 g of tumors excised from the P1 generation of mice were digested to obtained a single-cell suspension [5] and put in culture as described in paragraph 4.2.

4.4. Immunohistochemical Analysis

The mesothelial features of cultures were confirmed by immunohistochemical (IHC) staining carried out on cells at passage 1. Specifically, cells were centrifuged at 1200× g for 5 min, fixed overnight in 4% v/v formalin at 4 °C, and then paraffin-embedded. The following antibodies were used: BAP-1 (Santa-Cruz Biotechnology, Santa Cruz, CA, USA, sc-28383, 1:100); Pan-cytokeratin AE1/AE3 (Dako, Agilent, Santa Clara, CA, USA, GA053, 1:500); Wilms Tumor-1 antigen (WT1) cl.6FH2 (Thermo Fisher Scientific, Waltham, MA, USA, MA1-46028, 1:10); Calretinin (Thermo Fisher Scientific, RB-9002-R7, 1:100). Mesothelial origin was confirmed if positivity for at least one between calretinin and WT1 was detected, as well as in the case of positivity for pancytokeratin. The histological features are reported in Table 1.

4.5. IC_{50} Calculation

Cells were seeded in 96-well plates at a density of 2×10^3/well and serially diluted lurbinectedin (0.01 nM–100 nM) was added to the medium. After 72 h of treatment, IC_{50} was evaluated with CellTiter-Glo (Promega) according to the manufacturer's instructions, using a Cytation 3 Imaging Reader (Bio-Tek Instruments, Winooski, VT, USA).

4.6. Crystal Violet Assay

For long-term proliferation, cells were seeded at a density of 4×10^3/well in 12-well plates and treated with the indicated concentrations of lurbinectedin for 10 days. Subsequently, cells were fixed and stained with 5% w/v crystal violet solution in 66% v/v

methanol and washed. Crystal violet was eluted by adding 10% acetic acid into each well. Quantification was performed by measuring the absorbance (570 nm) with Cytation 3 Imaging Reader (Bio-Tek Instruments).

4.7. Soft-Agar Assay

For anchorage-independent cell growth assay, cells were suspended in 0.45% type VII low-melting agarose in medium supplemented with 10% FBS at 1×10^5 cells/well, plated on a layer of 0.9% agarose in 10% FBS medium in 6-well plates, and cultured for 20–30 days with the indicated concentrations of lurbinectedin.

4.8. Cell Cycle Analysis

Cells were plated at a density of 1.2×10^5/well in 6-well plates and treated with the indicated concentrations of lurbinectedin for 24 h. Subsequently, cells were washed in PBS, treated with RNAse (167 µg/mL), and stained for 15 min at RT with propidium iodide (33 µg/mL). The cell-cycle distribution in G0/G1, S, and G2/M phases was analyzed by FACSCalibur flow cytometer (Becton Dickinson, Franklin Lanes, NJ, USA) and calculated using the CellQuest program (Becton Dickinson).

4.9. Apoptosis Detection Assay

MPM cells were plated at a density of 1.2×10^5/well in 6-well plates and treated with the indicated concentrations of lurbinectedin for 72 h. Subsequently, floating and adherent cells were washed with PBS and stained with tetramethylrhodamine methylester perchlorate (TMRM) (200 nM) for 15 min at RT. The percentage of apoptosis was measured by FACSCalibur flow cytometer (Becton Dickinson) and calculated using the CellQuest program (Becton Dickinson).

4.10. Comet Assay

DNA damage was assessed by Single Cell Gel Electrophoresis assay (Comet assay) [43]. At least 100 nuclei were counted in each condition. The percentage of DNA in the tail was quantified using the CometScore software (TriTek Corp., Sumerduck, VA, USA).

4.11. Western Blot Analysis

Cells were washed with ice-cold PBS and incubated for 20 min on ice in 0.1% Triton X-100 lysis buffer (20 mM Tris HCl pH 7.4; 150 mM NaCl; 5 mM EDTA; 0.1% Triton X-100; 1 mM Phenylmethanesulfonyl fluoride; 10 mM NaF; 1 mM Na3VO4, supplemented with protease inhibitor cocktail). Cells were then centrifuged at $14,000 \times g$ for 15 min at 4 °C to remove any cellular debris. Protein lysates were subsequently quantified using DC protein assay (Bio-Rad), loaded in 4–12% NuPAGE Bis-Tris Protein Gels (Thermo Fisher Scientific) according to the manufacturer's instructions, and transferred onto Hybond ECL nitrocellulose membranes. Blocking was performed with 5% Nonfat dried milk (PanReac AppliChem, Darmstadt, Germany) for 45 min at RT. Membranes were then incubated O/N at 4°C with the following antibodies: BAP-1 (Santa Cruz Biotechnology, sc-28383); phospho(Ser345) Chk1 (Cell Signaling, Danvers, MA, USA, 2348); phospho(Thr68) Chk2 (Cell Signaling, 2197); phospho(Ser15) p53 (Cell Signaling, 9286); GAPDH (Cell Signaling, 5174); cleaved Caspase3 (Cell Signaling, 9661); phospho(Ser139)-Histone H2A.X (Cell Signaling, 9718); rabbit IgG, HRP-linked (Cell Signaling, 7074); mouse IgG, HRP-linked (Cell Signaling, 7076). Proteins were detected with horseradish peroxidase-conjugated secondary antibodies and Pierce™ ECL Western Blotting Substrate.

4.12. Image Processing

Image acquisition was performed with Leica dmire2 microscope and with Olympus BX51. Images were processed with the ImageJ software package (https://imagej.nih.gov/ij/ accessed on 16 April 2021).

4.13. Statistical Analysis

All values were expressed as mean ± SEM and derived from at least two independent experiments. Statistical analyses were performed using Microsoft Excel and GraphPad Prism 5. Graphs were generated using Microsoft Excel and GraphPad Prism. Two-tailed Student's t-test was used to evaluate statistical significance: $^{NS}\, p > 0.05$; * $p < 0.05$; ** $p < 0.01$; *** $p < 0.001$; **** $p < 0.0001$.

5. Conclusions

Overall, our work proves the efficacy of lurbinectedin at nanomolar concentration against primary MPM cells. Although obtained in a relatively small cohort, that however is representative of the different MPM phenotypes, our results are particularly encouraging and put the basis for investigating lurbinectedin in different therapeutic settings of MPM.

Supplementary Materials: The following are available online at https://www.mdpi.com/article/10.3390/cancers13102332/s1, Figure S1: Lurbinectedin effects on cell cycle distribution, Figure S2: Lurbinectedin treatment strongly impairs cell viability in MPM cell lines, Table S1: Histological features of the original tumors and clinical features of the corresponding patients.

Author Contributions: Conceptualization, C.R., R.T., G.V.S., F.P., P.B., and D.P.A.; methodology, F.P., D.P.A., M.F.L., D.M., L.R., F.N., M.G.P., A.P., F.D.N., C.G., F.B., V.C., F.G., A.S., F.L., R.L., P.A., and S.N.; writing—review and editing C.R., R.T., G.V.S., and P.B.; supervision, C.R., R.T., P.B., and G.V.S. All authors have read and agreed to the published version of the manuscript.

Funding: The research plan has received funding from AIRC under IG 2019—ID. 23760 project to G.V.S and IG 2019 ID. 21408 project to C.R. EX60% Funding 2019 to P.B.; ERA-Net Transcan-2-JTC 2017 (TOPMESO to F.B.). PharmaMar kindly provided the drug for the study without any influence on the conduction of the experiments.

Institutional Review Board Statement: The study was conducted according to the guidelines of the Declaration of Helsinki and approved by the Ethics Committee of San Luigi Hospital (#126/2016) and the Biological Bank of Mesothelioma, S. Antonio e Biagio Hospital, Alessandria, Italy (#9/11/2011). All animal procedures were performed in accordance with the national, institutional, and international law, policies, and guidelines (NIH guide for the Care and Use of Laboratory Animals -2011 edition-; European Economic Community (EEC) Council Directive 2010/63/UE; Italian Governing Law D. lg 26/2014). The animal study was approved by the Ethical Committee of the University of Turin and by the Italian Ministry of Health (400/2017-PR).

Informed Consent Statement: Informed consent was obtained from all subjects involved in the study.

Data Availability Statement: The data presented in this study are available in this article (and Supplementary Materials).

Acknowledgments: We are grateful to all patients and their families who participated in the study.

Conflicts of Interest: G.V.S. received honoraria from AstraZeneca, Eli Lilly, MSD, Pfizer, Roche, Johnson & Johnson, Takeda; consulting or advisory role for Eli Lilly, Beigene, and AstraZeneca, received institutional research funding from Eli Lilly and MSD and received travel, accommodations from Bayer. The Riganti and Taulli laboratories have received research support from PharmaMar. The other authors declare no conflict of interest. The funders had no role in the design of the study; in the collection, analyses, or interpretation of data; in the writing of the manuscript, or in the decision to publish the results.

References

1. Peto, J.; Decarli, A.; Vecchia, C.L.; Levi, F.; Negri, E. The European Mesothelioma Epidemic. *Br. J. Cancer* **1999**, *79*, 666–672. [CrossRef]
2. Chen, T.; Sun, X.-M.; Wu, L. High Time for Complete Ban on Asbestos Use in Developing Countries. *JAMA Oncol.* **2019**, *5*, 779–780. [CrossRef] [PubMed]
3. Yap, T.A.; Aerts, J.G.; Popat, S.; Fennell, D.A. Novel Insights into Mesothelioma Biology and Implications for Therapy. *Nat. Rev. Cancer* **2017**, *17*, 475–488. [CrossRef] [PubMed]

4. Kojima, M.; Kajino, K.; Momose, S.; Wali, N.; Hlaing, M.T.; Han, B.; Yue, L.; Abe, M.; Fujii, T.; Ikeda, K.; et al. Possible Reversibility between Epithelioid and Sarcomatoid Types of Mesothelioma Is Independent of ERC/Mesothelin Expression. *Respir. Res.* **2020**, *21*, 187. [CrossRef]
5. Salaroglio, I.C.; Kopecka, J.; Napoli, F.; Pradotto, M.; Maletta, F.; Costardi, L.; Gagliasso, M.; Milosevic, V.; Ananthanarayanan, P.; Bironzo, P.; et al. Potential Diagnostic and Prognostic Role of Microenvironment in Malignant Pleural Mesothelioma. *J. Thorac. Oncol.* **2019**, *14*, 1458–1471. [CrossRef] [PubMed]
6. Hegmans, J.P.J.J.; Hemmes, A.; Hammad, H.; Boon, L.; Hoogsteden, H.C.; Lambrecht, B.N. Mesothelioma Environment Comprises Cytokines and T-Regulatory Cells That Suppress Immune Responses. *Eur. Respir. J.* **2006**, *27*, 1086–1095. [CrossRef] [PubMed]
7. Veltman, J.D.; Lambers, M.E.H.; van Nimwegen, M.; Hendriks, R.W.; Hoogsteden, H.C.; Aerts, J.G.J.V.; Hegmans, J.P.J.J. COX-2 Inhibition Improves Immunotherapy and Is Associated with Decreased Numbers of Myeloid-Derived Suppressor Cells in Mesothelioma. Celecoxib Influences MDSC Function. *BMC Cancer* **2010**, *10*, 464. [CrossRef] [PubMed]
8. Ujiie, H.; Kadota, K.; Nitadori, J.; Aerts, J.G.; Woo, K.M.; Sima, C.S.; Travis, W.D.; Jones, D.R.; Krug, L.M.; Adusumilli, P.S. The Tumoral and Stromal Immune Microenvironment in Malignant Pleural Mesothelioma: A Comprehensive Analysis Reveals Prognostic Immune Markers. *Oncoimmunology* **2015**, *4*, e1009285. [CrossRef]
9. Chu, G.J.; van Zandwijk, N.; Rasko, J.E.J. The Immune Microenvironment in Mesothelioma: Mechanisms of Resistance to Immunotherapy. *Front. Oncol.* **2019**, *9*, 1366. [CrossRef]
10. Riganti, C.; Lingua, M.F.; Salaroglio, I.C.; Falcomatà, C.; Righi, L.; Morena, D.; Picca, F.; Oddo, D.; Kopecka, J.; Pradotto, M.; et al. Bromodomain Inhibition Exerts Its Therapeutic Potential in Malignant Pleural Mesothelioma by Promoting Immunogenic Cell Death and Changing the Tumor Immune-Environment. *Oncoimmunology* **2018**, *7*, e1398874. [CrossRef]
11. Cinausero, M.; Rihawi, K.; Sperandi, F.; Melotti, B.; Ardizzoni, A. Chemotherapy Treatment in Malignant Pleural Mesothelioma: A Difficult History. *J. Thorac. Dis.* **2018**, *10*, S304–S310. [CrossRef]
12. Baas, P.; Scherpereel, A.; Nowak, A.K.; Fujimoto, N.; Peters, S.; Tsao, A.S.; Mansfield, A.S.; Popat, S.; Jahan, T.; Antonia, S.; et al. First-Line Nivolumab plus Ipilimumab in Unresectable Malignant Pleural Mesothelioma (CheckMate 743): A Multicentre, Randomised, Open-Label, Phase 3 Trial. *Lancet* **2021**, *397*, 375–386. [CrossRef]
13. Nicolini, F.; Bocchini, M.; Bronte, G.; Delmonte, A.; Guidoboni, M.; Crinò, L.; Mazza, M. Malignant Pleural Mesothelioma: State-of-the-Art on Current Therapies and Promises for the Future. *Front. Oncol.* **2019**, *9*, 1519. [CrossRef]
14. Cantini, L.; Hassan, R.; Sterman, D.H.; Aerts, J.G.J.V. Emerging Treatments for Malignant Pleural Mesothelioma: Where Are We Heading? *Front. Oncol.* **2020**, *10*, 343. [CrossRef]
15. Hmeljak, J.; Sanchez-Vega, F.; Hoadley, K.A.; Shih, J.; Stewart, C.; Heiman, D.; Tarpey, P.; Danilova, L.; Drill, E.; Gibb, E.A.; et al. Integrative Molecular Characterization of Malignant Pleural Mesothelioma. *Cancer Discov.* **2018**, *8*, 1548–1565. [CrossRef]
16. Bueno, R.; Stawiski, E.W.; Goldstein, L.D.; Durinck, S.; de Rienzo, A.; Modrusan, Z.; Gnad, F.; Nguyen, T.T.; Jaiswal, B.S.; Chirieac, L.R.; et al. Comprehensive Genomic Analysis of Malignant Pleural Mesothelioma Identifies Recurrent Mutations, Gene Fusions and Splicing Alterations. *Nat. Genet.* **2016**, *48*, 407–416. [CrossRef] [PubMed]
17. Guo, G.; Chmielecki, J.; Goparaju, C.; Heguy, A.; Dolgalev, I.; Carbone, M.; Seepo, S.; Meyerson, M.; Pass, H.I. Whole-Exome Sequencing Reveals Frequent Genetic Alterations in BAP1, NF2, CDKN2A, and CUL1 in Malignant Pleural Mesothelioma. *Cancer Res.* **2015**, *75*, 264–269. [CrossRef] [PubMed]
18. Patil, N.S.; Righi, L.; Koeppen, H.; Zou, W.; Izzo, S.; Grosso, F.; Libener, R.; Loiacono, M.; Monica, V.; Buttigliero, C.; et al. Molecular and Histopathological Characterization of the Tumor Immune Microenvironment in Advanced Stage of Malignant Pleural Mesothelioma. *J. Thorac. Oncol.* **2018**, *13*, 124–133. [CrossRef]
19. Nasu, M.; Emi, M.; Pastorino, S.; Tanji, M.; Powers, A.; Luk, H.; Baumann, F.; Zhang, Y.-A.; Gazdar, A.; Kanodia, S.; et al. High Incidence of Somatic BAP1 Alterations in Sporadic Malignant Mesothelioma. *J. Thorac. Oncol.* **2015**, *10*, 565–576. [CrossRef]
20. Bott, M.; Brevet, M.; Taylor, B.S.; Shimizu, S.; Ito, T.; Wang, L.; Creaney, J.; Lake, R.A.; Zakowski, M.F.; Reva, B.; et al. The Nuclear Deubiquitinase BAP1 Is Commonly Inactivated by Somatic Mutations and 3p21.1 Losses in Malignant Pleural Mesothelioma. *Nat. Genet.* **2011**, *43*, 668–672. [CrossRef]
21. Carbone, M.; Flores, E.G.; Emi, M.; Johnson, T.A.; Tsunoda, T.; Behner, D.; Hoffman, H.; Hesdorffer, M.; Nasu, M.; Napolitano, A.; et al. Combined Genetic and Genealogic Studies Uncover a Large BAP1 Cancer Syndrome Kindred Tracing Back Nine Generations to a Common Ancestor from the 1700s. *PLoS Genet.* **2015**, *11*, e1005633. [CrossRef] [PubMed]
22. Testa, J.R.; Cheung, M.; Pei, J.; Below, J.E.; Tan, Y.; Sementino, E.; Cox, N.J.; Dogan, A.U.; Pass, H.I.; Trusa, S.; et al. Germline BAP1 Mutations Predispose to Malignant Mesothelioma. *Nat. Genet.* **2011**, *43*, 1022–1025. [CrossRef] [PubMed]
23. Carbone, M.; Harbour, J.W.; Brugarolas, J.; Bononi, A.; Pagano, I.; Dey, A.; Krausz, T.; Pass, H.I.; Yang, H.; Gaudino, G. Biological Mechanisms and Clinical Significance of BAP1 Mutations in Human Cancer. *Cancer Discov.* **2020**, *10*, 1103–1120. [CrossRef] [PubMed]
24. Lee, H.-S.; Lee, S.-A.; Hur, S.-K.; Seo, J.-W.; Kwon, J. Stabilization and Targeting of INO80 to Replication Forks by BAP1 during Normal DNA Synthesis. *Nat. Commun.* **2014**, *5*, 5128. [CrossRef]
25. Lee, H.-S.; Seo, H.-R.; Lee, S.-A.; Choi, S.; Kang, D.; Kwon, J. BAP1 Promotes Stalled Fork Restart and Cell Survival via INO80 in Response to Replication Stress. *Biochem. J.* **2019**, *476*, 3053–3066. [CrossRef]
26. Yu, H.; Pak, H.; Hammond-Martel, I.; Ghram, M.; Rodrigue, A.; Daou, S.; Barbour, H.; Corbeil, L.; Hébert, J.; Drobetsky, E.; et al. Tumor Suppressor and Deubiquitinase BAP1 Promotes DNA Double-Strand Break Repair. *Proc. Natl. Acad. Sci. USA* **2014**, *111*, 285–290. [CrossRef]

27. Nishikawa, H.; Wu, W.; Koike, A.; Kojima, R.; Gomi, H.; Fukuda, M.; Ohta, T. BRCA1-Associated Protein 1 Interferes with BRCA1/BARD1 RING Heterodimer Activity. *Cancer Res.* **2009**, *69*, 111–119. [CrossRef]
28. Santamaría Nuñez, G.; Robles, C.M.G.; Giraudon, C.; Martínez-Leal, J.F.; Compe, E.; Coin, F.; Aviles, P.; Galmarini, C.M.; Egly, J.-M. Lurbinectedin Specifically Triggers the Degradation of Phosphorylated RNA Polymerase II and the Formation of DNA Breaks in Cancer Cells. *Mol. Cancer Ther.* **2016**, *15*, 2399–2412. [CrossRef]
29. Poveda, A.; Del Campo, J.M.; Ray-Coquard, I.; Alexandre, J.; Provansal, M.; Guerra Alía, E.M.; Casado, A.; Gonzalez-Martin, A.; Fernández, C.; Rodriguez, I.; et al. Phase II Randomized Study of PM01183 versus Topotecan in Patients with Platinum-Resistant/Refractory Advanced Ovarian Cancer. *Ann. Oncol.* **2017**, *28*, 1280–1287. [CrossRef]
30. Vidal, A.; Muñoz, C.; Guillén, M.-J.; Moretó, J.; Puertas, S.; Martínez-Iniesta, M.; Figueras, A.; Padullés, L.; García-Rodriguez, F.J.; Berdiel-Acer, M.; et al. Lurbinectedin (PM01183), a New DNA Minor Groove Binder, Inhibits Growth of Orthotopic Primary Graft of Cisplatin-Resistant Epithelial Ovarian Cancer. *Clin. Cancer Res.* **2012**, *18*, 5399–5411. [CrossRef]
31. Leal, J.F.M.; Martínez-Díez, M.; García-Hernández, V.; Moneo, V.; Domingo, A.; Bueren-Calabuig, J.A.; Negri, A.; Gago, F.; Guillén-Navarro, M.J.; Avilés, P.; et al. PM01183, a New DNA Minor Groove Covalent Binder with Potent in Vitro and in Vivo Anti-Tumour Activity. *Br. J. Pharmacol.* **2010**, *161*, 1099–1110. [CrossRef] [PubMed]
32. Cruz, C.; Llop-Guevara, A.; Garber, J.E.; Arun, B.K.; Pérez Fidalgo, J.A.; Lluch, A.; Telli, M.L.; Fernández, C.; Kahatt, C.; Galmarini, C.M.; et al. Multicenter Phase II Study of Lurbinectedin in BRCA-Mutated and Unselected Metastatic Advanced Breast Cancer and Biomarker Assessment Substudy. *J. Clin. Oncol.* **2018**, *36*, 3134–3143. [CrossRef] [PubMed]
33. Benton, C.B.; Chien, K.S.; Tefferi, A.; Rodriguez, J.; Ravandi, F.; Daver, N.; Jabbour, E.; Jain, N.; Alvarado, Y.; Kwari, M.; et al. Safety and Tolerability of Lurbinectedin (PM01183) in Patients with Acute Myeloid Leukemia and Myelodysplastic Syndrome. *Hematol. Oncol.* **2019**, *37*, 96–102. [CrossRef]
34. Cote, G.M.; Choy, E.; Chen, T.; Marino-Enriquez, A.; Morgan, J.; Merriam, P.; Thornton, K.; Wagner, A.J.; Nathenson, M.J.; Demetri, G.; et al. A Phase II Multi-Strata Study of Lurbinectedin as a Single Agent or in Combination with Conventional Chemotherapy in Metastatic and/or Unresectable Sarcomas. *Eur. J. Cancer* **2020**, *126*, 21–32. [CrossRef] [PubMed]
35. Calvo, E.; Moreno, V.; Flynn, M.; Holgado, E.; Olmedo, M.E.; Criado, M.L.; Kahatt, C.; Lopez-Vilariño, J.A.; Siguero, M.; Fernandez-Teruel, C.; et al. Antitumor Activity of Lurbinectedin (PM01183) and Doxorubicin in Relapsed Small-Cell Lung Cancer: Results from a Phase I Study. *Ann. Oncol. Off. J. Eur. Soc. Med. Oncol.* **2017**, *28*, 2559–2566. [CrossRef] [PubMed]
36. Singh, S.; Jaigirdar, A.A.; Mulkey, F.; Cheng, J.; Hamed, S.S.; Li, Y.; Liu, J.; Zhao, H.; Goheer, A.; Helms, W.S.; et al. FDA Approval Summary: Lurbinectedin for the Treatment of Metastatic Small Cell Lung Cancer. *Clin. Cancer Res.* **2020**, *27*, 2378–2382. [CrossRef]
37. Metaxas, Y.; Früh, M.; Eboulet, E.I.; Grosso, F.; Pless, M.; Zucali, P.A.; Ceresoli, G.L.; Mark, M.; Schneider, M.; Maconi, A.; et al. Lurbinectedin as Second- or Third-Line Palliative Therapy in Malignant Pleural Mesothelioma: An International, Multi-Centre, Single-Arm, Phase II Trial (SAKK 17/16). *Ann. Oncol.* **2020**, *31*, 495–500. [CrossRef]
38. Soares, D.G.; Machado, M.S.; Rocca, C.J.; Poindessous, V.; Ouaret, D.; Sarasin, A.; Galmarini, C.M.; Henriques, J.A.P.; Escargueil, A.E.; Larsen, A.K. Trabectedin and Its C Subunit Modified Analogue PM01183 Attenuate Nucleotide Excision Repair and Show Activity toward Platinum-Resistant Cells. *Mol. Cancer Ther.* **2011**, *10*, 1481–1489. [CrossRef]
39. Minchom, A.; Aversa, C.; Lopez, J. Dancing with the DNA Damage Response: Next-Generation Anti-Cancer Therapeutic Strategies. *Ther. Adv. Med. Oncol.* **2018**, *10*, 1758835918786658. [CrossRef]
40. Cho, Y.-J.; Liang, P. S-Phase-Coupled Apoptosis in Tumor Suppression. *Cell. Mol. Life Sci.* **2011**, *68*, 1883–1896. [CrossRef]
41. Lee, S.Y.; Russell, P. Brc1 Links Replication Stress Response and Centromere Function. *Cell Cycle* **2013**, *12*, 1665–1671. [CrossRef] [PubMed]
42. Guazzelli, A.; Meysami, P.; Bakker, E.; Bonanni, E.; Demonacos, C.; Krstic-Demonacos, M.; Mutti, L. What Can Independent Research for Mesothelioma Achieve to Treat This Orphan Disease? *Expert Opin. Investig. Drugs* **2019**, *28*, 719–732. [CrossRef] [PubMed]
43. Freyria, F.S.; Bonelli, B.; Tomatis, M.; Ghiazza, M.; Gazzano, E.; Ghigo, D.; Garrone, E.; Fubini, B. Hematite Nanoparticles Larger than 90 Nm Show No Sign of Toxicity in Terms of Lactate Dehydrogenase Release, Nitric Oxide Generation, Apoptosis, and Comet Assay in Murine Alveolar Macrophages and Human Lung Epithelial Cells. *Chem. Res. Toxicol.* **2012**, *25*, 850–861. [CrossRef] [PubMed]

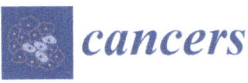

Systematic Review

Meta-Analysis of Survival and Development of a Prognostic Nomogram for Malignant Pleural Mesothelioma Treated with Systemic Chemotherapy

Rupesh Kotecha [1,2,*,†], Raees Tonse [1,†], Muni Rubens [1], Haley Appel [1], Federico Albrecht [3], Paul Kaywin [3], Evan W. Alley [4], Martin C. Tom [1,2] and Minesh P. Mehta [1,2]

1. Department of Radiation Oncology, Miami Cancer Institute, Baptist Health South Florida, Miami, FL 33176, USA; Mohammed.tonse@baptisthealth.net (R.T.); MuniR@baptisthealth.net (M.R.); HaleyA@baptisthealth.net (H.A.); MartinTo@baptisthealth.net (M.C.T.); MineshM@baptisthealth.net (M.P.M.)
2. Herbert Wertheim College of Medicine, Florida International University, Miami, FL 33199, USA
3. Department of Medical Oncology, Miami Cancer Institute, Baptist Health South Florida, Miami, FL 33176, USA; FedericoA@baptisthealth.net (F.A.); PaulKa@baptisthealth.net (P.K.)
4. Department of Medical Oncology, Cleveland Clinic Florida, Weston, FL 33331, USA; alleye@ccf.org
* Correspondence: rupeshk@baptisthealth.net; Tel.: +1-(786)-527-8140
† These authors given the equal contribution to the manuscript.

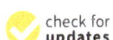

Citation: Kotecha, R.; Tonse, R.; Rubens, M.; Appel, H.; Albrecht, F.; Kaywin, P.; Alley, E.W.; Tom, M.C.; Mehta, M.P. Meta-Analysis of Survival and Development of a Prognostic Nomogram for Malignant Pleural Mesothelioma Treated with Systemic Chemotherapy. *Cancers* **2021**, *13*, 2186. https://doi.org/10.3390/cancers13092186

Academic Editors: Daniel L. Pouliquen and Joanna Kopecka

Received: 31 March 2021
Accepted: 30 April 2021
Published: 2 May 2021

Publisher's Note: MDPI stays neutral with regard to jurisdictional claims in published maps and institutional affiliations.

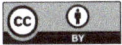

Copyright: © 2021 by the authors. Licensee MDPI, Basel, Switzerland. This article is an open access article distributed under the terms and conditions of the Creative Commons Attribution (CC BY) license (https://creativecommons.org/licenses/by/4.0/).

Simple Summary: Malignant pleural mesothelioma (MPM) is a rare cancer with an aggressive disease course. For patients who are medically inoperable or surgically unresectable, multi-agent systemic therapy remains an accepted standard-of-care around the world. Given the rare incidence of MPM and the disease's aggressive nature, novel clinical trial designs are required. The purpose of this meta-analysis is to provide baseline summative survival estimates as well as evaluate the influence of prognostic variables to provide comparative estimates for future trial designs. In this study, a nomogram model was created to estimate survival with treatment with platinum-pemetrexed using covariates known to be associated with survival, including median age, gender, ECOG performance status, tumor stage, and tumor pathology subtype. Collaborative efforts can drive the change in the right direction, and appreciable progress has to be facilitated and newer trial designs may need to pave the way for future innovations in this rare disease.

Abstract: (1) Purpose: Malignant pleural mesothelioma (MPM) is a rare cancer with an aggressive course. For patients who are medically inoperable or surgically unresectable, multi-agent systemic chemotherapy remains an accepted standard-of-care. The purpose of this meta-analysis is to provide baseline summative survival estimates as well as evaluate the influence of prognostic variables to provide comparative estimates for future trial designs. (2) Methods: Using PRISMA guidelines, a systematic review and meta-analysis was performed of MPM studies published from 2002–2019 obtained from the Medline database evaluating systemic therapy combinations for locally advanced or metastatic disease. Weighted random effects models were used to calculate survival estimates. The influence of proportions of known prognostic factors on overall survival (OS) were evaluated in the creation of a prognostic nomogram to estimate survival. The performance of this model was evaluated against data generated from one positive phase II study and two positive randomized trials. (3) Results: Twenty-four phase II studies and five phase III trials met the eligibility criteria; 2534 patients were treated on the included clinical studies. Ten trials included a platinum-pemetrexed-based treatment regimen, resulting in a pooled estimate of progression-free survival (PFS) of 6.7 months (95% CI: 6.2–7.2 months) and OS of 14.2 months (95% CI: 12.7–15.9 months). Fifteen experimental chemotherapy regimens have been tested in phase II or III studies, with a pooled median survival estimate of 13.5 months (95% CI: 12.6–14.6 months). Meta-regression analysis was used to estimate OS with platinum-pemetrexed using a variety of features, such as pathology (biphasic vs. epithelioid), disease extent (locally advanced vs. metastatic), ECOG performance status, age, and gender. The nomogram-predicted estimates and corresponding 95% CIs performed well when applied to recent randomized studies. (4) Conclusions: Given the rarity of MPM and the aggressive nature of the disease, innovative clinical trial designs with significantly greater randomization to experimental regimens can be performed using robust survival estimates from prior studies. This study provides baseline comparative values and also allows for accounting for differing proportions of known prognostic variables.

Keywords: mesothelioma; first line; meta-analysis; systematic review

1. Introduction

Malignant pleural mesothelioma (MPM) is a rare cancer with an aggressive disease course associated with poor prognosis [1]. Its incidence in the United States is approximately 3000 new cases diagnosed annually, but is still increasing in the rest of the world, particularly Asia and Europe [2]. Due to its insidious presentation, most patients are diagnosed with locally advanced or metastatic disease-unamenable to radical resection. For patients who are medically inoperable or surgically unresectable, multi-agent systemic chemotherapy remains a current standard-of-care with a median survival of approximately 12 months [3].

Although recent data from the CheckMate 743 trial have demonstrated improved outcomes with first-line immunotherapy [4], the combination of cisplatin and pemetrexed is commonly utilized in the front-line setting worldwide [5,6]. Carboplatin has similar efficacy to cisplatin, with a favorable toxicity profile and ease of administration; therefore, it has often been used in combination with pemetrexed for a large proportion of MPM patients, especially the elderly [7]. The purpose of this meta-analysis is to provide baseline summative survival estimates as well as evaluate the influence of basic prognostic variables to provide comparative estimates for future trial designs.

2. Methods

2.1. Selection of Articles

The Preferred Reporting Items for Systematic reviews and Meta-Analyses (PRISMA) criteria were followed in conducting this systematic review and meta-analysis [8]. The article selection was performed by searching the MEDLINE (PubMed) and Cochrane electronic bibliographic databases for first-line systemic therapy combinations for patients with locally advanced or metastatic MPM. To ensure a comprehensive initial search strategy, generic key words were used in the initial article screen: "mesothelioma" and "locally advanced" and "metastatic" and "first-line" and "systemic therapies" and "platinum/pemetrexed" and "experimental therapies". Full text articles published in the English language were considered and no publishing date restrictions were used through February 2021.

The initial query identified 447 reports that were subsequently screened by thorough review of the article titles and abstracts, as necessary. Inclusion criteria were publication in the English language, phase II and phase III clinical trials with 10 or more patients evaluable and with published outcomes on the efficacy endpoints of interest. Publications that were available in abstract only form and those in languages other than English were excluded. Case reports and limited case series, preclinical trials, studies using locoregional interventions alone, and studies using second-line therapies, were all excluded. A manual review of the references of the articles that were retrieved was performed to identify additional relevant publications. The search strategy used for this meta-analysis and the methodology for study inclusion is illustrated in Figure S1.

The studies were divided by treatment regimen: platinum-pemetrexed-based treatment and other experimental therapies. The demographic data abstracted for this analysis included year of publication, acronyms of the study or study title, duration of the study period, type of study (phase II/III), primary and secondary endpoints, number of patients included, median age, sex (male/female), ECOG Performance status (0,1,2), tumor stage (loco-regional disease; stage I–III and metastatic disease; stage IV), and tumor pathology (epithelioid, biphasic, sarcomatoid). Overall survival (OS), 1-year and 2-year OS rates, progression free survival (PFS), and objective response rate (ORR) were the outcomes evaluated. The radiological response data included patients having complete response (CR), partial response (PR), stable disease (SD), progressive disease (PD), and disease control rate (DCR). The toxicity summary included patients with grade 3–4 toxicities and was subdivided into toxicity category (i.e., general, blood and lymphatic system, cardiac, gastro-intestinal, infections, respiratory, and skin).

2.2. Outcome Measures and Statistical Analysis

The primary outcomes were OS and PFS; extracted medians of these variables were transferred into a logarithm scale [9]. The random-effects model described by DerSimonian and Laird [10] was used for this analysis. For primary and secondary outcomes, corresponding forest plots were created. Study heterogeneity was assessed using I^2 statistics. Values of 0–30%, 31–60%, 61–75%, and 76–100% indicated low, moderate, substantial, or considerable heterogeneity, respectively [11]. All analyses were performed in R (Version 4.0, R Foundation for Statistical Computing, Vienna, Austria). For identifying publication bias, funnel plots and the Egger test were used. Statistical significance of $p < 0.05$ indicated the presence of bias. To investigate the potential effects of each of the prognostic variables on OS, patient characteristics were also extracted from each study and included as predictors in the meta-regression model. Considered variables include median age, gender, ECOG performance status, tumor stage, and tumor pathology. The extent to which the meta-regression model explained heterogeneity of the effect among studies was quantified by the percentage reduction of between-study variability. Plot of residuals was used to check the adequacy of the meta-regression model. Nomograms were used to represent results of the meta-regression model, estimating survival time using the covariates. In developing the nomogram, we used model coefficients to assign points to characteristics and predictions from the model to map cumulative point totals. Finally, the nomogram was used to predict the overall survival outcomes reported in the positive phase II reports (STELLAR [12] study) and phase III studies (MAPS [13] and CheckMate 743 [4]) and compared to the original results to assess the model performance.

3. Results

Twenty-four phase II studies and five phase III trials were included in this meta-analysis with outcomes data collected on 2534 patients (Figure S1). Key patient characteristics, demographics, and treatment information were not uniformly or consistently reported across the literature. However, there was no publication bias detected ($p > 0.05$) across the included studies regarding the primary outcomes evaluated in this meta-analysis (Figure S2).

3.1. Demographic Data of Platinum-Pemetrexed Regimen

Ten trials (n = 1303 patients) included a platinum-pemetrexed-based treatment regimen with a median of 89 patients in each study (range: 11–302 patients) (Table 1). Across all studies, 81% were male, and the median age was 66 years (range: 59–72 years). The majority of patients (60%) had an ECOG status of 1. The patients diagnosed with loco-regional disease and metastatic disease were 35% and 47%, respectively. The majority of patients across all studies were epithelioid (80%), followed by biphasic (11%), and sarcomatoid (8%).

Table 1. Demographic data of malignant pleural mesothelioma patients treated with cisplatin/carboplatin and pemetrexed.

Author	Year	Acronymous	Duration	Type of Study	Treatment	Primary End Point	Secondary Endpoint	N	Median Age	Sex [No.(%)]		ECOG Performance Status [No.(%)]			Tumour Stage		Tumour Pathology		
										Male	Female	0	1	2	Loco-Regional (Stage I-III)	Metastatic (Stage IV)	Epithelioid	Biphasic	Sarcomatoid
Vogelzang et al. [6]	2003	NA	1999–2001	III	Cisplatin + Pemetrexed	OS	PFS, RR, duration of response	226	61	184 (81%)	42 (19%)	NA	NA	NA	73 (32%)	102 (45%)	154 (68%)	37 (16%)	18 (8%)
Ceresoli et al. [7]	2006	NA	2002–2005	II	Carboplatin + Pemetrexed	ORR	toxicity, TTP, and OS	102	65	76 (75%)	26 (25%)	33 (32%)	61 (60%)	8 (8%)	34 (33%)	49 (48%)	80 (78%)	8 (8%)	7 (7%)
Castagneto et al. [14]	2008	NA	2003–2005	II	Carboplatin + Pemetrexed	RR	OS, TTP, Toxicity	76	65	54 (71%)	22 (29%)	NA	NA	NA	27 (36%)	36 (48%)	57 (75%)	13 (17%)	3 (4%)
Katirtzoglou et al. [15]	2010	NA	2004–2007	II	Carboplatin + Pemetrexed	RR	OS, TTP	62	66	53 (86%)	9 (14%)	25 (40%)	37 (60%)	0	23 (37%)	17 (27%)	47 (76%)	NA	15 (24%)
Krug et al. [16]	2014	NA	NA	II	Cisplatin + Pemetrexed	PFS	OS, DCR, and safety/toxicity	23	66	20 (87%)	3 (13%)	7 (30%)	16 (70%)	0	NA	NA	16 (70%)	2 (9%)	11 (18%)
Buikhuisen et al. [17]	2016	NA	2009–2012	II	Cisplatin + Pemetrexed	RR	OS, PFS	11	59	10 (89%)	1 (11%)	NA	NA	NA	NA	NA	10 (89%)	1 (11%)	0
Zalcman et al. [13]	2016	MAPS	NA	III	Cisplatin + Pemetrexed	OS	PFS, QoL and safety	225	66	170 (76%)	55 (25%)	NA	NA	NA	NA	NA	182 (81%)	NA	NA
Tsao et al. [18]	2019	SWOG S0905	2011–2016	II	Cisplatin + Pemetrexed	PFS	OS, DCR, and safety/toxicity	47	72	40 (85%)	7 (15%)	NA	NA	NA	NA	NA	35 (74%)	12 (26%)	NA
Scagliotti et al. [19]	2019	LUME-Meso	2016–2018	III	Cisplatin + Pemetrexed	PFS	OS, ORR, DCR, QoL	229	66	169 (74%)	60 (26%)	98 (43%)	131 (57%)	NA	90 (39%)	105 (46%)	223 (97%)	6 (3%)	NA
Baas et al. [4]	2021	CheckMate 743	2016–2018	III	Cisplatin/Carboplatin + Pemetrexed	OS	PFS, ORR, DCR	302	69	233 (77%)	69 (23%)	124 (42%)	173 (57%)	NA	106 (35%)	149 (49%)	227 (75%)	39 (13%)	36 (12%)

Abbreviations: OS = overall survival; PFS = progression free survival; ORR = objective response rate; RR = response rate; TTP = time to progression; DCR = disease control rate; QoL = quality of life; ECOG = Eastern Cooperative Oncology Group; NA = not available.

3.2. Treatment Outcomes, Radiological Response, and Toxicity Summary Data of Platinum-Pemetrexed Regimen

Treatment with a platinum-pemetrexed-based regimen resulted in a pooled PFS of 6.7 months (95% CI: 6.2–7.2 months) and an OS of 14.2 months (95% CI: 12.7–15.9) (Figure 1A,B).

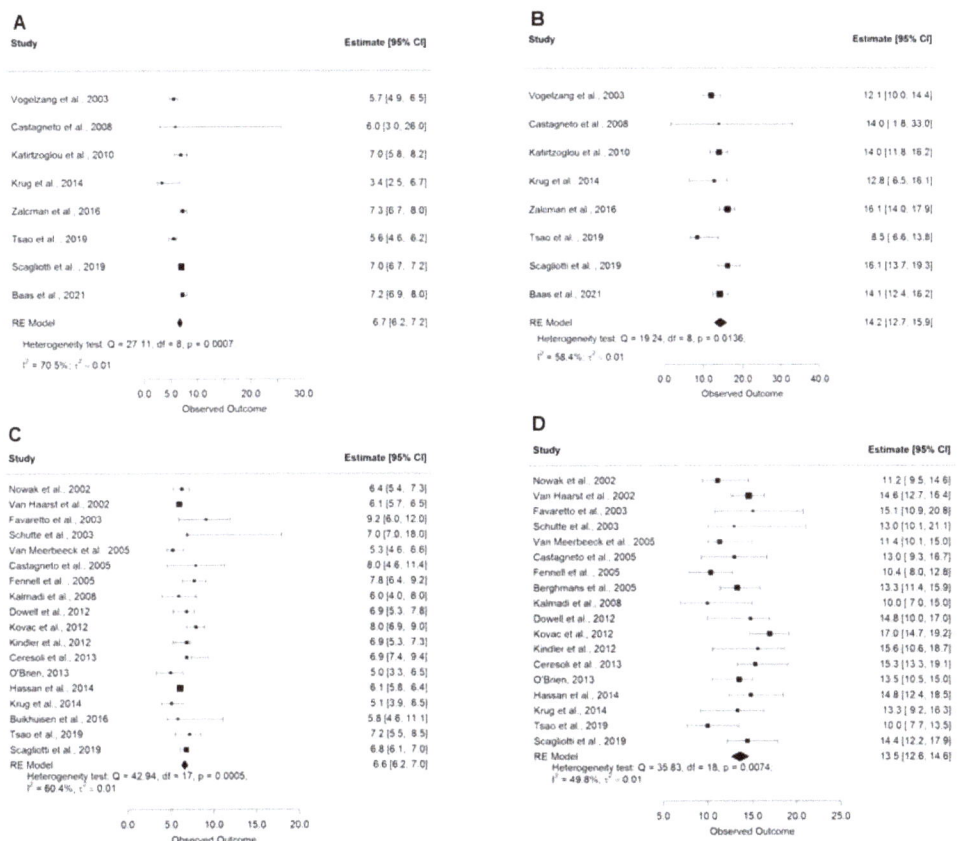

Figure 1. Forest plots demonstrating the (**A**) progression-free survival with platinum/pemetrexed; (**B**) overall survival with platinum/pemetrexed; (**C**) progression-free survival with other experimental therapies; and (**D**) overall survival with other experimental therapies. Squares indicate the proportions from individual studies and horizontal lines indicate the 95% confidence interval. The size of the data marker corresponds to the relative weight assigned in the pooled analysis using the random effects model. The diamond indicates the pooled proportion with 95% CI.

Across all studies, the proportion of ORR was 24% (95% CI: 12–35%) and DCR was 73% (95% CI: 56–90%) (Table 2). Across all patients, the proportion of individual response rates for CR was 1.5% (95% CI: 1–4%), 19% PR (95% CI: 10–27%), 53% SD (95% CI: 37–69%), and 31% PD (95% CI: 14–48%).

Table 2. Treatment outcomes, radiological response, and toxicity summary for malignant pleural mesothelioma patients treated with cisplatin/carboplatin and pemetrexed.

Author	Year	N	OS (Months)	1 Yr. Survival Rates	2 Yr. Survival Rates	PFS (Months)	Objective Response Rate (ORR)	Radiological Response Rate [N (%)]				Disease Control Rate (%)	Toxicity Summary (Grade 3 and 4) N (%)								
								Complete Response	Partial Response	Stable Disease	Progressive Disease		Blood and Lymphatic System Disorders			Cardiac Disorders	Gastrointestinal Disorders	Fatigue	Infections	Respiratory Disorders	Skin Disorders	Nausea and Vomiting
													Anemia	Neutropenia	Thrombocytopenia							
Vogelzang et al. [6]	2003	226	12.1	6	NA	5.7	41.3	NA	NA	NA	NA	NA	11 (5%)	NA	NA	NA	NA	NA	11 (5%)	NA	3 (1%)	33 (15%)
Ceresoli et al. [7]	2006	102	12.7	6.5	NA	6.5	19	2 (2%)	17 (17%)	48 (47%)	33 (33%)	67	12 (12%)	20 (20%)	8 (8%)	NA	3 (3%)	1 (1%)	NA	NA	NA	1 (1%)
Castagneto et al. [11]	2008	76	14	NA	NA	6	25	3 (4%)	16 (21%)	29 (38%)	28 (37%)	63	6 (8%)	25 (33%)	10 (13%)	NA	9 (12%)	NA	4 (5%)	NA	NA	NA
Katirtzoglou et al. [15]	2010	62	14	NA	NA	7	29	0	18 (29%)	34 (56%)	10 (16%)	85	6 (10%)	15 (24%)	5 (8%)	NA	2 (3%)	8 (13%)	1 (1%)	NA	3 (5%)	9 (15%)
Krug et al. [16]	2014	23	12.8	NA	NA	3.4	10	0	2 (10%)	10 (50%)	8 (40%)	60	1 (4%)	1 (4%)	NA	1 (4%)	1 (4%)	3 (13%)	NA	NA	NA	2 (9%)
Buikhuisen et al. [17]	2016	11	18.5	NA	NA	8.3	18	NA	2 (18%)	8 (73%)	NA	91	0	1 (5%)	0	0	0	0	0	0	NA	0
Zalcman et al. [13]	2016	225	16.1	NA	NA	7.3	NA	NA	NA	NA	NA	NA	30 (13%)	100 (44%)	21 (9%)	2 (1%)	3 (1%)	28 (13%)	7 (3%)	NA	NA	18 (8%)
Tsao et al. [8]	2019	47	8.5	NA	NA	5.6	20	NA	NA	NA	NA	NA	7 (15%)	9 (20%)	2 (4%)	0	0	6 (13%)	NAA	NA	NA	0
Scagliotti et al. [12]	2019	229	16.1	NA	NA	7	43	NA	98 (43%)	NA	NA	93	33 (14%)	54 (24%)	NA	NA	10 (4%)	17 (7%)	14 (6%)	NA	1 (1%)	15 (7%)
Baas et al. [4]	2021	302	14.1	8.1	3.8	7.2	43	0	129 (43%)	125 (41%)	14 (5%)	85	32 (11%)	43 (15%)	10 (3%)	NA	3 (2%)	5 (2%)	NA	NA	0	13 (4%)

Abbreviations: OS = overall survival; PFS = progression free survival; yr. = year; ORR = objective response rate; QoL = quality of life; NA = not available; N = number.

The pooled estimates of the treatment-related toxicity outcomes for patients who received a platinum-pemetrexed regimen (Figure 2A-I) with grade 3–4 blood and lymphatic system toxicities were anemia 10% (95% CI: 8–13%), neutropenia 22% (95% CI: 15–30%), and thrombocytopenia 7% (95% CI: 5–10%). Cardiac toxicity was seen in 1% (95% CI: 0–3%), gastro-intestinal toxicity in 3% (95% CI: 1–5%), fatigue in 6% (95% CI: 3–12%), infections in 5% (95% CI: 3–6%), skin toxicity in 1% (95% CI: 0–3%), and nausea and vomiting in 6% (95% CI: 3–10%).

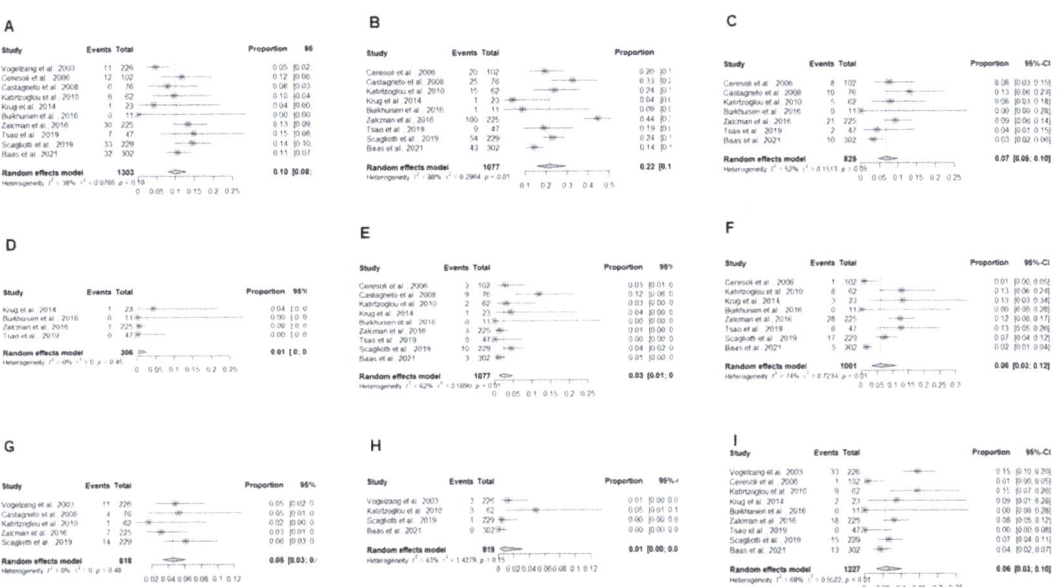

Figure 2. Forest plots demonstrating the toxicity outcomes for platinum/pemetrexed regimen based on toxicity category: (**A**) Anemia; (**B**) Neutropenia; (**C**) Thrombocytopenia; (**D**) Cardiac Toxicity; (**E**) Gastro-intestinal toxicity; (**F**) Fatigue; (**G**) Infections; (**H**) Skin toxicity; and (**I**) Nausea and vomiting. Squares indicate the proportions from individual studies and horizontal lines indicate the 95% confidence interval. The size of the data marker corresponds to the relative weight assigned in the pooled analysis using the random effects model. The diamond indicates the pooled proportion with 95% CI.

3.3. Demographic Data of Experimental Regimens

Nineteen trials tested 15 experimental chemotherapy regimens (*n* = 1231 patients) in negative phase II or III studies, with a median of 52 patients (range: 20–229 patients) in each study (Table A1). Across these studies, 75% were male, and the median age was 63 years (range: 55–72 years). Patients had an ECOG status of 0 (30%), 1 (60%), and 2 (10%). The patients diagnosed with loco-regional disease and metastatic disease were 39% and 34%, respectively. In these studies, the majority of patients had epithelioid subtype (76%), followed by biphasic (15%), and sarcomatoid (9%).

3.4. Outcomes, Radiological Response, and Toxicity Summary Data of Experimental Regimens

Treatment with these experimental regimens resulted in a pooled estimate of PFS of 6.6 months (95% CI: 6.2–7.0 months) and OS of 13.5 months (95% CI: 12.6–14.6 months) (Figure 1C,D). Across all studies, the proportion of ORR was 31% (95% CI: 26–36%) and the DCR was 76% (95% CI: 69–84%) (Table A2). Responses using these experimental therapies were low: overall proportions for CR were 0.7% (95% CI: 0.3–1.6%), 29% PR (95% CI: 24–34%), 48% SD (95% CI: 42–55%), 22% PD (95% CI: 13–29%).

The pooled toxicity estimates for patients who received experimental chemotherapy regimens (Figure 3A-I) resulted in blood and lymphatic system grade 3–4 toxicities, with anemia in 4% (95% CI: 2–7%), neutropenia in 21% (95% CI: 12–33%), and thrombocytopenia in 12% (95% CI: 6–24%). Cardiac toxicity was seen in 4% (95% CI: 2–9%), gastro-intestinal toxicity in 4% (95% CI: 2–7%), fatigue in 12% (95% CI: 10–15%), infections in 5% (95% CI: 3–7%), skin toxicity in 1% (95% CI: 0–3%), and nausea and vomiting in 9% (95% CI: 6–15%).

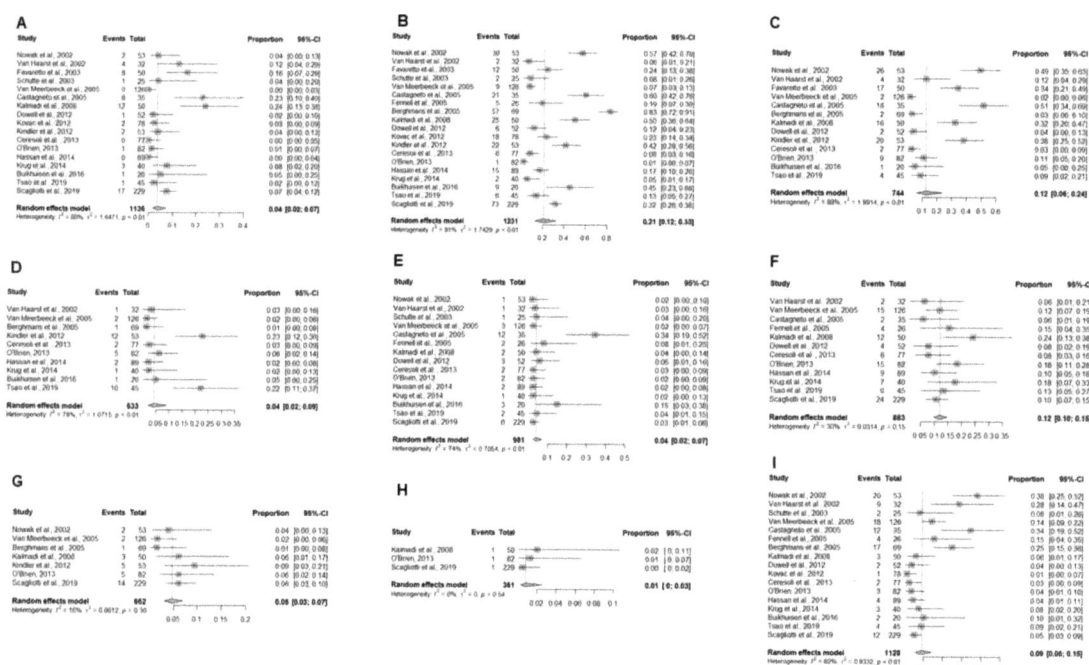

Figure 3. Forest plots demonstrating the toxicity outcomes for various experimental regimens: (**A**) Anemia; (**B**) Neutropenia; (**C**) Thrombocytopenia; (**D**) Cardiac Toxicity; (**E**) Gastro-intestinal toxicity; (**F**) Fatigue; (**G**) Infections; (**H**) Skin toxicity; and (**I**) Nausea and vomiting. Squares indicate the proportions from individual studies and horizontal lines indicate the 95% confidence interval. The size of the data marker corresponds to the relative weight assigned in the pooled analysis using the random effects model. The diamond indicates the pooled proportion with 95% CI.

3.5. Development of a Prognostic Nomogram to Estimate Survival

Meta-regression analysis was used to estimate survival with treatment with platinum-pemetrexed using covariates known to be associated with OS, including median age, gender, ECOG performance status, tumor stage, and tumor pathology subtype (Figure 4).

Unlike the aforementioned experimental regimens, two randomized phase III trials and one single-arm phase II trial have demonstrated promising outcomes in this disease entity. The Mesothelioma Avastin Plus Pemetrexed-cisplatin Study (MAPS) [13] evaluated cisplatin/pemetrexed/bevacizumab compared to cisplatin/pemetrexed, the STELLAR trial [12] evaluated the use of tumor-treating fields (TTFields) in addition to cisplatin/pemetrexed, and recently CheckMate 743 [4] evaluated nivolumab plus ipilimumab compared to cisplatin/carboplatin and pemetrexed. To evaluate the prognostic nomogram developed in this study, we compared the estimated outcomes using the patient populations enrolled onto these studies and the proportion of each of the covariates and compared the nomogram estimates with the published results. For the MAPS study, given the patient population in the experimental arm of the phase III study, the OS estimate from the nomogram was 15.76 months (95% CI: 13.96–17.81 months) compared to the reported 18.8 months in the study. Similarly, the OS estimate from the nomogram using the CheckMate 743 trial was 13.65 months (95% CI: 11.41–16.33 months) compared to

18.1 months reported in the experimental arm. Therefore, the results of the experimental arms of these two studies were outside the confidence interval estimate based on historical data and consistent with a positive outcome. For the STELLAR trial, the OS estimate from the nomogram was 16.95 months (95% CI: 10.49–27.38 months) and given the wide confidence interval, potentially could overlap with the 18.2 months reported in the study.

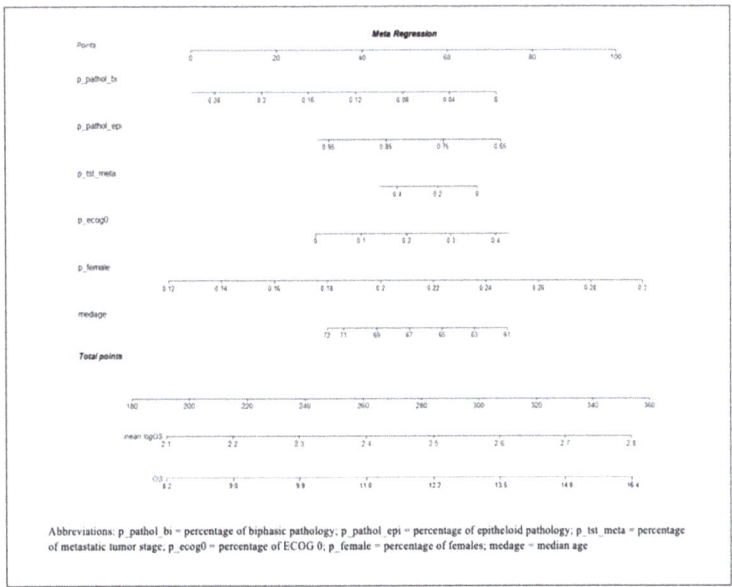

Figure 4. Nomogram model developed to predict overall survival (OS) in patients with malignant pleural mesothelioma treated with platinum/pemetrexed therapy. The mean log OS can be calculated by drawing a vertical line connecting the value of each variable with the point score at the top of the nomogram. The point scores for individual variables are then summed to get a total point score. This is then plotted along the total points line at the bottom of the nomogram. This line is projected to the mean log OS of the trial. Then the exponential of mean log OS is calculated to obtain the OS in months.

4. Discussion

Since 2003, chemotherapy with cisplatin/carboplatin and pemetrexed has been a standard first-line therapy for the majority of newly diagnosed patients who have locally advanced and metastatic MPM [6]. Over the past 15 years, multiple studies have established the outcomes for MPM patients treated with this regimen including single-arm phase II trials [7,14,15], the experimental arms of randomized trials compared to cisplatin alone [6], and the control arms of randomized trials testing novel experimental regimens [4,13,17–20]. In total, 1303 patients have been treated with this regimen across 10 studies, the data of which were abstracted in this systematic review and meta-analysis to determine pooled estimates of a PFS of 6.7 months and an OS of 14.2 months. In fact, a similar number—1231 patients—have been treated with experimental regimens who showed no improved outcomes compared to these historical estimates, underscoring the need for novel therapeutic development in this space. Moreover, despite advances in this field with the addition of bevacizumab and immunotherapy, doublet chemotherapy remains to be commonly used in most parts of the world where mesothelioma incidence continues to rise. Although the addition of bevacizumab to first-line chemotherapy has been added to the national guidelines [13], this regimen has not received FDA approval. Moreover, in CheckMate 743, nivolumab and ipilimumab were compared to pemetrexed-platinum, and although the OS was extended in the experimental arm, subgroup analysis yielded important caveats [4].

For example, for patients with epithelioid histologies (75% of those enrolled), the 12-month OS rates were not as striking (66% vs. 69%). Similarly, for those patients with a PDL-1 < 1%, the Kaplan-Meier curves crossed with longer follow-up, yielding an overall hazard ratio of 0.94. Hence, the role of first-line chemotherapy continues to be evaluated in ongoing trials.

Randomized controlled trials (RCTs) are deemed the gold standard of clinical research [21]. Randomization is often recommended for endpoints with a higher risk of confounding and selection bias, and it has been shown to improve the ability of phase II results to accurately predict phase III success [22,23]. However, modifications to traditional randomized trial designs have been performed to improve their performance in clinical practice. For example, the permuted block randomization has been widely used; however, in this design, there exists a compromise between effective imbalance control with a small block size and accurate allocation target with large block size [24]. Several alternative randomization designs have been proposed, such as the maximal procedure, brick tunnel randomization, and block urn designs [25–27]. However, for cancers such as mesothelioma, there are several logistical constraints for patients with rare diseases, as well as accrual/drop-out issues for those randomized to standard arms with known historically poor outcomes. Therefore, in other similar rare disease entities with robust historical survival estimates, there has been a resurgence in the consideration of alternative clinical trial designs [28]. Bayesian randomized designs and multi-arm multi-stage designs are two different approaches for improving reliability by using patient outcomes [29]. The Bayesian design allocates a greater proportion of prospective patients to well-performing treatments, whereas the multi-arm multi-stage designs use pre-specified stopping boundaries to discontinue novel treatments due to lack of efficacy. Although the Bayesian randomized designs have been shown to be more effective than traditional RCTs in multi-arm studies, their efficiency improvements in two-arm studies have been modest, especially if the rate of accrual outpaces the event rate, since the latter is required to modified the "prior" in a Bayesian concept [29]. Some studies examined the effects of phase II designs for binary endpoints on subsequent phase III trials, and found that randomization is useful when interstudy variability is high or there is a tendency to underestimate the control response [30]. Therefore, there is continued need to develop novel methods of clinical study and pooling historical data may help in future with future trial designs.

Meta-regression, the technique used in this study to develop the nomogram, is often used to assess the relationship between one or more covariates and a dependent variable. Similar approaches can be performed with a meta-analysis alone; however the covariates are at the level of the study rather than the level of the subject [31]. The differences that we need to address as we transition from using primary study data to meta-analysis for regression are similar to those for subgroup analyses. For example, in this meta-analysis, using meta-regression, we identified variables that were associated with OS and developed a nomogram to determine the influence of each of these on survival, including median age, gender, ECOG performance status, tumor stage, and tumor pathology. Using the nomogram, the overall survival was predicted as reported in the positive phase II and III studies and compared to the original result reported in these studies.

In the MAPS study [13], the patient population in the experimental arm of the phase III study showed an OS estimate from the nomogram to be 15.76 months (95% CI: 13.96–17.81 months), as compared to the 18.8 months that was reported in the original study. Similarly, for another phase III study (CheckMate 743) [4], the OS estimate from the nomogram was 13.65 months (95% CI: 11.41–16.33 months), as compared to 18.1 months reported in the study. Based on the nomogram model developed from historical estimates, the OS reported for the positive phase III trials are outside of the 95% confidence interval range of the historical estimates; however, the predicted OS from the nomogram was also similar to the OS from the control arms in the original studies, indicating good performance. Interestingly, in the single-arm phase II STELLAR study [12], the OS estimate from the nomogram was 16.95 months (95% CI: 10.49–27.38 months), compared to 18.2 months. The OS reported in this study falls within the range of the 95% confidence interval predicted from the nomogram. This demonstrates the importance of patient numbers in phase II trials, as the effectiveness of a phase II trial cannot be measured due to the wide confidence interval, prompting well-powered confirmatory studies. A well-designed phase II trial with complete reporting of the trial design, patient eligibility, study endpoints, and statistical analyses may be reliable and applicable in rare diseases, such as MPM [32].

There are important limitations to our analysis that should be noted. Formally, any categorical variable should have specific outcome-specific data to optimize the performance of the meta-regression. For example, for gender, male-specific OS and female-specific OS should be calculated. Unfortunately, this was difficult to extract from existing publications, since this level of detail is seldom reported. Similarly, Brims et al. [33] developed a prediction model for MPM using variables like Hb, weight loss, and albumin, which was unable to be extracted from existing publications for this study but would likely improve the performance of the survival estimates. However, in this study, we included percentages as continuous variables in the meta-regression. Furthermore, individual patient-level data can also be used to enhance any created model and should be pursued in subsequent studies. Given this promising approach with study-level data, further projects using individual patient-level data should be performed.

5. Conclusions

Given the rare incidence of MPM and the aggressive nature of the disease course, innovative clinical trial designs with significantly weighted randomization to experimental regimens can be utilized using robust survival estimates from prior studies. This study provides baseline comparative values and also allows for accounting for differing proportions of known prognostic variables. Collaborative efforts can drive change in the right direction, and appreciable progress has to be facilitated. Newer trial designs may be needed to pave the way for future innovations in this rare disease.

Supplementary Materials: The following are available online at https://www.mdpi.com/article/10.3390/cancers13092186/s1, Figure S1: PRISMA flow diagram showing the selection of studies for the systematic review of malignant pleural mesothelioma patients treated in the first-line setting with combination chemotherapy regimens, Figure S2: Funnel plots for (A) progression-free survival with platinum/pemetrexed, (B) overall survival with platinum/pemetrexed, (C) progression-free survival with other experimental therapies, and (D) overall survival with other experimental therapies to assess the potential for publication bias.

Author Contributions: Conception and Design: R.K., R.T. & M.R. Analysis: M.R. Critical Review of Manuscript: R.K., R.T., M.R., H.A., F.A., P.K., E.W.A., M.C.T., M.P.M. All authors have read and approved the manuscript.

Funding: This research received no specific grant from any funding agency in the public, commercial, or not-for-profit sectors.

Institutional Review Board Statement: Not applicable.

Informed Consent Statement: Not applicable.

Data Availability Statement: No new data were created or analyzed in this study. Data sharing is not applicable to this article.

Conflicts of Interest: R.K.: Honoraria from Accuray Inc., Elekta AB, Viewray Inc., Novocure Inc., Elsevier Inc. Institutional research funding from Medtronic Inc., Blue Earth Diagnostics Ltd., Novocure Inc., GT Medical Technologies, Astrazeneca, Exelixis, Viewray Inc; H.A.: Honoraria from Novocure Inc.; F.A.: Speaker's Bureau for Eli Lilly and Company and Boehringer Ingelheim; M.T.: Institutional research funding from Blue Earth Diagnostics Ltd; M.P.M.: Consulting for Karyopharm, Sapience, Zap, Mevion. Board of Directors: Oncoceutics. Other authors declare no conflict of interest.

Appendix A

Table A1. Demographic data for patients with malignant pleural mesothelioma treated with experimental therapies, negative on phase II/III studies.

Author	Year	Acronyms	Duration	Type of Study	Treatment	Primary End Point	Secondary Endpoint	N	Median Age	Sex [No.(%)] Male	Sex [No.(%)] Female	ECOG Performance Status [No.(%)] 0	1	2	Tumour stage Locally Advanced	Metastatic	Tumour Pathology Epithelioid	Biphasic	Sarcomatoid
Nowak et al. [14]	2002	NA	NA	II	Cisplatin + Gemcitabine	ORR	PFS, OS, QoL	53	63	45 (85%)	8 (15%)	17 (32%)	31 (59%)	5 (9%)	33 (62%)	13 (25%)	42 (79%)	2 (4%)	7 (13%)
Van Haarst et al. [15]	2002	NA	April 1999–Dec 1999	II	Cisplatin + Gemcitabine	ORR	PFS, OS, QoL	32	56	27 (86%)	5 (14%)	5 (14%)	26 (85%)	1 (1%)	15 (48%)	13 (41%)	26 (82%)	3 (9%)	3 (9%)
Favaretto et al. [36]	2003	NA	1996–2000	II	Carboplatin + Gemcitabine	RR	OS, PFS, Toxicity	50	60	34 (68%)	16 (32%)	11 (22%)	33 (66%)	6 (12%)	11 (22%)	12 (24%)	34 (68%)	13 (26%)	3 (6%)
Schutte et al. [37]	2003	NA	1999–2001	II	Oxaliplatin + Gemcitabine	ORR	OS, PFS, Toxicity	25	65	18 (72%)	7 (28%)	7 (28%)	13 (52%)	5 (20%)	13 (52%)	10 (25%)	16 (64%)	8 (32%)	1 (3%)
Van Meerbeeck et al. [38]	2005	NA	NA	III	Cisplatin + Raltitrexed	OS	PFS, RR, safety, QoL	126	59	104 (83%)	22 (17%)	32 (25%)	77 (61%)	17 (14%)	NA	NA	95 (75%)	18 (14%)	5 (4%)
Castagneto et al. [39]	2005	NA	1999–2001	II	Cisplatin + Gemcitabine	ORR	OS, PFS	35	61	21 (60%)	14 (40%)	33 (94%)		2 (6%)	8 (23%)	16 (46%)	22 (63%)	10 (29%)	3 (8%)
Fennell et al. [40]	2005	NA	NA	II	Oxaliplatin + Vinorelbine	ORR	OS, PFS	26	60	21 (87%)	5 (13%)	6 (16%)	15 (69%)	5 (13%)	6 (16%)	15 (79%)	13 (75%)	7 (18%)	5 (13%)
Berghmans et al. [41]	2005	NA	1998–2003	II	Cisplatin + Epirubicin	ORR	Toxicity and OS	69	62	59 (93%)	10 (7%)	NA	NA	NA	18 (12%)	23 (19%)	43 (74%)	6 (10%)	9 (16)
Kalmadi et al. [42]	2008	SWOG 9810	1999–2000	II	Cisplatin + Gemcitabine	OS	ORR, Toxicity	50	69	44 (88%)	6 (12%)	13 (26%)	27 (54%)	10 (20%)	NA	NA	25 (50%)	3 (6%)	4 (8%)
Dowell et al. [43]	2012	NA	NA	II	Cisplatin + Pemetrexed + Bevacizumab	PFS	RR, OS and toxicity	52	66	44 (85%)	8 (15%)	17 (33%)	35 (67%)	NA	NA	NA	32 (62%)	11 (21%)	7 (13%)
Kovac et al. [44]	2012	NA	2002–2008	II	Cisplatin + Gemcitabine	RR	OS, PFS, Toxicity	78	58	58 (74%)	20 (26%)	14 (18%)	51 (65%)	13 (17%)	38 (49%)	22 (29%)	56 (72%)	15 (19%)	4 (5%)
Kindler et al. [45]	2012	NA	2001–2005	II	Cisplatin + Gemcitabine + Bevacizumab	PFS	OS	53	62	39 (73%)	14 (27%)	24 (45%)	29 (55%)	NA	NA	NA	39 (74%)	14 (26%)	NA
Ceresoli et al. [46]	2013	NA	2007–2009	II	Carboplatin + Pemetrexed + Bevacizumab	PFS	Toxicity, RR and OS	77	67	49 (64%)	27 (36%)	58 (76%)	18 (24%)	NA	NA	NA	61 (80%)	6 (8%)	5 (7%)
O'Brien et al. [1]	2013	EORTC 08052	2007–2010	II	Cisplatin + Bortezomib	PFSR-18	ORR, OS, PFS and safety	82	55	55 (67%)	27 (33%)	NA	73 (89%)	NA	35 (43%)	28 (34%)	48 (59%)	11 (13%)	6 (7%)
Hassan et al. [48]	2014	NA	2009–2010	II	Cisplatin + Pemetrexed + Amatuximab	6 months PFS	ORR, OS, PFS and safety	89	67	69 (78%)	20 (22%)	NA	NA	NA	35 (39%)	43 (48%)	79 (89%)	10 (11%)	NA
Krug et al. [16]	2014	NA	NA	II	Cisplatin + Pemetrexed + CBP501	PFS	OS, DCR, and safety/toxicity	40	64	32 (80%)	8 (20%)	14 (35%)	25 (63%)	1 (3%)	NA	NA	30 (75%)	6 (15%)	4 (10%)
Buikhuisen et al. [17]	2016	NA	2009–2012	II	Cisplatin + Pemetrexed + Axitinib	RR	OS, PFS	20	63	15 (75%)	5 (25%)	NA	NA	NA	NA	NA	16 (80%)	2 (10%)	2 (10%)
Tsao et al. [18]	2019	SWOG S0905	2011–2016	II	Cisplatin + Pemetrexed + Cediranib	PFS	OS, DCR, and safety/toxicity	45	72	38 (84%)	7 (16%)	NA	NA	NA	NA	NA	34 (76%)	11 (24%)	NA
Scagliotti et al. [19]	2019	LUME-Meso	2016–2018	III	Cisplatin + Pemetrexed + Nintedanib	PFS	OS, ORR, DCR, QoL	229	66	165 (72%)	64 (28%)	99 (43%)	130 (57%)	NA	89 (39%)	113 (49%)	220 (96%)	9 (4%)	NA

Abbreviations: OS = overall survival; PFS = progression free survival; ORR = objective response rate; RR = response rate; TTP = time to progression; DCR = disease control rate; QoL = quality of life; ECOG = Eastern Cooperative Oncology Group; NA = not available.

Table A2. Treatment outcomes, radiological response, and toxicity summary for malignant pleural mesothelioma patients treated with experimental therapies, negative on phase II/III studies.

Author	Year	OS (Months)	1 yr. Survival Rates	2 yr. Survival Rates	PFS (Months)	Objective Response Rate (ORR %)	Radiological Response Rate (No. (%))				Disease Control Rate (%)	Toxicity summary (Grade 3 and 4) n (%)									
							Complete Response	Partial Response	Stable Disease	Progressive Disease		Anemia	Blood and Lymphatic System Disorders		Cardiac Disorders	Gastrointestinal Disorders	Fatigue	Infections	Respiratory Disorders	Skin Disorders	Nausea and Vomiting
													Neutropenia	Thrombocytopenia							
Nowak et al. [ ]	2002	17.3	NA	NA	6.4	33	0	17 (33%)	31 (60%)	4 (7%)	93	2 (7%)	30 (56%)	26 (49%)	NA	1 (2%)	NA	2 (4%)	NA	NA	20 (37%)
Van Haasst et al. [ ]	2002	14.6	NA	NA	6.1	16	0	4 (16%)	18 (72%)	3 (12%)	88	4 (13%)	2 (6%)	4 (13%)	1 (3%)	1 (3%)	2 (6%)	0	0	0	9 (29%)
Favaretto et al. [ ]	2003	15.1	8	4.5	9.2	26	0	13 (26%)	25 (50%)	12 (24%)	76	8 (16%)	12 (24%)	17 (34%)	0	0	0	0	0	0	0
Schutte et al. [ ]	2003	13	6.7	NA	7	40	0	10 (40%)	6 (24%)	9 (36%)	64	1 (4%)	2 (8%)	0	NA	1 (4%)	0	0	0	NA	2 (8%)
Van Meerbeeck et al. [ ]	2005	11.4	5.2	2.1	5.3	24	2 (2%)	24 (26%)	58 (63%)	NA	89	4 (3%)	9 (7%)	2 (2%)	2 (2%)	3 (2%)	15 (12%)	2 (2%)	0	NA	18 (14%)
Castagneto et al. [ ]	2005	13	NA	NA	8	26	0	9 (26%)	14 (40%)	11 (31%)	66	8 (24%)	21 (61%)	18 (52%)	NA	12 (35%)	NA	NA	NA	NA	12 (35%)
Fennell et al. [ ]	2005	10.4	2.8	NA	7.8	23	0	6 (23%)	17 (65%)	3 (12%)	88	NA	5 (18%)	NA	NA	2 (6%)	4 (12%)	NA	NA	NA	4 (12%)
Berghmans et al. [ ]	2005	13.3	6.6	NA	NA	19	0	12 (19%)	25 (40%)	24 (38%)	59	NA	57 (84%)	2 (3%)	1 (2%)	NA	NA	1 (2%)	2 (3%)	NA	17
Kalmadi et al. [ ]	2008	10	3	NA	6	12	1 (2%)	5 (10%)	25 (50%)	19 (38%)	62	12 (24%)	25 (50%)	16 (32%)	NA	2 (4%)	12 (24%)	3 (6%)	NA	1 (2%)	3 (6%)
Dowell et al. [ ]	2012	14.8	NA	NA	6.9	40	NA	NA	35	NA	35	1 (2%)	6 (11%)	2 (4%)	NA	3 (6%)	4 (8%)	NA	NA	NA	2 (4%)
Kovac et al. [ ]	2012	17	NA	NA	8	50	4 (5%)	35 (45%)	35 (45%)	4 (5%)	95	2 (3%)	18 (23%)	NA	NA	NA	NA	NA	NA	NA	1 (1%)
Kindler et al. [ ]	2012	15.6	9.1	4.8	6.9	25	0	13 (25%)	27 (51%)	12 (28%)	75	2 (4%)	22 (42%)	20 (38%)	12 (23%)	NA	NA	5 (10%)	NA	NA	NA
Ceresoli et al. [ ]	2013	15.3	9.5	3.9	6.9	34	NA	24 (34%)	44 (58%)	NA	92	3 (4%)	6 (8%)	2 (3%)	2 (3%)	2 (3%)	6 (8%)	NA	1 (1%)	NA	2 (3%)
O'Brien et al. [ ]	2013	13.5	7.5	NA	5	27	2 (2%)	21 (29%)	39 (49%)	16 (20%)	80	1 (1%)	1 (1%)	9 (11%)	5 (6%)	2 (2%)	15 (18%)	5 (6%)	NA	1 (1%)	3 (3%)
Hassan et al. [ ]	2014	14.8	NA	NA	6.1	33	0	33%	42%	8%	75	10 (11%)	15 (17%)	0%	2 (3%)	2 (3%)	9 (10%)	0	3 (4%)	0%	4 (5%)
Krug et al. [ ]	2014	13.3	NA	NA	5.1	31	0	12 (31%)	15 (38%)	NA	69	3 (8%)	2 (6%)	NA	1 (3%)	1 (3%)	7 (18%)	NA	NA	NA	3 (8%)
Buikhuisen et al. [ ]	2016	18.9	NA	NA	5.8	36	NA	8 (36%)	9 (43%)	NA	79	1 (5%)	9 (45%)	1 (5%)	1 (5%)	3 (15%)	0	NA	1 (5%)	NA	2 (10%)
Tsao et al. [ ]	2019	10	NA	NA	7.2	50	NA	NA	NA	NA	NA	1 (2%)	6 (13%)	4 (9%)	10 (22%)	2 (4%)	6 (13%)	NA	NA	NA	4 (9%)
Scagliotti et al. [ ]	2019	14.4	NA	NA	6.8	45	NA	103 (45%)	NA	NA	91	17 (7%)	73 (32%)	NA	NA	6 (3%)	24 (11%)	14 (6%)	NA	1 (1%)	12 (5%)

Abbreviations: OS = overall survival; PFS = progression free survival; yr. = year; ORR = objective response rate; QoL = quality of life; NA = not available; N = number.

References

1. Robinson, B.W.; Musk, A.W.; Lake, R.A. Malignant mesothelioma. *Lancet* **2005**, *366*, 397–408. [CrossRef]
2. Delgermaa, V.; Takahashi, K.; Park, E.-K.; Le, G.V.; Hara, T.; Sorahan, T. Global mesothelioma deaths reported to the World Health Organization between 1994 and 2008. *Bull. World Health Organ.* **2011**, *89*, 716–724. [CrossRef]
3. Kindler, H.L.; Ismaila, N.; Armato, S.G.; Bueno, R.; Hesdorffer, M.; Jahan, T.; Jones, C.M.; Miettinen, M.; Pass, H.; Rimner, A.; et al. Treatment of Malignant Pleural Mesothelioma: American Society of Clinical Oncology Clinical Practice Guideline. *J. Clin. Oncol.* **2018**, *36*, 1343–1373. [CrossRef]
4. Baas, P.; Scherpereel, A.; Nowak, A.K.; Fujimoto, N.; Peters, S.; Tsao, A.S.; Mansfield, A.S.; Popat, S.; Jahan, T.; Antonia, S.; et al. First-line nivolumab plus ipilimumab in unresectable malignant pleural mesothelioma (CheckMate 743): A multicentre, randomised, open-label, phase 3 trial. *Lancet* **2021**, *397*, 375–386. [CrossRef]
5. Scagliotti, G.V.; Shin, D.-M.; Kindler, H.L.; Vasconcelles, M.J.; Keppler, U.; Manegold, C.; Burris, H.; Gatzemeier, U.; Blatter, J.; Symanowski, J.T.; et al. Phase II Study of Pemetrexed With and Without Folic Acid and Vitamin B 12 as Front-Line Therapy in Malignant Pleural Mesothelioma. *J. Clin. Oncol.* **2003**, *21*, 1556–1561. [CrossRef]
6. Vogelzang, N.J.; Rusthoven, J.J.; Symanowski, J.; Denham, C.; Kaukel, E.; Ruffie, P.; Gatzemeier, U.; Boyer, M.; Emri, S.; Manegold, C.; et al. Phase III Study of Pemetrexed in Combination with Cisplatin Versus Cisplatin Alone in Patients with Malignant Pleural Mesothelioma. *J. Clin. Oncol.* **2003**, *21*, 2636–2644. [CrossRef] [PubMed]
7. Ceresoli, G.L.; Zucali, P.A.; Favaretto, A.G.; Grossi, F.; Bidoli, P.; Del Conte, G.; Ceribelli, A.; Bearz, A.; Morenghi, E.; Cavina, R.; et al. Phase II Study of Pemetrexed Plus Carboplatin in Malignant Pleural Mesothelioma. *J. Clin. Oncol.* **2006**, *24*, 1443–1448. [CrossRef] [PubMed]
8. Moher, D.; Liberati, A.; Tetzlaff, J.; Altman, D.G. Preferred Reporting Items for Systematic Reviews and Meta-Analyses: The PRISMA Statement. *PLoS Med.* **2009**, *6*, e1000097. [CrossRef]
9. Zang, J.; Xu, J.; Xiang, C.; He, J.; Zou, S. Multi-level Model Synthesis of Median Survival Time in Meta-analysis. *Epidemiology* **2015**, *26*, e2–e3. [CrossRef] [PubMed]
10. DerSimonian, R.; Laird, N. Meta-analysis in clinical trials. *Control. Clin. Trials* **1986**, *7*, 177–188. [CrossRef]
11. Higgins, J.P.T.; Thompson, S.G. Quantifying heterogeneity in a meta-analysis. *Stat. Med.* **2002**, *21*, 1539–1558. [CrossRef]
12. Ceresoli, G.L.; Aerts, J.G.; Dziadziuszko, R.; Ramlau, R.; Cedres, S.; van Meerbeeck, J.P.; Mencoboni, M.; Planchard, D.; Chella, A.; Crinò, L.; et al. Tumour Treating Fields in combination with pemetrexed and cisplatin or carboplatin as first-line treatment for unresectable malignant pleural mesothelioma (STELLAR): A multicentre, single-arm phase 2 trial. *Lancet Oncol.* **2019**, *20*, 1702–1709. [CrossRef]
13. Zalcman, G.; Mazieres, J.; Margery, J.; Greillier, L.; Audigier-Valette, C.; Moro-Sibilot, D.; Molinier, O.; Corre, R.; Monnet, I.; Gounant, V.; et al. Bevacizumab for newly diagnosed pleural mesothelioma in the Mesothelioma Avastin Cisplatin Pemetrexed Study (MAPS): A randomised, controlled, open-label, phase 3 trial. *Lancet* **2016**, *387*, 1405–1414. [CrossRef]
14. Castagneto, B.; Botta, M.; Aitini, E.; Spigno, F.; Degiovanni, D.; Alabiso, O.; Serra, M.; Muzio, A.; Carbone, R.; Buosi, R.; et al. Phase II study of pemetrexed in combination with carboplatin in patients with malignant pleural mesothelioma (MPM). *Ann. Oncol.* **2008**, *19*, 370–373. [CrossRef] [PubMed]
15. Katirtzoglou, N.; Gkiozos, I.; Makrilia, N.; Tsaroucha, E.; Rapti, A.; Stratakos, G.; Fountzilas, G.; Syrigos, K.N. Carboplatin plus pemetrexed as first-line treatment of patients with malignant pleural mesothelioma: A phase II study. *Clin. Lung Cancer* **2010**, *11*, 30–35. [CrossRef] [PubMed]
16. Krug, L.M.; Wozniak, A.J.; Kindler, H.L.; Feld, R.; Koczywas, M.; Morero, J.L.; Rodriguez, C.P.; Ross, H.J.; Bauman, J.E.; Orlov, S.V.; et al. Randomized phase II trial of pemetrexed/cisplatin with or without CBP501 in patients with advanced malignant pleural mesothelioma. *Lung Cancer* **2014**, *85*, 429–434. [CrossRef]
17. Buikhuisen, W.A.; Scharpfenecker, M.; Griffioen, A.W.; Korse, C.M.; Van Tinteren, H.; Baas, P. A randomized phase II study adding axitinib to pemetrexed-cisplatin in patients with malignant pleural mesothelioma: A single-center trial combining clinical and translational outcomes. *J. Thorac. Oncol.* **2016**, *11*, 758–768. [CrossRef]
18. Tsao, A.S.; Miao, J.; Wistuba, I.I.; Vogelzang, N.J.; Heymach, J.V.; Fossella, F.V.; Lu, C.; Velasco, M.R.; Box-Noriega, B.; Hueftle, J.G.; et al. Phase II trial of cediranib in combination with cisplatin and pemetrexed in chemotherapy-naïve patients with unresectable malignant pleural mesothelioma (SWOG S0905). *J. Clin. Oncol.* **2019**, *37*, 2537–2547. [CrossRef]
19. Scagliotti, G.V.; Gaafar, R.; Nowak, A.K.; Nakano, T.; van Meerbeeck, J.; Popat, S.; Vogelzang, N.J.; Grosso, F.; Aboelhassan, R.; Jakopovic, M.; et al. Nintedanib in combination with pemetrexed and cisplatin for chemotherapy-naive patients with advanced malignant pleural mesothelioma (LUME-Meso): A double-blind, randomised, placebo-controlled phase 3 trial. *Lancet Respir. Med.* **2019**, *7*, 569–580. [CrossRef]
20. Krug, L.M.; Pass, H.I.; Rusch, V.W.; Kindler, H.L.; Sugarbaker, D.J.; Rosenzweig, K.E.; Flores, R.; Friedberg, J.S.; Pisters, K.; Monberg, M.; et al. Multicenter phase II trial of neoadjuvant pemetrexed plus cisplatin followed by extrapleural pneumonectomy and radiation for malignant pleural mesothelioma. *J. Clin. Oncol.* **2009**, *27*, 3007–3013. [CrossRef]
21. Stephenson, J.; Imrie, J. Why do we need randomised controlled trials to assess behavioural interventions? *BMJ* **1998**, *316*, 611–613. [CrossRef]

22. Tang, H.; Foster, N.R.; Grothey, A.; Ansell, S.M.; Goldberg, R.M.; Sargent, D.J. Comparison of error rates in single-arm versus randomized phase II cancer clinical trials. *J. Clin. Oncol.* **2010**, *28*, 1936–1941. [CrossRef] [PubMed]
23. Sharma, M.R.; Stadler, W.M.; Ratain, M.J. Randomized phase II trials: A long-term investment with promising returns. *J. Natl. Cancer Inst.* **2011**, *103*, 1093–1100. [CrossRef]
24. Zhao, W. A better alternative to stratified permuted block design for subject randomization in clinical trials. *Stat. Med.* **2014**, *33*, 5239–5248. [CrossRef] [PubMed]
25. Berger, V.W.; Ivanova, A.; Deloria Knoll, M. Minimizing predictability while retaining balance through the use of less restrictive randomization procedures. *Stat. Med.* **2003**, *22*, 3017–3028. [CrossRef]
26. Zhao, W.; Weng, Y. Block urn design—A new randomization algorithm for sequential trials with two or more treatments and balanced or unbalanced allocation. *Contemp. Clin. Trials* **2011**, *32*, 953–961. [CrossRef]
27. Kuznetsova, O.M.; Tymofyeyev, Y. Brick tunnel randomization for unequal allocation to two or more treatment groups. *Stat. Med.* **2011**, *30*, 812–824. [CrossRef]
28. Sharma, M.R.; Karrison, T.G.; Jin, Y.; Bies, R.R.; Maitland, M.L.; Stadler, W.M.; Ratain, M.J. Resampling phase III data to assess phase II trial designs and endpoints. *Clin. Cancer Res.* **2012**, *18*, 2309–2315. [CrossRef] [PubMed]
29. Wason, J.M.S.; Trippa, L. A comparison of Bayesian adaptive randomization and multi-stage designs for multi-arm clinical trials. *Stat. Med.* **2014**, *33*, 2206–2221. [CrossRef]
30. Pond, G.R.; Abbasi, S. Quantitative evaluation of single-arm versus randomized phase II cancer clinical trials. *Clin. Trials* **2011**, *8*, 260–269. [CrossRef]
31. Lambert, P.C.; Sutton, A.J.; Abrams, K.R.; Jones, D.R. A comparison of summary patient-level covariates in meta-regression with individual patient data meta-analysis. *J. Clin. Epidemiol.* **2002**, *55*, 86–94. [CrossRef]
32. Tomblyn, M.R.; Rizzo, J.D. Are there circumstances in which phase 2 study results should be practice-changing? *Hematol. Am. Soc. Hematol. Educ. Progr.* **2007**, 489–492. [CrossRef]
33. Brims, F.J.H.; Meniawy, T.M.; Duffus, I.; de Fonseka, D.; Segal, A.; Creaney, J.; Maskell, N.; Lake, R.A.; de Klerk, N.; Nowak, A.K. A Novel Clinical Prediction Model for Prognosis in Malignant Pleural Mesothelioma Using Decision Tree Analysis. *J. Thorac. Oncol.* **2016**, *11*, 573–582. [CrossRef]
34. Nowak, A.K.; Byrne, M.J.; Williamson, R.; Ryan, G.; Segal, A.; Fielding, D.; Mitchell, P.; Musk, A.W.; Robinson, B.W.S. A multicentre phase II study of cisplatin and gemcitabine for malignant mesothelioma. *Br. J. Cancer* **2002**, *87*, 491–496. [CrossRef]
35. Van Haarst, J.M.W.; Baas, P.; Manegold, C.; Schouwink, J.H.; Burgers, J.A.; De Bruin, H.G.; Mooi, W.J.; Van Klaveren, R.J.; De Jonge, M.J.A.; Van Meerbeeck, J.P. Multicentre phase II study of gemcitabine and cisplatin in malignant pleural mesothelioma. *Br. J. Cancer* **2002**, *86*, 342–345. [CrossRef]
36. Favaretto, A.G.; Aversa, S.M.L.; Paccagnella, A.; Manzini, V.D.P.; Palmisano, V.; Oniga, F.; Stefani, M.; Rea, F.; Bortolotti, L.; Loreggian, L.; et al. Gemcitabine combined with carboplatin in patients with malignant pleural mesothelioma: A multicentric phase II study. *Cancer* **2003**, *97*, 2791–2797. [CrossRef] [PubMed]
37. Schuette, W.; Blankenburg, T.; Lauerwald, K.; Schreiber, J.; Bork, I.; Wollschlaeger, B.; Treutler, D.; Schneider, C.P.; Bonnet, R. A multicenter phase II study of gemcitabine and oxaliplatin for malignant pleural mesothelioma. *Clin. Lung Cancer* **2003**, *4*, 294–297. [CrossRef] [PubMed]
38. Van Meerbeeck, J.P.; Gaafar, R.; Manegold, C.; Van Klaveren, R.J.; Van Marck, E.A.; Vincent, M.; Legrand, C.; Bottomley, A.; Debruyne, C.; Giaccone, G. Randomized phase III study of cisplatin with or without raltitrexed in patients with malignant pleural mesothelioma: An intergroup study of the European organisation for research and treatment of cancer lung cancer group and the National Cancer Institute. *J. Clin. Oncol.* **2005**, *23*, 6881–6889. [CrossRef]
39. Castagneto, B.; Zai, S.; Dongiovanni, D.; Muzio, A.; Bretti, S.; Numico, G.; Botta, M. Cisplatin and gemcitabine in malignant pleural mesothelioma: A phase II study. *Am. J. Clin. Oncol. Cancer Clin. Trials* **2005**, *28*, 223–226. [CrossRef] [PubMed]
40. Fennell, D.A.; Steele, J.P.C.; Shamash, J.; Sheaff, M.T.; Evans, M.T.; Goonewardene, T.I.; Nystrom, M.L.; Gower, N.H.; Rudd, R.M. Phase II trial of vinorelbine and oxaliplatin as first-line therapy in malignant pleural mesothelioma. *Lung Cancer* **2005**, *47*, 277–281. [CrossRef]
41. Berghmans, T.; Lafitte, J.J.; Paesmans, M.; Stach, B.; Berchier, M.C.; Wackenier, P.; Lecomte, J.; Collon, T.; Mommen, P.; Sculier, J.P. A phase II study evaluating the cisplatin and epirubicin combination in patients with unresectable malignant pleural mesothelioma. *Lung Cancer* **2005**, *50*, 75–82. [CrossRef] [PubMed]
42. Kalmadi, S.R.; Rankin, C.; Kraut, M.J.; Jacobs, A.D.; Petrylak, D.P.; Adelstein, D.J.; Keohan, M.L.; Taub, R.N.; Borden, E.C. Gemcitabine and cisplatin in unresectable malignant mesothelioma of the pleura: A phase II study of the Southwest Oncology Group (SWOG 9810). *Lung Cancer* **2008**, *60*, 259–263. [CrossRef]
43. Dowell, J.E.; Dunphy, F.R.; Taub, R.N.; Gerber, D.E.; Ngov, L.; Yan, J.; Xie, Y.; Kindler, H.L. A multicenter phase II study of cisplatin, pemetrexed, and bevacizumab in patients with advanced malignant mesothelioma. *Lung Cancer* **2012**, *77*, 567–571. [CrossRef] [PubMed]
44. Kovac, V.; Zwitter, M.; Rajer, M.; Marin, A.; Debeljak, A.; Smrdel, U.; Vrankar, M. A phase II trial of low-dose gemcitabine in a prolonged infusion and cisplatin for malignant pleural mesothelioma. *Anticancer Drugs* **2012**, *23*, 230–238. [CrossRef] [PubMed]
45. Kindler, H.L.; Karrison, T.G.; Gandara, D.R.; Lu, C.; Krug, L.M.; Stevenson, J.P.; Jänne, P.A.; Quinn, D.I.; Koczywas, M.N.; Brahmer, J.R.; et al. Multicenter, double-blind, placebo-controlled, randomized phase II trial of gemcitabine/cisplatin plus bevacizumab or placebo in patients with malignant mesothelioma. *J. Clin. Oncol.* **2012**, *30*, 2509–2515. [CrossRef] [PubMed]

46. Ceresoli, G.L.; Zucali, P.A.; Mencoboni, M.; Botta, M.; Grossi, F.; Cortinovis, D.; Zilembo, N.; Ripa, C.; Tiseo, M.; Favaretto, A.G.; et al. Phase II study of pemetrexed and carboplatin plus bevacizumab as first-line therapy in malignant pleural mesothelioma. *Br. J. Cancer* **2013**, *109*, 552–558. [CrossRef]
47. O'Brien, M.E.R.; Gaafar, R.M.; Popat, S.; Grossi, F.; Price, A.; Talbot, D.C.; Cufer, T.; Ottensmeier, C.; Danson, S.; Pallis, A.; et al. Phase II study of first-line bortezomib and cisplatin in malignant pleural mesothelioma and prospective validation of progression free survival rate as a primary end-point for mesothelioma clinical trials (European Organisation for Research and Treatment. *Eur. J. Cancer* **2013**, *49*, 2815–2822. [CrossRef] [PubMed]
48. Hassan, R.; Kindler, H.L.; Jahan, T.; Bazhenova, L.; Reck, M.; Thomas, A.; Pastan, I.; Parno, J.; O'Shannessy, D.J.; Fatato, P.; et al. Phase II clinical trial of amatuximab, a chimeric antimesothelin antibody with pemetrexed and cisplatin in advanced unresectable pleural mesothelioma. *Clin. Cancer Res.* **2014**, *20*, 5927–5936. [CrossRef] [PubMed]

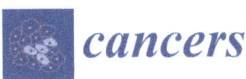

Commentary

Precision Therapy for Mesothelioma: Feasibility and New Opportunities

Sean Dulloo [1,2], Aleksandra Bzura [2] and Dean Anthony Fennell [1,2,*]

1. Medical Oncology, University Hospitals of Leicester NHS Trust, Leicester LE1 5WW, UK; sean.dullo@uhl-tr.nhs.uk
2. Mesothelioma Research Programme, Leicester Cancer Research Centre, University of Leicester, Leicester LE2 7LX, UK; ab973@leicester.ac.uk
* Correspondence: df132@leicester.ac.uk

Simple Summary: Mesothelioma remains a lethal cancer. Personalized treatment is lacking. Emerging insights into the genomic and epigenomic landscape of mesothelioma highlight promising opportunities for precision therapy, where are discussed.

Abstract: Malignant pleural mesotheliomas (MPMs) are characterised by their wide variation in natural history, ranging from minimally to highly aggressive, associated with both interpatient and intra-tumour genomic heterogeneity. Recent insights into the nature of this genetic variation, the identification of drivers, and the emergence of novel strategies capable of targeting vulnerabilities that result from the inactivation of key tumour suppressors suggest that new approaches to molecularly strategy therapy for mesothelioma may be feasible.

Keywords: mesothelioma; histotype; Hippo pathway; NF2; BAP1; CDKN2A; PTCH1; SETD2; MTAP

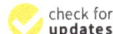

Citation: Dulloo, S.; Bzura, A.; Fennell, D.A. Precision Therapy for Mesothelioma: Feasibility and New Opportunities. *Cancers* **2021**, *13*, 2347. https://doi.org/10.3390/cancers 13102347

Academic Editors: Daniel L. Pouliquen and Joanna Kopecka

Received: 7 April 2021
Accepted: 3 May 2021
Published: 13 May 2021

Publisher's Note: MDPI stays neutral with regard to jurisdictional claims in published maps and institutional affiliations.

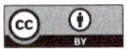

Copyright: © 2021 by the authors. Licensee MDPI, Basel, Switzerland. This article is an open access article distributed under the terms and conditions of the Creative Commons Attribution (CC BY) license (https://creativecommons.org/licenses/by/4.0/).

1. Introduction

Over the last decade, multiple landmark next-generation sequencing studies of MPM have shed light on the spectrum of recurrently mutated cancer genes [1–4]. These studies have revealed a preponderance of tumour suppressor gene alterations and dominance of copy number alterations with a relatively low mutation burden of around two mutations per megabase. The absence of a bone fide tyrosine kinase proto-oncogene activating mutations as seen in other cancers (e.g., epidermal growth factor receptor or anaplastic lymphoma kinase, or ROS1 in lung adenocarcinoma), limits the opportunities to target gain-of-function somatic alterations directly. However, emerging insights into the biology of MPM highlight opportunities for targeting vulnerabilities that may emerge due to tumour suppressor inactivation, and potentially, oncogenic processes (Figure 1).

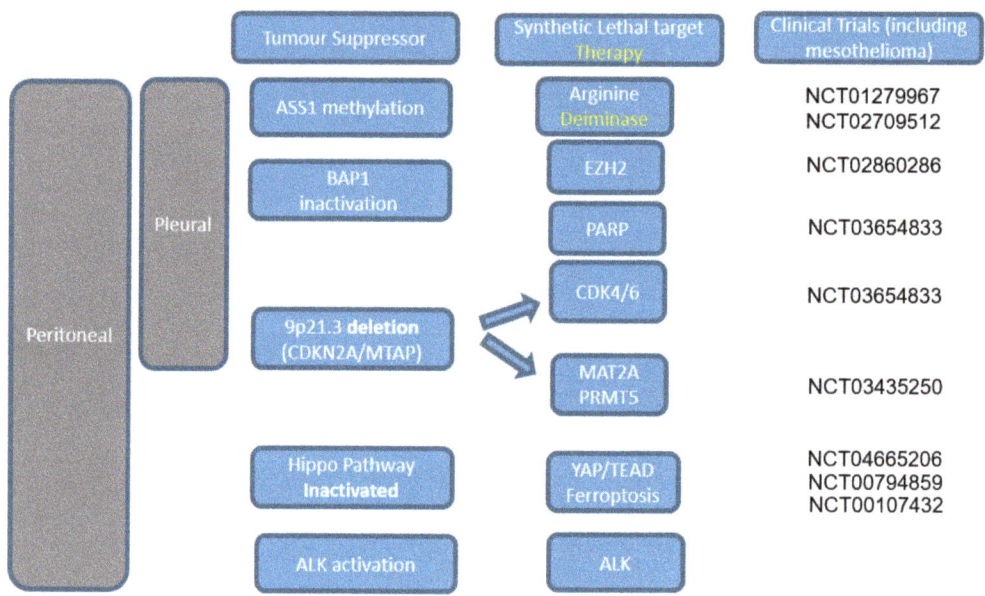

Figure 1. Potentially actionable somatic alterations involving common tumour suppressors in pleural or periotoneal mesothelioma, or oncogene (ALK) in peritoneal mesothelioma. Trials shown on the right are evauating these strategies and are denoted by their trials.gov identifier.

2. Histology, Prognosis, and Molecular Stratification of Therapy

To date, the most commonly used classification of MPM has been histopathological, encompassing prognostically distinct subtypes spanning epithelioid (the most frequent and associated with a better prognosis) to biphasic and sarcomatoid (the latter being the most aggressive). Genomic comparisons of these subtypes do not reveal mutually exclusive somatic alterations, with all harbouring, to some extent, the three most common tumour suppressors at 9p21.3 (CDKN2A), 3p21 (BAP1), or 22q (NF2).

However, phenotypically there is a clear gradient of epithelial–mesenchymal transition or EMT [5–7] which may underpin chemotherapy resistance and the most aggressive behaviour of mesenchymal-like sarcomatoid MPMs. Patients with sarcomatoid MPM tend to have the worst outcomes with median survival ranging between 3.5 to 8 months [8], considerably shorter than for epithelioid subtype [9]. To date, although EMT exhibits plasticity, targeting EMT to revert a mesenchymal-to-epithelial phenotype has proven to be challenging [10].

The MPM histological spectrum may offer opportunities for stratified therapy. One approach has been to target epithelioid MPMs by taking advantage of the differential expression of mesothelin, which is commonly lacking in sarcomatoid MPMs. For example, the antibody-dependent conjugate anetumab ravtansine has demonstrated clinical activity [11–13] in a molecularly stratified treatment context. Conversely biphasic and sarcomatoid MPMs harbour epigenetic silencing of argininosuccinate synthetase1 (ASS1) which can be therapeutically exploited [9,14–16]. ASS1 catalyses the condensation of citrulline with aspartate to form argininosuccinate. Cells that lacking ASS1 expression exhibit a vulnerability to arginine deprivation owing to a dependency (they are unable to convert endogenous citrulline–known as *auxotrophy*). In vitro, deprivation induces apoptosis which translates to clinical efficacy [9,16]. In the clinical trial called Arginine Deaminase and Mesothelioma (ADAM) study, patients were randomised in a 2:1 ratio to ADI-PEG20 (weekly intramuscular dose) versus best supportive care. The primary endpoint was progression-free survival. The trial met its primary endpoint with a superior outcome with a Hazard ratio of 0.56 [9] confirming proof of concept.

A correlation between ASS1, and platinum/antifolate sensitivity was investigated in preclinical models [17,18]. The Phase 1 dose-escalation study involving ADI-PEG 20 in combination with pemetrexed and cisplatin has shown seven (out of nine) MPM patients having partial responses (78%) of which three had sarcomatoid/biphasic histology [14]. This phase 1 subsequently led to the development of the randomised phase 2/3 trial called ATOMIC MESO, randomising ADI-PEG20 or placebo with cisplatin and pemetrexed (ADICiSPem) non-epithelioid MPM patients which most commonly lack ASS1 [19].

3. Targeting Hippo Pathway Mutations—Disrupting an Oncogenic Pathway?

One of the most frequent pathways to be inactivated in MPM involves Hippo signalling, a pathway that regulates organ size. The most common somatic alterations involve the neurofibromatosis 2 gene (NF2 22q12) and the large tumour suppressor gene 2 (LATS2, 13q11-12) [20]. NF2 encodes merlin which recruits LATS1/2 kinases which phosphorylate the downstream effectors of the Hippo pathway, yes-associated protein (YAP), and its paralogue TAZ (WW domain-containing transcription regulator 1, or WWTR1). Inhibition of YAP/TAZ prevents their nuclear entry and ability to activate an oncogenic transcriptional programme in partnership with TEA domain transcription factor (TEAD) [21,22]. Therefore, Hippo pathway mutations de-repress a bone fide oncogenic pathway in MPM that is associated with shorter survival.

Recent analysis exploring the evolution of MPM has revealed that Hippo pathway inactivation involving NF2 almost always occurs as a secondary event during early clonal evolution, preceded by another other driver alteration [23]. Using a deep learning methodology to explore phylogenetic data obtained from multiregional sequencing of MPMs, it was repeated evolution was revealed across the cohort. This suggests that Hippo inactivation is deterministic, highlighting its significance as a potential biomarker for novel therapeutic strategies.

Early preclinical studies demonstrated a correlation between merlin loss and upregulation of focal adhesion kinase (FAK); inhibition of FAK was associated with the selective killing of merlin deficient cell lines, highlighting a potential synthetic lethal relationship [24,25]. This concept was then tested in a merlin-stratified, global randomised phase 2 trial called COMMAND [26–28], comparing maintenance defactinib or placebo. This study was, however, negative. Further preclinical studies revealed a novel function of FAK as an enhancer of regulatory T cell immunosuppression, leading to a phase 1 trial of defactinib and the PD1 inhibitor pembrolizumab, which includes an MPM cohort [29,30].

Alternative approaches to target Hippo-inactivated MPMs are emerging. Preclinical studies have highlighted potential sensitivity to SRC or BCR/Abl inhibition [31]. TEAD inhibitors are currently in development and could directly disable transcriptional oncogenic signalling [32]. Preclinical studies have identified that Hippo inactivation leads to a vulnerability to ferroptosis, a form of iron-dependent cell death. TEAD signalling upregulates ferroptosis modulators ACSL4 and TFRC, leading to enhanced sensitivity to agents such as sorafenib or sulphasalazine that can modify glutamate transport and cellular redox state [33,34].

4. BAP1 Inactivation

BRCA1 associated protein 1(BAP1) is a frequently inactivated tumour suppressor gene in MPM, which is also rarely associated with germline mutation [35]. Mechanisms through which BAP1 inactivation occurs include mutation, copy number loss, or translocations [4]. BAP1 deubiquitinates histone 2A lysine 119, and BAP1 deletion causing an increase in H3K27me3 associated with repression of enhancer of zeste 2 polycomb repressive complex 2 subunit (EZH2) activation. This suggests that small-molecule EZH2 inhibition could be an effective therapy in *BAP1*-mutant cancers. Based on this model, EZH2 inhibition was tested in BAP1 inactivated MPMs [36].

The EZH2 inhibitor tazemetostat was administered to patients with BAP1 inactivated MPM (loss of nuclear expression). The primary endpoint was disease control (i.e., stable disease, complete or partial response) at 12 weeks. The study enrolled 74 patients with the primary endpoint being met at 51%, demonstrating disease control at 12 weeks, with 25% continuing to 24 weeks. Interestingly, 2 of the 61 patients had confirmed partial responses [37]. Based on these data, EZH2 inhibitors might have antitumour activity; however, larger trials would be needed to support these findings.

Nuclear BAP1 regulates homologous recombination (HR) repair via interaction with RAD51 and BRCA1/BARD1 complex [38–40], in contrast to its cytoplasmic function in which it modulates calcium signalling mediated cell death [38]. Recruitment to DNA double-strand break sites is mediated via phosphorylation of BAP1, and the role of BAP in DNA damage response involves its catalytic activity [41].

Synthetic lethality associated with BRCA1/2 and PARP inhibition is well established and widely used for targeting homologous recombination deficient cancers. Cells harbouring HR deficiency switch to base excision repair, which is assisted by PARP, to repair DNA single-strand breaks [42]. PARP inhibitors trap PARP on DNA, resulting in catastrophic accumulation of double-strand breaks due to stalling and collapse of DNA replication forks, triggering cell death. The synthetic lethality interaction is observed in the clinic, in tumours harbouring somatic biallelic inactivation in BRCA1/2, leading to approval of PARP inhibitors in BRCA1/2 cancers [43]. A recent panel sequencing study of MPM reported a 36.9% involvement of HR pathway mutations, and this was deemed the most commonly mutated pathway in MPM [44], warranting evaluation of PARP inhibition in MPM.

Recently a phase 2a trial evaluated the use of rucaparib in patients with BAP1 or BRCA1 deficient MPM-*MPM Stratified Therapy 1* (MiST1) [45]. The primary endpoint for this trial was 12-week disease control which was met with a disease control rate of 58% (95% CI 37–77) with evidence of durable partial responses lasting more than a year, with manageable toxicity. In another study, olaparib (NCT03531840) reported 81% disease control at 6 weeks, with evidence of partial responses (4%) of which one responder harboured an MRE11A mutation [46]. Niraparib is being explored in patients with Trial (NCT03207347) in BAP1 and other DNA damage repair-deficient neoplasms, including MPM.

Evidence to support BAP1 as a bone fide predictor of sensitivity to PARP inhibition is lacking. One study recently identified that the sensitivity of MPM cells is not dependent on BAP1 but is enhanced by temozolomide in cells with high Schlafen 11 and low O6–methylguanine –DNA methyltransferase expression [47]. On the other hand, a novel MPM-specific splice isoform of BAP1 has been identified, lacking a portion of the catalytic domain, and which had decreased deubiquitinating activity compared to its full-length counterpart [48]. Cells expressing more than 20% of BAP1Δ were found to be more sensitive to olaparib than wild-type BAP1 MPM [48]. Coiled-coil domain containing 6 (CCDC6) interacts with BAP1 and has been reported to regulate both homologous recombination and PARP inhibitor sensitivity. Loss of expression of CCDC6 led to increased preclinical sensitivity to PARP inhibitors and is observed in around 30% of MPMs [32].

PARP inhibitors are proinflammatory and activate cytosolic DNA sensing by cyclic GMP–AMP synthase (cGAS) mediated activation of the endoplasmic reticulum-associated stimulator of interferon genes (STING) pathway [49,50]. The cyclic GMP–AMP synthase/stimulator of IFN genes (cGAS/STING) pathway [51] is responsible for sensing of damaged cytosolic DNA leading to activation of innate immune responses via initiation of signalling cascade involving the cytoplasmic DNA sensor cGAS, in concert with STING and TBK1, and transcription factors, such as IRF3 and NF-κB, that collectively induce a type I IFN response [51]. Therefore, the disruption of nuclear DNA integrity, via endogenous or exogenous factors, activates cGAS/STING pathway, leading to immunotherapy response [52]. Combining PARP inhibitors with immune checkpoint inhibitors in MPM is therefore rational and is being explored in the MIST 5 trial.

5. 9p21.3 Deletion

Homozygous deletion of 9p21, the locus harbouring the *p16ink4a* tumour suppressor is a frequent somatic alteration [53]. This deletion occurs within a cluster of genes that include CDKN2B, CDKN2A, and MTAP in up to 72% of MPMs [54]. CDKN2A regulates two important cell cycle proteins p16ink4a (an inhibitor of cyclin-dependent kinases 4 and 6), and p14ARF, an inhibitor of MDM2 which prevents p53 degradation. Restoring p16ink4a function is feasible with small-molecule CDK4/6 inhibition (to phenocopy p16ink4a). Preclinical studies of CDK4/6 inhibitors have reported evidence of nanomolar potency of palbociclib against MPM xenografts [55]. The MIST2 trial has completed accrual testing abemaciclib in p16ink4a negative MPM (results to be presented at the American Society of Clinical Oncology Conference in 2021).

Adenoviral mediated p14ARF gene transfection has been reported to induce G1 cell cycle arrest and apoptosis which was dependent upon the expression of p53 [56]. The heterodimerisation of MDM2 with its homologue, MDMX protein, enhances p53 ubiquitination and degradation. Phase 1 clinical study has investigated AMG 232, a selective MDM2 inhibitor that restores p53 tumour suppression by blocking the MDM2–p53 interaction with picomolar affinity [57] appears to be safe and could provide a strategy to target CDKN2A deleted MPMs, which harbour wild-type p53.

Methylthioadenosine phosphorylase (MTAP), encoded at the 9p21.3 locus is an enzyme essential in the methionine salvage pathway. MTAP converts methylthioadenosine, a product of polyamine synthesis, to adenine and methylthioribose-1-phosphate. The former is used for AMP and the latter for methionine synthesis [54]. MTAP deficiency leads to a dependency on de novo purine synthesis. The first attempt to target MTAP MPM involved L-alanosine (an inhibitor of de novo purine synthesis); however, there were no reported objective responses [58]. However, recently, it has been shown that loss of MTAP leads to elevation of its substrate methylthioadenosine (MTA). This partially inhibits protein arginine methyltransferase 5 (PRMT5) creating a vulnerability to further inhibition [59]. The old antibiotic quinacrine has been recently reported to silence PRMT5 transcriptionally, phenocopying siRNA-mediated inhibition of cell growth [60]. Inhibition of PRMT5 causes defective mRNA splicing and inactivation of MDM4, leading to p53 activation as a major pathway leading to impaired cell growth [61,62]. Interestingly, this pathway is also used by CDK 4/6 inhibitors [63]. An alternative approach being currently explored is the inhibition of MAT2A, the enzyme involved in the synthesis of the PRMT5 substrate, S-adenosyl methionine. MAT2A inhibition appears to be MTAP dependent and also disrupts mRNA splicing. This is approach is being explored in a phase 1 clinical trial with the agent AG-270.

6. Anaplastic Lymphoma Kinase (ALK)

ALK rearrangement in NSCLC is well studied and has multiple targeted treatment options with a good prognosis in these patients. In the recent few years, there has been evidence of ALK rearrangements in mesothelioma in the peritoneal subtype. One study that was carried out in pleural MPM identified 25 out of 128 patients (19.5%) with overexpressed ALK transcripts; however, only 10 expressed the ALK protein, and all were negative for ALK rearrangement by fluorescence in situ hybridisation (FISH) [64]. In contrast to the MPM findings, ALK rearrangement tends to be more prevalent in patients with peritoneal MPM, which was confirmed by FISH. ALK positivity was divided into focal weak (no ALK rearrangement) and diffuse strong (ALK rearrangement detected). Sequencing of these samples identified ALK fusion partners STRN, TPM1, ATG16L1 [65]. This has been translated into clinical practice, where the use of ceritinib in a patient with STRN–ALK-rearranged malignant peritoneal mesothelioma showed response as early as 6 weeks into treatment [65].

7. PTCH-1

The hedgehog signalling pathway is involved in embryonic development and is inactivated in the adult mesothelium. Hedgehog ligands (Hh) bind to the transmembrane receptor Patched (PTCH1), which subsequently removes the inhibitory influence of the G-protein-coupled receptor smoothened (SMO). SMO activation leads to the induction of glioma-associated protein (GLI 1) and hedgehog interacting protein (Hhip) [66]. PTCH1 has been shown to be positively selected in the MPM [67] suggesting its role as a relatively rare driver (6%). Targeting the Ptch1 could play an important role in targeting the hedgehog signalling pathway. Vismodegib has recently shown activity in a patient with relapsed malignant MPM harbouring PTCH1F1147fs mutation. This patient had a durable response to Vismodegib [68].

8. Conclusions

Given the long latency of pleural malignant MPM and ongoing use of asbestos in several non-Western countries, malignant pleural MPM will remain a global health issue during the 21st century. Consequently, there is a pressing need for novel, effective, targeted treatments to improve patient outcomes. Targeted therapy is currently in its infancy for mesothelioma, but emerging developments preclinically and clinically are showing some promise. In summary, targeting altered tumour suppressors in MPM remains a challenge due to the need to identify and action vulnerabilities capable of inducing synthetic lethality; however, promising developments suggest that this may be feasible for the more common somatic alterations in this cancer.

Funding: This research received no external funding.

Institutional Review Board Statement: Not applicable.

Informed Consent Statement: Not applicable.

Data Availability Statement: Not applicable.

Conflicts of Interest: D.A.F. Research Funding Eli Lilly, GSK, Bergen Bio, MSD, Clovis Oncology, BMS, Boehringer Ingelheim, Astex Therapeutics, Bayer Oncology Honoraria Targovax, Inventiva, BMS, Bayer, Boehringer Ingelheim, Novocure, Lab 21. S.D. and A.B. declare no conflict of interest.

References

1. Hmeljak, J.; Sanchez-Vega, F.; Hoadley, K.A.; Shih, J.; Stewart, C.; Heiman, D.; Tarpey, P.; Danilova, L.; Drill, E.; Gibb, E.A.; et al. Integrative Molecular Characterization of Malignant Pleural Mesothelioma. *Cancer Discov.* **2018**, *8*, 1548–1565. [CrossRef]
2. Testa, J.R.; Cheung, M.; Pei, J.; Below, J.E.; Tan, Y.; Sementino, E.; Cox, N.J.; Dogan, A.U.; Pass, H.I.; Trusa, S.; et al. Germline BAP1 mutations predispose to malignant mesothelioma. *Nat. Genet.* **2011**, *43*, 1022–1025. [CrossRef]
3. Bott, M.; Brevet, M.; Taylor, B.S.; Shimizu, S.; Ito, T.; Wang, L.; Creaney, J.; Lake, R.A.; Zakowski, M.F.; Reva, B.; et al. The nuclear deubiquitinase BAP1 is commonly inactivated by somatic mutations and 3p21.1 losses in malignant pleural mesothelioma. *Nat. Genet.* **2011**, *43*, 668–672. [CrossRef]
4. Bueno, R.; Stawiski, E.W.; Goldstein, L.D.; Durinck, S.; De Rienzo, A.; Modrusan, Z.; Gnad, F.; Nguyen, T.T.; Jaiswal, B.S.; Chirieac, L.R.; et al. Comprehensive genomic analysis of malignant pleural mesothelioma identifies recurrent mutations, gene fusions and splicing alterations. *Nat. Genet.* **2016**, *48*, 407–416. [CrossRef]
5. Blum, Y.; Meiller, C.; Quetel, L.; Elarouci, N.; Ayadi, M.; Tashtanbaeva, D.; Armenoult, L.; Montagne, F.; Tranchant, R.; Renier, A.; et al. Dissecting heterogeneity in malignant pleural mesothelioma through histo-molecular gradients for clinical applications. *Nat. Commun.* **2019**, *10*, 1333. [CrossRef]
6. Merikallio, H.; Paakko, P.; Salmenkivi, K.; Kinnula, V.; Harju, T.; Soini, Y. Expression of snail, twist, and Zeb1 in malignant mesothelioma. *APMIS* **2013**, *121*, 1–10. [CrossRef]
7. Fassina, A.; Cappellesso, R.; Guzzardo, V.; Dalla Via, L.; Piccolo, S.; Ventura, L.; Fassan, M. Epithelial-mesenchymal transition in malignant mesothelioma. *Mod. Pathol.* **2012**, *25*, 86–99. [CrossRef]
8. Galetta, D.; Catino, A.; Misino, A.; Logroscino, A.; Fico, M. Sarcomatoid mesothelioma: Future advances in diagnosis, biomolecular assessment, and therapeutic options in a poor-outcome disease. *Tumori* **2016**, *102*, 127–130. [CrossRef]
9. Szlosarek, P.W.; Steele, J.P.; Nolan, L.; Gilligan, D.; Taylor, P.; Spicer, J.; Lind, M.; Mitra, S.; Shamash, J.; Phillips, M.M.; et al. Arginine Deprivation With Pegylated Arginine Deiminase in Patients With Argininosuccinate Synthetase 1-Deficient Malignant Pleural Mesothelioma: A Randomized Clinical Trial. *JAMA Oncol.* **2017**, *3*, 58–66. [CrossRef]
10. Davis, F.M.; Stewart, T.A.; Thompson, E.W.; Monteith, G.R. Targeting EMT in cancer: Opportunities for pharmacological intervention. *Trends Pharmacol. Sci.* **2014**, *35*, 479–488. [CrossRef]
11. Hassan, R.; Thomas, A.; Alewine, C.; Le, D.T.; Jaffee, E.M.; Pastan, I. Mesothelin Immunotherapy for Cancer: Ready for Prime Time? *J. Clin. Oncol.* **2016**, *34*, 4171–4179. [CrossRef]

12. Golfier, S.; Kopitz, C.; Kahnert, A.; Heisler, I.; Schatz, C.A.; Stelte-Ludwig, B.; Mayer-Bartschmid, A.; Unterschemmann, K.; Bruder, S.; Linden, L.; et al. Anetumab ravtansine: A novel mesothelin-targeting antibody-drug conjugate cures tumors with heterogeneous target expression favored by bystander effect. *Mol. Cancer Ther.* **2014**, *13*, 1537–1548. [CrossRef]
13. Hassan, R.; Blumenschein, G.R., Jr.; Moore, K.N.; Santin, A.D.; Kindler, H.L.; Nemunaitis, J.J.; Seward, S.M.; Thomas, A.; Kim, S.K.; Rajagopalan, P.; et al. First-in-Human, Multicenter, Phase I Dose-Escalation and Expansion Study of Anti-Mesothelin Antibody-Drug Conjugate Anetumab Ravtansine in Advanced or Metastatic Solid Tumors. *J. Clin. Oncol.* **2020**, *38*, 1824–1835. [CrossRef] [PubMed]
14. Beddowes, E.; Spicer, J.; Chan, P.Y.; Khadeir, R.; Corbacho, J.G.; Repana, D.; Steele, J.P.; Schmid, P.; Szyszko, T.; Cook, G.; et al. Phase 1 Dose-Escalation Study of Pegylated Arginine Deiminase, Cisplatin, and Pemetrexed in Patients With Argininosuccinate Synthetase 1-Deficient Thoracic Cancers. *J. Clin. Oncol.* **2017**, *35*, 1778–1785. [CrossRef] [PubMed]
15. Delage, B.; Fennell, D.A.; Nicholson, L.; McNeish, I.; Lemoine, N.R.; Crook, T.; Szlosarek, P.W. Arginine deprivation and argininosuccinate synthetase expression in the treatment of cancer. *Int. J. Cancer* **2010**, *126*, 2762–2772. [CrossRef]
16. Szlosarek, P.W.; Klabatsa, A.; Pallaska, A.; Sheaff, M.; Smith, P.; Crook, T.; Grimshaw, M.J.; Steele, J.P.; Rudd, R.M.; Balkwill, F.R.; et al. In vivo loss of expression of argininosuccinate synthetase in malignant pleural mesothelioma is a biomarker for susceptibility to arginine depletion. *Clin. Cancer Res.* **2006**, *12*, 7126–7131. [CrossRef]
17. Nicholson, L.J.; Smith, P.R.; Hiller, L.; Szlosarek, P.W.; Kimberley, C.; Sehouli, J.; Koensgen, D.; Mustea, A.; Schmid, P.; Crook, T. Epigenetic silencing of argininosuccinate synthetase confers resistance to platinum-induced cell death but collateral sensitivity to arginine auxotrophy in ovarian cancer. *Int. J. Cancer* **2009**, *125*, 1454–1463. [CrossRef]
18. Allen, M.D.; Luong, P.; Hudson, C.; Leyton, J.; Delage, B.; Ghazaly, E.; Cutts, R.; Yuan, M.; Syed, N.; Lo Nigro, C.; et al. Prognostic and therapeutic impact of argininosuccinate synthetase 1 control in bladder cancer as monitored longitudinally by PET imaging. *Cancer Res.* **2014**, *74*, 896–907. [CrossRef]
19. Szlosarek, P.W.; Baas, P.; Ceresoli, G.L.; Fennell, D.A.; Gilligan, D.; Johnston, A.; Lee, P.; Mansfield, A.S.; Nolan, L.; Nowak, A.K.; et al. ATOMIC-Meso: A randomized phase 2/3 trial of ADI-PEG20 or placebo with pemetrexed and cisplatin in patients with argininosuccinate synthetase 1-deficient non-epithelioid mesothelioma. *J. Clin. Oncol.* **2017**, *35*, TPS8582. [CrossRef]
20. Miyanaga, A.; Masuda, M.; Tsuta, K.; Kawasaki, K.; Nakamura, Y.; Sakuma, T.; Asamura, H.; Gemma, A.; Yamada, T. Hippo pathway gene mutations in malignant mesothelioma: Revealed by RNA and targeted exon sequencing. *J. Thorac. Oncol.* **2015**, *10*, 844–851. [CrossRef]
21. Sato, T.; Sekido, Y. NF2/Merlin Inactivation and Potential Therapeutic Targets in Mesothelioma. *Int. J. Mol. Sci.* **2018**, *19*, 988. [CrossRef]
22. Zhang, L.; Ren, F.; Zhang, Q.; Chen, Y.; Wang, B.; Jiang, J. The TEAD/TEF family of transcription factor Scalloped mediates Hippo signaling in organ size control. *Dev. Cell* **2008**, *14*, 377–387. [CrossRef]
23. Zhang, M.; Luo, J.L.; Sun, Q.; Harber, J.; Dawson, A.G.; Nakas, A.; Busacca, S.; Sharkey, A.J.; Waller, D.; Sheaff, M.T.; et al. Clonal architecture in mesothelioma is prognostic and shapes the tumour microenvironment. *Nat. Commun.* **2021**, *12*, 1751. [CrossRef]
24. Shapiro, I.M.; Kolev, V.N.; Vidal, C.M.; Kadariya, Y.; Ring, J.E.; Wright, Q.; Weaver, D.T.; Menges, C.; Padval, M.; McClatchey, A.I.; et al. Merlin deficiency predicts FAK inhibitor sensitivity: A synthetic lethal relationship. *Sci. Transl. Med.* **2014**, *6*, 237ra68. [CrossRef]
25. Poulikakos, P.I.; Xiao, G.H.; Gallagher, R.; Jablonski, S.; Jhanwar, S.C.; Testa, J.R. Re-expression of the tumor suppressor NF2/merlin inhibits invasiveness in mesothelioma cells and negatively regulates FAK. *Oncogene* **2006**, *25*, 5960–5968. [CrossRef]
26. Fennell, D.A.; Baitei, E.Y. Mesothelioma: Hippo pathway as a target, lessons from COMMAND. *Oncotarget* **2019**, *10*, 3996–3997. [CrossRef]
27. Fennell, D.A.; Taylor, P.; Gilligan, D.; Nakano, T.; Scherpereel, A.; Pavlakis, N.; van Meerbeeck, J.P.; Aerts, J.; Nowak, A.K.; Kindler, H.; et al. Reply to K. Masuda et al. *J. Clin. Oncol.* **2019**, *37*, 2294–2295. [CrossRef]
28. Fennell, D.A.; Baas, P.; Taylor, P.; Nowak, A.K.; Gilligan, D.; Nakano, T.; Pachter, J.A.; Weaver, D.T.; Scherpereel, A.; Pavlakis, N.; et al. Maintenance Defactinib Versus Placebo After First-Line Chemotherapy in Patients With Merlin-Stratified Pleural Mesothelioma: COMMAND-A Double-Blind, Randomized, Phase II Study. *J. Clin. Oncol.* **2019**, *37*, 790–798. [CrossRef]
29. Serrels, A.; Lund, T.; Serrels, B.; Byron, A.; McPherson, R.C.; von Kriegsheim, A.; Gomez-Cuadrado, L.; Canel, M.; Muir, M.; Ring, J.E.; et al. Nuclear FAK controls chemokine transcription, Tregs, and evasion of anti-tumor immunity. *Cell* **2015**, *163*, 160–173. [CrossRef]
30. Serrels, B.; McGivern, N.; Canel, M.; Byron, A.; Johnson, S.C.; McSorley, H.J.; Quinn, N.; Taggart, D.; Von Kriegsheim, A.; Anderton, S.M.; et al. IL-33 and ST2 mediate FAK-dependent antitumor immune evasion through transcriptional networks. *Sci. Signal.* **2017**, *10*, eaan8355. [CrossRef]
31. Yang, H.; Hall, S.R.R.; Sun, B.; Zhao, L.; Gao, Y.; Schmid, R.A.; Tan, S.T.; Peng, R.W.; Yao, F. NF2 and Canonical Hippo-YAP Pathway Define Distinct Tumor Subsets Characterized by Different Immune Deficiency and Treatment Implications in Human Pleural Mesothelioma. *Cancers* **2021**, *13*, 1561. [CrossRef]
32. Kurppa, K.J.; Liu, Y.; To, C.; Zhang, T.; Fan, M.; Vajdi, A.; Knelson, E.H.; Xie, Y.; Lim, K.; Cejas, P.; et al. Treatment-Induced Tumor Dormancy through YAP-Mediated Transcriptional Reprogramming of the Apoptotic Pathway. *Cancer Cell* **2020**, *37*, 104–122.e12. [CrossRef]
33. Wu, J.; Minikes, A.M.; Gao, M.; Bian, H.; Li, Y.; Stockwell, B.R.; Chen, Z.N.; Jiang, X. Intercellular interaction dictates cancer cell ferroptosis via NF2-YAP signalling. *Nature* **2019**, *572*, 402–406. [CrossRef]

34. Fennell, D. Cancer-cell death ironed out. *Nature* **2019**, *572*, 314–315. [CrossRef]
35. Farzin, M.; Toon, C.W.; Clarkson, A.; Sioson, L.; Watson, N.; Andrici, J.; Gill, A.J. Loss of expression of BAP1 predicts longer survival in mesothelioma. *Pathology* **2015**, *47*, 302–307. [CrossRef]
36. LaFave, L.M.; Beguelin, W.; Koche, R.; Teater, M.; Spitzer, B.; Chramiec, A.; Papalexi, E.; Keller, M.D.; Hricik, T.; Konstantinoff, K.; et al. Loss of BAP1 function leads to EZH2-dependent transformation. *Nat. Med.* **2015**, *21*, 1344–1349. [CrossRef]
37. Zauderer, M.G.; Szlosarek, P.; Moulec, S.L.; Popat, S.; Taylor, P.; Planchard, D.; Scherpereel, A.; Jahan, T.; Koczywas, M.; Forster, M.; et al. Phase 2, multicenter study of the EZH2 inhibitor tazemetostat as monotherapy in adults with relapsed or refractory (R/R) malignant mesothelioma (MM) with BAP1 inactivation. *J. Clin. Oncol.* **2018**, *36*, 8515. [CrossRef]
38. Affar, E.B.; Carbone, M. BAP1 regulates different mechanisms of cell death. *Cell Death Dis.* **2018**, *9*, 1151. [CrossRef]
39. Ismail, I.H.; Davidson, R.; Gagne, J.P.; Xu, Z.Z.; Poirier, G.G.; Hendzel, M.J. Germline mutations in BAP1 impair its function in DNA double-strand break repair. *Cancer Res.* **2014**, *74*, 4282–4294. [CrossRef]
40. Nishikawa, H.; Wu, W.; Koike, A.; Kojima, R.; Gomi, H.; Fukuda, M.; Ohta, T. BRCA1-associated protein 1 interferes with BRCA1/BARD1 RING heterodimer activity. *Cancer Res.* **2009**, *69*, 111–119. [CrossRef]
41. Yu, H.; Pak, H.; Hammond-Martel, I.; Ghram, M.; Rodrigue, A.; Daou, S.; Barbour, H.; Corbeil, L.; Hebert, J.; Drobetsky, E.; et al. Tumor suppressor and deubiquitinase BAP1 promotes DNA double-strand break repair. *Proc. Natl. Acad. Sci. USA* **2014**, *111*, 285–290. [CrossRef]
42. Helleday, T. The underlying mechanism for the PARP and BRCA synthetic lethality: Clearing up the misunderstandings. *Mol. Oncol.* **2011**, *5*, 387–393. [CrossRef] [PubMed]
43. Ledermann, J.; Harter, P.; Gourley, C.; Friedlander, M.; Vergote, I.; Rustin, G.; Scott, C.L.; Meier, W.; Shapira-Frommer, R.; Safra, T.; et al. Olaparib maintenance therapy in patients with platinum-sensitive relapsed serous ovarian cancer: A preplanned retrospective analysis of outcomes by BRCA status in a randomised phase 2 trial. *Lancet Oncol.* **2014**, *15*, 852–861. [CrossRef]
44. Patel, M.; Elliott, A.; Liu, S.V.; Kim, C.; Raez, L.E.; Feldman, R.; Pai, S.G.; Wozniak, A.J.; Nagasaka, M.; Lopes, G.; et al. Genomic landscape and immune phenotype of malignant pleural mesothelioma. *J. Clin. Oncol.* **2020**, *38*, 9056. [CrossRef]
45. Fennell, D.A.; King, A.; Mohammed, S.; Branson, A.; Brookes, C.; Darlison, L.; Dawson, A.G.; Gaba, A.; Hutka, M.; Morgan, B.; et al. Rucaparib in patients with BAP1-deficient or BRCA1-deficient mesothelioma (MiST1): An open-label, single-arm, phase 2a clinical trial. *Lancet Respir. Med.* **2021**, in press. [CrossRef]
46. Hassan, R.; Mian, I.; Wagner, C.; Mallory, Y.; Agra, M.; Padiernos, E.; Sengupta, M.; Morrow, B.; Wei, J.S.; Thomas, A.; et al. Phase II study of olaparib in malignant mesothelioma (MM) to correlate efficacy with germline and somatic mutations in DNA repair genes. *J. Clin. Oncol.* **2020**, *38*, 9054. [CrossRef]
47. Rathkey, D.; Khanal, M.; Murai, J.; Zhang, J.; Sengupta, M.; Jiang, Q.; Morrow, B.; Evans, C.N.; Chari, R.; Fetsch, P.; et al. Sensitivity of Mesothelioma Cells to PARP Inhibitors Is Not Dependent on BAP1 but Is Enhanced by Temozolomide in Cells With High-Schlafen 11 and Low-O6-methylguanine-DNA Methyltransferase Expression. *J. Thorac. Oncol.* **2020**, *15*, 843–859. [CrossRef]
48. Parrotta, R.; Okonska, A.; Ronner, M.; Weder, W.; Stahel, R.; Penengo, L.; Felley-Bosco, E. A Novel BRCA1-Associated Protein-1 Isoform Affects Response of Mesothelioma Cells to Drugs Impairing BRCA1-Mediated DNA Repair. *J. Thorac. Oncol.* **2017**, *12*, 1309–1319. [CrossRef]
49. Shen, J.; Zhao, W.; Ju, Z.; Wang, L.; Peng, Y.; Labrie, M.; Yap, T.A.; Mills, G.B.; Peng, G. PARPi Triggers the STING-Dependent Immune Response and Enhances the Therapeutic Efficacy of Immune Checkpoint Blockade Independent of BRCAness. *Cancer Res.* **2019**, *79*, 311–319. [CrossRef]
50. Burdette, D.L.; Monroe, K.M.; Sotelo-Troha, K.; Iwig, J.S.; Eckert, B.; Hyodo, M.; Hayakawa, Y.; Vance, R.E. STING is a direct innate immune sensor of cyclic di-GMP. *Nature* **2011**, *478*, 515–518. [CrossRef]
51. Chen, Q.; Sun, L.; Chen, Z.J. Regulation and function of the cGAS-STING pathway of cytosolic DNA sensing. *Nat. Immunol.* **2016**, *17*, 1142–1149. [CrossRef]
52. Mackenzie, K.J.; Carroll, P.; Martin, C.A.; Murina, O.; Fluteau, A.; Simpson, D.J.; Olova, N.; Sutcliffe, H.; Rainger, J.K.; Leitch, A.; et al. cGAS surveillance of micronuclei links genome instability to innate immunity. *Nature* **2017**, *548*, 461–465. [CrossRef]
53. Takeda, M.; Kasai, T.; Enomoto, Y.; Takano, M.; Morita, K.; Kadota, K.; Nonomura, A. 9p21 deletion in the diagnosis of malignant mesothelioma, using fluorescence in situ hybridization analysis. *Pathol. Int.* **2010**, *60*, 395–399. [CrossRef]
54. Illei, P.B.; Rusch, V.W.; Zakowski, M.F.; Ladanyi, M. Homozygous deletion of CDKN2A and codeletion of the methylthioadenosine phosphorylase gene in the majority of pleural mesotheliomas. *Clin. Cancer Res.* **2003**, *9*, 2108–2113. [PubMed]
55. Aliagas, E.; Martínez-Iniesta, M.; Hernández, M.; Alay, A.; Cordero, D.; Solé, X.; Rivas, F.; Ureña, A.; Vilariño, N.; Munoz-Pinedo, C.; et al. MA23.02 CDK4/6 Inhibitors Show Antitumor Effects in Preclinical Models of Malignant Pleural Mesothelioma. *J. Thorac. Oncol.* **2019**, *14*, S343. [CrossRef]
56. Yang, C.T.; You, L.; Yeh, C.C.; Chang, J.W.; Zhang, F.; McCormick, F.; Jablons, D.M. Adenovirus-mediated p14(ARF) gene transfer in human mesothelioma cells. *J. Natl. Cancer Inst.* **2000**, *92*, 636–641. [CrossRef]
57. Gluck, W.L.; Gounder, M.M.; Frank, R.; Eskens, F.; Blay, J.Y.; Cassier, P.A.; Soria, J.C.; Chawla, S.; de Weger, V.; Wagner, A.J.; et al. Phase 1 study of the MDM2 inhibitor AMG 232 in patients with advanced P53 wild-type solid tumors or multiple myeloma. *Investig. New Drugs* **2020**, *38*, 831–843. [CrossRef]
58. Kindler, H.L.; Burris, H.A., 3rd; Sandler, A.B.; Oliff, I.A. A phase II multicenter study of L-alanosine, a potent inhibitor of adenine biosynthesis, in patients with MTAP-deficient cancer. *Investig. New Drugs* **2009**, *27*, 75–81. [CrossRef]

59. Kryukov, G.V.; Wilson, F.H.; Ruth, J.R.; Paulk, J.; Tsherniak, A.; Marlow, S.E.; Vazquez, F.; Weir, B.A.; Fitzgerald, M.E.; Tanaka, M.; et al. MTAP deletion confers enhanced dependency on the PRMT5 arginine methyltransferase in cancer cells. *Science* **2016**, *351*, 1214–1218. [CrossRef]
60. Busacca, S.; Zhang, Q.; Sharkey, A.; Dawson, A.G.; Moore, D.A.; Waller, D.A.; Nakas, A.; Jones, C.; Cain, K.; Luo, J.-l.; et al. Transcriptional perturbation of protein arginine methyltransferase-5 exhibits MTAP-selective oncosuppression. *Sci. Rep.* **2021**, *11*, 7434. [CrossRef]
61. Gerhart, S.V.; Kellner, W.A.; Thompson, C.; Pappalardi, M.B.; Zhang, X.P.; Montes de Oca, R.; Penebre, E.; Duncan, K.; Boriack-Sjodin, A.; Le, B.; et al. Activation of the p53-MDM4 regulatory axis defines the anti-tumour response to PRMT5 inhibition through its role in regulating cellular splicing. *Sci. Rep.* **2018**, *8*, 9711. [CrossRef]
62. Bezzi, M.; Teo, S.X.; Muller, J.; Mok, W.C.; Sahu, S.K.; Vardy, L.A.; Bonday, Z.Q.; Guccione, E. Regulation of constitutive and alternative splicing by PRMT5 reveals a role for Mdm4 pre-mRNA in sensing defects in the spliceosomal machinery. *Genes Dev.* **2013**, *27*, 1903–1916. [CrossRef] [PubMed]
63. AbuHammad, S.; Cullinane, C.; Martin, C.; Bacolas, Z.; Ward, T.; Chen, H.; Slater, A.; Ardley, K.; Kirby, L.; Chan, K.T.; et al. Regulation of PRMT5-MDM4 axis is critical in the response to CDK4/6 inhibitors in melanoma. *Proc. Natl. Acad. Sci. USA* **2019**, *116*, 17990–18000. [CrossRef] [PubMed]
64. Monch, D.; Bode-Erdmann, S.; Kalla, J.; Strater, J.; Schwanen, C.; Falkenstern-Ge, R.; Klumpp, S.; Friedel, G.; Ott, G.; Kalla, C. A subgroup of pleural mesothelioma expresses ALK protein and may be targetable by combined rapamycin and crizotinib therapy. *Oncotarget* **2018**, *9*, 20781–20794. [CrossRef]
65. Ruschoff, J.H.; Gradhand, E.; Kahraman, A.; Rees, H.; Ferguson, J.L.; Curioni-Fontecedro, A.; Zoche, M.; Moch, H.; Vrugt, B. STRN -ALK Rearranged Malignant Peritoneal Mesothelioma With Dramatic Response Following Ceritinib Treatment. *JCO Precis. Oncol.* **2019**, *3*. [CrossRef] [PubMed]
66. Felley-Bosco, E.; Opitz, I.; Meerang, M. Hedgehog Signaling in Malignant Pleural Mesothelioma. *Genes (Basel)* **2015**, *6*, 500–511. [CrossRef]
67. Martincorena, I.; Raine, K.M.; Gerstung, M.; Dawson, K.J.; Haase, K.; Van Loo, P.; Davies, H.; Stratton, M.R.; Campbell, P.J. Universal Patterns of Selection in Cancer and Somatic Tissues. *Cell* **2017**, *171*, 1029–1041. [CrossRef]
68. Popat, S.; Sharma, B.; MacMahon, S.; Nicholson, A.G.; Sharma, R.K.; Schuster, K.; Lazdunski, L.L.; Fennell, D. Durable Response to Vismodegib in PTCH1 F1147fs Mutant Relapsed Malignant Pleural Mesothelioma: Implications for Mesothelioma Drug Treatment. *JCO Precis. Oncol.* **2021**, *5*, 39–43. [CrossRef]

MDPI
St. Alban-Anlage 66
4052 Basel
Switzerland
Tel. +41 61 683 77 34
Fax +41 61 302 89 18
www.mdpi.com

Cancers Editorial Office
E-mail: cancers@mdpi.com
www.mdpi.com/journal/cancers

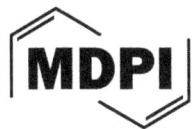

www.ingramcontent.com/pod-product-compliance
Lightning Source LLC
LaVergne TN
LVHW070214100526
838202LV00015B/2044